The Macula

A Comprehensive Text and Atlas

The Macula

A Comprehensive Text and Atlas

LAWRENCE A. YANNUZZI, MD

Director of Retinal Services
Manhattan Eye, Ear and Throat Hospital
Affiliated with The New York Hospital-Cornell Medical Center
New York, New York

KURT A. GITTER, MD

Director, Touro Infirmary
Eye Research Laboratory
Clinical Professor, Department of Opthalmology
Louisiana State University School of Medicine
New Orleans, Louisiana
Consultant United States Public Health Service Hospital,
New Orleans, Louisiana

HOWARD SCHATZ, MD

Director, Retina Research Fund
St. Mary's Hospital and Medical Center
Associate Clinical Professor of Ophthalmology
University of California Medical Center
San Francisco, California

THE WILLIAMS & WILKINS COMPANY
Baltimore

Made in the United States of America

Library of Congress Cataloging in Publication Data
Main entry under title:

The Macula: a comprehensive text and atlas.

Updated contributions of a meeting held in March, 1976, in New York, sponsored by the New York Eye Bank for Sight Restoration and Manhattan Eye, Ear, and Throat Hospital.
Includes index.
1. Macula lutea—Diseases—Diagnosis—Congresses. 2. Fluorescence angiography—Congresses. 3. Retina—Diseases—Diagnosis—Congresses. I. Yannuzzi, Lawrence A. II. Gitter, Kurt A., 1937- III. Schatz, Howard. IV. Eye-Bank for Sight Restoration. V. New York (City). Manhattan Eye, Ear, and Throat Hospital.

RE661.M3M33 617.7′3 78-8971
ISBN 0-683-09322-3

Composed and printed at the
Waverly Press, Inc.
Mt. Royal and Guilford Aves.
Baltimore, Md. 21202, U.S.A.

Preface

Macular disease is a major cause of blindness in patients of all ages and is currently the number one cause of new blindness in patients over 60 years of age. Since the advent of fluorescein angiography and argon laser photocoagulation, the diagnosis and treatment of macular disease has come to represent a substantial segment of ophthalmology. In fact, the study of macular disease has emerged as a distinct subdivision of the retinal service in a number of major ophthalmologic institutions. This is largely because of the vast differences between "medical retina" (the diagnosis and treatment of macular disease) and "surgical retina" (the surgical treatment of rhegmatogenous retinal detachments).

As a result of this new interest, numerous symposia and conferences have been held in recent years for the purpose of disseminating new information related to the diagnosis and treatment of macular disease. It was at such a meeting, sponsored by the New York Eye Bank for Sight Restoration and the Manhattan Eye, Ear and Throat Hospital and held in New York City in March of 1976, that this book on the macula found its roots. The faculty of this meeting was composed of a group of ophthalmologists who shared a common interest and expertise in macular diseases.

Nearly 350 ophthalmologists attended the macular course in New York, and a large number expressed interest in obtaining written material on the subject matter. Accordingly, the lecture material served as a basis for the text contained herein. The talks were updated and modified, and additional chapters were added to include material vital to a comprehensive and current text and atlas on macular disease.

The more common disorders associated with macular dysfunction are reviewed with reference to the clinical findings, the natural course, the histopathologic features where known, and the treatment. The strong emphasis on fluorescein angiography suggests that knowledge of the fundamentals of this important diagnostic test is critically important to the understanding of the pathophysiology of macular disease and its treatment. A basic knowledge of the clinico-histopathologic features of macular disease is best achieved through an understanding of fluorescein angiography, which will also help the clinician develop a rational approach to photocoagulation therapy.

The text is intended primarily for residents in ophthalmology and for ophthalmologists who have had no formal training in macular diseases, who have had little opportunity to observe the lesser known manifestations of macular diseases, or who contemplate utilizing photocoagulation therapy. The authors have edited all chapters by individual contributors, modifying the text and providing additional photographs where necessary. Strict editorial guidelines to maintain absolute uniformity were not imposed by the authors so that individual contributors' styles might be preserved. Thus, variations in organization exist from chapter to chapter.

The three of us have enjoyed a close friendship for nearly ten years, originating from a common interest in diseases of the macula. Over the years, we have enjoyed working with and learning from each other, and it has indeed been a pleasure for us to collaborate on this volume. We owe a great deal to many, including the contributing authors, the physicians who have referred patients from whom we have learned so much, and our residents who have been constant sources of inspiration through their inquisitive and provocative thoughts. We wish to thank, in particular, Tom Burton, MD and Maurice Rabb, MD for their work on the scientific exhibit which formed the basis for Chapter 4; Robert Wallyn, MD for his clinical work leading to the data reported in Chapter 13; Ron E. Smith, MD for reviewing Chapter 28; Walter Schachat, MD for his editorial comments; Laurie Sisco, Rob Wolfson, Alvin Meyerowitz and Karen Schomaker for photographic and technical assistance; Sylvia Grossman, Roxanne Peterson and Lorraine Fisher for secretarial assistance. We owe special thanks to Cynthia Fazzini who worked faithfully and diligently for many hours editing the text, verifying and standardizing the bibliography, and coordinating the material submitted by the contributors. Above all, we wish to thank William S. Farkas, our most skilled ophthalmic-biological photographer who was unfaltering during the extremely challenging task of printing and labelling the photographs needed for completion of the book.

Lawrence A. Yannuzzi, MD
New York, New York

Kurt A. Gitter, MD
New Orleans, Louisiana

Howard Schatz, MD
San Francisco, California

March 28, 1978

DEDICATION

To Our Parents

Gerald and Jo Yannuzzi
Morris and Maria Gitter
Lawrence and Beatrice Schatz

Contributors

William H. Annesley, Jr., MD
Chief, Department of Ophthalmology
Lankenau Hospital
Philadelphia, Pennsylvania

Alan H. Barnert, MD
Attending Surgeon, Manhattan Eye, Ear and Throat Hospital
New York, New York

Charles R. Beyrer, MD
Associate Clinical Professor of Ophthalmology
State University of New York at Stony Brook
Stony Brook, New York

James R. Brinkley, Jr., MD
Fellow in Retinal-Vitreous Diseases
Department of Ophthalmology
University of Southern California
School of Medicine
Estelle Doheny Eye Foundation
Los Angeles, California

Thomas C. Burton, MD
Associate Professor of Ophthalmology
University of Iowa Hospitals and Clinics
Iowa City, Iowa

Ronald E. Carr, MD, MSc (ophthalmology)
Professor of Ophthalmology
New York University Medical Center
New York, New York

Brian J. Curtin, MD
Surgeon Director and Chief of the Sprague Myopia Clinic
Manhattan Eye, Ear and Throat Hospital, affiliated with the New York Hospital-Cornell Medical Center
New York, New York

Eleanor E. Faye, MD
Medical Director, Lighthouse Low Vision Service
New York Association for the Blind
Attending Surgeon, Manhattan Eye, Ear and Throat Hospital, affiliated with The New York Hospital-Cornell Medical Center, New York, NY

Jay L. Federman, MD
Associate Professor, Department of Ophthalmology
Thomas Jefferson University Medical School
Senior Assisting Surgeon, Retinal Service, Wills Eye Hospital
Philadelphia, Pennsylvania

Stuart L. Fine, MD
Associate Professor of Ophthalmology
Assistant Professor of Emergency Medicine
The Johns Hopkins Medical Institutions
Baltimore, Maryland 21205

Yale L. Fisher, MD
Ultrasonography Laboratory
Associate Attending Surgeon, Manhattan Eye, Ear and Throat Hospital
affiliated with The New York Hospital-Cornell Medical Center, New York, New York

Conrad L. Giles, MD
Clinical Associate Professor
Kresge Eye Institute
Wayne State University College of Medicine
Detroit, Michigan

Kurt A. Gitter, MD
Director, Touro Infirmary
Eye Research Laboratory
New Orleans, Louisiana

William M. Haining, FRCSE
Head, Department of Ophthalmology
University of Dundee, Scotland

Lee M. Jampol, MD
Associate Professor of Ophthalmology
University of Illinois Eye and Ear Infirmary
Chicago, Illinois

Johnny Justice, Jr.
Assistant Professor of Ophthalmology
Cullen Eye Institute
Baylor College of Medicine
Houston, Texas

Francis A. L'Esperance, Jr., MD
Associate Professor of Clinical Ophthalmology
Columbia University College of Physicians and Surgeons
New York, New York

G. Richard O'Connor, MD
Director, Francis I. Proctor Foundation
Professor of Ophthalmology
University of California
San Francisco, California

Arnall Patz, MD
Professor of Ophthalmology and The Seeing Eye Research Professor
Director, Retinal Vascular Center
The Johns Hopkins Medical Institutions
Baltimore, Maryland

Maurice F. Rabb, MD
Director of the Fluorescein Angiography Laboratory
Michael Reese Hospital
Professor of Clinical Ophthalmology
University of Illinois Eye and Ear Infirmary
Chicago, Illinois

Ronald L. Radius, MD
Fellow of Ophthalmology, Wilmer Eye Institute
The Johns Hopkins Medical Institutes
Baltimore, Maryland

Emanuel S. Rosen, MD, BSc, FRCSE, FRPS
Consultant Ophthalmic Surgeon
Manchester Royal Eye Hospital
Honorary Lecturer in Ophthalmology
University of Manchester

Stephen J. Ryan, MD
Director, Estelle Doheny Eye Foundation
Professor and Chairman, Department of Ophthalmology
University of Southern California
Los Angeles, California

Jerry A. Shields, MD
Senior Assistant Surgeon, Oncology Unit, Retina Service
Wills Eye Hospital, Philadelphia, Pennsylvania
Associate Professor of Ophthalmology
Thomas Jefferson University Hospital, Philadelphia, Pennsylvania

Howard Schatz, MD
Director, Retina Research Fund
St. Mary's Hospital and Medical Center
Associate Clinical Professor of Ophthalmology,
University of California Medical Center
San Francisco, California

Terrance L. Tomer
Director of Diagnostic Photography
Wills Eye Hospital, Philadelphia, Pennsylvania

Murray A. Wolkstein, MD
Assistant Clinical Professor of Ophthalmology
Mount Sinai School of Medicine
New York, New York

Lawrence A. Yannuzzi, MD
Director of Retinal Services,
Manhattan Eye, Ear and Throat Hospital,
affiliated with The New York Hospital-Cornell Medical Center,
New York, New York

Myron Yanoff, MD
Chairman and Professor, Department of Ophthalmology
University of Pennsylvania, Philadelphia, Pennsylvania
Director, Scheie Eye Institute, Philadelphia, Pennsylvania

Contents

Part IV MISCELLANEOUS DISEASES

Part V PHOTOCOAGULATION THERAPY OF MACULAR DISEASE

PART I

Introduction

CHAPTER 1

Macular Pathology

Myron Yanoff, M.D.

Terminology

The *anatomic macula* can be defined as that part of the retina where the ganglion cells are greater than one cell in thickness (Fig. 1.1). Everywhere else in the retina, outside of the macula, the ganglion cell layer consists of a single row of continuous cells (Fig. 1.2). Histologically, the multilayered ganglion cells are found almost from the temporal edge (and often to the temporal edge) of the optic disc extending temporally for a distance of 4–5 disc diameters (about 6.0–7.5 mm), and almost completely between the superior and inferior vascular arcades (Fig. 1.3). Clinically, the area of the anatomic-histologic macula (also called the area centralis) is often referred to as the *posterior pole* (table 1.1).

The *anatomic fovea* (fovea centralis) can be defined as that part of the retina where there is sudden change in its internal surface so that a slope (clivus)-directed internally, then flat, then externally forms an elongated, narrow-based pit. The diameter across the pit is approximately 1.5 mm, i.e., about the same size as the horizontal diameter of the optic disc. Clinically, the start of the slope causes a precipitous change in the reflex from the retinal surface appearing as a ring (Fig. 1.4). The area of the pit, the anatomic fovea is commonly referred to clinically as the macula.

The *anatomic foveola* is the floor of the fovea (Fig. 1.5). The shape of the floor, much like a concave mirror, often produces a reflected spot of light overlying it in the vitreous. This is called the clinical foveal light reflex. The size, shape, and intensity of the light reflex depends on the slope and shape of the foveola. Occasionally, a normal foveola may be shaped so as to produce no light reflex. The presence or absence of a light reflex, therefore, is not an important clinical observation in determining pathology in this area unless, of course, a light reflex noted previously disappears. The anatomic foveola is often clinically called the fovea, and measures approximately 0.33 mm in diameter. It is slightly smaller than, and contained within, the retinal avascular zone which measures approximately 0.5 mm in diameter (Fig. 1.6). In this discussion, as well as in the rest of this text, the anatomic fovea will be referred to as the macula and the anatomic foveola will be referred to as the fovea because of their widespread use in clinical ophthalmology.

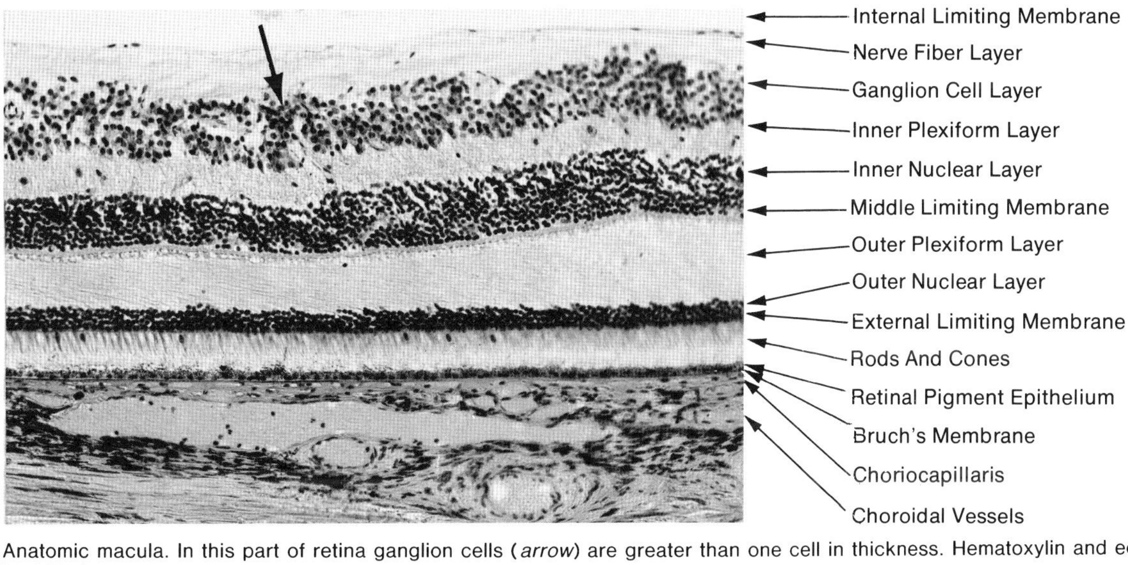

Figure 1.1 Anatomic macula. In this part of retina ganglion cells (*arrow*) are greater than one cell in thickness. Hematoxylin and eosin. ×115. (AFIP neg. 64-6651).

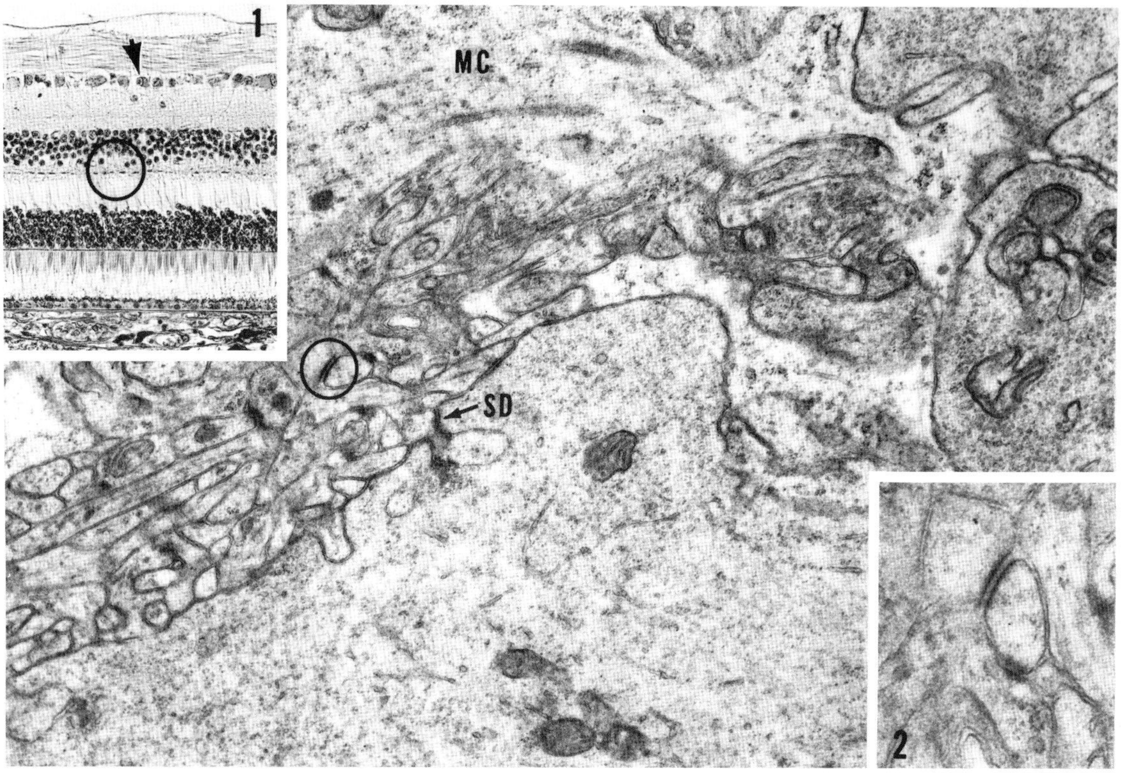

Figure 1.2. Retina outside of anatomic macula. Single continuous row of ganglion cells are shown (*arrow, inset 1*). Blood vessels are present in inner half of retina only, extending externally to the middle limiting membrane (*dotted line extending out from center of circle, inset 1*). Membrane (*main figure*) consists of desmosome-like densities (*circle, inset 2*) attaching adjacent neurites to one another within outer plexiform layer. *MC*, Müller cell; *SD*, synaptic density. *Main figure*, ×18,000; *inset 1*, hematoxylin and eosin, ×130, AFIP neg. 61-1960; *inset 2*, ×32,400. (*Main figure* from B. S. Fine: Retinal structure: light and electron microscopic observations. *In* New and Controversial Aspects of Retinal Detachment, ed. by A. McPherson, p. 16, 1968, © Hoeber, New York. *Insets 1 and 2* from B. S. Fine and M. Yanoff: Ocular Histology: A Text and Atlas, 1972, © Harper & Row, New York; all were reprinted with permission.)

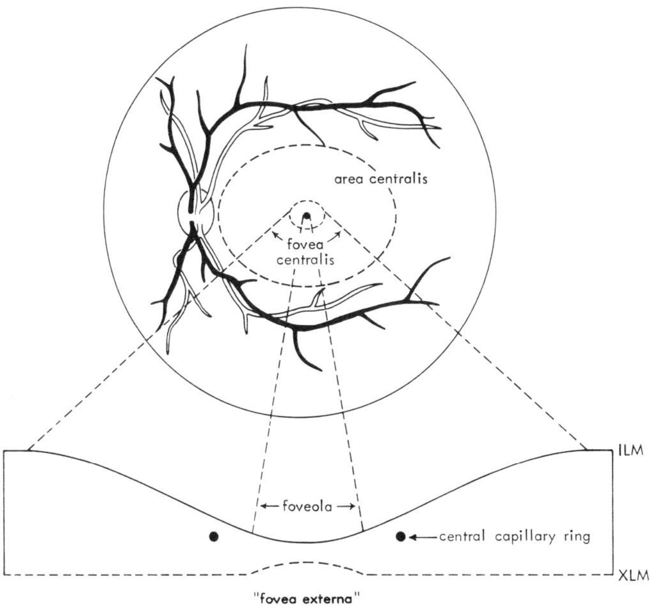

Figure 1.3. Anatomic macula, also called area centralis or posterior pole. Anatomic fovea and foveola contained within center of anatomic macula. *ILM*, internal limiting membrane; *XLM*, external limiting membrane. (AFIP neg. 75-14575; courtesy Dr. Ben S. Fine).

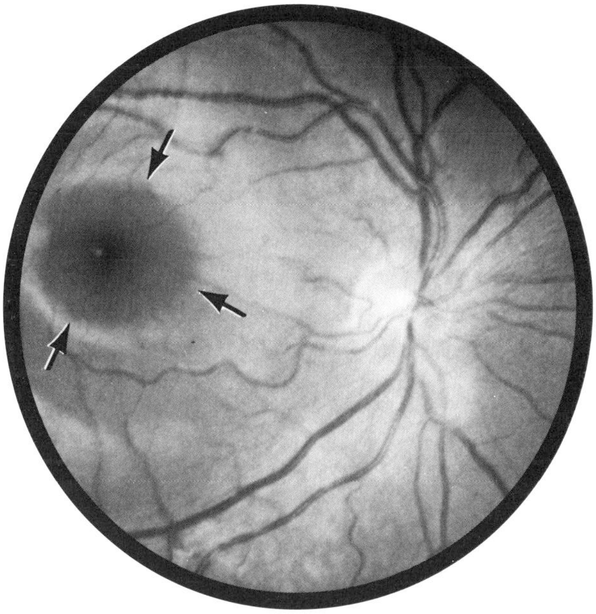

Figure 1.4. Start of slope of anatomic fovea (*arrows*) causes change in reflex from retinal surface.

Table 1.1. Anatomic and clinical equation of terms

Anatomic	Clinical
Area centralis (histologic macula): 6.0–7.5 mm	Posterior Pole
Fovea (centralis): 1.5 mm (i.e., 1 disc diameter)	Macula
Foveola: 0.33 mm (avascular zone: 0.5 mm)	Fovea

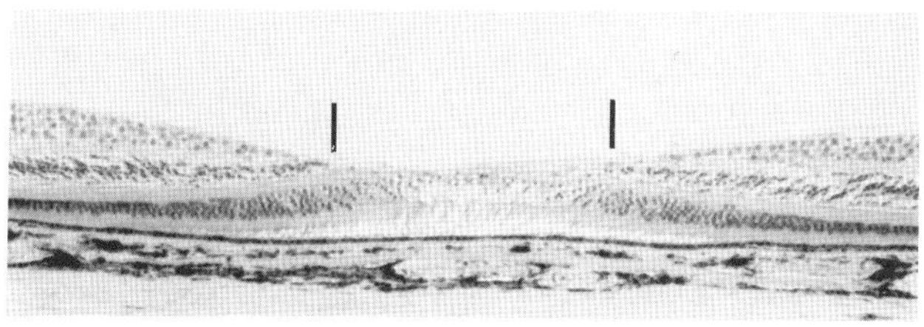

Figure 1.5. Anatomic foveola (*between lines*) is floor of anatomic fovea. Hematoxylin and eosin. ×63.

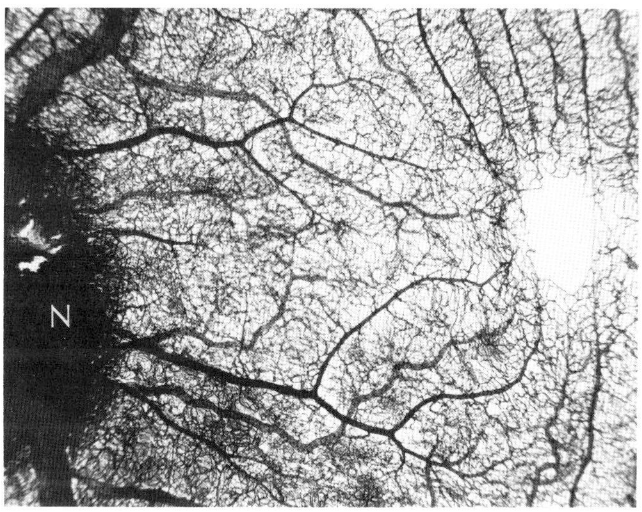

Figure 1.6. Trypsin digestion of retina. Avascular zone to *right*, optic nerve (*N*) to *left*. Periodic acid-Schiff. ×22. (From M. Yanoff: *In* Adler's Textbook of Ophthalmology, 8th ed., ed. by H. G. Scheie and D. M. Albert, 1969, © W. B. Saunders, Philadelphia; reprinted with permission.)

The Normal Macula

It is known that the macula shows less fluorescence than any other part of the retina (Fig. 1.7). There are at least four reasons for this dark zone of the macula: (1) the shape of the cells of the macular retinal pigment epithelium (RPE); (2) the pigment content of the macular RPE; (3) the yellow pigment in the sensory retina of the macula (xanthophyll); and (4) the perifoveal retinal capillary-free zone.

The cells of the macular RPE are narrower, taller, and more regular (i.e., highly uniform) than cells of the RPE elsewhere. (Fig. 1.8). Extramacular RPE, therefore, tends to be wide, low, and irregular, especially toward the periphery. Cells of the macular RPE contain pigment granules throughout their cytoplasm, whereas cells of the extramacular RPE contain granules concentrated mainly within their apical cytoplasm. There are, therefore, more pigment granules per unit area in the macula than elsewhere in the retina.

The macular RPE pigment granules are also different from pigment granules elsewhere (Fig. 1.8). Extramacular RPE contains melanin granules. Pure lipofuscin granules and a mixture of lipofuscin and melanin granules (compound granules) are most prominent in the macular RPE. Lipofuscin has more orange color then melanin; therefore, it is a more efficient fluorescein filter than melanin alone. Less blue excitatory light penetrates to produce choroidal fluorescence and less choroidal fluorescence passes through to the film plane in areas which contain lipofuscin-laden retinal pigment epithelial cells.

Finally, a yellow pigment (xanthophyll), presumably a soluble protein, is found in the macula probably mainly in the outer plexiform layer of the retina. The yellow color imparted to the macula by this pigment is responsible for the term *macula lutea.* The author has observed the yellow pigment in freeze-dried eyes, from rhesus monkeys and from humans (normal donor eyes), in an area that corresponds almost exactly to the macula. Microscopic study of cross-sections, indicates that the yellow color is located within the external plexiform layer and tends to disappear with time following enucleation.

Xanthophyll in the sensory retina acts like lipofuscin and melanin in the pigment epithelium to screen out excitatory light directed toward the choroidal circulation and fluorescing light emerging from it. These three major factors, combined with the perifoveal retinal capillary-free zone, serve collectively to produce the normal dark zone characteristically present in the macula on a fluorescein angiogram.

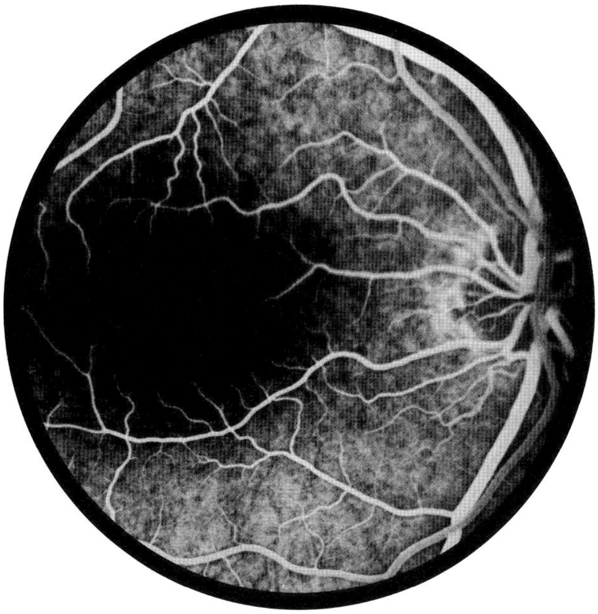

Figure 1.7. Clinical macula (anatomic fovea) shows less fluorescence than remainder of retina. (Courtesy of Terrance L. Tomer.)

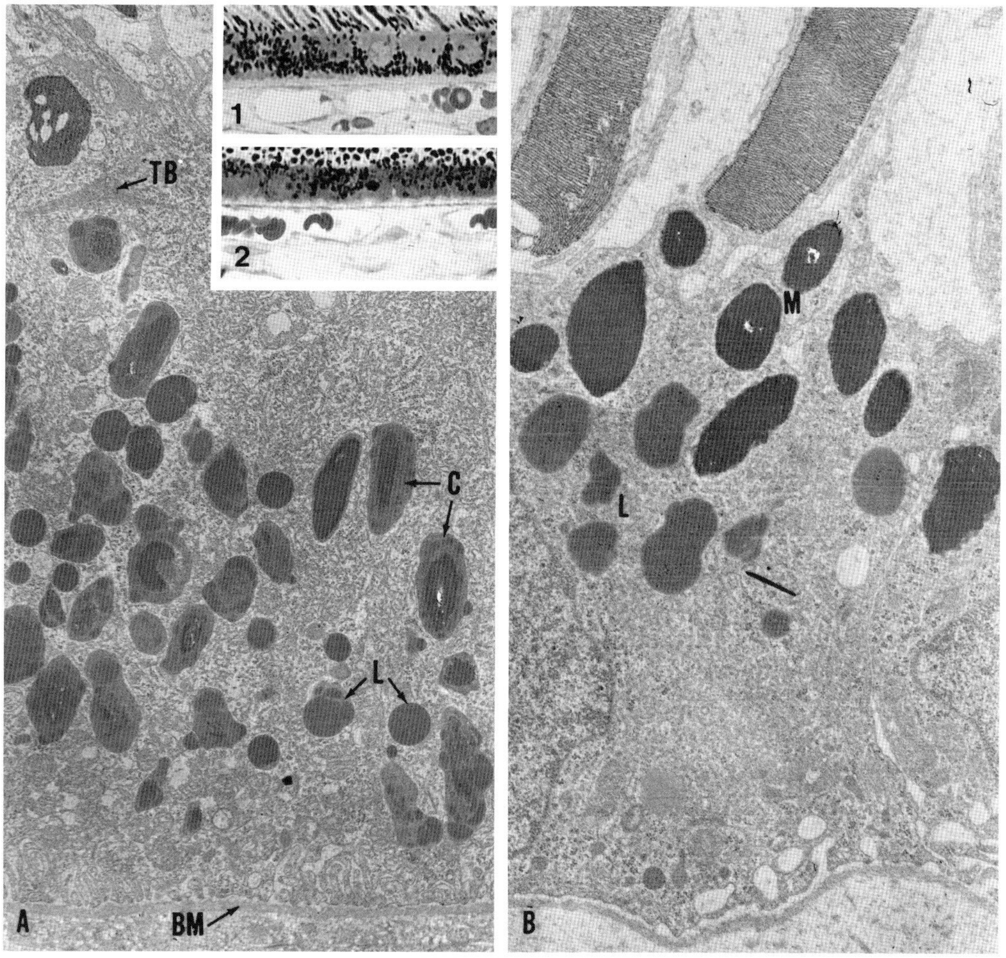

Figure 1.8. *A*, electron micrograph of retinal pigment epithelium (RPE) of anatomic macular area similar to that in *inset 1*. Body and base of cell are occupied by lipofuscin (*L*) and compound (*C*) granules. *BM*, basement membrane of RPE; *TB*, terminal bar (zonula adherens portion). *Main figure*, ×6,000; *inset 1*, 1.5 μ PD ×400, AFIP neg. 71-4896; *inset 2*, 1.5 μ PD ×400, AFIP neg. 71-4897. *B*, electron micrograph of RPE of nonmacular area, similar to nasal retina shown in *inset 2* in *A*, shows fewer granules, located mostly within apical cytoplasm. Ratio of lipofuscin (*L*) to melanin granules (*M*) lower here than in macula. ×12,300. (From B. S. Fine and M. Yanoff: Ocular Histology: A Text and Atlas, 1972, © Harper & Row, New York; reprinted with permission.)

The vasculature of the sensory retina consists of a "closed" system. The capillaries have no fenestrations, contain endothelial cells whose cytoplasm makes up the walls of the capillaries, and are incompletely covered by pericytes (Fig. 1.9). Only the inner half of the retina up to the middle limiting membrane contains vessels. The large vessels are restricted to the nerve fiber and ganglion cell layers. The capillaries present in the nerve fiber, ganglion cell, inner plexiform, inner nuclear, and the innermost aspect of the outer plexiform layers form two distinct plexuses: a superficial capillary plexus located in the nerve fiber and ganglion cell layers; and a deep plexus located in the inner nuclear and inner edge of the outer plexiform layer. The inner plexiform layer contains relatively few capillaries. The outer half of the retina depends on the choriocapillaris and the inner half of the retina for its blood supply. The avascular zone of the sensory retina surrounding the fovea depends on the choriocapillaris along with the surrounding retinal vessels for its nourishment. A separate radial peripapillary capillary network surrounds the disc and the inferior and superior temporal vascular arcades, but is not present in the macula. Because the retinal vasculature is a closed system, under normal conditions fluorescein does not leak out of the retinal vessels.

The RPE is juxtaposed between the sensory retina and the choroid. Because of its pigment content, it acts as a filter to screen out, in part, underlying choroidal fluorescence, especially in the macular area where there is both an increased pigment content and the presence of lipofuscin in addition to the ubiquitous melanin discussed previously. The limiting plasma membranes of the apical villi of the RPE are separated from the retinal photoreceptors by a typical intercellular space which becomes exaggerated greatly when fluid collects there, e.g., in pathologic states like idiopathic central serous chorioretinopathy. Adjacent RPE cells are attached one to another by terminal bars which possess both zonula occludens and zonula adherens portions (Fig. 1.10). The zonula occludens consist of dense adjacent cell membranes so closely applied that the intercellular space appears more or less obliterated, thus obstructing completely, under normal conditions, the flow of serum (and fluorescein) from the choroid *between* the cells of the RPE and into the subsensory retinal space. A similar bond exists in the outer plexiform layer of the retina serving to prevent passage of subretinal fluid into the middle and inner layers of the retina.

The choriocapillaris of the choroid is an open vasculature that consists of an interconnecting network (not a continuous network), and is formed by fenestrated endothelial cells, showing fenestrations on both its inner and outer walls (Fig. 1.11). The total area of fenestrations, however, is greatest in the inner walls. Because of the open vasculature, fluorescein leaks out of the choriocapillaris in abundance to fill the choroid and later stains the underlying sclera.

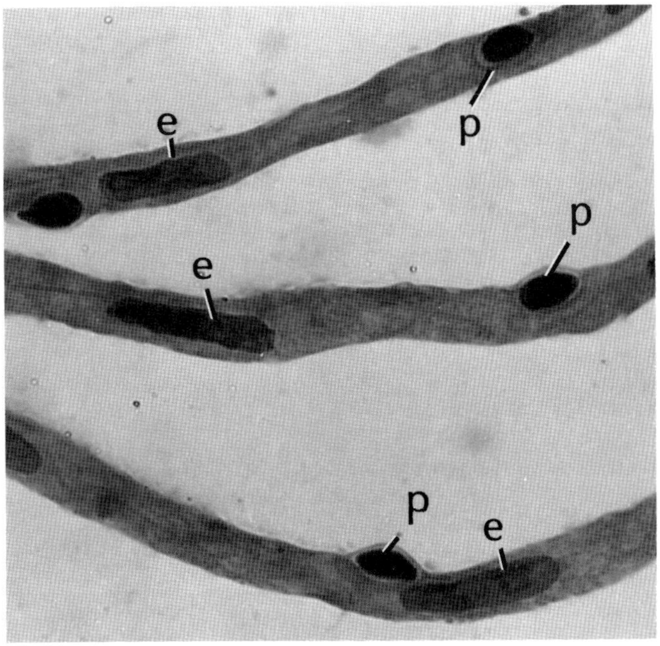

Figure 1.9. Trypsin digestion of retina. Capillaries show endothelial cells (*e*) and pericytes (*p*). Periodic acid-Schiff. ×630. (SEI 74-718; from M. Yanoff and B. S. Fine: Ocular Pathology: A Text and Atlas, 1972, © Harper & Row, New York; reprinted with permission.)

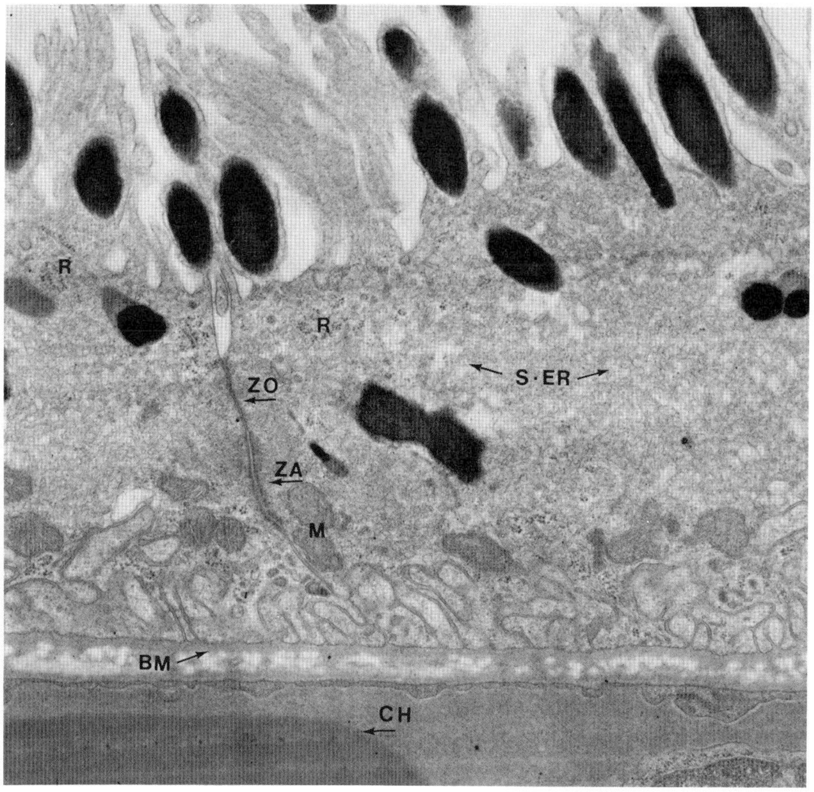

Figure 1.10. RPE shows thin basement membrane (*BM*) along base of cell. Terminal bar attachment girdle, consisting of both a zonula occludens (*ZO*) and zonula adherens (*ZA*) portion, is present between adjacent cells. Mitochondria (*M*) are present in basilar cytoplasm. *R*, free and attached ribosomes; *S · ER,* agranular endoplasmic reticulum; *CH*, choriocapillaris. ×22, 500. (From B. S. Fine: Retinal structure: light and electron microscopic observations. *In* New and Controversial Aspects of Retinal Detachment, ed. by A. McPherson, 1968, © Hoeber, New York; reprinted with permission.)

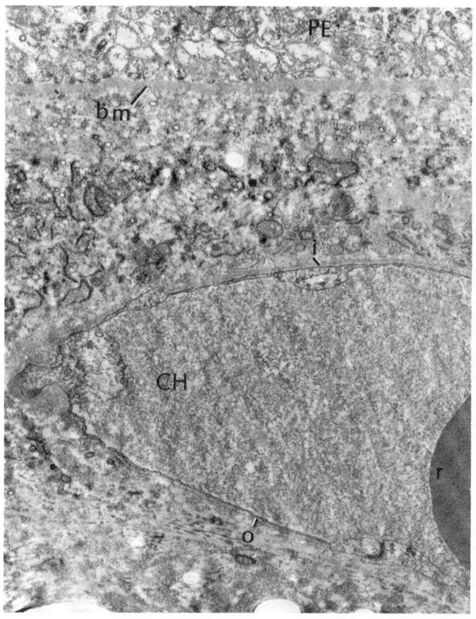

Figure 1.11. Choriocapillaris (*CH*) shows fenestrations on both inner (*i*) and outer (*o*) walls. *bm*, basement membrane of retinal pigment epithelium (*PE*); *r*, red blood cell; from 48-year-old woman who had normal eye removed as part of exenteration. ×14,000. (Courtesy of Dr. Ben S. Fine.)

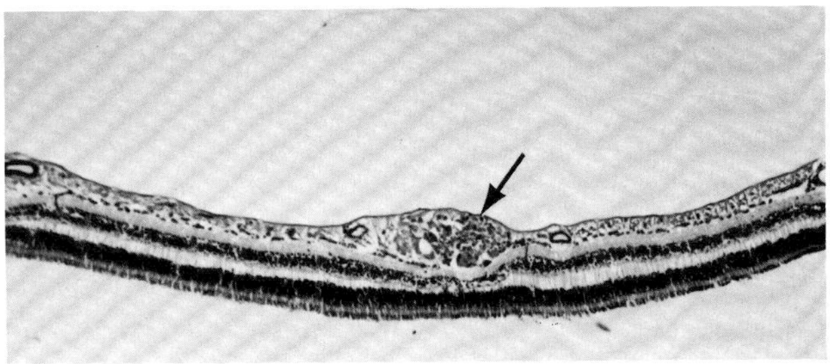

Figure 1.12. Cytoid bodies (*arrow*) in nerve fiber layer of retina from patient with systemic lupus erythematosus. Periodic acid-Schiff. ×28. (SEI 74-1015.)

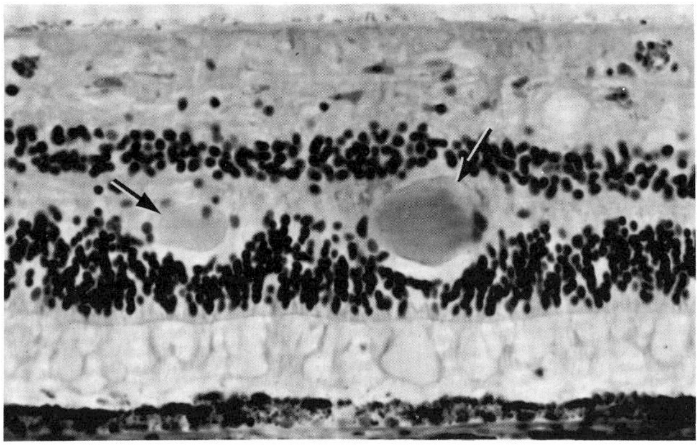

Figure 1.13. Intraretinal collections of fluid (*arrows*) in outer plexiform layer from patient with diabetes mellitus. Hematoxylin and eosin. ×160. (From M. Yanoff: *Am J Ophthalmol, 67:* 21, 1969; reprinted with permission.)

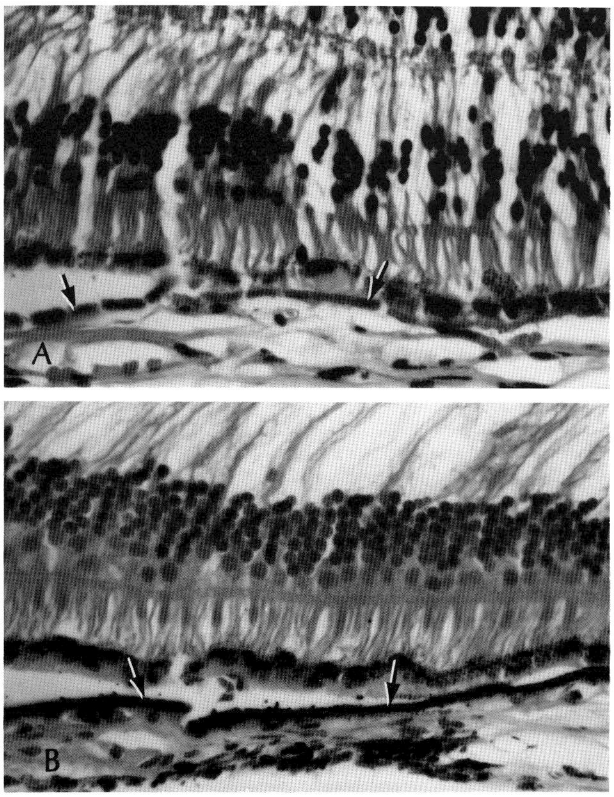

Figure 1.14. In nonexudative-macular degeneration Bruch's membrane (*arrows*) is basophilic in hematoxylin and eosin-stained sections (*A*) and stains positively with von Kossa stain for calcium (*B*). Breaks in Bruch's membrane are artifacts but show fragility of membrane. *A*, hematoxylin and eosin, ×250, SEI 74-660; *B*, von Kossa, ×250; SEI 74-661; *A* and *B*, from M. Yanoff and B. S. Fine: Ocular Pathology: A Text and Atlas, 1975, © Harper & Row, Hagerstown, Md.; reprinted with permission.)

Histopathologic-Fluorescein Angiographic Correlations

Arteriolar obstruction of the superficial capillary plexus of the retina may result in a microinfarct of the nerve fiber layer, i.e., a cotton wool spot (Fig. 1.12). Because of the nonperfusion of the area and of relative mechanical blockage of fluorescence, a cotton wool spot appears hypofluorescent. Other pathologic superficial or deep intraretinal collections of solid substances such as blood or pigment will also block normal choroidal fluorescence and result in areas of hypofluorescence. Leakage of the superficial capillary plexus in general is not too important because of the rich surrounding capillary bed which reabsorbs the excess fluid rapidly. Obstruction of the deep capillary plexus of the retina is relatively unimportant from a clinical-diagnostic point of view. Leakage, however, from the deep plexus, as occurs in diabetic retinopathy, other vaso-occlusive disorders, or in the Irvine-Gass syndrome of cystoid macular edema, "spills over" into the avascular outer retinal layers where reabsorption from the vascularized inner retinal layers and from the choriocapillaris takes place slowly. Hence, if leakage from the deep plexus is significant, fluid collects in the outer retinal layers, predominantly but not exclusively, in the outer plexiform layer in the form of microcystoid spaces. The spaces form as compressed adjacent nerve fibers and/or Müller's fibers jointly serve as their walls. The leaking vessels appear increasingly hyperfluorescent throughout the angiogram series as fluorescein pools into the cystoid spaces. On the other hand, intrasensory retinal collection of fluid itself, may block underlying choroidal fluorescence and appear hypofluorescent, especially when rich in lipoproteins (lipophilic exudates (Fig. 1.13)).

Leakage with the typical signs of increasing size and intensity of fluorescence may occur from the choriocapillaris, through Bruch's membrane, into the subretinal pigment epithelial space, i.e., detachment of the RPE. Because the subretinal pigment epithelial fluid is in direct continuity with the choriocapillaris and the freely permeable Bruch's membrane, hyperfluorescence is seen in the early stages of

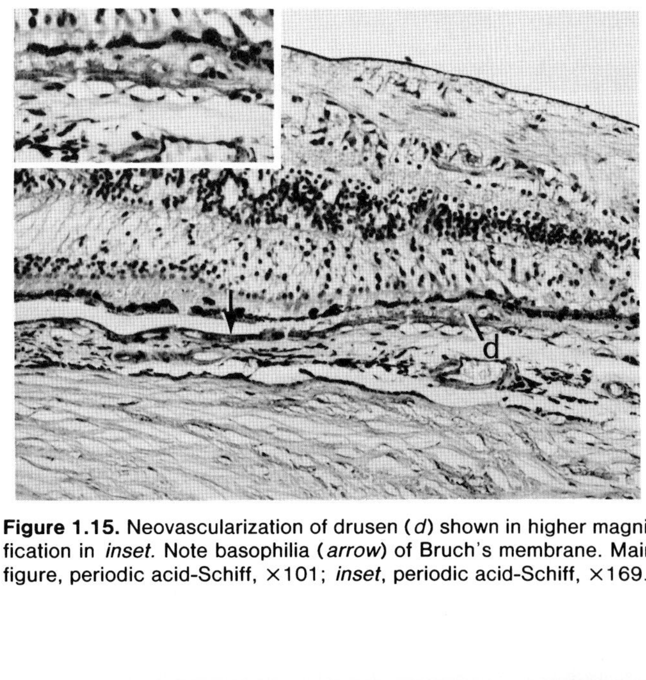

Figure 1.15. Neovascularization of drusen (*d*) shown in higher magnification in *inset.* Note basophilia (*arrow*) of Bruch's membrane. Main figure, periodic acid-Schiff, ×101; *inset*, periodic acid-Schiff, ×169.

the angiogram delineating the entire extent of the retinal pigment epithelial detachment. When a retinal pigment epithelial leak results in a detachment of the sensory retina, i.e., central serous chorioretinopathy, the pigment epithelial leak is evident early in the angiogram as a hyperfluorescent beacon of light but the subsensory retinal detachment becomes hyperfluorescent slowly and fills incompletely with fuzzy borders due to the indirect path which the dye has made through the RPE into the subsensory retinal space.

It is reasonable to expect a detachment of the sensory retina rather than intraretinal edema from fluid flowing through a break in the RPE. A detachment occurs most likely because of the nature of the external limiting membrane of the retina. This membrane is composed of attachment sites of adjacent photoreceptors and Müller cells. The attachments are terminal bars that contain zonula adherens, but not zonula occludens. The tight adherens of cells in the outer part of the sensory retina probably markedly restrict the flow of fluid from the subretinal area into the retina; thus, a sensory retinal detachment results as the fluid, unable to penetrate the sensory retina, collects under it. A loose adherence between the sensory retina and the pigment epithelium itself may also contribute to this phenomenon.

A solid tumor mass such as that produced by hemorrhage, inflammation, or neoplasm, which is avascular or only slightly vascular, will tend to be hypofluorescent depending on its size, density, and location. For example, blood just under the internal limiting membrane of the retina will block out totally underlying fluorescence of the retinal and choroidal circulations. A hemorrhage underneath the RPE, or in the subsensory retinal space, will block out all choroidal fluorescence but not retinal fluorescence; a hemorrhage in the choroid which does not involve the choriocapillaris (or a suprachoroidal nevus which characteristically does not involve the choriocapillaris) will block out large choroidal vessels but not the choriocapillaris or the retinal circulation.

Newly formed capillaries are very fragile and much more permeable than mature vessels. Fluid, and even erythrocytes, leak readily from the new vessels. The newly formed capillaries most likely allow fluid to escape because of incomplete formation of endothelial cell junctions, so that the tight zone (zonula occludens of a terminal bar) is not present or is not developed fully. The neovascularized areas may be contiguous with areas of hemorrhage, offering an excellent opportunity to study differences between hypo- and hyperfluorescence.

Nonexudative or dry macular degeneration shows certain clinical and histologic features. The clinical characteristics consist mainly of drusen, increased translucency, and mottled pigmentation. Histologically, drusen and basophilia (calcification) of Bruch's membrane are noted (Fig. 1.14). In addition, neovascularization of drusen (Fig. 1.15) or subpigment epithelial neovascularization (Fig. 1.16) may be seen. If no hemorrhage or neovascularization is present, the overlying sensory retina may remain normal or may undergo simple atrophy, i.e., nonexudative or dry involutional macular degeneration. With hemorrhage, generally from a neovascularized subpigment epithelial membrane,

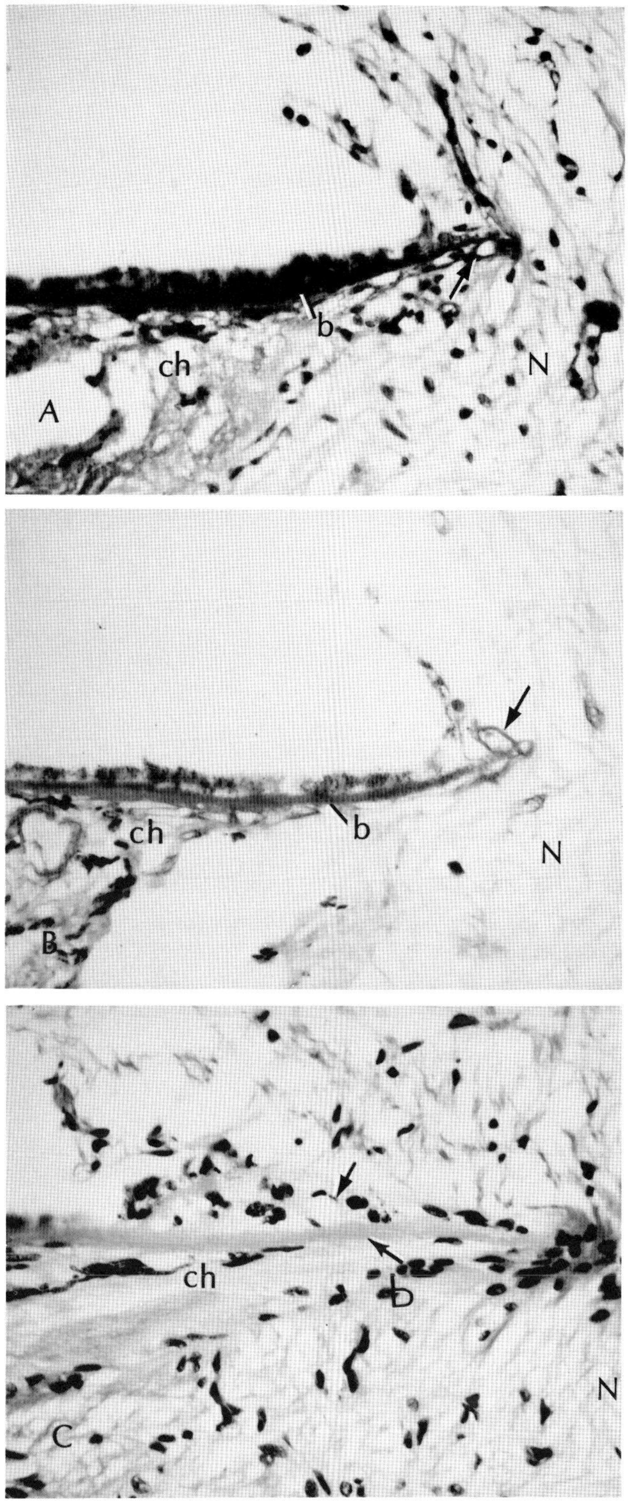

Figure 1.16. Subpigment epithelial neovascularization. Serial microscopic sections show blood vessels (*arrow*) under Bruch's membrane at edge of optic nerve (*A*), turning "corner" (*arrow*) around edge of Bruch's membrane (*B*), and between Bruch's membrane and retinal pigment epithelium (*C*). *Ch*, choroid; *b*, Bruch's membrane; *N*, optic nerve. *A*, periodic acid-Schiff, ×250; *B*, periodic acid-Schiff without hematoxylin, ×250; *C*, hematoxylin and eosin, ×250.

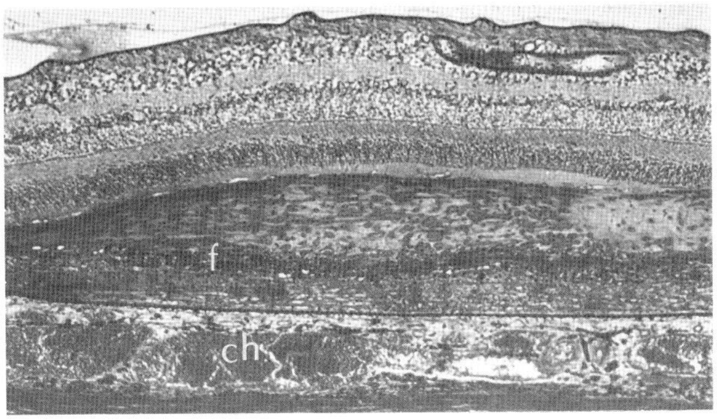

Figure 1.17. Large fibrous plaque (*f*) present under neurosensory retina. *Ch*, choroid. Trichrome. ×40. (SEI 74-491; from M. Yanoff and B. S. Fine: Ocular Pathology: A Text and Atlas, 1975, © Harper & Row, Hagerstown, Md.; reprinted with permission.)

organization and fibrosis occur along with degeneration of the overlying sensory retina, i.e., exudative or wet involutional macular degeneration (Fig. 1.17). Retinal pigment epithelial serous and hemorrhagic detachments, sensory retinal detachments, intraretinal cystoid change, subretinal and intraretinal exudation, subretinal hemorrhage and scar formation are also manifestations of this form of degeneration and may all occur during the evolution of the disciform process.

From a fluorescein angiographic perspective, the state of the RPE and its potential to undergo change are critical. It may detach in a micro way to form drusen or more extensively as pigment epithelial detachments, some of which are complicated by subpigment epithelial neovascularization. Subpigment epithelial turbid fluid may be sufficiently opaque to shield these vessels. The pigment epithelium may also become sufficiently hyperpigmented to shield a subtle subpigment epithelial neovascularized membrane. The

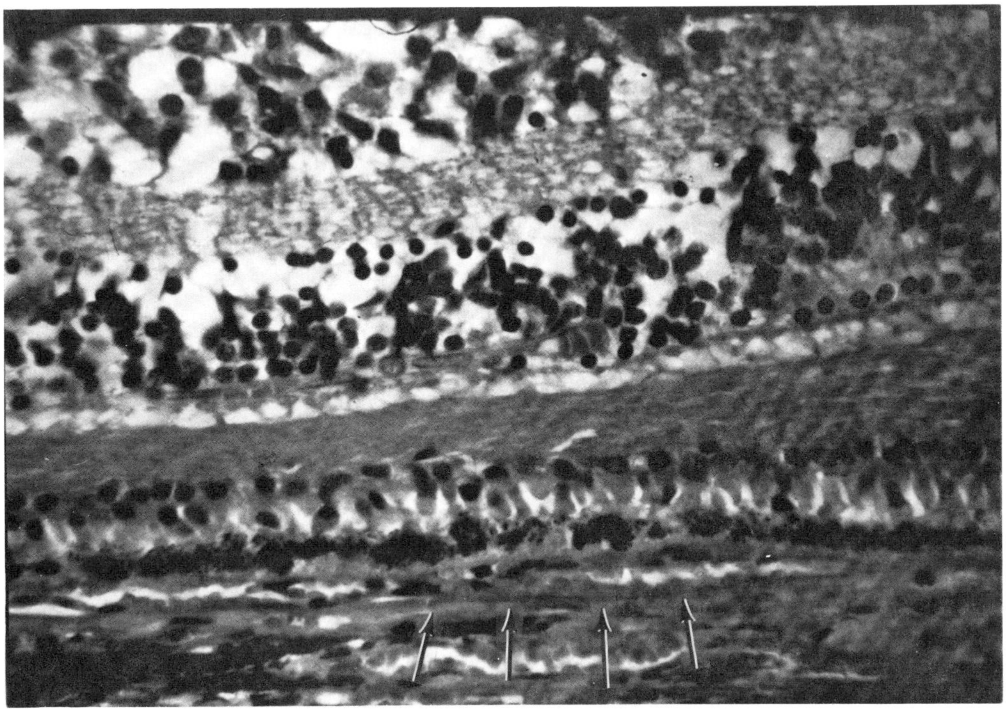

Figure 1.18. Subpigment epithelial neovascularization between Bruch's membrane (*arrows*) and the RPE, in a case of angioid streaks with minimal change in the RPE and sensory retina, implying good vision and a relatively normal fluorescein angiogram. (Courtesy of Brooks Crawford, M.D.)

presence of minimal scarring and the absence of a detachment produce a nonexudative response on the fluorescein angiogram. Preservation of the outer segments of the sensory retina are compatible with these changes, creating a situation in which the eye may function well in the presence of subpigment epithelial neovascularization. Likewise, the fluorescein angiogram may be unable to identify these fine vascular membranes through the pigment epithelium, because of the absence of an exudative response (Fig. 1.18). Thus, subpigment epithelial neovascularization, a dreaded macular manifestation associated with an increasing number of disorders, may be present in visually asymptomatic eyes and not recognizable on either clinical or fluorescein angiographic examination. This possibility poses a number of problems in the full diagnosis and treatment of macular diseases associated with this histopathologic change.

Suggested Readings

Fine, B.S.: Retinal structure: light and electron microscopic observations. *In* New and Controversial Aspects of Retinal Detachment, ed. by A. McPherson, Hoeber, New York, 1968, p. 16.

Friedman, A.H., Gartner, S., and Modi, S.S.: Drusen of the optic disc. A retrospective study in cadaver eyes. *Brit J Ophthalmol, 59:* 413, 1975.

Fine, B.S. and Yanoff, M.: Ocular Histology: A Text and Atlas, Harper & Row, New York, 1972, pp. 29, 30, 48–55, 88–103, 187–189.

Gass, J.D.M.: Pathogenesis of disciform detachment of the neuroepithelium. I-VI. *Am J Ophthalmol, 63:* 573, 1967.

Gass, J.D.M.: Drusen and disciform macular detachment and degeneration. *Arch Ophthalmol, 90:* 206, 1973.

Schatz, H., Burton, T., Yannuzzi, L., and Rabb, M.: Fundus Fluorescein Angiography: A Comprehensive Text and Atlas, C. V. Mosby, St. Louis, 1978.

Wise, G.N., Dollery, C.T., and Henkind, P.: The Retinal Circulation, Harper & Row, New York, 1971, pp. 22–30, 456–498.

Yanoff, M.: Ocular pathology of diabetes mellitus. *Am J Ophthalmol, 67:* 21, 1969.

Yanoff, M.: Anatomy. *In* Adler's Textbook of Ophthalmology, 8th ed., ed. by H.G. Scheie and D.M. Albert, W.B. Saunders, Philadelphia, 1969, p. 66.

Yanoff, M., and Fine, B.S.: Ocular Pathology: A Text and Atlas, Harper & Row, Hagerstown, 1975, pp. 391, 394, 421–431.

CHAPTER 2

Macular Function Tests

Murray A. Wolkstein, M.D., and Ronald E. Carr, M.D.

In diagnosing macular disease as well as in following the course of such diseases, some form of subjective or objective testing is necessary. There is a wide range of such tests, running from the relatively simple visual acuity measurement to more sophisticated psychophysical and electrophysiologic studies. One or more of these tests can be important in determining the extent of macular damage, in following the course of a macular disease, in diagnosing a disease which may not be ophthalmoscopically visible, in determining if a macular change is only part of a more widespread retinal disorder, and in the differentiation of hysteria or malingering from early macular degeneration.

This chapter will initially review certain aspects of the anatomy of the macula that seem appropriate for a better understanding of these tests, will then discuss the more commonly used tests of macular function as well as some recent innovations which may prove useful in the future, and lastly will give some clinical examples in which certain of those test procedures were important in the evaluation of the patient.

Anatomic Definitions

Some of the terms for the areal subdivisions of the posterior retina are clearly defined and precise, whereas others are not. Because of this, a short anatomic review is included to more clearly define various regions to be mentioned in the body of this chapter.

The fovea refers to the concave, central 1.5 mm of retina corresponding to 5 degrees of central visual field. It lacks the inner retinal layers; namely, the nerve fiber layer, the ganglion cell layer, the bipolar cell layer, and the middle limiting membrane. The center of the fovea is located about 3.0–4.25 mm temporal to the optic disc and slightly inferior to the horizontal meridian from the center of the disc. Because of the heaping up of the ganglion cells at its periphery, the foveal reflex is seen ophthalmoscopically. The central 0.4–0.65 mm is avascular and devoid of capillaries. The foveola is the central 0.33 mm of the fovea. It appears ophthalmoscopically as a reddish spot with a yellowish punctate or curvilinear, glinting reflex, the foveolar reflex. This region contains only cones. The clinician conventionally refers to the foveola as the fovea.

The term "macula" is used differently by various authors and indeed the differences in describing the anatomic, histologic, and clinical macular areas often seem justified.

Histologists have defined the macular region in terms of three other criteria: (1) the ganglion cell layer is more than one cell thick; (2) the Henle fibers are obliquely arranged; and (3) the concentration of cones is large.

Other commonly used histologic terms to subdivide the posterior retina are parafovea and perifovea. Others have defined these in terms of the number of rows of ganglion cells. The fovea contains no ganglion cells. The parafovea is a 0.5-mm belt surrounding the fovea containing five to eight rows of ganglion cells whereas the perifovea is a band 1.5 mm in width outside the parafovea containing two to four rows of ganglion cells. Some authors use the term macula to define the area within the outer border of the perifovea, a zone 5.5 mm in diameter.

The term macula as used in this chapter shall be a clinical one and will refer to that area temporal to the disc in which the foveal pit constitutes the center, and the entire region encompasses an area of approximately one disc diameter. This clinical designation seems more appropriate when speaking of macular disease.

A common misconception is that the central retinal area contains only cones. However, it is only the central 0.4–0.6 mm that is rod free and this region contains about 25,000 total cones [1]. The remainder of the fovea contains on the average about one rod per cone. Cone density is maximal at the foveola and falls off rapidly to a low constant level outside the central 10 degrees. Conversely, rod density increases markedly outside the foveal region to a maximum at approximately 20 degrees nasal to fixation and 15 degrees temporal (Fig. 2.1).

Some authors have tried to correlate visual acuity with specific areas of retina. The acuity range within the foveola or central 1.0 degree is found to be between 20/10 and 20/25, whereas at the edge of this rod free zone, acuities range from 20/20 to 20/50. The range at 2.5 degrees from fixation is 20/40 to 20/70; at 5 degrees, 20/60 to 20/80; and at 10 degrees, 20/100 to 20/200.

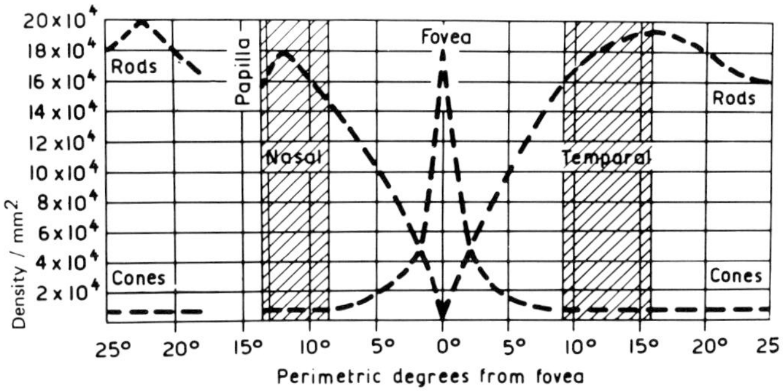

Figure 2.1. Photoreceptor concentration. The concentration of rods and cones with respect to retinal locus is graphically presented. The cone concentration is maximal at the fovea and rapidly falls to a low constant value outside of 10 degrees from fixation. The maximal rod concentration occurs 20 degrees nasal and 15 degrees temporal to fixation. No rods are present in the central 1–2 degrees. (Adapted from G.A. Osterberg: *Acta Ophthalmol,* suppl. VI, 1935.)

MACULAR FUNCTION TESTS

Retinal function testing can be divided into psychophysical and physiologic methods. A psychophysical test is subjective. A physical stimulus is presented to the patient and the patient indicates verbally or by other subjective means his detection of the stimulus. Physiologic methods are objective. A stimulus is presented and a response parameter is measured by electrophysiological or other means.

I. Psychophysical Tests
   A. Visual acuity
   B. Color vision
   C. Dark adaptation
   D. Perimetry
   E. Amsler grid
   F. Photostress test
   G. Tests dependent on macular pigment
   H. Grating psychophysics
   I. Foveal flicker sensitivity
II. Electrophysiologic Tests
   A. Electroretinography (ERG)
   B. Electrooculography (EOG)
   C. Visually evoked response (VER)

PSYCHOPHYSICAL TESTS

Visual Acuity

Visual acuity measurement is the most common test of foveal function. The eye must first be refracted to best correction for acuity to be a significant measure of foveolar performance. Acuity is measured by the visual resolution of a letter, symbol, or a pattern. The smaller the visual angle subtended by the parts of the test letter correctly seen by the observer, the better the resolution of his visual system.

A second factor involved in acuity measurement is contrast. One definition of contrast is the difference in the luminance between dark and light parts of the test area (dark letters and the white surround of a Snellen chart) divided by the mean luminance. Visual resolution of single figures generally suffers when contrast is markedly diminished.

The Snellen Chart

Since the early 1900's, the Snellen chart has been almost universally used by ophthalmologists for acuity measurement. The Snellen score is expressed as a fraction. The numerator is the test distance and the denominator is determined by the size of the smallest letter correctly identified. The numerical value of the denominator is the distance at which the height of this smallest identified test letter subtends 5 minutes of visual angle on the retina. Each component of this letter subtends 1 minute at this distance. For example, a 20/50 Snellen score means that the test is performed at 20 feet, the smallest letter correctly identified subtends 5 minutes of visual angle at 50 feet, and each component line subtends 1 minute at 50 feet. The reciprocal of the Snellen fraction gives the visual angle, in minutes, which is subtended by each component at the test distance. Therefore, the reciprocal of 20/50 (0.4) is 2.5; the component lines of the smallest correctly read letter subtends 2.5 minutes at the 20-foot test distance and the total letter height subtends 12.5 minutes.

Some Snellen charts are constructed of white cardboard with black letters and are illuminated by a light source. Alternatively, black letters and a light surround are projected on a screen. Both systems provide background luminances well into the photopic range where small changes in contrast or background luminance have little effect on acuity scores.

The Landolt C

The Landolt C chart is composed of a series of letter "C's" of decreasing size in which the position of the gap in the C is variable. Each test line is labeled with the distance at which the height of the C subtends 5 minutes. At each distance the width of the curved line composing the C subtends 1 minute and the gap, likewise, subtends 1 minute. The score is expressed as a fraction, analogous to the Snellen fraction. The Landolt C, like the Snellen test, is performed at high contrast levels.

Grating Acuity

Gratings constructed of alternating black and white bars have been used since the 18th century to measure visual acuity. The acuity score is determined by the finest grating that can be detected at near 100% contrast; i.e., when the bars are black and white.

In the past it was believed that grating acuity was in close agreement with acuity obtained by methods employing single figures such as the Snellen test. For example, the expected visual resolution for a patient with 20/20 acuity was a 1-minute component of a 20/20 Snellen letter and also a 1-minute bar of grating. In recent years, however, a dissociation of grating and Snellen acuity has been observed in patients with lesions of the central nervous system [2] and in cases of presumed maculopathy of tapeto-retinal degenerations [3]. Unlike the traditional Snellen and Landolt C tests, gratings have been used to determine a patient's contrast sensitivity as well as his visual resolution. This technique will be described later in this chapter. It is presently a research tool requiring a complex stimulus and recording apparatus.

Optokinetic Nystagmus

Optokinetic nystagmus (OKN) is not a subjective (psychophysical) test, but since it is used to measure acuity, it shall be discussed under this section.

An OKN drum containing alternating stripes is rotated in front of the observer. This normally elicits a jerky nystagmus if the observer's visual system can resolve the stripes. The visual angle can be calculated from the width of this finest effective stripe and the distance between the test drum and the subject. The stimulus visual angle can be varied by using drums of decreasing bar width. Another method decreases the visual angle by increasing the test distance. However, doing this also decreases the total drum or total target size resulting in a smaller retinal area being stimulated and, therefore, a weaker stimulus for OKN. The correlation of OKN acuity with that of single figure methods is not always reliable.

Alternatively, stationary targets of variable size can be placed in front of the rotating drum. If the subject is able to resolve and fixate on the stationary target, the OKN reflex will not occur. Acuity is calculated from the visual angle subtended by the smallest target that stops the OKN. OKN tests require some patient cooperation, and an unwilling subject can often stare through the moving stripes.

Color Vision

Useful trichromatic color vision is thought to be processed by the central 30–60 degrees of the visual field. Hereditary dystrophies of the posterior pole, nonhereditary maculopathies, and certain optic nerve conditions often result in acquired color defects. One must likewise be aware that a maculopathy may also develop in a patient with a previously existing and unrelated congenital color defect.

As a rule, congenital trichromatic color deficiencies, are not particularly rare, affect males, are symmetric, involve the red-green color system, and occur as isolated visual defects. By contrast, acquired dyschromatopsias are asymmetric, are accompanied by other visual dysfunctions and most commonly show irregularities in color testing not usually seen in the congenital varieties. Examples of acquired color defects are the blue-yellow dyschromatopsia of central serous chorioretinopathy and retinitis pigmentosa, or the red-green defect of acquired cone degeneration or optic neuritis.

Color defectives have specific areas of intrinsic desaturation in the visual spectrum. Desaturation means that a hue appears washed out, grayish, or whitish. For example, deep red is saturated; pink of the same hue (wavelength) and intensity is desaturated. Points of minimum saturation, known as neutral points, are characteristic for each type of color defect. A hue at the neutral point appears grayish and the complementary color for this neutral point also appears desaturated. Consequently, the color defective has difficulty differentiating the color at the neutral point from its complement or from gray. Thus, the neutral point and its complement are color confusion pairs. If each of these complements is mixed with the same amount of a third color, two other color confusion pairs result. Many color tests take advantage of this phenomenon and either the test object and the background are color confusion pairs or the test object is a neutral point color and the background is gray. Tests utilizing these factors are called color confusion tests and in the clinical sphere include the Ishihara test plates, the Farnsworth Panel D-15, the American Optical Hardy-Rand-Rittler peudoisochromatic plates (AOHRR), and the Sloan Achromatopsia Test.

Color Confusion Tests

Ishihara Plates. This test is based on color confusion in the red-green color blind patient. The color of the test symbol and the background is of such hue, saturation, and intensity so as to be confused by protans (red blind) and deutans (green blind).

Farnsworth Panel D-15. This test is also based on zones of color confusion. The subject is asked to arrange a series of 15 colored caps such that each succeeding cap appears most similar in appearance to the previous cap. The D-15 Panel classifies the moderate and severe color defective into protan (red blind), deutan (green blind), and tritan (blue blind) axes of confusion. Mild color defectives score normally.

AOHRR Plates. The AOHRR plates have colored symbols and a gray background. The hues of the colored symbols occur at the neutral points of color defective patients. The saturation of the test symbol colors is progressively increased in successive plates. The color blind patient has difficulty discerning the test symbol from the gray background. This test is useful for screening and categorizing red-green and blue-yellow defectives in terms of severity of the defect and the axis of confusion. It cannot differentiate a dichromat (a patient with only two cone pigments) from an anomalous trichromat (one with three cone pigments).

Sloan Achromatopsia Test. This test presents to the observer a series of highly saturated colors which he is asked to match to a series of gray shades. The achromat, or totally color blind patient, makes characteristic matches while a dichromat or trichromat cannot make any match.

Hue Discrimination Tests

Hue (wavelength) discrimination for the color defective and normal is best at spectral zones of intrinsic desaturation and poorest at zones of best saturation (Pitt's law). The results are diagnostic for the type of dyschromatopsia. The color blind subject exhibits characteristic spectral regions of poor hue discrimination which differ from the normal subject since the intrinsic saturation for the color defective differs from the normal.

Farnsworth-Munsell 100 Hue Test. The subject arranges

85 colored caps (4 separate boxes each containing about 20 caps) such that each succeeding cap is closest in hue to the preceding cap. The F-M 100 Hue test is based entirely on hue discrimination and not on color confusion pairs as the caps are balanced for saturation and intensity. The test rates the degree of color discrimination in normal subjects in addition to measuring zones of poor hue discrimination in color defectives. Specific zones of poor hue discrimination identify the nature of the dyschromatopsia. This test takes longer to perform and is more taxing on a patient than the previous ones.

All of the tests mentioned so far should be performed under the standard illumination of the MacBeth lamp.

Nagel Anomaloscope

This test is based on color matching. It is considered by some authorities to be the best examination for the accurate classification of red-green defects. The subject must match a standard yellow light in color and brightness with a mixture of red and green. Normal subjects give a narrow matching range, the so-called Rayleigh match. Characteristic matching patterns are elicited for the different types of red-green dyschromatopsias and achromats.

There are other anomaloscopes now available which classify blue-yellow defects in addition to the red-green variety. Some of these intruments have larger test areas than the Nagel anomaloscope and are therefore more easily used by patients with macular dysfunction.

Recent Innovations in Color

Gunkel [4] recently introduced a new color test apparatus. The visual spectrum is arranged in a color circle. Each circumferential meridian of the circle is of constant saturation and changing hue. Each radial meridan exhibits constant hue, but progressively decreasing saturation toward the center of the circle. The very central point is seen as white. In the view box, the patient sees a patch from any region of the color circle and indicates whether he sees a hue or just gray or white. In this manner, a two-dimensional area of color neutrality is plotted on a color circle diagram. This instrument seems to be a promising new diagnostic tool although it has not been used extensively in the clinical setting as yet.

Dark Adaptation

Dark adaptometry is a test whereby retinal sensitivity can be followed over time.

The eye is exposed to a standard light bleach (pre-adaptation). This precedes the plotting of the dark adaptation curve. Following the bleach, the patient fixates on a test light located 12–15 degrees eccentric to the stimulus light which itself can be varied in diameter. This retinal locus is in an area of good cone-rod mix. The intensity of the test light is slowly increased from below threshold until the patient detects it. The minimal intensity for detection is the threshold at this point in time. By taking a threshold reading every minute a curve of the changing threshold versus time of dark adaptation is obtained. The curve is normally biphasic with a "rod-cone break" at about 10 minutes. The primary or early branch concerns mainly cone adaptation and the secondary branch, rod adaptation (Fig. 2.2). Additional information can be derived by varying the size of the test stimulus so as to derive an area-intensity function.

In addition to a complete curve at a single retinal location, a retinal profile of "final adaptation thresholds" can be obtained at a series of retinal loci after full dark adaptation. Thus, one can look at the sensitivity of a variety of retinal areas. Such a test can be done by modifying a standard adaptometer (Goldmann-Weekers) or by using certain of the standard perimeters.

With regard to the macular region, this test can likewise be modified so that foveal function can be studied as well as parafoveal areas. Often the sensitivity of such studies can be enhanced by using red light stimuli, a color to which the cones show maximal sensitivity. In testing the foveal area a monophasic function is derived which is indicative of cone function (Fig. 2.2).

Perimetry

Dynamic Perimetry

Dynamic perimetry offers another, more commonly used method for the evaluation of the central visual field. Central or paracentral scotomata are often elicited in posterior pole disease and the plotting of several isopters by variation of test object, color, size, and intensity help to better characterize field defects. Macular disease is sometimes part of a generalized pathologic process, and in such cases peripheral fields may also show abnormalities.

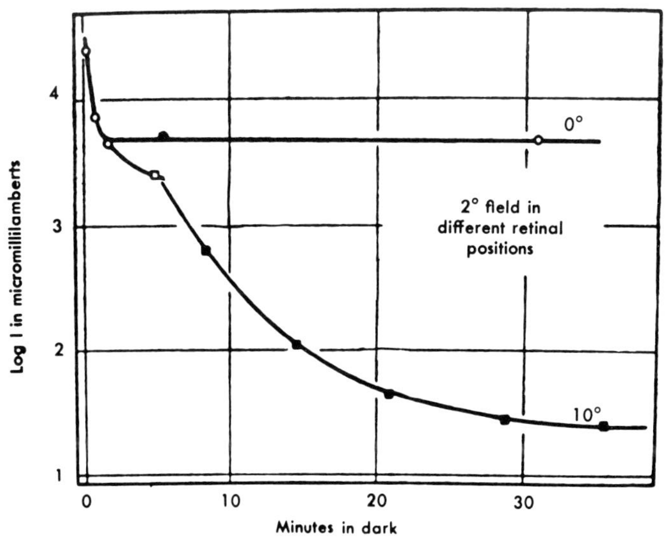

Figure 2.2. Dark adaptation. After a standard pre-adaptation bleach, a dark adaptation curve is obtained with a 2 degree white target. The bottom curve is taken from a point 10 degrees inferior to fixation, an area of good rod-cone mixture. A biphasic curve results with the primary branch reflecting rod adaptation. The rod-cone break occurs at about 10 minutes. The uppermost curve was taken at fixation. The central 2 degrees of retina contains cones primarily. Therefore, a monophasic curve is obtained.

Static Perimetry

Static perimetry differs from dynamic perimetry in that it measures the detection of a static target at a specific point in the visual field. The luminance of the target is slowly increased until it is detected. Each target is presented for 1 second followed by a 2- to 3-second rest. A standard steady photopic background luminance is maintained in the perimeter bowl. The luminance necessary for detection of the target is plotted along several diagonal meridians. Each meridian crosses the fixation point and, thus, a sensitivity curve is obtained for each meridian. While this test has been used in the past primarily for the study of glaucoma patients, careful static perimetry of the central 2–4 degrees offers promise as a sensitive index for the diagnosis of early maculopathy [3].

Flicker Perimetry

Flicker perimetry measures the critical fusion frequency to a small (about 2 degrees) white flickering light at different positions in the visual field. The peak luminance of the test light is a constant in the photopic range and the flicker frequency in flashes per second is gradually increased. The critical fusion frequency is the lowest frequency at which the subject perceives the light to be nonflickering. From the results a flicker field is plotted that can be compared to a normal plot.

Amsler Grid

The Amsler grid is a qualitative nonspecific test that can be helpful in detecting scotomata and visual distortion. When distortion of the grid lines is seen, it is nonspecific in terms of locus in the visual system except to state that the scotoma is either central or paracentral in visual field projections. This is an easy and rapid screening test.

Photostress Test

The clinical observation that some patients with macular edema had prolonged afterimages provided the impetus in the development of the light or photostress test. In this test after visual acuity is determined, a light is shined into the eye for a specific period. After the light is extinguished, the time to return to baseline acuity is then measured and compared to a normal eye regression curve. The intensity and duration of the light stress should be standardized by each clinician so that reliable deviations from the norm can be determined. The test is rather nonspecific inasmuch as patients with many forms of macular disease and also some patients with optic nerve disease may require a much longer time than normal to recover their pretest acuity. It is of interest, however, that the presence of macular edema will lead to greatest prolongation. While standards of abnormalcy and age regression curves have been determined for this test, there are no specific guidelines as to the cause of prolonged afterimages or to the types of maculopathies which might cause this phenomenon.

Tests Dependent on Macular Pigment

Two tests are believed to depend on the arrangement of the yellow pigment in the inner retinal layers of the macula lutea. These are the Haidinger's brushes and the Maxwell's spot.

Haidinger's Brushes

The subject looks through a polarizer at a surface illuminated with blue light. If his macula is normal, he will see two hourglass-shaped brushes radiating from the fixation point. The axis of the brushes is parallel to the vector of light transmitted by the polarizer. Because of adaptation to stationary brushes, the polarizer is rotated and then the brushes will persist and be observed to rotate continually.

It is hypothesized that there is differential absorption of radially and tangentially polarized blue light due to the arrangement of the pigment molecules. This differential absorption results in the perception of the Haidinger's brushes by a normal macula. If the yellow pigment arrangement is disrupted by pathology in the inner retinal layers, the brushes will not be seen. This test is commonly used as a screening test for retinal pathology in strabismus patients with amblyopia.

Maxwell's Spot

A subject with a normal macula will see a 3-degree dark ring surrounding fixation upon looking through a blue filter at a brightly illuminated white surface. Usually a smaller dark spot is seen at the fixation point itself. The dark ring and the spot will fade as the eye adapts to the blue light. These can be restored by readapting to a yellow light; i.e., by having the subject look through a yellow filter for a moment. Following this, the dark ring and spot will again be elicited by the blue filter.

Some visual physiologists believe that perception of the Maxwell's spot depends on the screening of the photoreceptors by the macular pigment while others believe that variations in the relative numbers of different types of color receptors in the foveal region explain this phenomenon.

Two other tests, grating psychophysics and foveal flicker sensitivity, are not clinically available in most centers. These tests may be characterized as research modalities, but they eventually may play an important role in the diagnosis of macular disorders.

Grating Psychophysics

Fourier's analysis is a mathematical tool which has been found to be valuable in the study of information processing in neural systems. It is especially easy to apply this technique to systems in which the output can be characterized as the sum of sinusoidal inputs; i.e., linear systems. Traditional gratings constructed of alternating discrete dark and light bars have a changing luminance described by a square wave function. In order to explore spatial processing by the visual system with Fourier's techniques, gratings have been introduced with bar luminance constantly changing to follow a sine wave function. Discrete edges are not seen in such gratings (Fig. 2.3).

A grating detection test is performed by having the patient fix on the center of a sinusoidal grating, preferably small enough to fall within the macular region. The mean luminance of the grating is held constant at all times. The pattern is alternated at a regular rate with a homogeneous screen of the same mean luminance. The patient indicates when he can or cannot see the on-off bar pattern. This test has been applied to visual problems resulting from cerebral and, more recently, retinal pathology [2, 3].

The number of pairs of dark and light bars per degree of visual angle is termed the "spatial frequency" of the grating. The "cut-off frequency" is the highest detectable spatial frequency at 100% contrast; i.e., the finest detectable grating with black and white bars. For lower spatial frequencies, contrast provides a measure of grating detectability. Contrast is defined as the luminance difference between the dark and light bars divided by twice the mean luminance of the pattern. The minimum contrast required to detect a given grating is the contrast threshold, and its inverse value is the contrast sensitivity. The plot of the latter as a function of the spatial frequency is a "contrast sensitivity curve." Abnormalities of a patient's contrast sensitivity are best demonstrated by a normalized plot called a "visuogram." This is a plot of the ratio of the patient's contrast sensitivity to that of the average normal subject's at corresponding spatial frequencies.

The contrast sensitivity curves of normal subjects with 20/20 Snellen acuity show little intersubject variability and change predictably with visual blurring due to refractive error. The bar width at the cut-off frequency correlates closely with the component width of the smallest Snellen letter correctly identified. However, in patients with cerebral lesions involving the visual pathways and with the presumed maculopathy of retinitis pigmentosa, the curve is no longer predictable from the visual acuity measurement.

Figure 2.3. Sinusoidal gratings. Sinusoidal gratings of two different spatial frequencies are demonstrated. Spatial frequency is the number of pairs of dark and light bars per degree of visual angle. The higher the spatial frequency, the finer the grating.

That is, different types of contrast sensitivity loss can be seen in different patients with the same Snellen acuity score [2]. In the presumed maculopathy of retinitis pigmentosa, a dissociation has been found between the cut-off frequency of the grating and the Snellen acuity score in addition to an increasing contrast sensitivity loss at the high spatial frequencies [3] (Fig. 2.4 and 2.5).

Foveal Flicker Sensitivity

There has been a rebirth of interest in the variation of foveal sensitivity to flicker as a function of temporal frequency. A small flickering test light is superimposed on a constant background luminance. The luminance of the flickering test light is sinusoidally modulated; i.e., it increases and decreases in a sinusoidal fashion above and below the mean luminance resulting in maximum and minimum peak luminances. The mean luminance of the

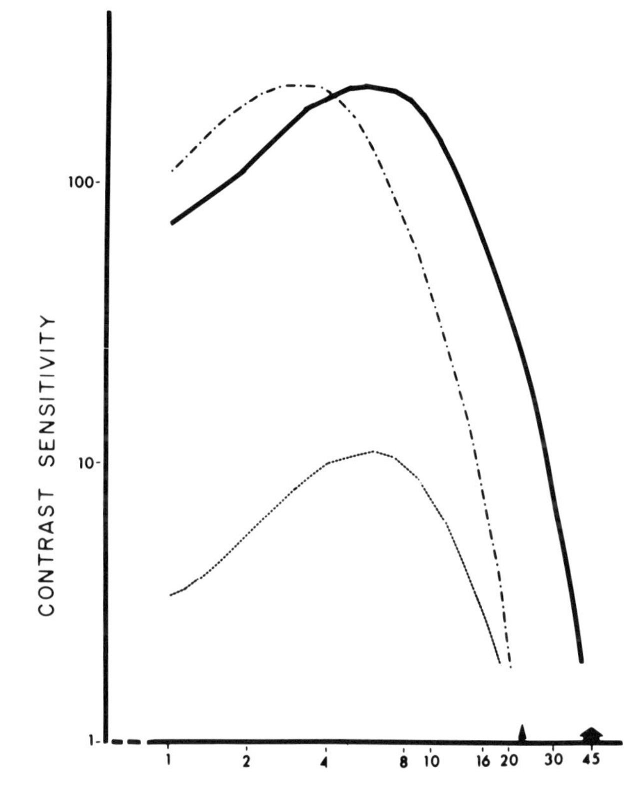

Figure 2.4. Grating contrast sensitivity. The *solid line* shows the grating contrast sensitivity curve of the average normal with 20/20 Snellen acuity. It extrapolates to a cut-off frequency of 45 cycles/degree (*broad solid arrow*). The *upper dotted curve* shows an increasing loss of contrast sensitivity at high spatial frequencies and can be viewed as a shift of the normal curve to the left. The *lower dotted curve* shows a level or constant loss of contrast sensitivity for all spatial frequencies and can be viewed as a shift of the normal curve inferiorly. Both *dotted curves* have similar extrapolated cut-off frequencies of 22.5 (*fine arrow*) corresponding to 20/40 Snellen acuity. It is obvious that the contrast sensitivity function is not predictable from the Snellen score. (From I. Bodis-Wollner and S. Diamond: *Brain, 99:* 695, 1976; reprinted with permission.)

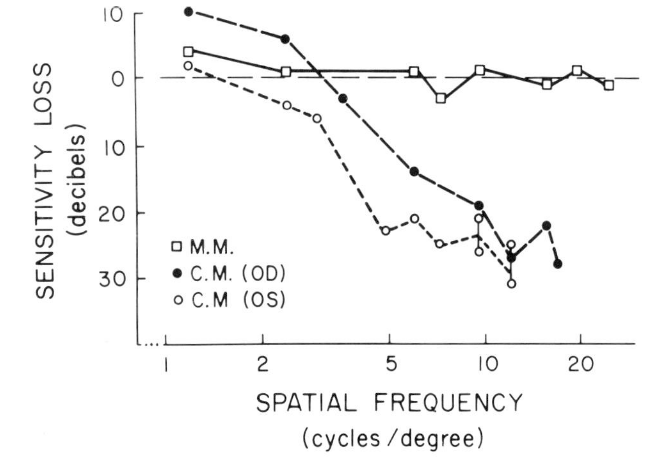

Figure 2.5. Visuogram plot of grating contrast sensitivity. A visuogram is a normalized plot of grating contrast sensitivity. Sensitivity loss is expressed in decibels similar to an audiogram. M.M. has retinitis pigmentosa, 20/20- Snellen acuity and a normal visuogram. C.M. also has retinitis pigmentosa and 202/0- Snellen acuity, but her visuogram shows an increasing loss of contrast sensitivity at high spatial frequencies. Her cut-off frequencies (cycles/degree), 17, OD and 12 OS, are much lower than the 45 cycles/degree expected for 20/20 Snellen acuity. (From M. Wolkstein, A. Atkin, and I. Bodis-Wollner: Grating acuity in two sisters with tapetoretinal degeneration. *In* ERG, VER and Psychophysics, ed. by T. Lawwill, XIV ISCERG Symposium in Louisville, Kentucky, *Doc Ophthalmol, 13:* 1976; reprinted with permission.)

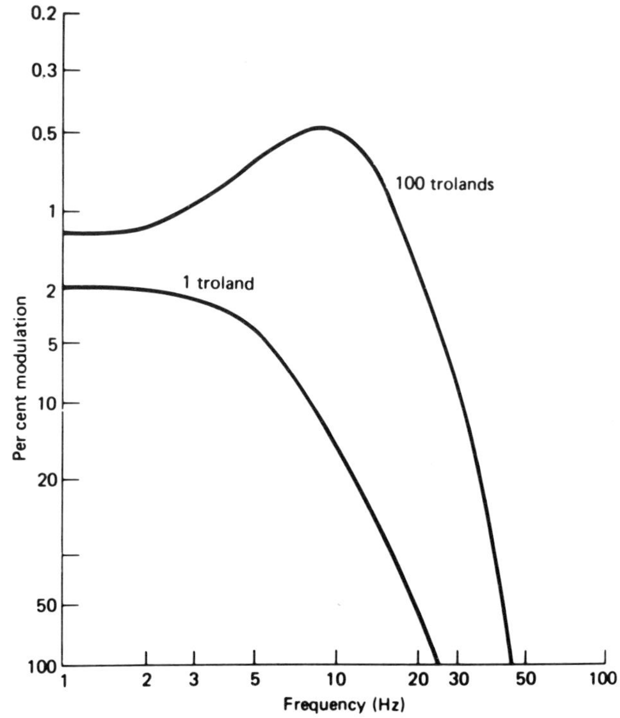

Figure 2.6. Foveal flicker sensitivity curves. Foveal flicker sensitivity curves are obtained using a sinusoidally modulated 0.5–2 degree flickering light. The mean luminance of the test light and the equiluminant surround is constant for each curve (100 trolands in the *upper* and 1 troland in the *lower*). At each temporal flicker frequency (plotted on the *abscissa* in Hz), the smallest per cent modulation is determined for perception of the foveally presented flickering test light. (Modified from H. DeLange: *J Opt Soc Am, 48:* 777, 1958.)

test light is equal to that of the surround. The test spot is usually 0.5–2.0 degrees in size for foveal flicker sensitivity.

For each temporal frequency value (cycles per second or Hz), the threshold is the minimum modulation depth at which detection of flicker occurs. The reciprocal of the threshold is the sensitivity. A flicker sensitivity curve can then be plotted as a function of temporal frequency of the flickering test light [5] (Fig. 2.6). For each curve the mean luminance of the test light and the equiluminant surround is a constant. The patient's flicker sensitivity curve can be compared with what is normally expected. Recently, fall-offs in sensitivity were found at high temporal flicker frequencies in certain retinal disorders, even when visual acuity was normal [6]. Flicker sensitivity studies may prove to be another fruitful avenue of research into the clinical diagnosis of macular disorders.

ELECTROPHYSIOLOGICAL TESTS

Electroretinography (ERG)

The usual clinical electroretinogram is the recording of the electrical potential waveform generated by the total (preganglionic) retina in response to a diffuse light stimulus. The test is performed using a corneal contact lens electrode which records changes in the corneo-retinal potential with each light stimulus. The clinically important components are the initial corneal negative a-wave and the second positive b-wave. The a-wave is believed to emanate from the inner segments of the photoreceptors and the b-wave from Müller cells in the bipolar region. The peak amplitudes and latencies as well as waveform shape are considered in the interpretation of the ERG. Since the ERG monitors preganglionic retinal activity, a patient due to optic atrophy may have a normal ERG.

A series of colored and white light stimuli of variable intensity are used under dark-adapted and light-adapted conditions. Pure cone waves and pure rod waves may be isolated by using scotopically or photopically balanced red and blue stimuli. Cone function may also be isolated using a stimulus which flickers at 30 flashes per second since rods will follow flicker only up to a rate of 15–20 cycles per second. Rod function may be isolated by using very dim blue stimuli under dark adapted conditions (Fig. 2.7).

Since the ERG is a mass retinal response, an isolated lesion of the macula would not be expected to affect this test. Conversely, widespread retinal disease processes sometimes may clinically appear to be localized macular lesions and, in such cases, the ERG is an invaluable test for a precise diagnosis.

One area undergoing investigation at present is the recording of a *focal ERG* from the macular region using computer summation techniques. One difficulty in recording the small responses that would be elicited from such a small area is the scattered light stimulation of peripheral regions. To overcome this problem, a background adapting light to dampen the response of outlying receptors has proved effective [7] as has the use of an alternating stripe stimulus so designed that the total light flux is always the

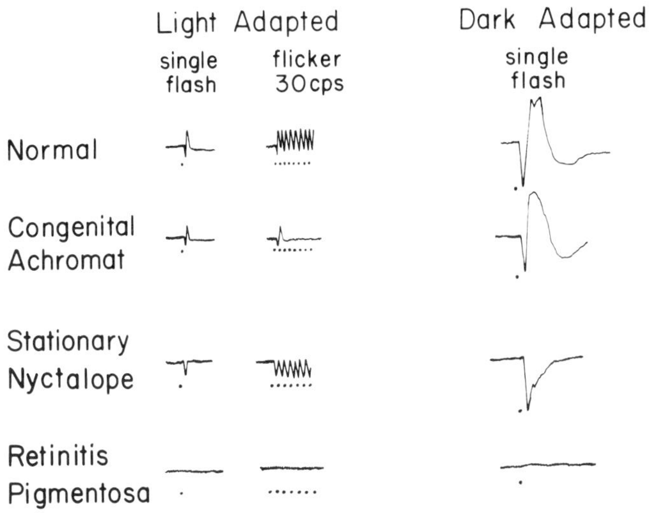

Figure 2.7. Electroretinography. Photopic (light-adapted) and scotopic (dark-adapted) ERGs using full field stimulation. In the congenital achromat there is absence of the photopic flicker response indicating abnormal cone function. In the stationary nightblind, due to a block in neural transmission in the bipolar cell regions, there is an absence of the b-wave. In retinitis pigmentosa there is an absence of all responses indicative of a widespread photoreceptor degeneration.

same and the only variable is the modulating pattern of stripes over the area to be studied [8]. Other problems, such as patient fixation, and precise focusing of pattern stimuli onto the retina, require further work. It has not been possible as yet to record a response when the stimulus was less than 2 degrees. This test, with further investigation, may prove to be of inestimable value in studying the overall function of the macular areas.

Electrooculography (EOG)

The electrooculogram measures the changes in the corneoretinal potential of the eye under varying conditions of illumination. To record this, two electrodes are placed on the skin, one at the lateral canthus and the other at the medial canthus. The subject is asked to shift fixation back and forth between two red lights that turn on and off sequentially in an alternating fashion. The angular distance between the lights and consequently the eye movement excursion is generally 30 degrees. Since the corneoretinal potential is positive with regard to the cornea, the EOG recording is positive when the patient's cornea (gaze) is turned toward the canthus with the recording electrode. The record is negative when the eye turns to the opposite direction (toward the reference electrode). Several measurements are taken every minute for a total of 12 minutes in darkness and then 12 minutes in the light. A plot of the average amplitude value for each minute against time normally shows a minimum trough value during the dark period and a maximum peak value in the light (Fig. 2.8).

The dark trough of the standing potential is believed to depend on the integrity of the pigment epithelial-outer segment region. The light rise depends on the function of the mid-retinal layers in addition to the outer retina-pigment epithelial complex. While the absolute value of the corneoretinal potential is quite variable, the light peak/dark trough ratio is found to be a reliable parameter of retinal function and the normal lower range is about 170% (calculated by taking the ratio of the maximum light-adapted to the minimum dark-adapted response and multiplying it by 100).

Since the EOG is likewise a reflection of the totality of retinal responsiveness, it usually goes hand in hand with the ERG. Thus, normalcy of one will indicate normalcy of the other. Likewise, if only a small region of the retina is affected, the EOG would not be expected to be abnormal.

There are, however, several clinical conditions known at present in which these statements do not hold. In both vitelliform macular dystrophy (Best's disease) as well as the very rare butterfly dystrophy, the EOG is abnormal in most cases. Of interest is the fact that the ERG is completely normal and there are no other findings which would indicate any widespread abnormality of the RPE-photoreceptor complex. A similar dichotomy between the EOG and ERG has been seen in occasional cases of fundus flavimaculatus and generalized drusen. This perplexing issue remains unsolved.

The Visually Evoked Response (VER)

The visually evoked response [9] is a measure of the electrical potential generated in response to a visual stimulus. It is recorded with scalp electrodes placed over the occipital lobe region, a cortical area with primarily a macular representation. The major contribution to the VER has been found to emanate from stimulation of the foveal region. Consequently, this test is of great value in the study of macular disease.

There are many different techniques of foveal stimulation in VER testing. One method makes use of a diffuse light

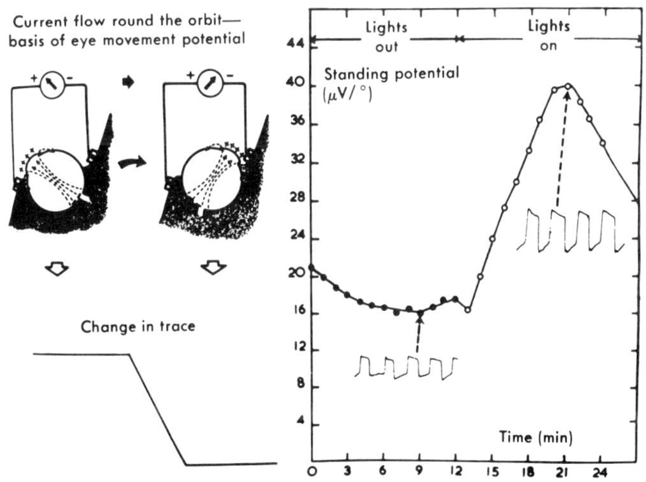

Figure 2.8. Electro-oculography. For the EOG, electrodes are secured at the temporal and nasal canthal regions. When the normal eye turns toward the recording electrode, a positive deflection is obtained. When the eye turns away from the recording electrode and toward the reference electrode, the deflection is negative. An EOG curve is shown at the right. The light peak (maximum)/dark trough (minimum) value is the EOG ratio. (From G.B. Arden and M.R. Fojas: *Arch Ophthal 68:* 369, 1962; reprinted with permission.)

stimulus which flashes intermittently, but the size of the flash, electrode positioning, and recording techniques vary from laboratory to laboratory. There is significant interindividual variability in waveform shape, amplitude, and peak latencies and there is, likewise, intraindividual variability at different test times. Another problem is that peripheral retinal activity evoked by reflected stray light may contaminate the flash VER.

The flash VER is most useful in the assessment of suspected monocular pathology. The eye with unexplained visual loss is compared with the normal eye in the same patient. The whole visual pathway from retina to the occipital lobe is being monitored, so an abnormal monocular result can occur from either retinal or optic nerve disease.

A second technique avoids stray light stimulation of extrafoveal retina by employing a patterned stimulus, the center of which is used for subject fixation. One such pattern presents alternating dark and light bars in the form of a sinusoidal grating. The light bars become dark and the dark bars become light with the pattern reversing at a constant rate. The dark and light bars are always 180 degrees out of phase. The size of the pattern can be varied but the test area should be small enough to ensure foveal stimulation primarily. The mean luminance of the pattern is held constant, but the spatial frequency and the contrast of the grating pattern can be varied. This technique gives very reproducible waveforms and, therefore, is quite useful in evaluating either macular or optic nerve disease.

A third technique employs a checker board pattern stimulator with alternation of dark and light checks. The checks may be uniform or increase in size from center to periphery (Fig. 2.9).

The usefulness of the VER in detecting lesions of the macula must be tempered by the fact that the ultimate record reflects neural transmission along the entirety of the visual pathway from retina to occipital lobe. Therefore, an abnormality anywhere along the system may give an abnormal VER. The use of patterned stimuli for evoking the VER has eliminated many of the vagaries of recording and this is a preferable technique in most instances. This technique might be substituted for the flash VER in the case of dense cataracts, an opaque vitreous, or in monocular lesions where the normal fellow eye is available for comparative study.

The combination of VER and focal ERG provides a definite advantage in attempting to differentiate macular disease from optic nerve disease, for in the former both the VER and focal ERG will be abnormal, while in the latter the focal ERG will be normal.

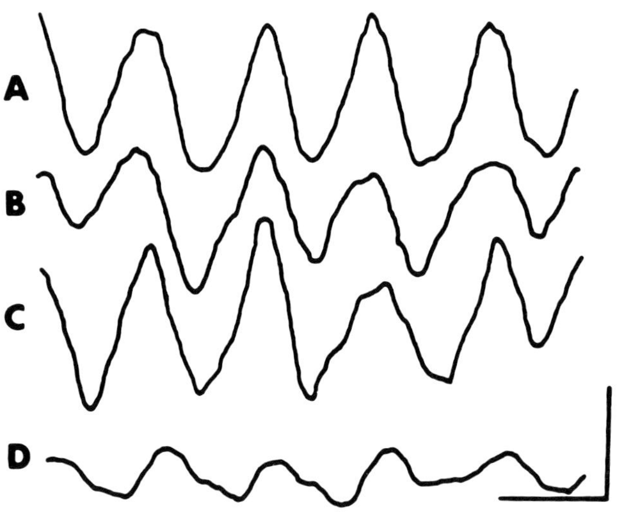

Figure 2.9. Checkerboard pattern VER. Pattern reversal VERs for 15 degree checks as a function of a decrease in field size. The field size was reduced from 12 degrees to 3 degrees without any significant change in amplitude: *A*, 12 degrees; *B*, 6 degrees; *C*, 3 degrees. *D*, the eye was stimulated with a 12 degree field that had the central 3 degrees blanked out. This provides evidence that the majority of the VER complex arises from the macular area. *Vertical line*, 10 μv; *horizontal line*, 100 msec. (From S. Sokol: *Surv Opthalmol, 21:* 18, 1976; reprinted with permission.)

CLINICAL APPLICATIONS

The following case reports illustrate how certain macular function tests can be of value in the overall diagnosis and management of patients with macular disease.

Case 1

An 18-year-old girl complained of a progressive decrease in visual acuity over the past 3 years but denied particular difficulty seeing in dim illumination. Her father had retinitis pigmentosa for many years, and the patient was also labeled with the same diagnosis by the referring physician. She worked as an usher in a prominent theater and was worried that her prognosis of nightblindness would jeopardize her chosen vocation.

Best corrected vision was 20/50 OD and 20/40 OS. Funduscopic examination revealed normal discs and vessels, a mild pigment mottling at the fovea, and pigment clumps plus yellow flecks around the posterior pole and in the mid-periphery.

A work-up revealed normal color tests, central scotomata OU with normal peripheral fields, a normal peripheral dark adaptation curve, a normal ERG, and an EOG LP/DT ratio of 165%.

Diagnosis: Fundus flavimaculatus with macular degeneration.

The diagnosis of retinitis pigmentosa is ruled out by the normal peripheral dark adaptation, normal visual fields, and a normal ERG. Occasionally, in fundus flavimaculatus, there may be a slight reduction in the EOG.

Case 2

A 7-year-old boy complained of difficulty seeing the blackboard in school. A previous consultant noted a moderate decreased visual acuity to 20/50 OU, and discrete lesions at both foveas consisting of hyper- and hypopigmentation. The discs, vessels, and peripheral examinations were otherwise normal. A provisional diagnosis of juvenile macular degeneration was made. Because the child cried when brought to the local moviehouse and refused to play outside during warm summer evenings, a second opinion was sought by the parents.

The child was too unreliable for psychophysical tests. However, an ERG was performed and found to be extinguished.

Diagnosis: Tapetoretinal Degeneration

Four years later, the patient was found to have early ring scotomata on visual field testing and elevated dark adaptation thresholds. He was also developing midperipheral pigment spicules on fundus examination. This case of so-called inverse retinitis pigmentosa is important to recognize since the visual prognosis of a generalized tapetoretinal degeneration is obviously much different from that of a macular degeneration.

Case 3

A 9-year-old girl complained of blurred vision for the past 1½ years. A previous work-up revealed normal color vision, normal funduscopic examination, and a normal fluorescein angiogram. Her vision was 20/30, although she read the Snellen chart with difficulty and hesitation. It was recommended that the parents seek psychiatric consultation for the girl. The parents sought a second opinion.

A repeat work-up revealed normal color vision, visual fields, Amsler grid, ERG, and EOG. A pattern VER, however, was markedly depressed in amplitude and a focal ERG showed diminished amplitudes.

Diagnosis: Early Macular Degeneration

Two years later, the typical metallic sheen of Stargardt's maculopathy was seen on fundus examination. In certain cases of juvenile macular degeneration the subjective symptom of decreased vision may antedate the ophthalmoscopically observable changes. The abnormal VER demonstrates an abnormality affecting macular fibers somewhere along the visual pathway and the ERG abnormality localizes the change to the retina. Macular function testing established an explanation for this patient's visual symptomatology and eliminated the need for psychiatric counseling.

Case 4

A 35-year-old visual field technician tripped while at work. He claims he could not see well with his right eye after the fall and sought compensation.

An examination revealed 20/100 OD and 20/20 OS. Retinal examination and fluorescein angiography was normal. The visual fields showed a central scotoma, which was doubled in size when the test distance and object size was doubled. Static perimetry showed central depression in sensitivity. Color tests, Amsler grid, ERG, EOG, foveal dark adaptation, pattern VER, and focal ERG were all normal.

Diagnosis: Malingering

An ophthalmologist finally was able to catch this intelligent, deceptive technician using a biprism. The technician subsequently quit his job in a huff. While malingering is a diagnosis of exclusion, the normalcy of the VER and ERG cast doubt on the reliability of this patient.

Case 5

A 35-year-old female noted a sudden decrease of visual acuity in the left eye occurring about 1 year prior to being seen. Funduscopic examination at that time revealed normal discs, maculae, and posterior pole vessels. However, pigmentation and venous sheathing were observed in the equatorial region, OU. Goldmann field testing revealed multiple scotomata in the mid-periphery. A diagnosis of retinitis pigmentosa was entertained.

During the past year, the patient noted some improvement in acuity. On present exam, her Snellen acuity was 20/20 in each eye. Color tests were completely normal. However, her perception of brightness and color was reportedly dimmer in the left eye. The ERG and the EOG were normal. The focal ERG was also normal, but the flash and pattern VER showed an increased latency in the waveform peaks in the left eye when compared to the right eye.

Diagnosis: Retrobulbar Neuritis Secondary to a Demyelinating Process

On further questioning, the patient admits that her OS vision deteriorates when she takes a hot bath. The use of VER latencies in optic nerve disease is important. Even in cases with an acuity of 20/20 and no ophthalmoscopic evidence of nerve changes, the latency may be delayed, thus demonstrating a conduction abnormality.

Case 6

A 30-year-old patient came to New York to pursue a career in a large corporation. A screening examination elicited a history of difficulty seeing in the dark and somewhat decreased vision ever since the patient could remember. The company ophthalmologist made a diagnosis of retinitis pigmentosa and advised the patient of his future progressive visual deterioration.

The patient sought a second opinion which would include electroretinographic testing. He was found to be moderately myopic with a best corrected vision of 20/40 OU. His visual fields and color vision were normal. An ERG showed a negative photopic single flash response, and after dark adaptation, an increase of the negative response but a continued absence of the positive wave. The a-wave latencies were normal. Dark adaptation showed a 2.5 log unit elevation of his peripheral final thresholds and a normal foveal threshold.

Diagnosis: Congenital Stationary Nightblindness with Myopia

The poor acuity and poor night vision in such patients may often lead the unaware to the mistaken diagnosis of retinitis pigmentosa. The typical ERG changes of congenital stationary nightblindness lead to the correct diagnosis.

Conclusion

The thoughtful ophthalmologist can make use of many simple office procedures for the evaluation of a patient with visual symptoms. In addition, a proper line of questioning will often provide helpful clues toward the diagnosis. The ophthalmologist's consideration of the total clinical picture (history, visual acuity, color testing, Amsler grid, visual fields, and the photostress test) can aid in determining the proper specialized retinal function tests for a diagnosis.

Modern psychophysic and electrophysiologic methods are valuable aids in the diagnosis of macular disease. Misdiagnoses have too often been made in cases of decreased vision in eyes with apparent pathology only at the macula or with no detectable funduscopic abnormalities. Conversely, improper grave diagnoses have been erroneously assigned to eyes solely because of the ophthalmoscopic appearance. Macular function testing is especially important in avoiding incorrect diagnoses in such cases. Hopefully, recent innovations in macular testing will better elucidate the pathologic physiology of the visual pathways and offer new tools for the early diagnosis of macular disease.

References

1. Østerberg, G.A.: Topography of the layer of rods and cones in the human retina. *Acta Ophthalmol,* suppl. VI, 1935.
2. Bodis-Wollner, I., and Diamond, S.: The measurement of spatial contrast sensitivity in cases of blurred vision associated with cerebral lesions. *Brain, 99:* 695, 1976.
3. Wolkstein, M., Atkin, A., and Bodis-Wollner, I.: Grating acuity in two sisters with tapetoretinal degeneration. *In* ERG, VER and Psychophysics, ed. by T. Lawwill, XIV ISCERG Symposium in Louisville, Kentucky, *Doc Ophthalmol, 13:* 1976.
4. Gunkel, R.D., and Kollarits, F.J.: A chromaticity diagram for defects in color vision. *In* ERG, VER and Psychophysics, ed. by T. Lawwill, XIV ISCERG Symposium in Louisville, Kentucky, *Doc Ophthalmol, 13:* 1976.
5. DeLange, H.: Research into the dynamic nature of the human fovea-cortex systems with intermittent and modulated light. I. Attenuation characteristics with white and colored light. *J Opt Soc Am, 48:* 777, 1958.
6. Tyler, C.W.: Flicker frequency response functions in the diagnosis of retinal disorders. Presented at ARVO Meeting, Sarasota, Fla., 1976.
7. Biersdorf, W.R., and Diller, D.A.: Local electroretinogram in macular degeneration. *Am J Ophthalmol, 68:* 296, 1969.
8. Lawwill, T.: The bar-pattern electroretinogram for clinical evaluation of the central retina. *Am J Ophthalmol, 78:* 121, 1974.
9. Sokol, S.: Visually evoked potentials: theory, techniques and clinical applications. *Surv Ophthalmol, 21:* 18, 1976.

CHAPTER 3

Fundus Photography and Angiography

Johnny Justice, Jr.

Fundus Photography

Ocular fundus photography as a clinical aid in the documentation of intraocular diseases has been available since the early part of this century. Since that time, ocular fundus photography has evolved quietly but steadily, primarily because of the efforts of Bedell [1], Allen [2], and others [3–5]. Improved cameras, better films, stereo techniques, and fluorescein angiography have advanced the fundus photograph beyond its documentary role to that of a frequently vital, pretherapeutic and posttherapeutic procedure. Thus, with the increasing significance of fundus photography in ophthalmological care, the importance of instrumentation technology and technique deserves special emphasis. This section will discuss the fundus photographer, equipment, care and maintenance of equipment, methodology, artifacts of illumination, stereo fundus photography, film, and processing procedures.

THE FUNDUS PHOTOGRAPHER

Fundus photography is now sufficiently specialized to require the full-time concentration of the photographer. A background in photography is important, but is not a prerequisite for choosing this occupation. While gaining technical skills, the photographer must also develop familiarity with the clinical pathology of the fundus. The performance of his technical duties relates directly to his understanding of the lesions examined and the ways in which their special pecularities can be shown angiographically. The growth and significance of an ophthalmic photography laboratory not only depend on the photographer's skill but, more important, on his interest and enthusiasm. Many ophthalmologists perform their own fundus photography; however, despite the ophthalmologist's interest in recording and further defining disorders of the retina and choroid, it is usually a photographer who is responsible for the excellence of this service.

EQUIPMENT AVAILABLE FOR FUNDUS PHOTOGRAPHY

Several instruments are currently available for fundus photography. The author has had the opportunity to use most of these instruments and will attempt to evaluate them in regard to engineering and, more important, in regard to quality of the photographs produced.

(1) The West German Zeiss fundus camera produces excellent photographs. This instrument is significantly more expensive than its competitors.

(2) The new, improved Topcon fundus camera is a reasonably priced instrument that delivers excellent photographs and has an accessory power supply that allows the photographer to take angiograms at up to three frames per second. In addition, this instrument has a unique timing device that allows the photographer a view of the digital timer.

(3) The Olympus fundus camera, also moderately priced, provides excellent photographs, but it is unavailable in the United States.

(4) The Kowa fundus camera is the least expensive. Unfortunately, this important factor affects the comparative quality of its photographs. However, good photographs can be obtained despite somewhat greater technical difficulties that are particularly obvious when the patient's cooperation is less than ideal. The difficulties have been in the light source. A newer model is now in production, but currently unavailable for evaluation.

(5) The Nikon 45° fundus camera is an expensive instrument with great potential for photographing a wider view of the fundus. The quality of the photographs is good.

(6) The East German Zeiss fundus camera is more moderately priced than the West German Zeiss fundus camera and takes good photographs. Service, however, is poor in the United States.

(7) The Clinitex 100° fundus camera, a contact lens camera, has potential. To this date, however, its photographs are not comparable to those taken with other instruments, in terms of overall resolution.

(8) The Pomerantz 120° fundus camera is also a contact lens camera with great potential. However, the author has not had the opportunity of evaluating this unique instrument.

(9) The Donaldson simultaneous stereo fundus camera is moderately priced, is ideal for color fundus photography, but cannot be used for fluorescein angiography.

(10) The Canno fundus camera, currently in production has the unique feature of a zoom lens.

CARE AND MAINTENANCE OF EQUIPMENT

Most fundus cameras are fairly sturdy instruments and require a minimal amount of care and maintenance. The objective lens should be covered by the lens cap when not in use, even during office hours. The entire instrument should be covered at night and on weekends and holidays. In spite of these efforts to maintain a clean instrument, foreign matter on the lens is a constant problem for the photographer. Children have an uncanny interest in touching the objective lens, leaving fingerprints and smudges. Cleaning the front surface of the objective lens can be easily done by the photographer. Kodak lens cleaner and a cotton-tipped applicator covered with a good quality lens tissue can be used on a routine basis without any damage to the surface of the lens. However, the removal of the objective lens by the photographer to clean its back surface is a serious mistake. This should be done only by a qualified manufacturer's representative. Dust spots and smudges on the back surface of the lens are particularly noticeable in eyes with high myopia. The photographer should be able to replace viewing lamps, electronic flashtubes, and fuses when they become ineffective. Power supply problems should be referred to an electronics expert, preferably a manufacturer's technician.

BASIC TECHNIQUES

Top quality fundus photographs are dependent on many details of production. The most important for the photographer to follow are:

(1) Make sure that the pupil is widely dilated. The author uses one drop of 1% Mydriacyl followed by one drop of 10% Neo-synephrine. These are quick acting drugs of short duration. Usually, the pupils are well dilated in 20–30 minutes. Cyclogel is an excellent cycloplegic for photography. In fairness to the patient, however, it is not recommended that the pupils remain dilated much longer than is necessary. An 8-mm pupil is ideal, but both single frame and stereo photography can be carried out with pupils that are considerably smaller.

(2) Set the focusing eyepiece on the proper setting. Out-of-focus photographs will result if the focusing eyepiece is not properly set by the photographer. Even if no one else uses the camera, the setting should be checked each time. Initially, consistently sharp photographs are difficult to obtain for many young photographers because of their accommodation problem. In these instances, a cycloplegic refraction is sometimes helpful. Practice makes perfect, and persistence pays dividends.

(3) Make sure that the correct camera body with the proper film is attached to the instrument. To avoid mistakes, attach the appropriate film label to the camera back.

(4) Check the shutter speed for the proper electronic flash synchronization. Shutter speeds in the range of 1/30 to 1/60 can be used. Faster shutter speeds on most camera backs will result in partially exposed photographs.

(5) Insert the synchronization cable in the proper electronic flash connection on the camera body.

(6) Take an identification photograph of the patient's name, the date photography is performed, and other pertinent information. All subsequent photographs will pertain to that patient. To avoid errors and angry referring ophthalmologists, all photographs should be appropriately labeled as rapidly as possible after their return from processing.

(7) Inform the patient about the procedure.

(8) Seat the patient comfortably at the instrument with his chin on the chin rest and his forehead against the headrest.

(9) Instruct the patient to look at the fixation device.

(10) Focus the filament of the viewing lamp on the cornea.

(11) After properly focusing the filament of the viewing lamp, look through the eyepiece and bring the retinal vessels into focus.

(12) When the image is in propr focus and the specific area of interest is in view, release the shutter.

(13) Wind the camera immediately, so that it will be ready to take the next photograph.

ARTIFACTS OF ILLUMINATION

From a technical standpoint, manipulation of the "joystick" is the single most vital aspect of fundus photography. This sensitive control mechanism is most directly related to rather common artifacts of illumination.

If the fundus camera is too close to the eye, a bright crescent-shaped light will appear at the edge of the photograph (Fig. 3.1,*A* and *D*). When the camera is too far from the eye, a low-contrast photograph (blue-gray) will be produced (Fig. 3.1,*B* and *E*). Optimal illumination is achieved within a small zone between these two extremes at a distance from the eye determined by its own optics (Fig. 3.1,*C* and *F*). To determine the optimal position of the camera, it is useful to routinely focus the projected filament image of the viewing lamp directly on the cornea. Then, while the fundus is viewed, small anterior posterior excursions of the joy-stick will provide the artifact-free viewing ready for final focusing and photographing.

STEREO FUNDUS PHOTOGRAPHY

Stereo fundus photography is the best way of documenting blurred disc margins, optic nervehead cupping, and the degree of retinal elevation from serous or solid detachments. As long as a standard stereo technique is used, comparative serial photographs of this type can be invaluable in the appraisal of change in the appearance of a lesion. Stereo fundus photographs can be obtained by three methods:

(1) The cornea-induced parallax method, advocated by Bedell [1] in 1929, produces excellent stereo photographs by using standard fundus camera equipment alone. The first photograph is taken through the temporal side of the pupil and the other through the nasal side. A lateral shift of

Figure 3.1. Artifacts of illumination: *A*, the camera is too close to the subject; *B*, the camera is too far from the subject; *C*, the camera is at the proper distance, and the filament is focused on the cornea; *D*, note the crescent-shaped artifact; *E*, a low-contrast photograph with blue haze (if color film is used); and *F*, a properly illuminated fundus photograph.

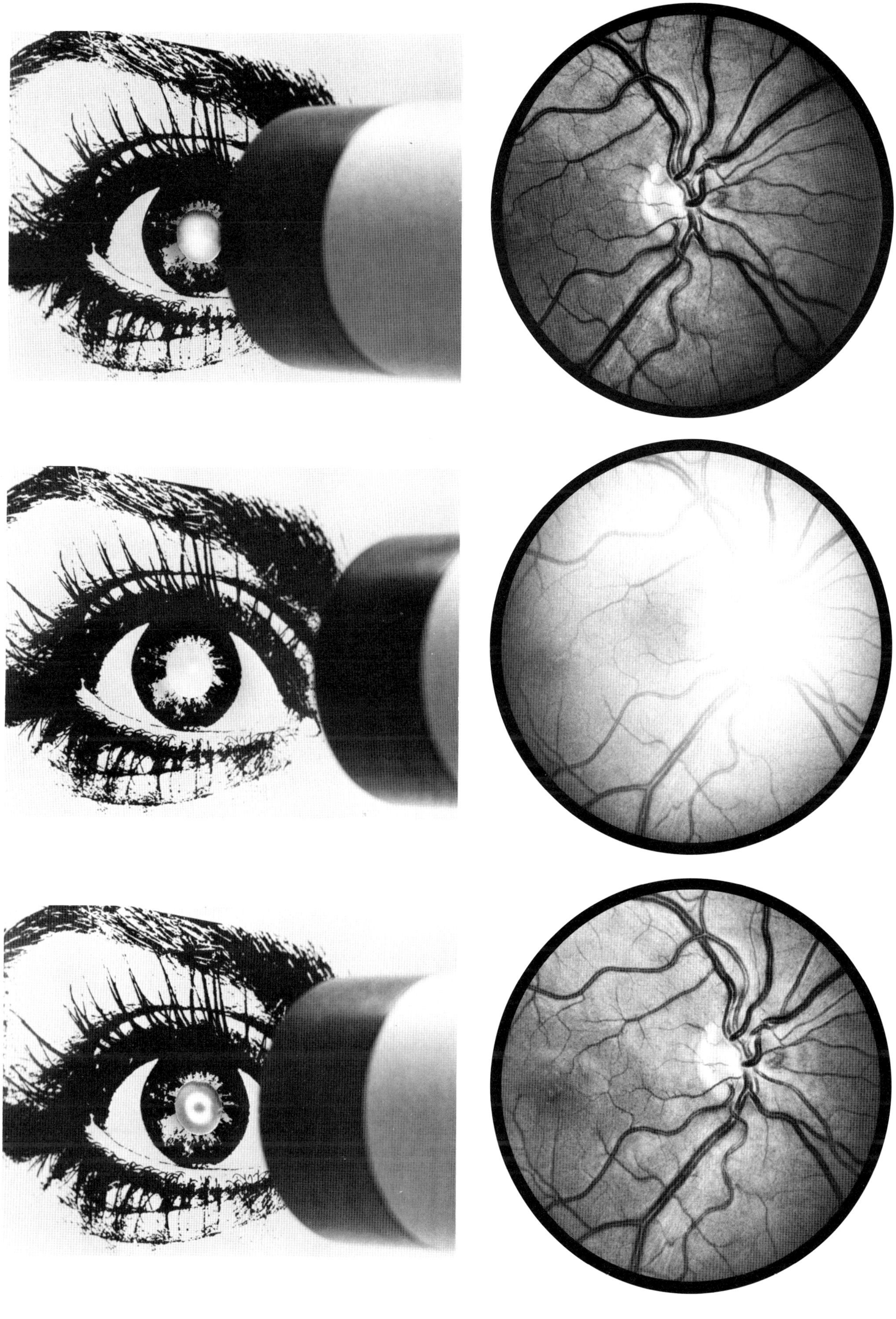

A

D

B

E

C

F

3.5 mm is recommended for optimum stereopsis, but any lateral shift will create a stereo photograph.

(2) A very effective manually operated stereoscopic separator, designed by Allen [4] in 1965, is now available commercially with motor drive. Certain patients with early cataracts, corneal opacities, or vitreous haze require manual alignment of the camera as described in the previous paragraph.

(3) The Donaldson simultaneous stereo fundus camera takes beautiful stereo photographs and is now available.

FILM AND PROCESSING

Until recently, Kodachrome II daylight film has been used by most ophthalmic photographers in the U.S.A. Unfortunately, Kodachrome films must be developed in a Kodak laboratory. Because of the 5- to 7-day delay in receiving the processed films, the author has switched to Ektachrome-X daylight film, which can be processed either locally or in one's own darkroom. A warming filter, Kodak Wrattan 81 EF, together with a 0.20 Kodak neutral density filter is placed over a large opening in the rotating diaphragm. The quality of the photographs is excellent, although resolution is not quite as good as that obtained using Kodachrome II.

Recently, Kodak discontinued Kodachrome II and replaced it with Kodachrome 25. This change aroused great concern in the field of ophthalmic photography. Complaints have been that the film is much too red, and early experiments with filtration have proved futile.

Agfachrome has been recommended as a substitute for Kodachrome II, but a similar delay in processing exists with this film. Ektachrome-X has proved to be an acceptable substitute, especially if rapid retrieval is a consideration.

Fluorescein Angiography

The photographer or ophthalmologist can usually make the transition to fluorescein angiography from routine fundus photography with relative ease. If the techniques for obtaining a good fundus photograph are followed, a good angiogram will result. This section will discuss filters for fluorescein angiography, methodology, film and developing, and the importance of a rapid angiography service for high quality angiograms.

FILTERS FOR FLUORESCEIN ANGIOGRAPHY

Novotny and Alvis [6] first described a practical method of fluorescein angiography in 1961. Since then, other investigators have published improvements in their techniques [3, 7, 8]. In 1966, Hodge and Clement's [9] description of the use of an interference filter, an excitor filter with a peak transmission of 80% at 4700 Angstroms, was the most significant technical contribution since the advent of fluorescein angiography. However, their choice of Ilford 109 (yellow) as a barrier filter allowed too much overlap (pseudofluorescence). Haining and Lancaster [10] showed, in 1968, that the advantages of the interference filter are better exploited when both excitor and barrier filters are of this type. Their B-4 excitor and B-5 barrier filters allowed minimal pseudofluorescence. In 1976, Delori [11] described a set of interference filters (excitor and barrier) designed specifically to study choroidal circulation. After using these filters for the past year, the author finds that they are unsurpassed for the choroidal circulation and are excellent for retinal vessel fluorescence as well (Fig. 3.2).

The most exciting feature of this truly excellent set of filters is that the photographer can better visualize fluorescein passing through the retinal and choroidal vessels. This set of filters offers three advantages: (1) better visualization during angiography allows the photographer to obtain better illumination and thus, eliminates the rather common artifacts of illumination that frequently appear during angiography; (2) active leakage sights can be detected visually, allowing the photographer to give the referring ophthalmologist a preliminary report; (3) there is better penetration of the ocular media because of the use of longer wave lengths for excitation. Improvement in filter combinations for fluorescein angiography will surely come to the forefront in the future, but at the present, the Delori (SE 40 excitor filter and SE 50 barrier filter) combination available for Spectrotech, Inc. is recommended as an international standard.

Many of the absorption filters used in black and white angiography are suitable for color fluorescein angiography [3, 7]. The excitor filter must have a transmission range of 400–500 nm with some additional transmission in the red part of the spectrum [12, 13]. The resolution and reproductibility of color fluorescein angiography are not comparable in quality to that of black and white angiography.

METHODOLOGY

After making the proper choice of excitor-barrier filters for the photographer's particular fundus camera, he should routinely follow several steps:

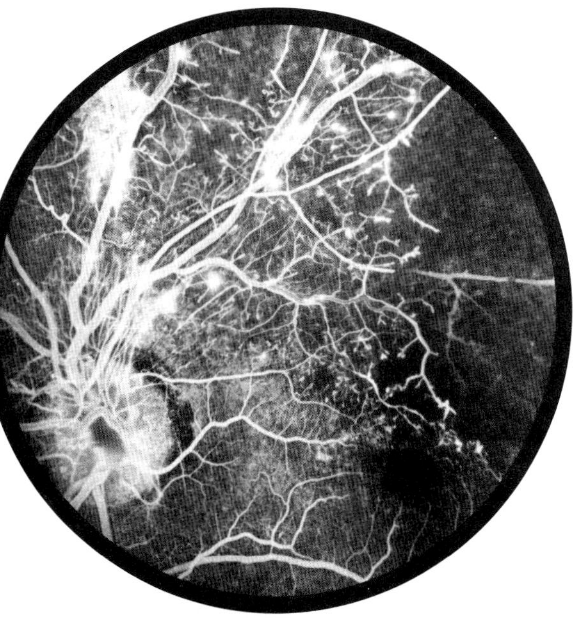

Figure 3.2. Note the details of the choroidal and retinal vessel fluorescence in this eye with vein occlusion, capillary avascularity, and neovascularization.

(1) Always take stereo color fundus photographs of both eyes (when possible) prior to fluorescein angiography. Angiography frequently demonstrates pathologic changes in the fellow eye that may have been overlooked or are not visible ophthalmoscopically. In addition, after fluorescein injection, the leakage of fluorescein beneath the retina, into the retina, into the vitreous, and into the aqueous obscures fundal detail. This detracts from the quality of stereo color fundus photographs.

(2) Explain in detail to the patient the entire procedure. It is especially important that the patient is aware that his/her urine will be discolored for 24–36 hours following the fluorescein injection. The skin color is sometimes yellowed or jaundiced in appearance. The author explains the possibility of reactions to intravenous fluorescein to the patient and obtains a signed consent form. However, the latter is not required by most institutions and private offices.

(3) Make sure the proper camera back with the appropriate barrier filter and appropriate film is properly attached to the fundus camera.

(4) Take a photograph of the patient's name, the date the study is performed, and any other useful information that will be helpful when the study is being reviewed.

(5) Seat the patient comfortably at the instrument.

(6) Follow instructions for obtaining quality fundus photographs.

(7) Take a red-free fundus stereo photograph with green filter (Kodak Wratten #58) at the disc and macula.

(8) Before the fluorescein injection, the illumination diaphragm should be changed to the appropriate excitor filter and a control photograph taken.

(9) Extend the patient's right or left arm across the armrest. The fluorescein should be injected as rapidly as possible into the anticubital vein. Use 3 cc of 25% or 5 cc of 10% fluorescein for maximum fluorescence. Assuming that the technique of photography is good, the contrast and quality of the angiogram depend primarily on the rapidity of injection.

(10) Activate the timer simultaneously with the injection of dye.

(11) Take rapid sequential stereo angiograms at one per second, starting approximately 7 seconds after the injection of fluorescein. This should continue for about 20 seconds. Then angiograms should be taken every 10–20 seconds for 1 minute, then at 5 minutes and 15 minutes postinjection. Be sure to take stereophotographs of the disc and macula in each eye during the mid and late stages of the study.

FILM AND DEVELOPING

There are many films and developers available for use in fluorescein angiography. The author uses Kodak Tri-X film (Tx 135-36) and develops it in Kodak D-11 developer, stock solution for 6 minutes at 72°F. An 8 × 10 contact print is made on Kodak Ektamatic SC paper, and an 8 × 10 enlargement is printed of a specific angiogram so that

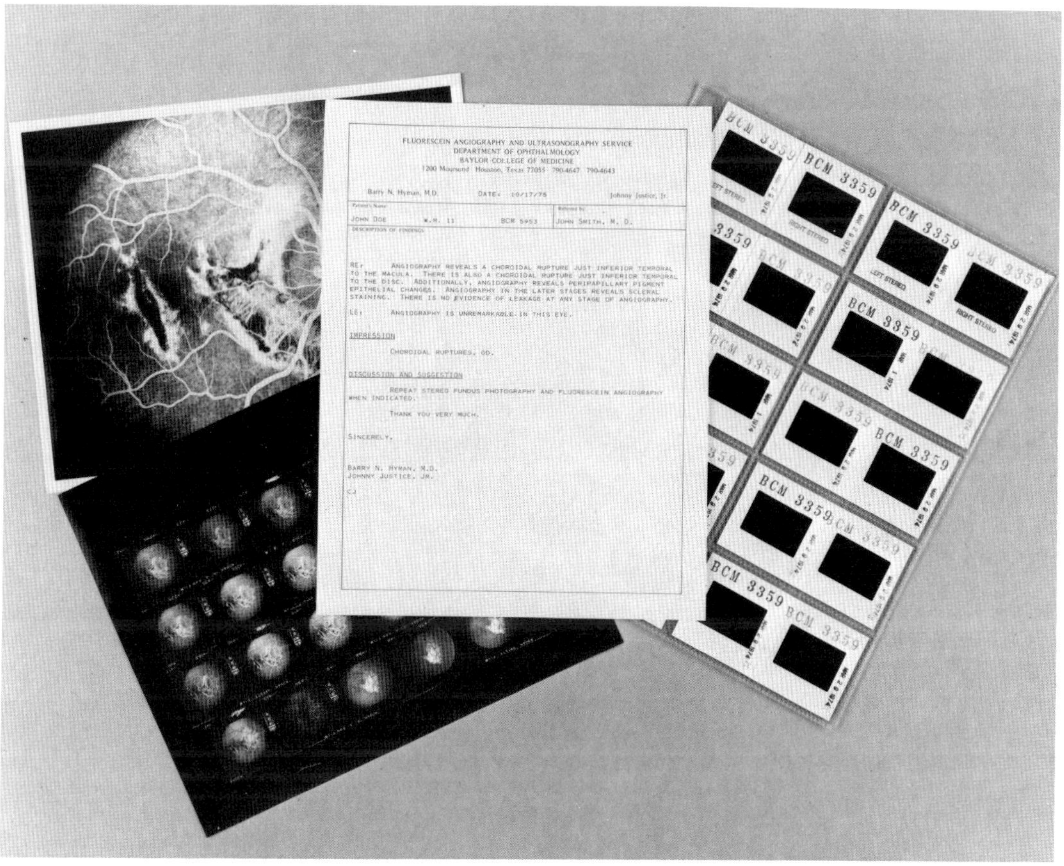

Figure 3.3. Complete fluorescein angiography report: a typewritten report, an 8 × 10 contact sheet, an 8 × 10 enlargement of a specific angiogram, and stereo color fundus photographs.

minute details can be seen in high magnification. The prints are developed by the stabilization technique (Kodak Ektamatic processor).

RAPID ANGIOGRAPHY SERVICE

Obviously, the best angiograms can be obtained if the pupil is well dilated and if there is no opacity in the optical media such as lesions of the cornea, cataractous changes in the lens, or vitreous abnormalities. The application of a topical anesthetic, topical fluorescein, applanation and Schiotz tonometry, and other ophthalmologic testing that disturb the corneal epithelium is not recommended prior to and on the same day that fluorescein angiography is being performed. Unfortunately, many patients have to travel long distances to see an ophthalmologist, so the convenience of the patient has to be considered. Consequently, most of the angiograms performed in our laboratory are carried out on the same day as the aforementioned procedures. Although these situations are not ideal, adequate angiography can be performed. If at all possible, however, the patient should be rescheduled for angiography at a later date.

It is usual for the author to send a complete fluorescein angiographic report (Fig. 3.3) 2–3 days following a fluorescein study. This package includes: (1) a typewritten report, (2) an 8 × 10 contact sheet of the entire study, (3) one or more 8 × 10 enlargements of specific angiograms, and (4) stereo color fundus photographs.

Film is processed at the end of the day and a report dictated the following morning. The reports are typed and usually signed on the same day. The Medical Illustration Department at Baylor College of Medicine also provides 1-day processing on Ektachrome-X color film. Color slides are labeled and stereo slides are mounted less than 48 hours following fluorescein angiography.

The most important aspect of a fluorescein angiography service is speed with quality angiograms and accurate interpretations. The role of fundus photography has extended beyond that of a documentary service to one with specific diagnostic value. Thus, ocular fundus photography and angiography relate directly to patient care and are essential parts of the sophisticated armamentarium of any clinical ophthalmologic unit.

The author acknowledges Little, Brown & Co. for permission to use portions of a previous report published in the *International Ophthalmology Clinics* of 1976.

References

1. Bedell, A.J.: Photographs of the Fundus Oculi, F. A. Davis, Philadelphia, 1929.
2. Allen, L.: Ocular fundus photography: suggestions for achieving consistently good pictures and instructions for stereoscopic photography. *Am J Ophthalmol, 57:* 13, 1964.
3. Justice, J., Jr.: The basic techniques of fundus photography and fluorescein angiography. *In* Proceedings of the International Symposium on Fluorescein Angiography, ed. by K. Shimizu, Igaku Shoin Ltd, Tokyo, 1974.
4. Allen, L., Kirkendall, W.M., Snyder, W.B., and Frazier, O.: Instant positive photographs and stereograms of ocular fundus fluorescence. *Arch Ophthalmol, 75:* 192, 1965.
5. Wong, D.: The fundamentals of ocular fundus photography and retinal fluorescence photography. *In* Photography Applications in Science, Technology and Medicine, Winter 1968–1969.
6. Novotny, H.R., and Alvis, D.L.: A method of photographing fluorescence in circulating blood in the human retina. *Circulation, 24:* 82, 1961.
7. Justice, J., Jr., and Sever, R.J.: Techniques of fluorescein fundus photography. *In* Neuro-Ophthalmology: Symposium of the University of Miami and the Bascom Palmer Eye Institute, ed. by J.L. Smith, C.V. Mosby, St. Louis, 1965, p. 82.
8. Machemer, R., Norton, E.W.D., Gass, J.D.M., and Choromokos, E.: Pseudofluorescence: a problem in interpretation of fluorescein angiograms. *Am J Ophthalmol, 70:* 1, 1970.
9. Hodge, J.V., and Clement, R.S.: Improved method for fluorescence angiography of the retina. *Am J Ophthalamol, 61:* 1400, 1966.
10. Haining, W.M., and Lancaster, R.C.: Advanced techniques for fluorescein angiography. *Arch Ophthalmol, 79:* 10, 1968.
11. Delori, F., Ben Sira, I., and Trempe, C.: Fluorescein angiography with an optimized filter combination. *Am J Ophthalmol, 82:* 559, 1976.
12. Allen, L., and Frazier, O.: The results of test on broad-band filter combinations for fluorescein angiography. *In* Proceedings of the International Symposium on Fluorescein Angiography, ed. by K. Shimizu, Igaku Shoin Ltd, Tokyo, 1972.
13. Hyvärinen, L., and Hochheimer, B.F.: Filter systems in fluorescein angiography. *Int Ophthalmol Clin, 14* (3): 49, 1974.

CHAPTER 4

Interpretation of Fluorescein Angiograms

Lawrence A. Yannuzzi, M.D., Howard Schatz, M.D., and Kurt A. Gitter, M.D.

The pathway to accurate interpretation of fluorescein angiograms lies in the full knowledge of the prerequisites. These include a review and understanding of fundus histopathology, fluorescein photography, fluorescein angioscopy, the normal fluorescein angiogram, and abnormal forms of fluorescence.

Fundus Histopathology

The fluorescein angiogram is a better, more dynamic depiction of the underlying histopathology than that provided by any other diagnostic ophthalmic aid currently available. Recognition of the histopathologic manifestations of the chorioretinal diseases studied by fluorescein angiography is enhanced by a thorough knowledge of the microscopic characteristics of the fundus. Certain tissue layers in particular warrant emphasis because they serve as landmarks on the angiogram, localizing intracellular or extracellular fluorescein more precisely (Fig. 4.1). These layers include: (1) internal limiting membrane; (2) retinal circulation (superficial and deep); (3) outer plexiform layer of retina; (4) retinal pigment epithelium; (5) choroidal circulation (choriocapillaris and larger vessels); and (6) sclera.

INTERNAL LIMITING MEMBRANE

The internal limiting membrane often has subtle irregularities in its appearance, which are not evident on the fluorescein angiogram. Consequently, an abnormal eye may very well display a normal angiogram. Fine, delicate irregularities in the internal limiting membrane may not be discernible on a fluorescein photograph and are best perceived on a red-free or monochromatic photograph, which accentuates such disturbances by increasing contrast (Fig. 4.2, *A* and *B*). Monochromatic photography has thus far proved most helpful in depicting a number of superficial retinal disorders, such as early preretinal membrane disease and juvenile retinoschisis involving the macula. Changes are evident on these photographs in the region of the internal limiting membrane preceding the development of any associated retinal vascular or even deeper retinal changes. Atrophy in the nerve fiber layer can also be recorded by this technique. Like color stereo photography, these monochromatic photographs enhance the overall diagnostic capability of fluorescein angiography by clarifying, in some instances, the perplexing enigma of an abnormal eye with a normal angiogram. These photographs should be considered as an essential part of every angiographic study.

RETINAL CIRCULATION

The superficial retinal circulation involving the larger retinal vessels is easily recognized in its pathologic expression on the angiogram. In essence, retinal vascular changes in this area speak for themselves, demonstrating occlusive and proliferative disease with secondary permeability abnormalities that are not part of the normal retinal architecture. Localization of abnormalities to this particular circulation is easily achieved on the angiogram because of the absence of any intervening tissues in eyes with clear media. Alterations in this vasculature are usually apparent monocularly by ophthalmoscopy, although, as in all attempts to localize and identify specific pathophysiologic changes, stereoscopic fluorescein angiographic evaluation is more sensitive and accurate. Flame-shaped hemorrhages and cotton wool spots are vascular manifestations localized to the superficial layers of the retina which are evident without the aid of the fluorescein angiograms. However, the recognition of noncystoid retinal edema in the superficial retina, as seen in the perivascular spaces in certain retinal inflammatory or occlusive disease, the perifoveal capillary free zone, capillary nonperfusion, collateralization, shunt and neovascularization formation, is simplified on the angiogram (Fig. 4.3).

The deeper retinal circulation, located in the inner nuclear layer, is responsible for the usual retinal permeability defects that lead to accumulation of edema in the outer plexiform layer that lies adjacent to it (Fig. 4.4). Leakage from these capillaries accumulates readily in the outer plexiform layer producing cystoid edema, while more extensive changes extend beyond the outer plexiform layer in the more superficial layers producing so-called noncystoid edema (Fig. 4.5, *A* and *B*). This circulation is also the site of dot and blot hemorrhages seen in certain retinal vascular disorders. Small hemorrhages in the deep capillary circulation are easily localized on the fluorescein angiogram as they produce no effect on the fluorescence of the overlying superficial circulation.

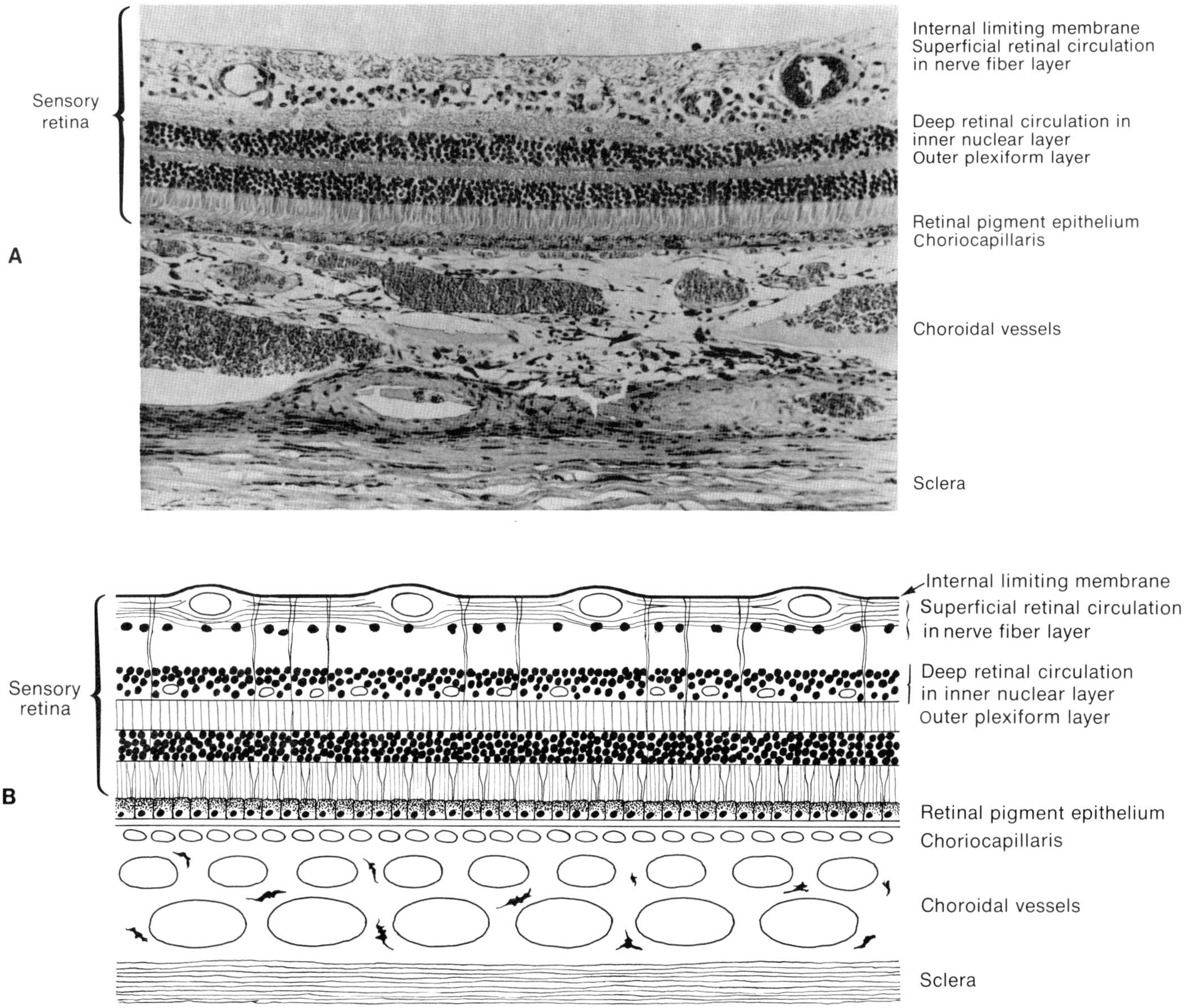

Figure 4.1. *A*, histopathology of a normal fundus in the posterior pole showing the layers that are critical in interpretation of fluorescein angiography. (Courtesy of Martin H. Vogel, M.D.) *B*, schematic representation of same. (From H. Schatz, T. Burton, L. Yannuzzi, and M. Rabb: Interpretation of Fundus Fluorescein Angiography, 1978, © C. V. Mosby Co., St. Louis; reprinted with permission.)

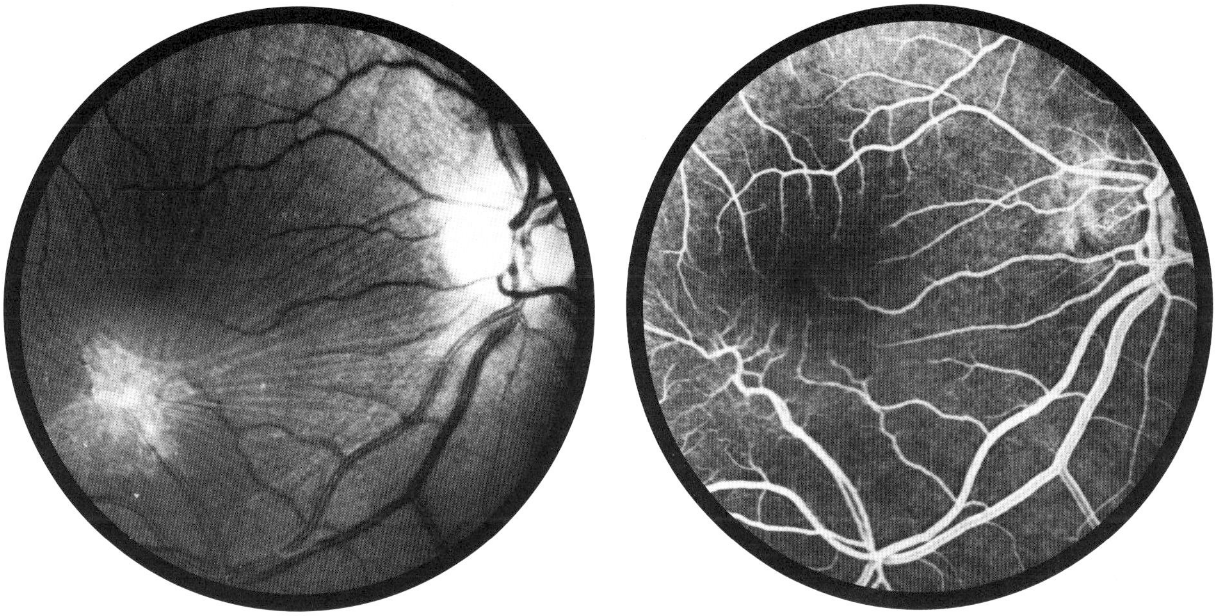

Figure 4.2. *A*, monochromatic red-free (560 nm, yellow-green) photograph of the macula showing an extensive preretinal membrane with numerous retinal folds radiating from a central area of gliosis. *B*, early venous phase fluorescein angiogram of the same patient. There is little evidence of the membrane except for slight retinal vascular prominence and tortuosity and slight obscuration of these vessels by the membrane itself.

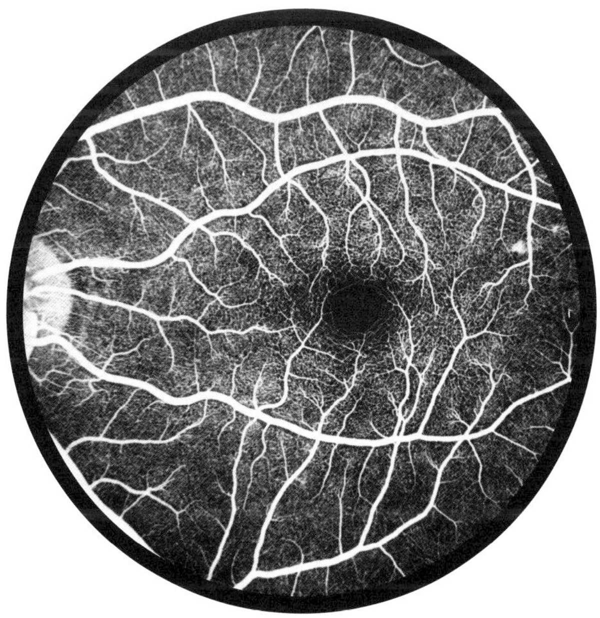

Figure 4.3. Late venous phase angiogram showing the details of the retinal circulation in the macula.

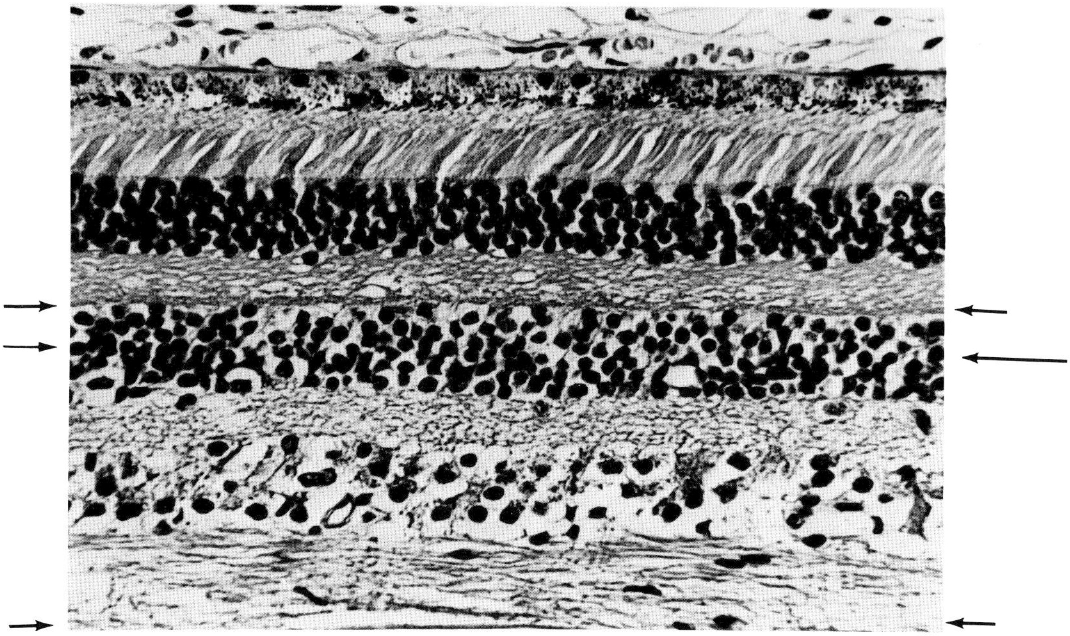

Figure 4.4. Normal retina, posterior pole, showing site of deep retinal circulation (*large arrows*). The vascular portion of the retina extends from the nerve fiber layer, the site of superficial retinal circulation, to the inner nuclear layer, the site of the deep retinal circulation. This is approximately from the internal limiting membrane to the middle limiting membrane (*small arrows*). ×40. (Courtesy, Martin H. Vogel, M.D.)

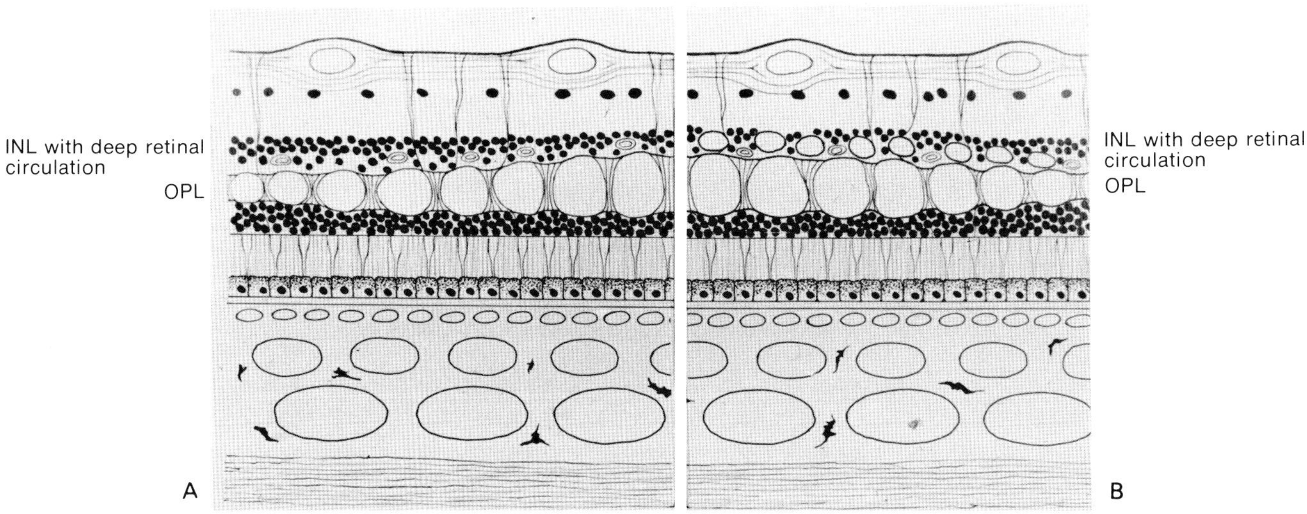

Figure 4.5. Intraretinal edema. *A,* accumulation of intraretinal edema in the outer plexiform layer (OPL) originating from the deep retinal circulation producing cystoid macular edema. *B,* more widespread edema extending beyond the outer plexiform layer to accumulate in the inner nuclear layer (INL), producing so-called noncystoid edema. (From H. Schatz, T. Burton, L. Yannuzzi, and M. Rabb: Interpretation of Fundus Fluorescein Angiography, 1978, C. V. Mosby Co., St. Louis; all reprinted with permission.)

OUTER PLEXIFORM LAYER

The outer plexiform layer represents the only true potential interstitial space in the retina. Because of its virtually anterior-posterior alignment outside the macular region, fluid accumulation in the spaces produces discrete spherical or globular changes from compression of adjacent fibers and/or Müller cells (cystoid edema). This intraretinal edema outside of the macular region has a classic "honeycombed" appearance on the fluorescein angiogram and is referred to as *cystoid retinal edema.* On the other hand, in the macular region, the outer plexiform layer takes on a more oblique orientation. Consequently, edema accumulation here produces a more stellate configuration surrounding the foveal region, known as *cystoid macular edema* (Fig. 4.6, *A* and *B*). This edema is a nonspecific manifestation produced by a variety of retinal, choroidal, and vitreous disorders.

In retinal vascular and certain vitreous disorders, the

Outer plexiform layer

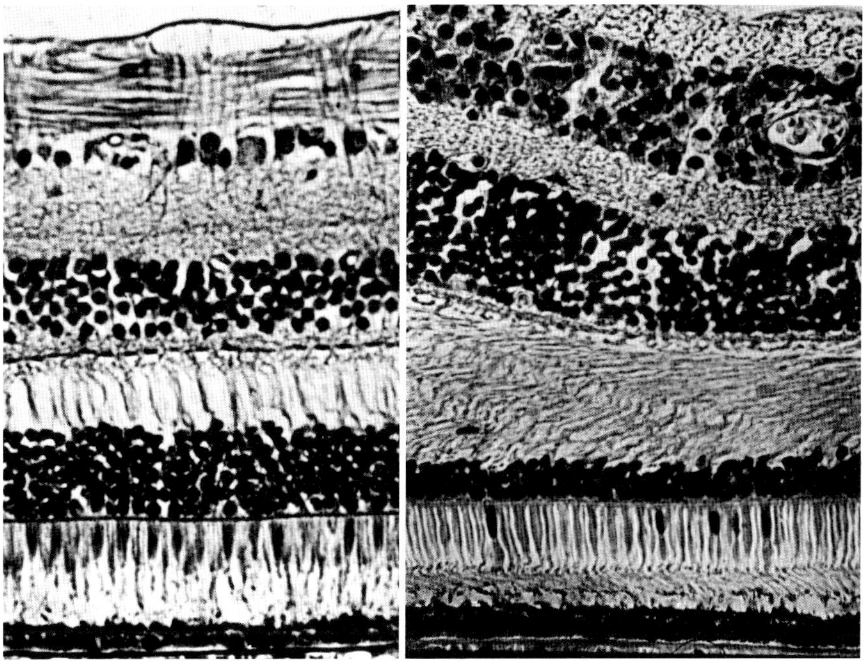

Outer plexiform layer

A

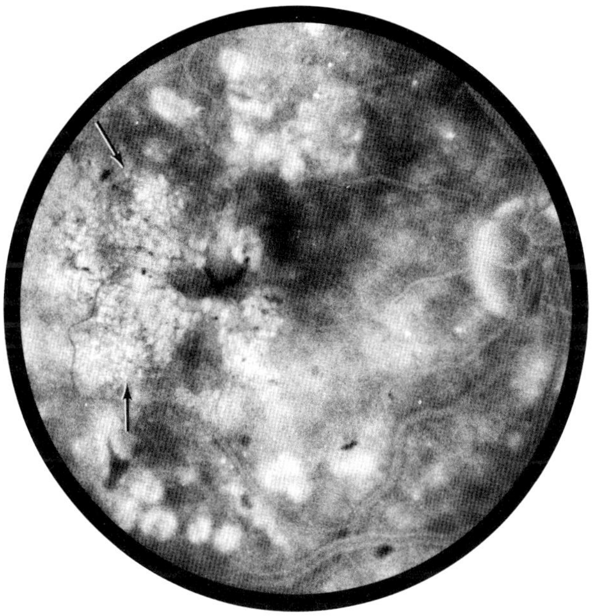

B

Figure 4.6. *A*, comparison of the outer plexiform layer (OPL) in the normal retina (*left*) and in the normal macula (*right*). In the retina, the fibers are vertically aligned perpendicular to the internal limiting membrane. Intraretinal fluid accumulates in spherical shapes as Müller fibers and/or adjacent nerve fibers become compressed to form the walls of the cysts. This is referred to as cystoid retinal edema and has a honeycombed appearance on fluorescein angiogram. In the macular region the fibers in the outer plexiform layer are more obliquely oriented as they radiate from the fovea. Intraretinal fluid accumulation forms a more stellate configuration surrounding the foveal region, known as cystoid macular edema. ×275. (*Right photo,* courtesy of AFIP Acc. 321406.) *B,* fluorescein angiogram demonstrating cystoid retinal edema (*arrows*) and cystoid macular edema surrounding the fovea in diabetic retinopahy.

abnormal deep capillaries become increasingly more hyperfluorescent as fluorescein pools into the outer plexiform layer. The more superficial retinal vessels fluoresce normally overlying the deeper leaking capillaries and serve as a stereoscopic aid to the exact localization of the abnormally permeable capillaries. These changes are preceded briefly by a period of hypofluorescence from the blockage of the choroidal circulation by the intraretinal edema itself. As the larger retinal vessels empty during the late stages of the angiogram, they may produce a dark silhouette appearance that overlies the deep late hyperfluorescence in the outer plexiform layer. This finding also serves as an aid to the exact localization of the fluid accumulation. Certain choroidal factors, such as subpigment epithelial neovascularization, tumors, and inflammation, may also be associated with intraretinal edema. The leaking retinal capillaries are not as prominent in these conditions since fluid probably originates subretinally, penetrating the normally impermeable external limiting membrane. Reduced contrast from subretinal hyperfluorescence, also present in these disorders, makes the intraretinal edema less evident on the fluorescein angiogram.

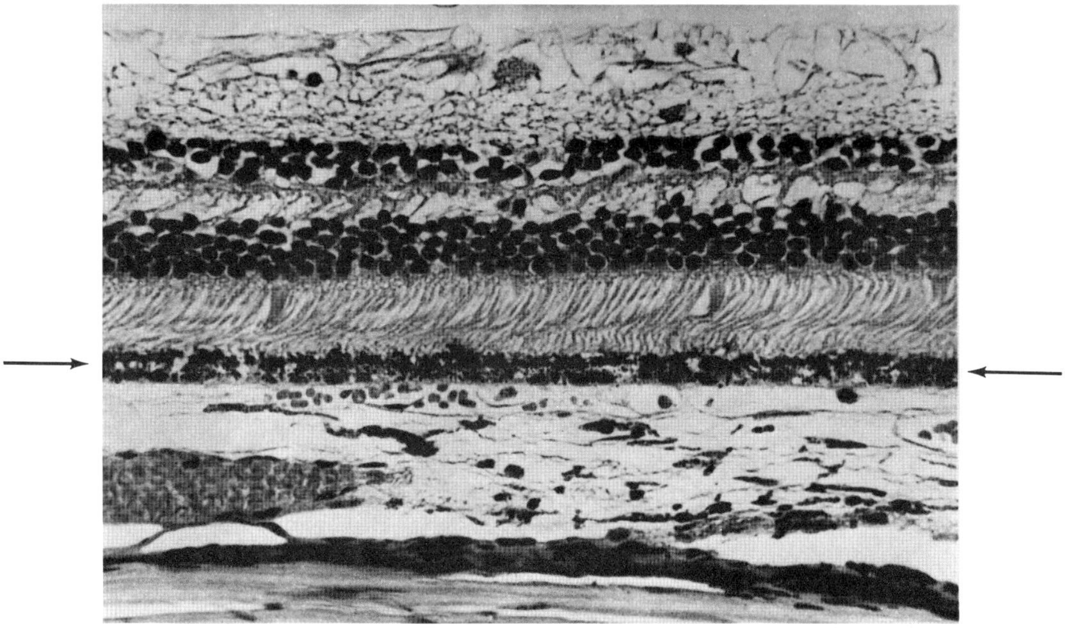

Figure 4.7. Normal retinal pigment epithelium (*arrows*). The essence of fluorescein angiography is the visualization of two circulations, the retinal and the choroidal, separated by a barrier of irregular density, the retinal pigment epithelium. ×40. (Courtesy of Martin H. Vogel, M.D.)

RETINAL PIGMENT EPITHELIUM

The retinal pigment epithelium is a critical layer because of its capacity to alter normal fluorescence. It has a broad potential for change including loss of pigment, atrophy, hyperpigmentation, hypertrophy, proliferation, migration, and serous as well as hemorrhagic detachment. In the normal eye it is essentially a filter of irregular density separating the choroidal and retinal circulations (Fig. 4.7). In the macular region, the cells are more densely packed, more columnar, and more heavily pigmented. The retinal pigment epithelium in the macular region has a higher percentage of lipofuscin-laden pigment granules than elsewhere in the retina. These characteristics combined with the presence of the intraretinal yellow pigment, xanthophyll, and the perifoveal retinal capillary-free zone, serve collectively to produce the characteristic dark zone of the macula (Fig. 4.8). It is, however, principally the characteristics of the pigment epithelium in the macula that produce this effect by diminishing the amount of excitatory light reaching the choroidal circulation and fluorescing the light emerging from it toward the film plane.

Either reduction of the pigment or the absence of the retinal pigment epithelium itself, serves to expose the underlying choroidal circulation producing transmitted fluorescence or the so-called pigment epithelial "window" defect. The understanding and recognition of transmitted fluorescence is a salient feature to fluorescein angiography interpretation. As stated above, it is due predominantly to a defect in the retinal pigment epithelium which produces an accentuation to the normal underlying choroidal fluorescence. It also implies an intact choriocapillaris (Fig. 4.9). Without a normally perfusing choriocapillaris, there would be no choroidal circulation to accentuate except for the larger choroidal vessels. When the retinal pigment epithelium is absent or void of pigment, and there is combined atrophy of the choriocapillaris, transmitted fluorescence will not be seen on the fluorescein angiogram. Rather, filling of the larger choroidal vessels and ultimately late staining of the sclera adjacent to any intact choriocapillaris will occur. Transmitted fluorescence is also a form of early hyperfluorescence that appears coincidental with the filling of the choroidal circulation. It changes very little in the course of the angiogram except in terms of its intensity as the choriocapillaris fills. It is most important that, in the late stage of the angiogram, it disappears as fluorescein empties from the choroidal circulation. It is an early, nonexudative form of hyperfluorescence that contrasts sharply to the later hyperfluorescence that is seen from leak.

Serous detachment of the retinal pigment epithelium, with or without associated subretinal neovascularization, is associated with late hyperfluorescence or leak as fluorescein accumulates beneath the detachment in the late phase angiogram.

The pigment epithelium may also undergo change which may reduce normal fluorescence. Pigment proliferation and migration, for example, can serve to obscure or block the view of the underlying choroidal fluorescence producing a form of hypofluorescence called blocked fluorescence.

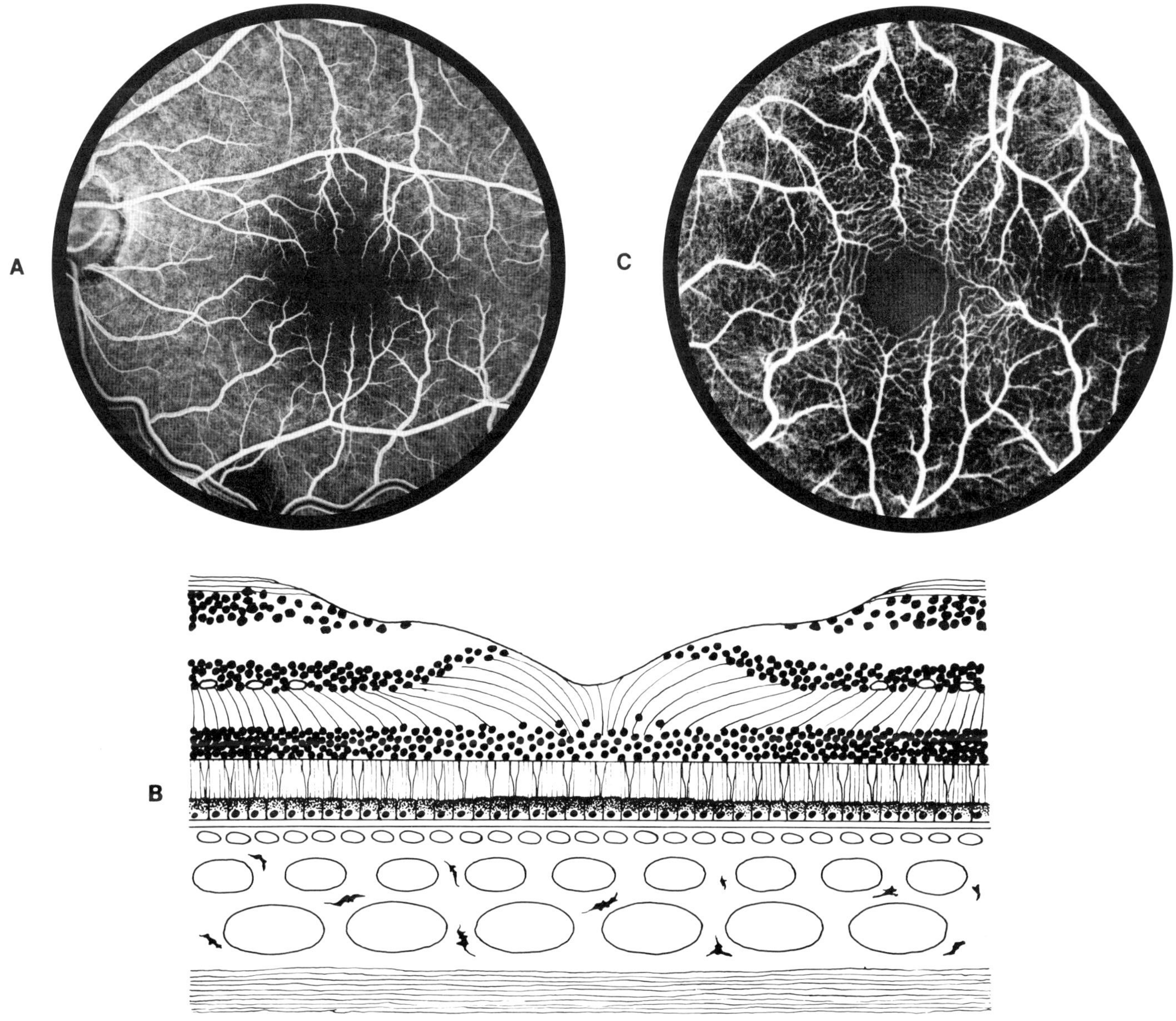

Figure 4.8. *A*, the dark zone of the macula. The macular region remains dark on angiography principally because of the character of the retinal pigment epithelium, which has more densely packed cells that are more columnar, more heavily pigmented, and contain a higher percentage of lipofuscin-laden pigment granules than elsewhere in the retina. In addition, the intraretinal yellow pigment, xanthophyll, and the perifoveal retinal capillary-free zone also serve to augment the macular dark zone. *B*, schematic representation of the macula illustrating the variations in the pigment epithelium. *C*, the perifoveal capillary-free zone. This zone, which is free of retinal capillaries, varies in size from 50–500 μ in diameter and contributes to the overall dark zone of the macula. (From H. Schatz, T. Burton, L. Yannuzzi, and M. Rabb: Interpretation of Fundus Fluorescein Angiography, 1978, © C. V. Mosby Co., St. Louis; reprinted with permission.)

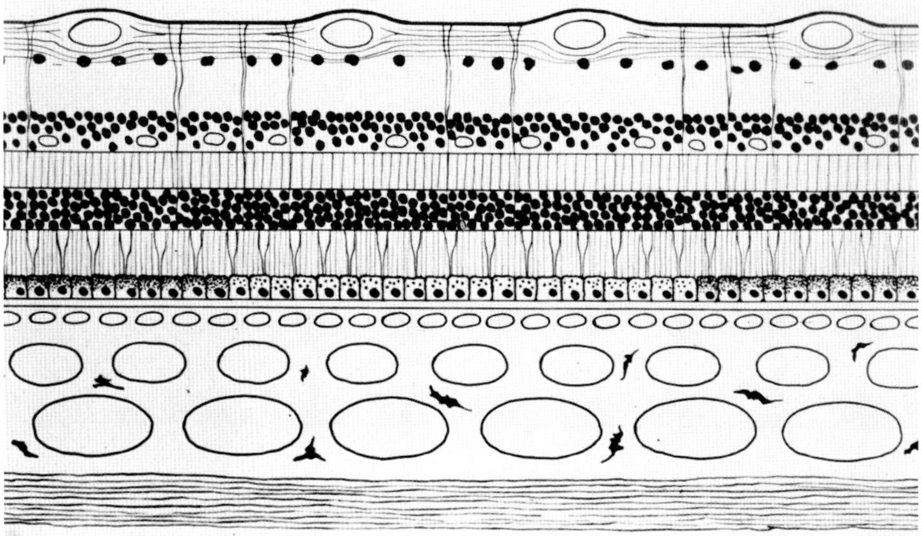

Figure 4.9. Schematic representation of transmitted fluorescence, or the so-called pigment epithelial "window" defect. The retinal pigment epithelium has reduced pigmentation, exposing the underlying choroidal circulation. Transmitted fluorescence is merely an accentuation of the underlying choroidal circulation due to defects in the retinal pigment epithelium. It also implies an intact choriocapillaris; otherwise, large choroidal vessels would be seen in place of the "ground glass" appearance of the normally fluorescent choriocapillaris. (From H. Schatz, T. Burton, L. Yannuzzi, and M. Rabb: Interpretation of Fundus Fluorescein Angiography, 1978, © C. V. Mosby Co., St. Louis, reprinted with permission.)

CHOROIDAL CIRCULATION

The choroidal circulation (Fig. 4.10) is visible outside the macular region and can be studied on the angiogram, particularly in eyes with reduced overall pigment in the pigment epithelium; i.e., as in an albinotic or myopic fundus (see chapter 19: Myopia). The choroidal circulation usually fills shortly before the retinal circulation, probably because of a shorter route to the eye or a lower end-capillary pressure compared to the retinal circulation. It fills in a patchy or heterogeneous fashion in the normal eye (Fig. 4.11). Thus, choroidal tumors, inflammations, and degenerative processes including neovascularization can be studied angiographically.

SCLERA

On the angiogram the sclera is important only in so far as it is visible in the fundus. The tendency of fluorescein to diffuse freely into it produces late hyperfluorescence or leak. This form of leak is physiologic in nature and is seen wherever sclera is visible in the fundus. Since it occurs into tissue, it is arbitrarily referred to as "staining." Staining of the sclera must be differentiated from more pathologic changes that may be present in the subsensory retinal area. The silhouette pattern of large choroidal vessels in the late phase angiogram overlying staining of the sclera is a familiar monocular clue to the localization of this form of late hyperfluorescence. When these larger choroidal vessels are not seen in silhouettes, the late hyperfluorescence is not due to staining of the sclera, but instead, to hyperfluorescence of some other subretinal manifestation such as a fibrous membrane.

Photographic and Darkroom Techniques

In evaluation of a fluorescein angiogram, photographic modification and artifacts are often encountered due to accidental contingencies or poor technique, either in the actual photography or in the darkroom procedures. Insufficient dye concentrations, systemic factors that tend to conjugate the dye into less fluorescent albumin bonds, the hematocrit, the ocular media, fixation and stereo devices, and the clarity of the optical system of the fundus camera are but a few of the numerous factors which serve to influence the overall photographic result. The filters employed, particularly because of their capability for mutual exclusion, are extremely important as a potential source of pseudofluorescence, a factor that must be taken into account by the interpreter in his overall evaluation of the study. Crescent and diffuse reflexes from poor alignment and focusing produce easily recognizable irregularities. High myopia, aphakia, and marked astigmatism, as well as attempts at peripheral photography, all introduce focusing difficulties and characteristic changes on the angiogram.

Darkroom procedures may result in a myriad of irregularities. Poor quality photographs may result from poor developing or printing techniques or choice of materials. Excessive contrast with elimination of fine capillary detail is a frequent problem. Negatives that have been handled carelessly can be scratched or can pick up dirt particles, artifactually altering the final product. These potential changes must all be recognized in the interpretation of a fluorescein angiogram.

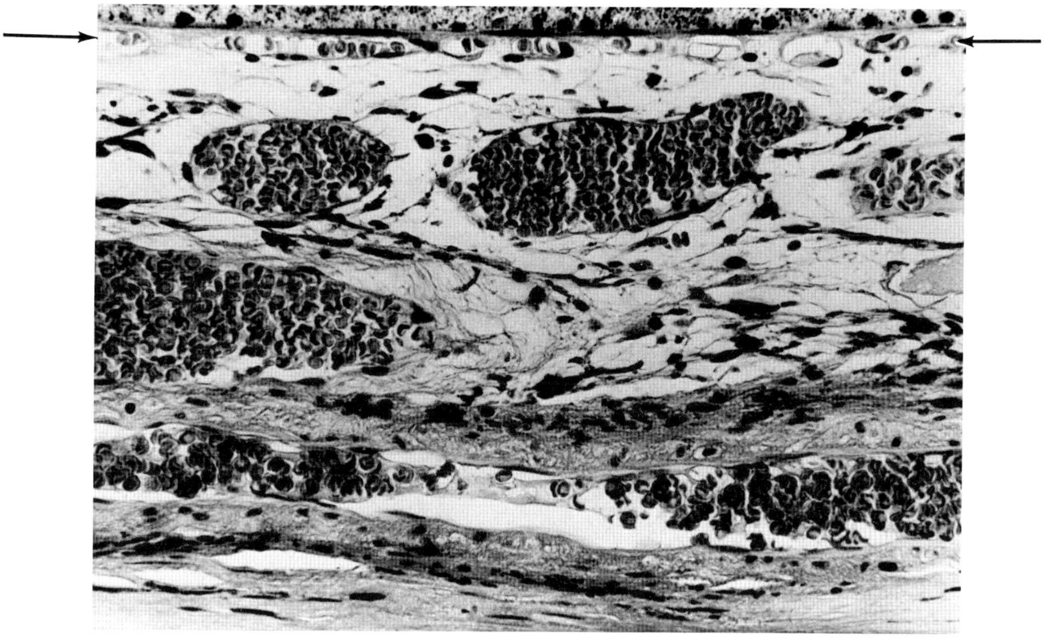

Figure 4.10. Normal choroidal circulation. The choriocapillaris (*arrows*) lies just beneath Bruch's membrane and the retinal pigment epithelium. The larger choroidal vessels are often visible in an albinotic or myopic fundus when there is reduced pigmentation in the retinal pigment epithelium. ×40. (Courtesy of Martin H. Vogel, M.D.)

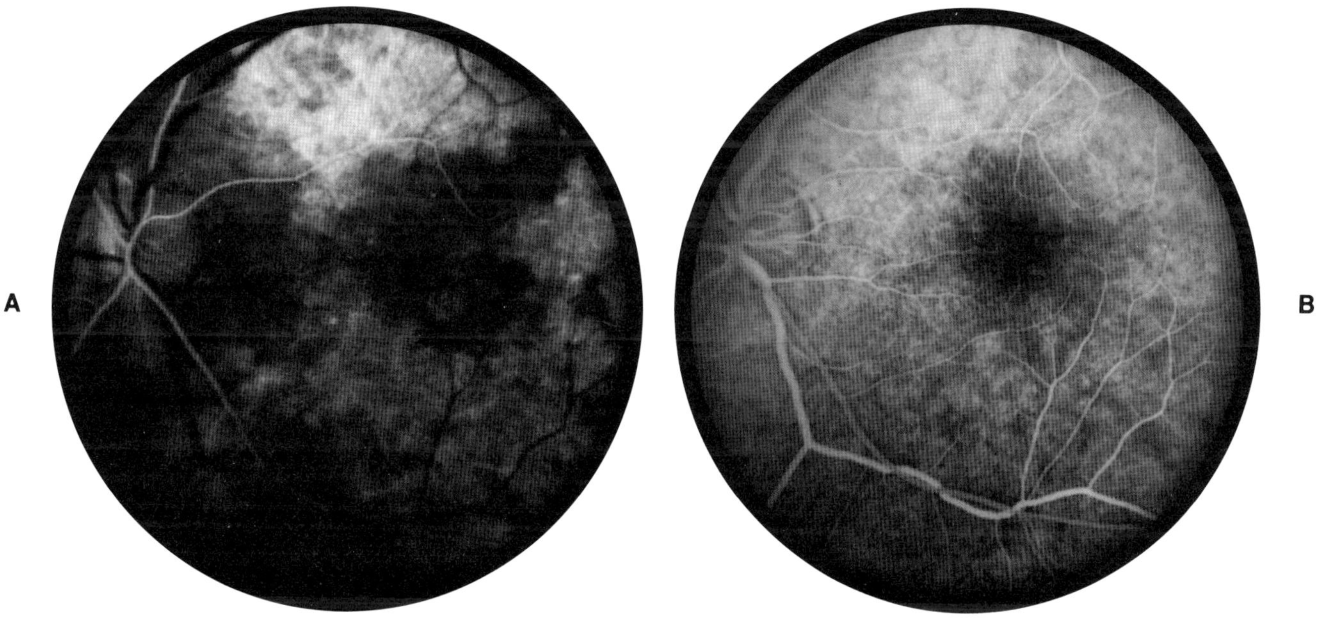

Figure 4.11. *A*, arterial phase angiogram. Note the geographic areas of hypofluorescence in the macula and peripapillary area. *B*, late venous phase angiogram. The areas of hypofluorescence have disappeared as the choriocapillaris fills with dye. Patchy irregular filling of the choriocapillaris is frequently seen in the normal eye.

Fluorescein Angioscopy

The importance of fluorescein angioscopy, or the ophthalmoscopic evaluation of the fundus utilizing the same dual filter system employed in fluorescein angiography, must not be underestimated in its capacity to reveal pathology overlooked in the photographic series. Its principal importance lies in its ability to detect peripheral fundus pathology, particularly lesions associated with secondary manifestations in the macula. Even a very skillful photographer can sometimes fail to recognize a small area of peripheral nonperfusion (see chapter 9: Peripheral Retinal Occlusive Disease), a leak in central serous chorioretinopathy outside the immediate posterior pole (see chapter 13: Central Serous Chorioretinopathy), or a subtle peripheral seafan. Many localized detachments of the macula have proved to have eccentric sources of leakage from the level of the pigment epithelium but remote from the immediate macula area. These can be initially detected with angioscopy and ultimately documented with photography. Peripheral seafans in sickle retinopathy, pre- and posttreatment, can be recognized easily from late pooling into the vitreous with angioscopy utilizing the indirect ophthalmoscope. It is important to realize, however, that this is not a technique that is sufficient in itself. When fluorescein angiography is indicated, fluorescein angioscopy is a good complement, rather than a substitute. One exception may be the search for cystoid macular edema after cataract surgery (Irvine-Gass syndrome), but only when photography is not available for definitive documentation of the edema.

The indirect ophthalmoscope can be used for fluorescein angioscopy by placing an appropriate excitatory filter (blue) over the light source and preferably, although not necessarily, by utilizing a barrier filter (yellow) over the viewing piece. This is essentially the same technique used in fundus fluorescein photography. The same form of examination can be carried out with the slit-lamp biomicroscope and the Goldmann lens. There is no substitute for the stereopsis and the increased magnification provided by this technique in examining the macula. The cobalt blue filter available on older slit lamps should be replaced by the preferred interference excitatory filters now conventionally provided with many of the newer slit lamps. The yellow filter may be placed anywhere in front of the examiner's eyes even in the form of spectacles. Incorporating the yellow filter into the examination enhances appreciation of true fluorescing surfaces by eliminating the excess of residual blue light emerging from the fundus. In a sense, this is a dynamic form of color fluorescein angiography with no possibility of pseudofluorescence when ideal filter combinations are employed. The better optics provided by the Goldmann lens makes it preferable to the Hruby lens. It is important to recall, however, that the Goldmann lens is a contact lens and even a relatively nonviscous solution can disturb the corneal clarity making it difficult to take sharply focused photographs after this examination.

Normal Angiogram

The fluorescein angiogram is essentially a dynamic record of the two fundus circulations, retinal and choroidal, that are separated by pigment epithelium which varies in its density. The patchy irregular filling of the choroidal circulation usually precedes the retinal filling phases of the angiogram. It is manifested as a faint, heterogeneous fluorescence in the posterior pole excluding the macula. The macula itself remains dark throughout the normal angiogram for reasons discussed above. When the choroidal circulation fills completely, it takes on an intensely bright and diffuse "ground glass" appearance that gradually fades as the choroid empties. Cilioretinal vessels, if present, also fill during the choroidal phase of the angiogram because of their choroidal origin.

The choroidal retinal vasculature filling phases have served as a convenient means of classification of the various stages of the angiogram. These stages are: (1) choroidal phase; (2) arteriole phase (filling of retinal arterioles); (3) arteriovenous phase (early laminar filling of veins); (4) early venous phase (dye concentration in arteriole equal to that of venule); (5) late venous phase (dye concentration in venule greater than arteriole); and (6) late phase (dye visibly gone from retinal and choroidal circulations) (Fig. 4.12). In the late phase angiogram staining of the lamina cribrosa and sclera are the only forms of normal visible hyperfluorescence. A faint hyperfluorescence of the posterior pole preceding the choroidal filling phase (retrobulbar fluorescence) from arrival of the dye to the retrobulbar structures appears to be seldom documentable and of little clinical importance.

Figure 4.12. Normal fluorescein angiogram. *A*, the choroidal phase. This is the first manifestation following intravenous fluorescein, which is seen as a diffuse, patchy, heterogeneous fluorescence in the posterior pole excluding the macula. If a cilioretinal vessel is present, it also fills at this stage in the angiogram. *B*, retinal arteriole phase. Dye first appears in the retinal arterioles in this stage of the angiogram. *C*, arteriovenous phase. Early laminar filling in the veins is evident in this stage of the angiogram. *D*, early venous phase. The early venous phase occurs when the retinal arteriolar fluorescence is equal to the venules. The choriocapillaris also has a diffuse "ground glass" appearance. In the late venous phase, fluorescence of the retinal venules is greater than the arterioles. *E*, late phase angiogram. Fluorescein is visibly gone from the retinal and choroidal circulation leaving fluorescence from staining of the lamina cribrosa and visible sclera.

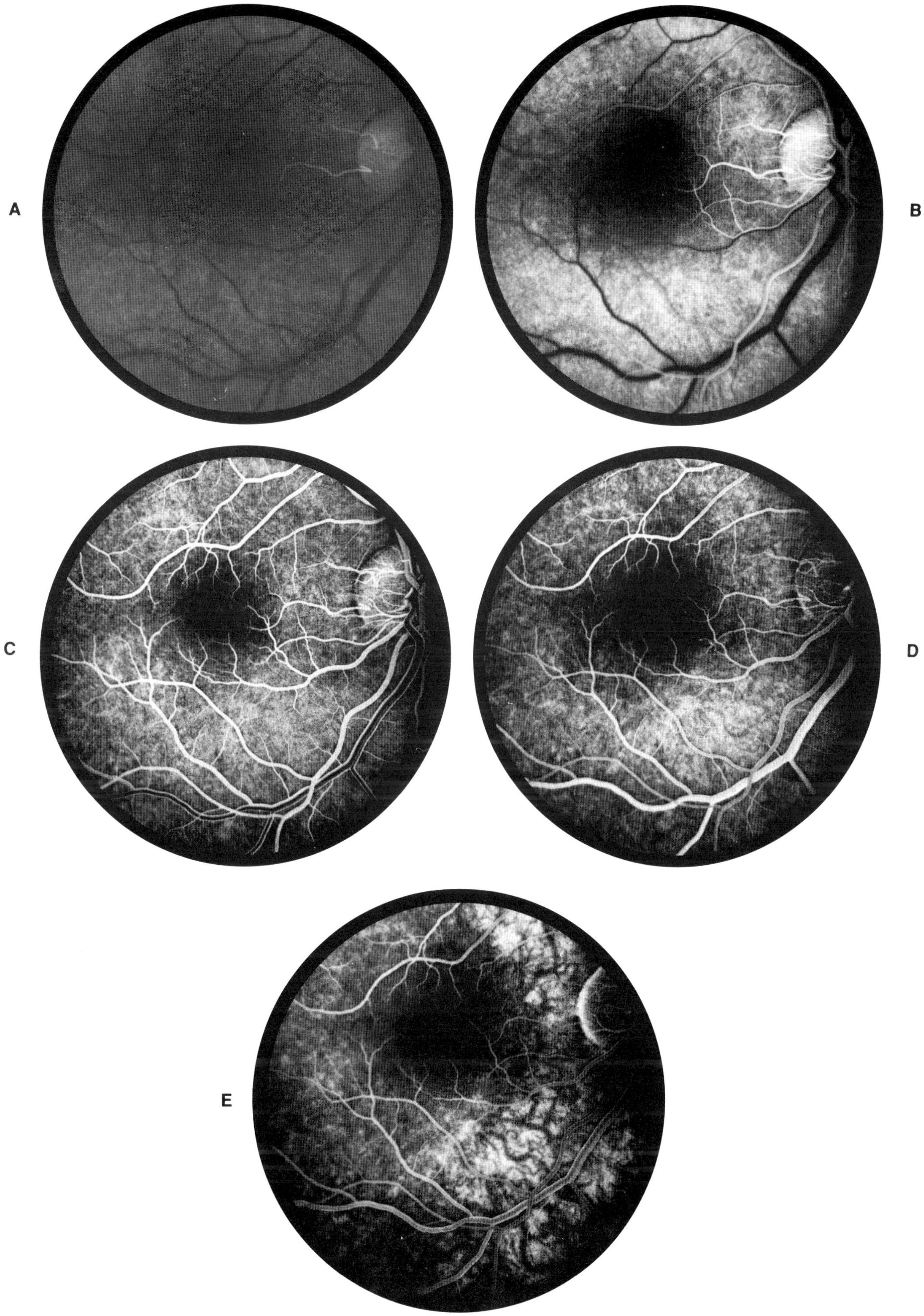

Figure 4.12

Abnormal Fluorescence

Following familiarization with the prerequisites suggested above, the training in the interpretation of the fluorescein angiograms can proceed utilizing the schematic guide to the interpretation of fluorescein angiograms (Fig. 4.13). It is designed to provide a simple comprehensive means for detecting and reporting all abnormal fundus fluorescence. It simplifies and defines all angiographic terminology, thereby providing a common language for reporting findings. The guide states clearly that there are only two types of abnormal fluorescence: hypofluorescence and hyperfluorescence. From this basic assumption a logical progression follows to determine more specifically the exact location and nature of the pathologic factor producing the abnormal fluorescence.

The first step in the use of the schematic guide is to decide whether the abnormal fluorescence is "hypo," which means abnormally reduced fluorescence, or "hyper," which means abnormally increased fluorescence. Once this initial, basic differentiation is made, a systematic series of decisions follow, designed to arrive at a proper diagnosis or appreciation of the related histopathologic manifestations.

When hypofluorescence appears on an angiogram, only two possibilities exist: (1) fluorescein is present in the two circulations of the fundus but it is blocked by some tissue or fluid barrier. This is called blocked fluorescence; or (2) fluorescein never reached the fundus as in a perfusion abnormality. This is called a vascular filling defect.

When hyperfluorescence appears, there are three major reasons for its presence: (1) there is an increase in the visibility of the normal choroidal fluorescence; referred to as "transmitted fluorescence" or so-called pigment epithelial window defect; (2) there are irregularities in the vascular fluorescence; called abnormal vessels; or (3) there are alterations in the normal permeability barriers in the fundus; this is called leak. When leak occurs into tissue, it is referred to as staining; when it occurs into an anatomic space, it is called pooling. Of minor importance are the preinjection forms of hyperfluorescence known as pseudofluorescence and autofluorescence.

Practical use of the schematic guide to the interpretation of fluorescein angiograms will be discussed by first evaluating examples of hypofluorescence. The reader in each case should study the photographs and refer to the schematic guide to determine increasingly more specifically the type of abnormality present.

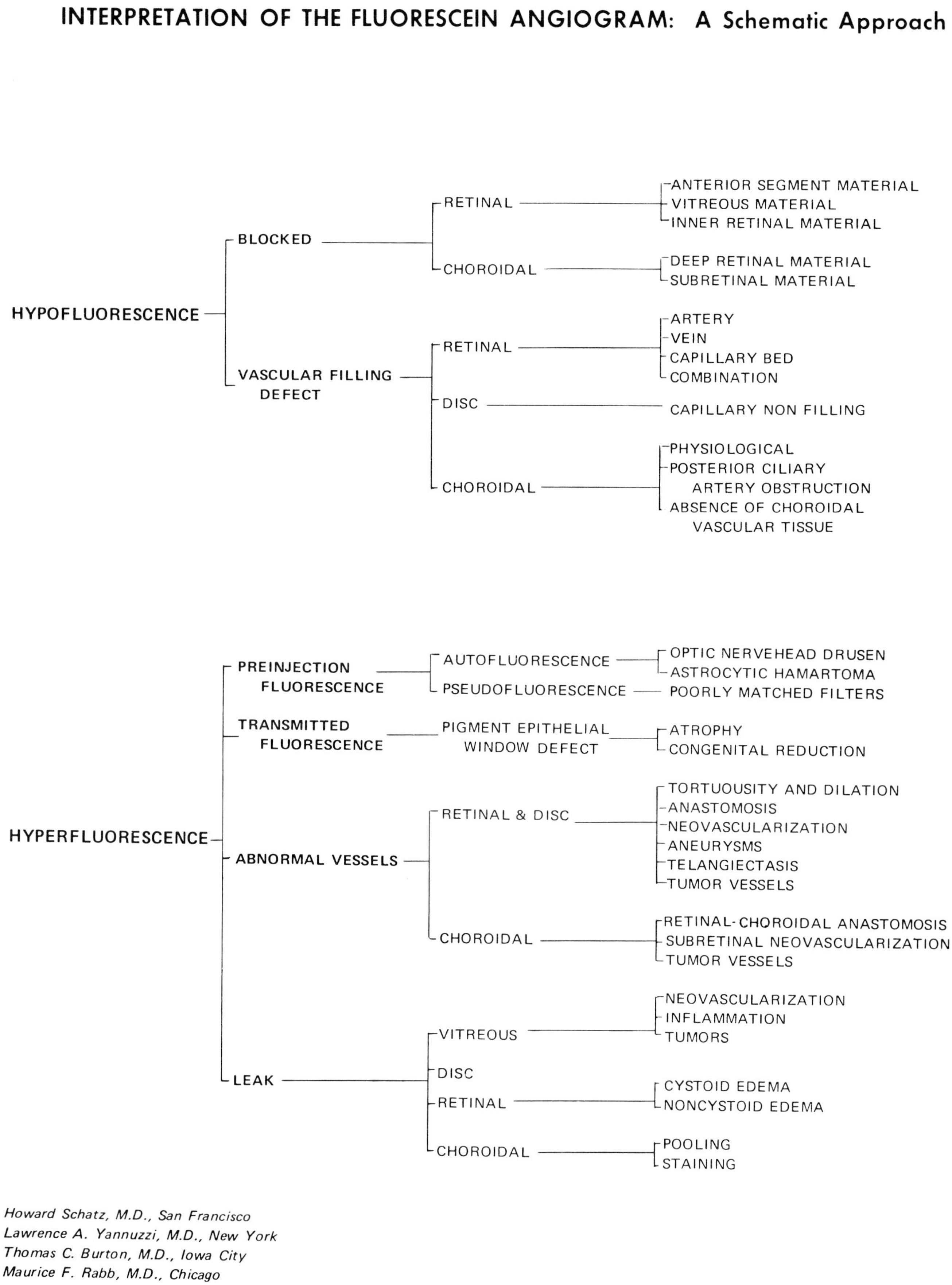

Figure 4.13. Schematic guide to the interpretation of fluorescein angiograms as suggested by H. Schatz, T. Burton, L. Yannuzzi and M. Rabb.

Hypofluorescence

BLOCKED FLUORESCENCE

Examine the first fluorescein angiographic photograph and decide if there are any areas of hypo- or hyperfluorescence present (Fig. 4.14*A*). Note the area of hypofluorescence in the macula. As suggested by the schematic guide, this indicates either blocked fluorescence or a vascular filling defect; to determine which, the ophthalmoscopic view is studied (Fig. 4.14*B*). On the color photograph there is an area of hemorrhage which corresponds in size, shape, and location to the hypofluorescence. Therefore, the hypofluorescence on the angiographic photograph is due to blocked fluorescence.

The next question posed by the schematic guide is designed to determine the exact site of the blockage; i.e., preretinal, retinal, or subretinal. One way to establish this is to determine which circulations in the fundus (superficial and deep retinal and choroidal) are being blocked. In this case, all of the fundus circulations are blocked, localizing the hemorrhage to the preretinal area. Now that the nature and site of the histopathologic factor have been established, a more accurate differential diagnosis can be made. In this case, the preretinal hemorrhage developed following a Valsalva maneuver.

In examining the fluorescein angiogram of the next case (Fig. 4.15*A*), begin by looking for areas of abnormal hypo- or hyperfluorescence. A relatively large area of hypofluorescence is seen surrounding the disc. As suggested by the schematic guide, this is caused by either blocked fluorescence or a vascular filling defect. To determine more precisely the cause, examine the color photograph (Fig. 4.15*B*). A light-yellowish material corresponds exactly to the angiographic picture of the hypofluorescent area around the disc. Therefore, the hypfluorescence seen on the angiogram is due to blocked fluorescence.

The next step is to examine the retinal and choroidal vasculature in order to localize the blocking material in the fundus. In this case the yellowish material overlies the retinal vessels. The material is composed of myelinated nerve fibers. Since these fibers are not totally opaque, the large and small retinal vessels as well as the disc vasculature are not completely blocked. Thus, in this case, the correla-

A 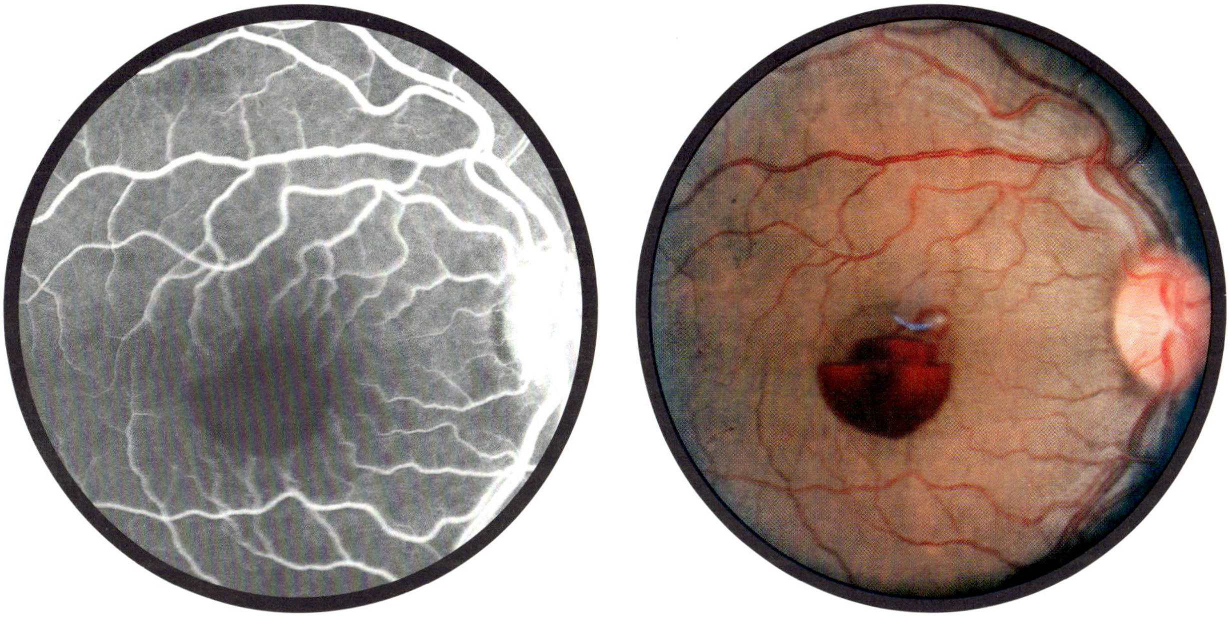 B

Figure 4.14. *A,* early venous phase angiogram. Note hypofluorescence in the macula. *B,* color photograph on the same patient. Note the presence of hemorrhage in the macula which corresponds in size and shape to the area of hypofluorescence present on the fluorescein angiogram. This form of hypofluorescence is, therefore, blocked fluorescence. Since the large retinal vessels are not seen, the hemorrhage is localized to the preretinal area, which in this case, was due to a Valsalva maneuver.

A 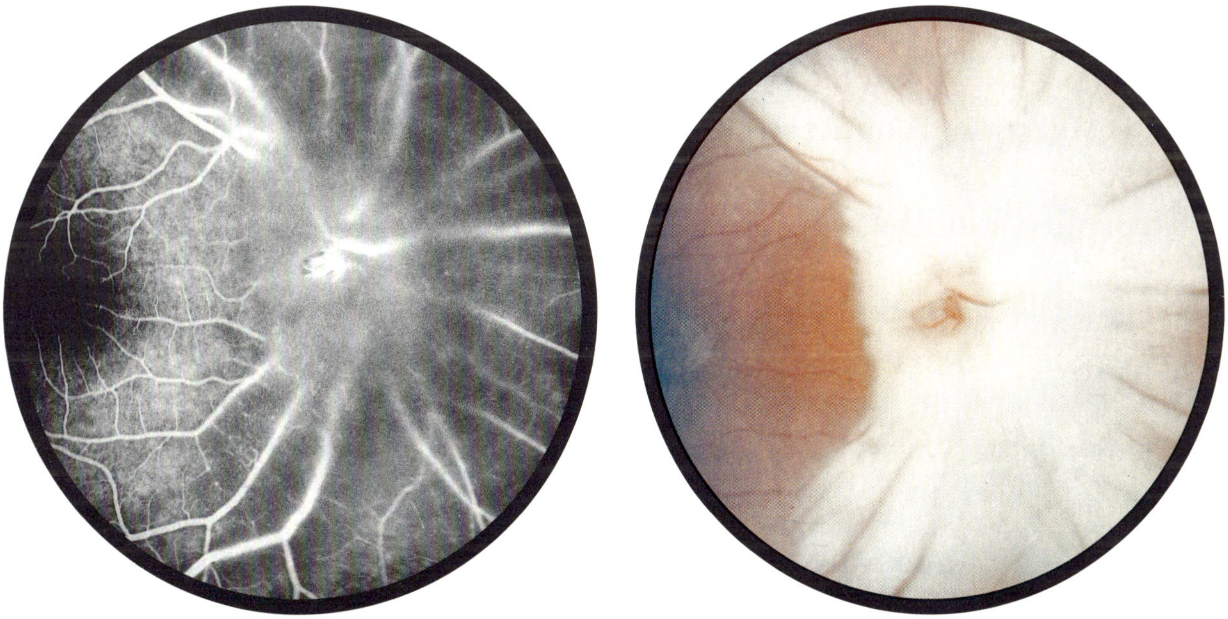 B

Figure 4.15. *A,* early venous phase fluorescein angiogram. Note the area of hypofluorescence surrounding the disc. *B,* color photograph on the same patient. Note the light yellowish material that surrounds the disc corresponding exactly to the zone of hypofluorescence. The hypofluorescence, therefore, is due to blocked fluorescence. The large retinal vessels in some areas are completely eliminated, while in others they are merely obscured. This localizes the blocking factor to the site of the retinal vessels, the nerve fiber layer. In this case, the blocked fluorescence is due to myelinated nerve fibers.

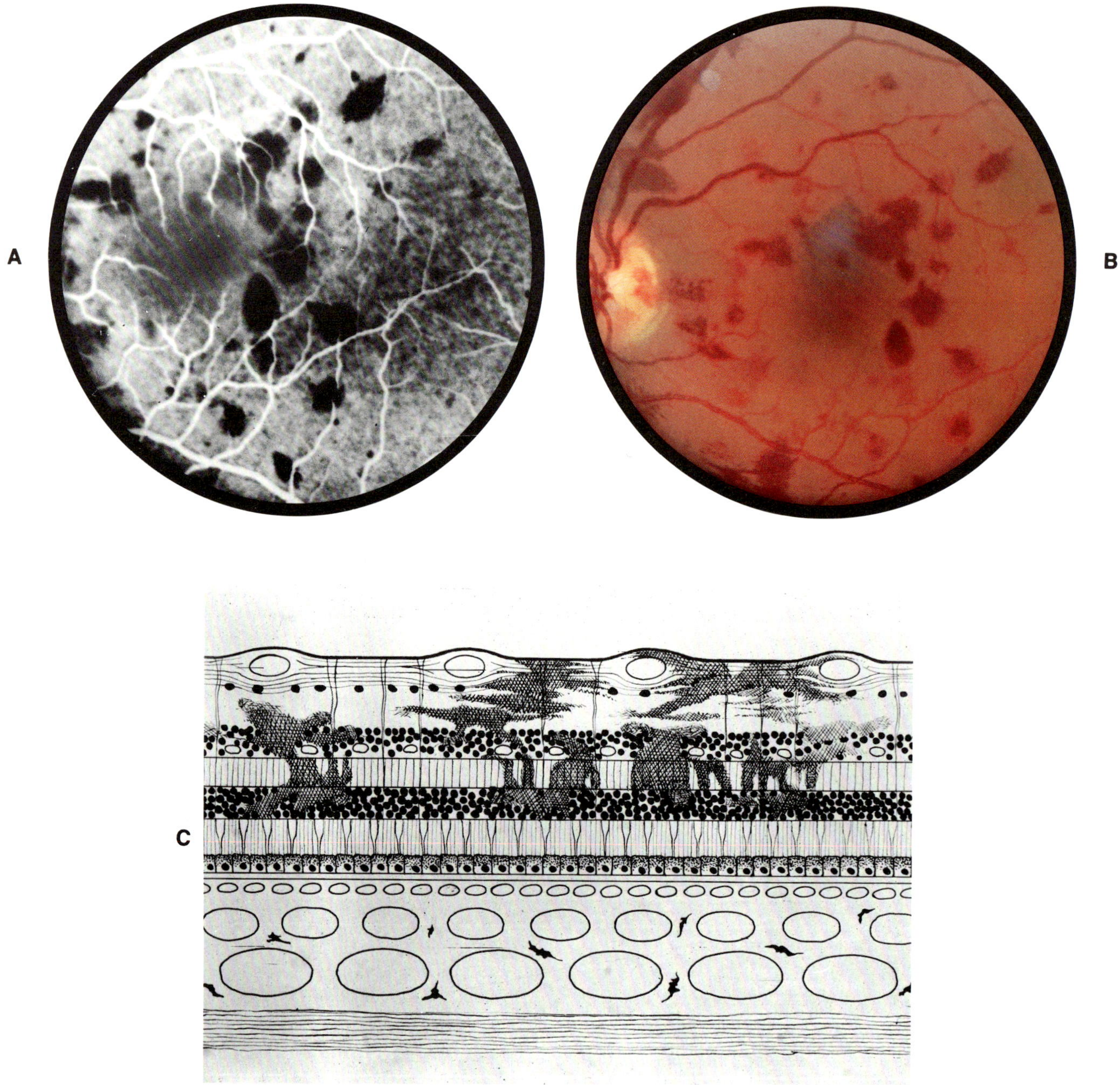

Figure 4.16. *A,* early venous phase fluorescein angiogram. Note the multiple areas of hypofluorescence scattered throughout the posterior pole. *B,* color photograph on the same patient. At the site of each area of hypofluorescence there is a corresponding hemorrhage which is identical in size and shape. The hypofluorescence, therefore, represents blocked fluorescence. Examination of the retinal vessels aids in determining the site of the hemorrhages. In most instances, the superficial larger retinal vessels are not blocked localizing hemorrhages to the deep capillary plexus of the retina. In a few areas, larger vessels are not visible or obscured, indicating that these hemorrhages are in the superficial circulation in the nerve fiber layer. In this case, the multiple hemorrhages originating from both retinal circulations developed in a patient with heparin toxicity. *C,* schematic representation of the same patient showing how retinal hemorrhages (*hatching*) may produce blocked fluorescence of the deep capillary plexus circulation of both the superficial and deep circulations depending on their location. (From H. Schatz, T. Burton, L. Yannuzzi, and M. Rabb: Interpretation of Fundus Fluorescein Angiography, 1978, © C. V. Mosby Co., St. Louis; reprinted with permission.)

tion of the angiogram with the color photograph aids in defining the specific type of hypofluorescence present and enhances the histopathologic understanding of the case.

Study the fluorescein angiogram of the next case and note multiple areas of hypofluorescence in the posterior pole (Fig. 4.16*A*). Are these due to blocked fluorescence or vascular filling defects? A comparison of the color photograph (Fig. 4.16*B*) indicates that there is a corresponding hemorrhage at the site of each area of hypofluorescence. Therefore, the hypofluorescence is blocked fluorescence.

The next question according to the schematic guide relates to where the blocking factors (the hemorrhages) are located. Is the choroidal circulation or the combined choroidal and retinal circulations blocked? Examination of the hypofluorescence reveals, in each case, that the choroidal circulation is blocked. In most instances the superficial larger retinal vessels are not blocked localizing the hemorrhage to the deep capillary circulation of the retina. In a few areas, the larger vessels are not visible or obscured indicating that these hemorrhages originated from the superficial circulation in the nerve fiber layers.

The schematic representation of this case (Fig. 4.16*C*) illustrates how the deep retinal hemorrhages block the choroidal and the deep retinal circulation, while the superficial hemorrhages block the superficial retinal circulation as well. Thus, the angiogram aids in localizing the hemorrhages within the retina in this case of heparin toxicity.

Examine the next angiogram for areas of abnormal hypo- or hyperfluorescence (Fig. 4.17*A*). Note the large area of hypofluorescence just below the macula. Again, the hypofluorescence present here must be due to either blocked fluorescence or a vascular filling defect. In order to determine which type, it is necessary to examine the color photograph (Fig. 4.17*B*). The color photo of the macula shows yellowish material that corresponds exactly in shape, size, and location to the hypofluorescence seen on the angiogram. Therefore, the hypofluorescence is blocked fluorescence.

Now it is necessary to decide whether the hypofluorescence involves the retinal vasculature and/or the choroidal vasculature to determine a more accurate localization of the blocking material. Note that on the angiogram the retinal vessels are visible overlying the hypofluorescent material. Therefore, the yellowish material is located under the retinal vessels in front of the choroidal vasculature. This is a case of Best's vitelliform maculopathy. The yellowish material, producing a pseudohypopyon because of its fluid level configuration, is a type of egg yolk formation in the macula.

A

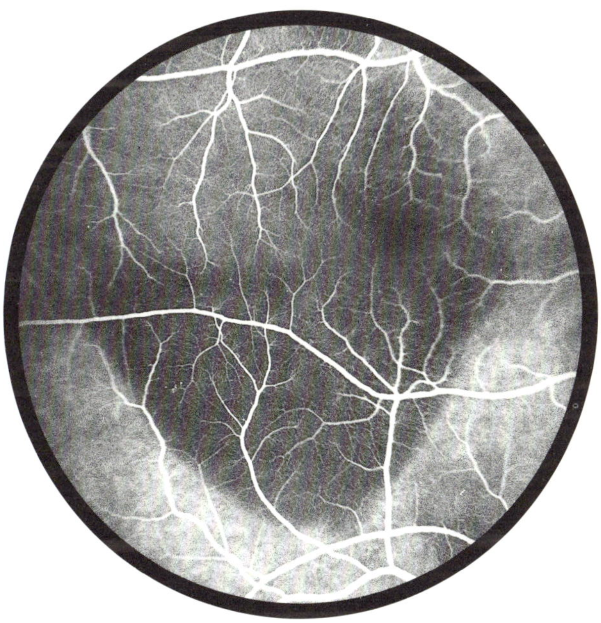

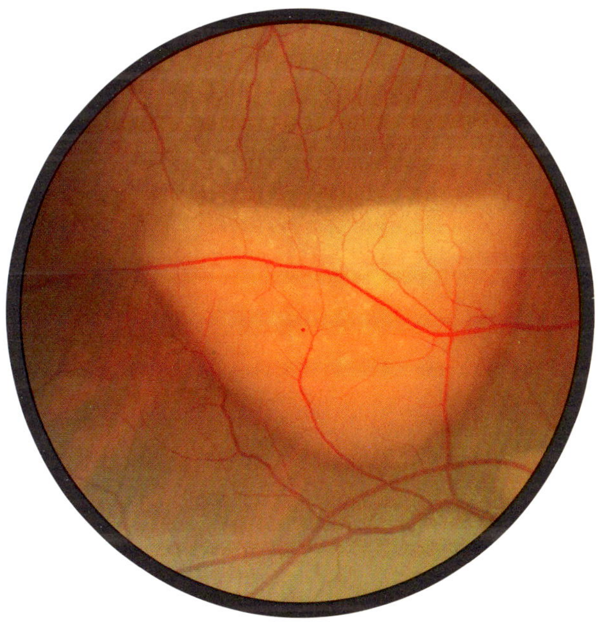

B

Figure 4.17. *A*, early venous phase fluorescein angiogram. Note the area of hypofluorescence just below the macula. (From H. Schatz, T. Burton, L. Yannuzzi, and M. Rabb: Interpretation of Fundus Fluorescein Angiography, 1978, © C. V. Mosby Co., St. Louis; reprinted with permission.) *B*, color photograph on the same patient. Note the yellowish material which corresponds exactly in size and shape to the hypofluorescence seen on the angiogram. Therefore, the hypofluorescence is blocked fluorescence. In localizing the site of the histopathologic factor producing the hypofluorescence, the retinal vasculature is noted to fluoresce normally overlying it. Therefore, the yellowish material was located under the retina in front of the choroidal vasculature. This is a case of Best's vitelliform maculopathy, producing a pseudohypopyon from a fluid level configuration.

VASCULAR FILLING DEFECT

Examine this fluorescein angiogram (Fig. 4.18*A*) for areas of abnormal hypo- or hyperfluorescence. An area of hypofluorescence can be seen in the macula. An examination of the color photograph must be made to determine whether this is blocked fluorescence or a vascular filling defect (Fig. 4.18*B*). In the color photograph there is a dark lesion which corresponds exactly to the hypofluorescent area seen on the angiogram. Therefore, this is blocked fluorescence. When there is blocked fluorescence the next step is to determine whether the retinal and/or choroidal vessels are blocked.

In the angiogram the retinal vessels are seen to overly the hypofluorescence; therefore, the pigmented lesion in this case is located under the retina. This is a typical angiogram for a choroidal nevus. The nevus blocks the choroidal vasculature because of its dense pigmentation. Occasionally, the nevus will be largely suprachoroidal and the choriocapillaris will be only partly involved (Fig. 4.19, *A* and *B*). In such cases, the blocked fluorescence will be limited to the large choroidal vessels as the partially intact choriocapillaris fluoresces normally above the nevus. A schematic representation of such a choroidal nevus (Fig. 4.19*C*) suggests that some choriocapillaris fluorescence may exist at the site of the lesion. This is particularly evident when atrophy exists in the overlying retinal pigment epithelium.

A

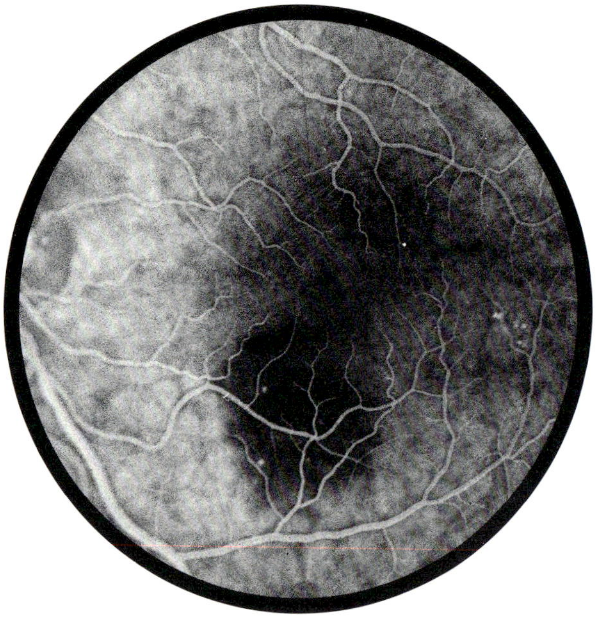

B

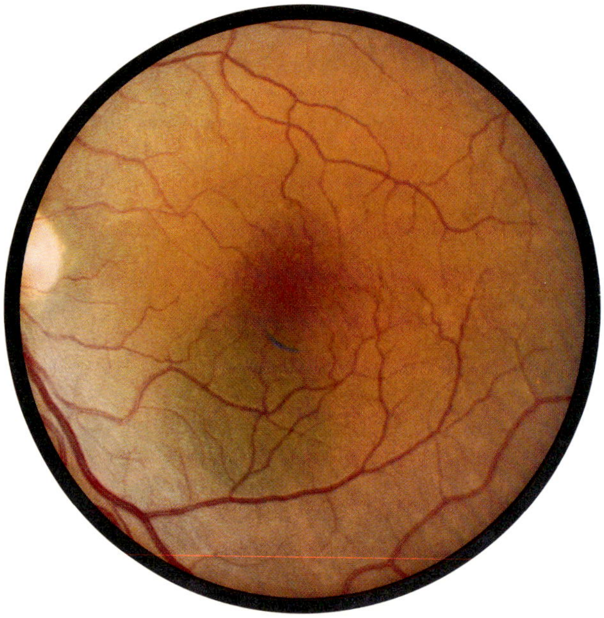

Figure 4.18. *A*, early venous phase fluorescein angiogram. Note the hypofluorescence in the inferior macula. *B*, color photograph on the same patient. Note the dark area in the macula that corresponds exactly to the hypofluorescent area seen on the angiogram, indicating this is blocked fluorescence. In the angiogram the retinal vessels are seen to overly the hypofluorescence; therefore, the pigmented lesion in this case is located under the retina. This is a typical angiogram for a choroidal nevus. The nevus blocks the choroidal vasculature because of its dense pigmentation. The hyperfluorescent dots correspond to drusen.

A

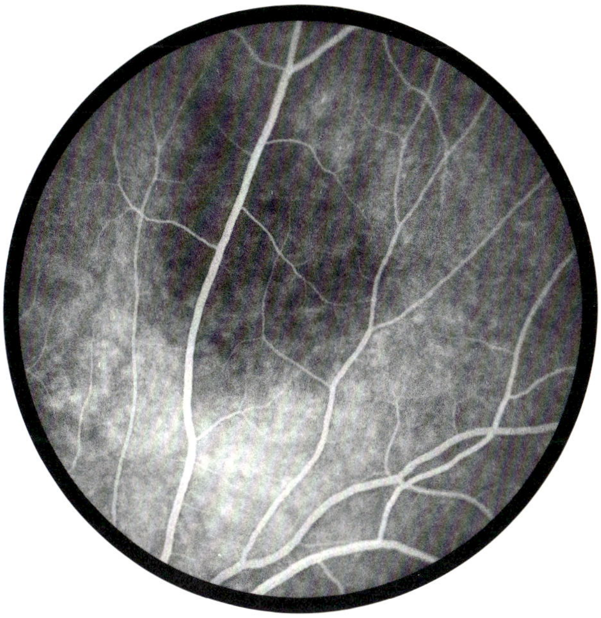

B

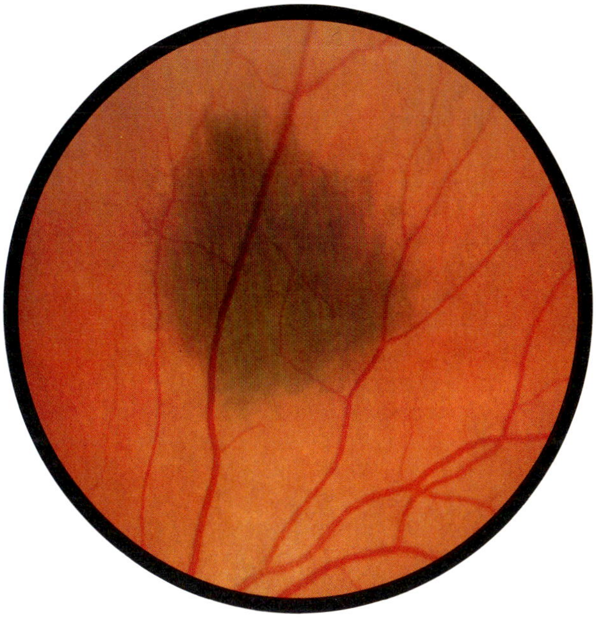

C

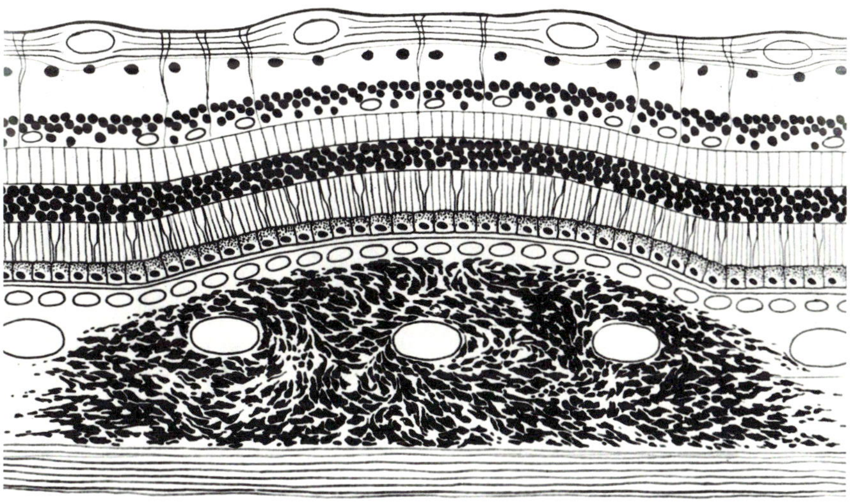

Figure 4.19. *A,* early venous phase angiogram of a choroidal nevus. In this case some of the choriocapillaris overlying the nevus is still intact and fluorescing. Only the larger choroidal vessels are blocked. *B,* color photograph of the same patient. *C,* schematic representation of the same case. (From H. Schatz, T. Burton, L. Yannuzzi, and M. Rabb: Interpretation of Fundus Fluorescein Angiography, 1978, © C. V. Mosby Co., St. Louis; reprinted with permission.) This suggests that the larger choroidal vessels are blocked by the densely pigmented nevus while some choriocapillaris remains intact. Atrophic changes in the overlying retinal pigment epithelium may also serve to accentuate the intact choriocapillaris on the angiogram.

Begin evaluating the next case by defining areas of abnormal hypo- or hyperfluorescence (Fig. 4.20*A*). Note that in this angiogram, although there are patent large retinal vessels nasal to the disc, there are large intervening spaces of hypofluorescence. A correlation of the color photograph (Fig. 4.20*B*) must now be made to determine if there is material blocking fluorescence or if this hypofluorescence is due to a vascular filling defect. There is no evidence of blocking material on the color photograph which corresponds to the hypofluorescence; therefore, this must be a vascular filling defect.

With vascular filling defects, the next step as suggested by the schematic guide, is to decide what circulation is involved—the retinal, the choroidal, or the disc. In this case, although the large retinal vessels can be seen in the nasal retina, the small retinal vasculature is absent, indicating that this is an area of retinal capillary nonperfusion. This angiogram is typical of a patient with a retinal vascular occlusive disease and associated capillary nonperfusion. In this case of radiation retinopathy, the fluorescein angiogram was essential in determining the state of the capillary bed which otherwise could not be determined by ophthalmoscopy alone.

Examine the angiogram in the next case for areas of abnormal hypo- or hyperfluorescence (Fig. 4.21*A*). Note that a vessel just inferior and temporal to the macula is not filled while all other vessels are normally fluorescing. This is clearly a vascular filling defect. According to the schematic guide, it must be established whether the vascular filling defect involves the retinal vessels, the choroidal vessels, or the disc. In this case, the hypofluorescence follows the geographic distribution of a retinal vein.

After establishing that a vascular filling defect is present and that it involves the retinal circulation, the next question is to determine whether the occlusion is total or partial. There is eventual filling of this vein as seen in the late stage of the angiogram (Fig. 4.21*B*). This photo also demonstrates delayed emptying of the involved vein and possibly some late hyperfluorescence from staining of its wall. This case illustrates the typical hypofluorescent findings of delayed filling and emptying in a branch retinal vein occlusion, except the site of occlusion was not at an arteriovenous crossing. In general, the large caliber retinal vessels (venules and arterioles) are readily identifiable on fluorescein angiograms when they are involved in occlusive disease, as perfusion is either delayed or absent along the geographic course of the hypofluorescent vessels. Comparison to the color photograph only confirms the presence or absence of accompanying blocking factors (Fig. 4.21*C*).

A complete retinal vascular filling defect is illustrated in

A

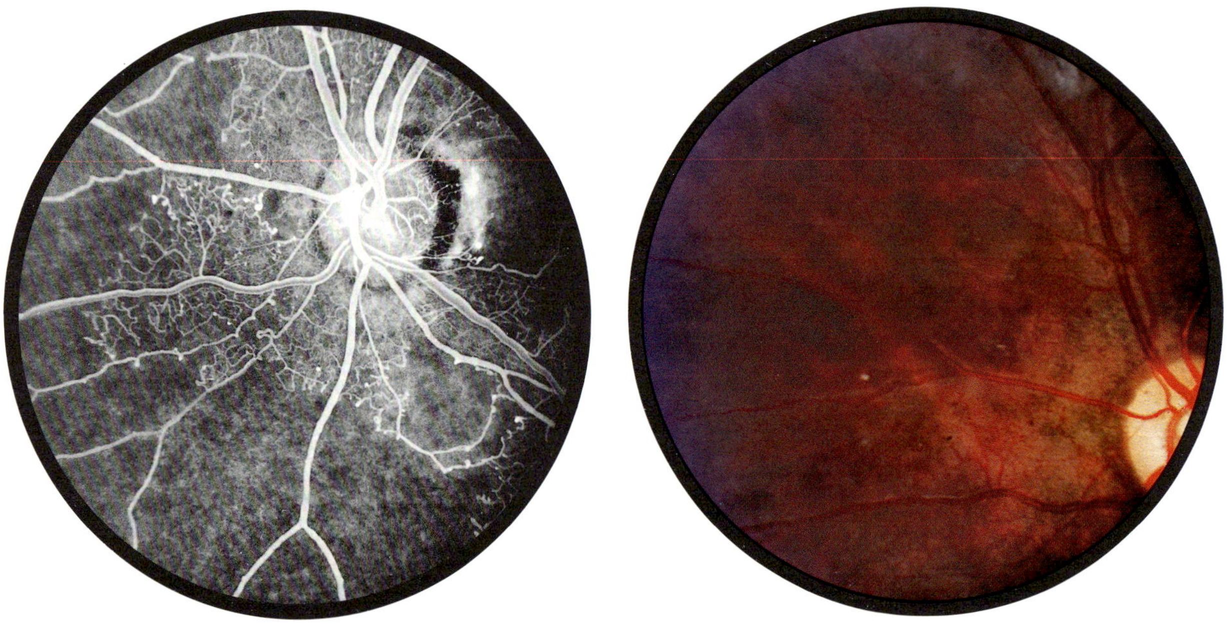

B

Figure 4.20. *A*, early venous phase fluorescein angiogram. Note the areas of hypofluorescence between larger, patent retinal vessels. (From H. Schatz, T. Burton, L. Yannuzzi, and M. Rabb: Interpretation of Fundus Fluorescein Angiography, 1978, © C. V. Mosby Co., St. Louis; reprinted with permission.) *B*, color photograph on the same patient. There is no evidence of blocking material on the color photograph that corresponds to the hypofluorescence; therefore, this is a vascular filling defect. In this case, although the larger retinal vessels are seen, the smaller retinal vasculature is absent, indicating an area of retinal capillary nonperfusion. This is a patient with radiation retinopathy and associated capillary nonperfusion.

A

B

C

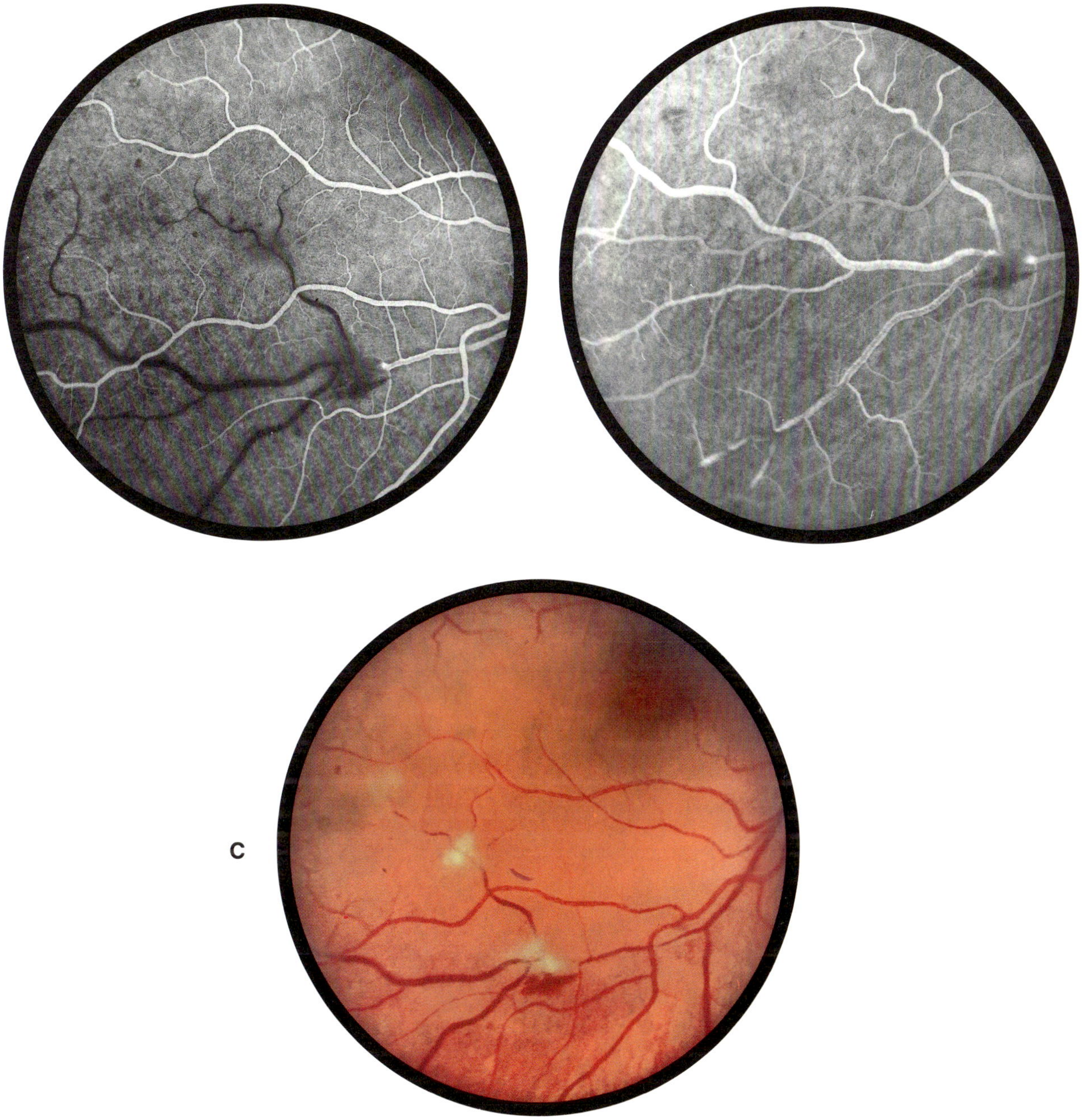

Figure 4.21. *A,* early venous phase angiogram. Note the hypofluorescence of a solitary, large retinal vessel just inferior and temporal to the macular region. The associated hypofluorescence follows the geographic pattern of a retinal vessel. This hypofluorescence, therefore, is due to a vascular filling defect involving a retinal vein. *B,* late venous phase angiogram on the same patient. There is eventual late filling of this vein, indicating that the vascular filling defect is not complete. *C,* color photograph on the same patient. Note the absence of any tissue or fluid barrier that corresponds to the hypofluorescence on the angiogram except for a small area of hemorrhage and exudate at the site of the occlusion. Comparison to the color photograph in a large retinal vascular filling defect only confirms the presence or absence of the accompanying blocking factors. In this case of ocular sarcoidosis, the fluorescein angiogram illustrates the typical hypofluorescent findings of the late filling and emptying in a branch retinal vein occlusion except that the site of the occlusion was not at an A/V crossing.

A

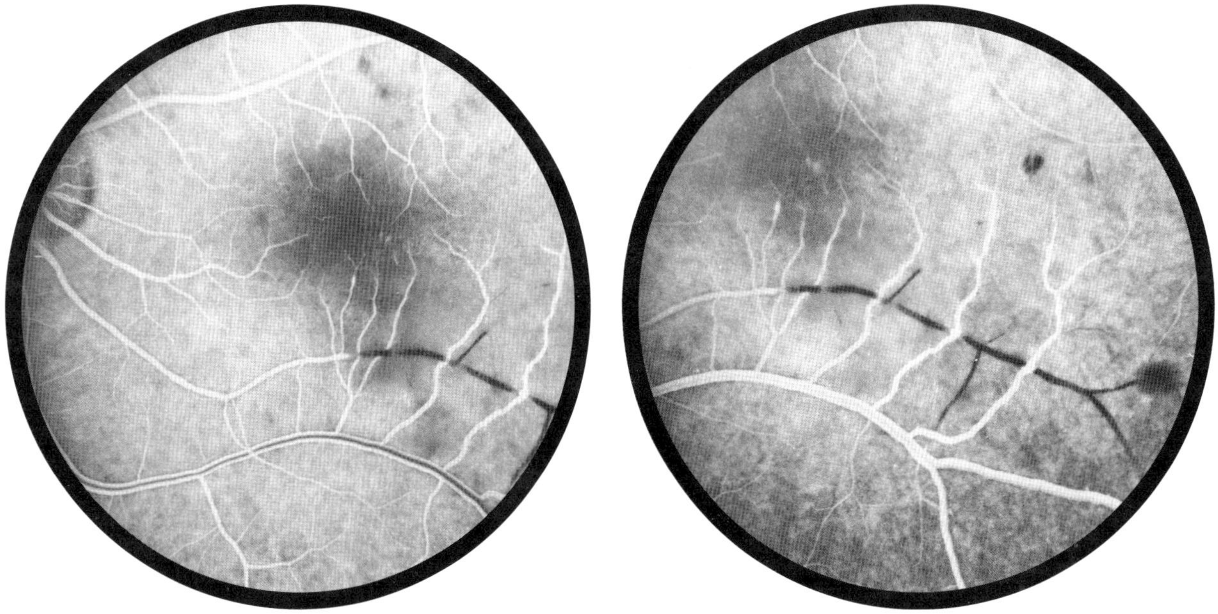

B

Figure 4.22. *A,* arteriovenous phase fluorescein angiogram. Note the hypofluorescence along the course of a retinal arteriole beginning just below the macula. *B,* late venous phase angiogram on the same patient. Note that the retinal arteriole has a complete vascular filling defect as dye does not perfuse beyond the occlusion site in the late stages of the angiogram. This is a case of retinal branch arterial occlusion in systemic lupus erythematosus.

(Fig. 4.22,). The involved retinal arteriole is hypofluorescent in its course beginning just below the macula. In the late venous phase of the angiogram, a complete filling defect is evident as the dye does not perfuse the peripheral end of the vessel. In this case of systemic lupus erythematosus, then, there is a complete branch retinal arteriole occlusion.

Note the area of hypofluorescence supratemporal to the disc in the next case (Fig. 4.23*A*). Is this blocked fluorescence or vascular filling defect? There is nothing on the color photograph which corresponds to the area of hypofluorescence (Fig. 4.23*B*); therefore, this is a vascular filling defect. Next, does the filling defect involve the vessels of the retina, choroid, or disc? Note that the retinal vessels are present and overlie an area of hypofluorescence. This is, therefore, a choroidal vascular filling defect. Is this choroidal and disc vascular filling defect complete or incomplete? To answer this question, a later phase of the angiogram must be examined (Fig. 4.23*C*). This photo reveals that the hypofluorescent area has completely disappeared. The vascular filling defect present here is therefore not complete. These are the typical fluorescein angiographic findings of patchy choroidal filling, a finding which is usually physiologic and seen frequently on angiograms.

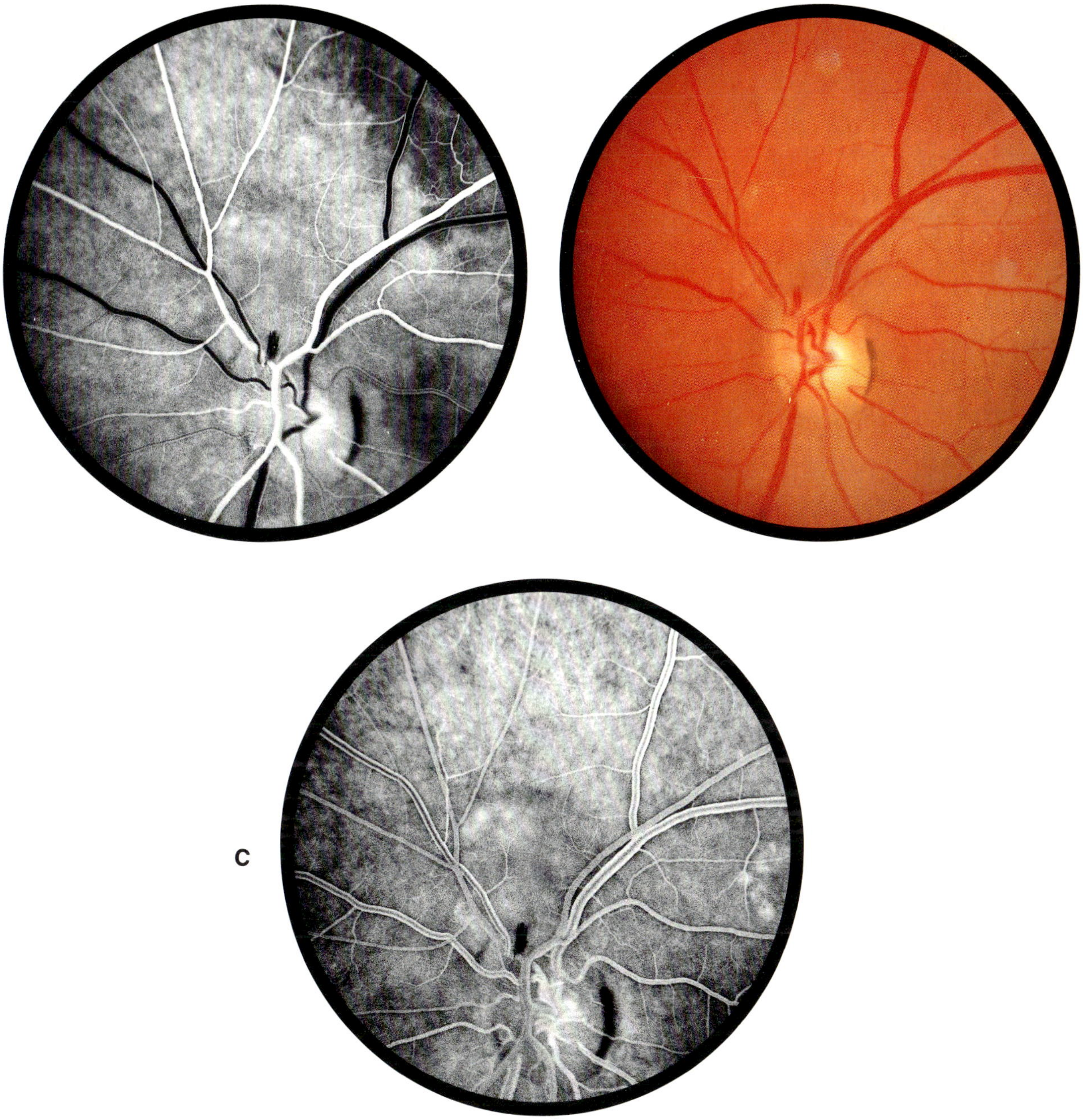

Figure 4.23. *A*, arterial phase angiogram. Note the hypofluorescence supratemporal to the disc. *B*, color photograph on the same patient. There is no tissue or fluid density which corresponds to the area of hypofluorescence evident on the fluorescein angiogram. Therefore, this is a vascular filling defect. *C*, late venous phase angiogram, same patient. The retinal vessels have continued to fill and empty normally. The area of hypofluorescence evident in the early stage of the angiogram has now completely disappeared. The vascular filling defect present here is, therefore, not complete and it involves the choroidal circulation. These are typical fluorescein angiographic findings of patchy choroidal filling, which are physiologic and frequently encountered on angiograms.

Hyperfluorescence

The next group of cases will demonstrate the schematic approach to the fluorescein angiographic interpretation of hyperfluorescence and its major causes. Transmitted fluorescence, or so-called pigment epithelial window defect, abnormal vessels involving the retina or choroid and leak are the three major types of hyperfluorescence. Transmitted fluorescence and abnormal vessels are seen as early hyperfluorescence in the filling phases of the angiogram because of their vascular nature. Late hyperfluorescence on the other hand is always due to leak. Of minor importance are two forms of preinjection fluorescence, known as autofluorescence and pseudofluorescence, and noted on the angiogram before the intravenous injection of fluorescein. These will also be briefly discussed.

TRANSMITTED FLUORESCENCE

Again, the first step in the interpretive process is to define areas of abnormal hypo- or hyperfluorescence. In the first case note the hyperfluorescence in the macula (Fig. 4.24, *A–C*). As suggested by the schematic guide it is necessary next to determine which of the three major causes of hyperfluorescence is present, transmitted fluorescence or so-called pigment epithelial window defect, abnormal vessels, or leak. Note that there is early hyperfluorescence as seen in Fig. 4.24*A*, but it gradually fades away in the late stages (Fig. 4.24*C*). Since there is no late hyperfluorescence there is no leak. The early hyperfluorescence must be due either to transmitted fluorescence or to abnormal vessels. Since no abnormal vessels can be seen on the angiogram, the hyperfluorescence is due to transmitted fluorescence or so-called pigment epithelial window defect. The pigment epithelium in the involved area is atrophic, allowing normal choroidal fluorescence from the filling of the choriocapillaris to be seen more clearly. The hyperfluorescence appears early as the choriocapillaris fills (Fig. 4.24*A*), increases slightly during the midphases of the angiogram (Fig. 4.24*B*), and disappears as the choriocapillaris empties (Fig 4.24*C*). This phenomenon of "now you see it, now you don't" is the typical pattern of transmitted fluorescence. It is a form of early hyperfluorescence produced by atrophy of the retinal pigment epithelium in an area where there is an intact choriocapillaris. This type of hyperfluorescence is not produced purely by a "window" in the pigment epithelium. It also necessitates the presence of normal choriocapillaris which appears accentuated in its fluorescing characteristics because of the reduced masking effect of the abnormal or absent pigment epithelium.

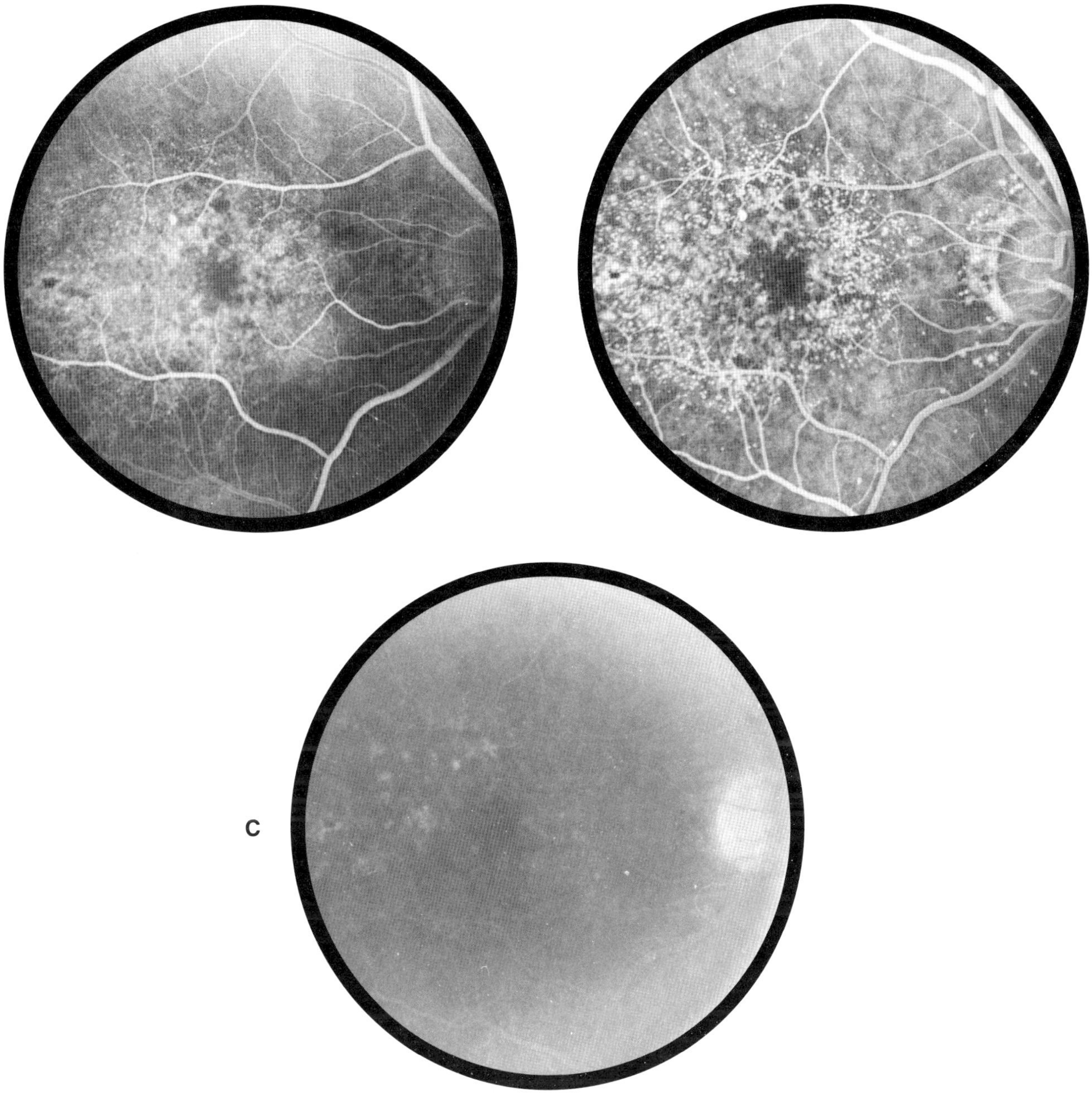

Figure 4.24. *A*, arterial phase angiogram. Note the diffuse patchy hyperfluorescence in the macula. *B*, late venous phase angiogram. The hyperfluorescence has increased in intensity but has not changed in size or shape. *C*, late phase angiogram. The hyperfluorescence has largely faded as the choriocapillaris empties. There is no late hyperfluorescence; therefore, there is no leak. This is a form of early hyperfluorescence which appears early, coincidental with the choroidal filling, increases in intensity but not size during the midphases of the angiogram, and disappears in the late phase of the study. This early hyperfluorescence is typical of transmitted fluorescence (so-called pigment epithelial window defect) secondary to atrophic changes in the retinal pigment epithelium.

ABNORMAL VESSELS

Note in the next angiogram the area of hyperfluorescence on the disc (Fig. 4.25). In this case the angiogram demonstrates that hyperfluorescence occurs early and has a vascular pattern. Therefore, this is early hyperfluorescence due to abnormal vessels. Once it is determined that the hyperfluorescence is due to abnormal vessels, the next step suggested by the schematic guide is to determine the involved vasculature, retinal, choroidal, or disc.

This is clearly a case of disc neovascularization. It has the typical features of an early lacy-like hyperfluorescence at the disc which obscures the underlying adjacent retinal vessels. In the late phases of the angiogram these vessels will also reveal a late hyperfluorescence which is due to leak into the vitreous and which has a "cotton-ball" appearance. This case of disc neovascularization developed in a patient with diabetic retinopathy. Thus, hyperfluorescence from abnormal vessels, like transmitted fluorescence, is a form of early hyperfluorescence as the abnormal vessels begin to fluoresce in the filling phases of the angiogram.

There is an area of hyperfluorescence in the next case which involves the entire macula area (Fig. 4.26*A*). The lacy pattern to the hyperfluorescence indicates that it is due to abnormal vessels. The next question is to identify the involved vasculature. In Figure 4.26*B*, the inferotemporal retinal vein is fed by small connective channels from the superior temporal retinal artery, thus circumventing the vascular flow to the retinal vasculature and representing a congenital arteriovenous shunt. These are usually benign lesions that cause no leakage or visual abnormality. The small hyperfluorescent dots are due to transmitted fluorescence at the site of drusen.

Again, in the next case the first step in the fluorescein angiographic interpretative process is to define areas of abnormal hypo- or hyperfluorescence. Note the area of hyperfluorescence in the center of the macula (Fig. 4.27*A*). The hyperfluorescence is seen early, and it is irregular and lacy in character. This suggests that it is vascular in origin and due to abnormal vessels. Some normal retinal vessels are seen to overlie the lesions; therefore, it is subretinal or choroidal in origin. This is a case of subretinal neovascularized membrane formation. Note (Fig. 4.27*B*) that there is marked late hyperfluorescence or leak associated with these vessels resulting in a sensory retinal detachment. The multiple hyperfluorescent dots are due to transmitted fluorescence at the site of drusen.

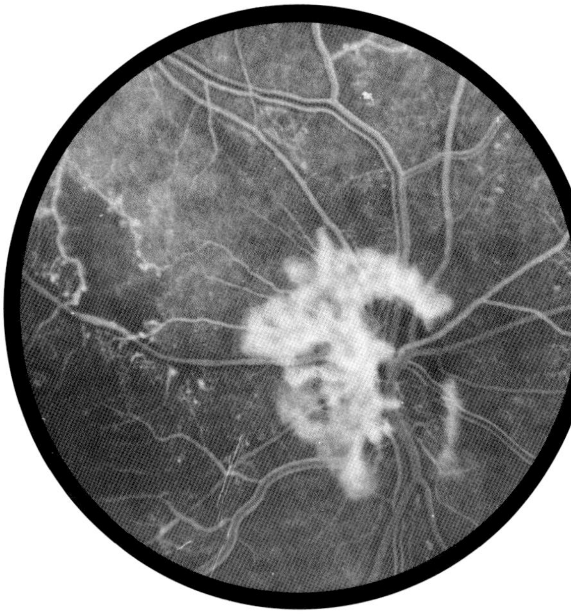

Figure 4.25. Arteriovenous phase angiogram. Note the lacy-like hyperfluorescence overlying the disc. This is a typical form of early hyperfluorescence secondary to abnormal vessels. In this case the abnormal vessels are due to disc neovascularization in a patient with diabetic retinopathy.

A

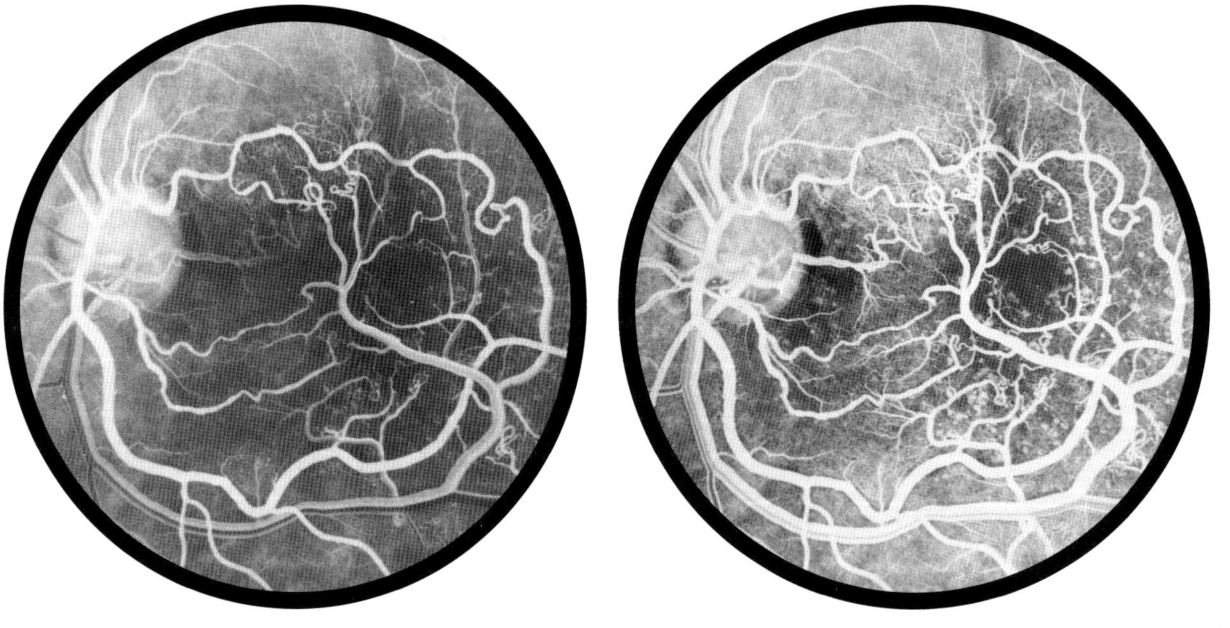

B

Figure 4.26. *A*, arteriovenous phase angiogram. Note the early hyperfluorescence due to abnormal vessels. *B*, early venous phase angiogram, same patient. Note the connecting channels originating from the supratemporal artery and feeding the inferior temporal vein, circumventing the retinal capillary bed. These abnormal vessels represent congenital arteriovenous shunts.

A

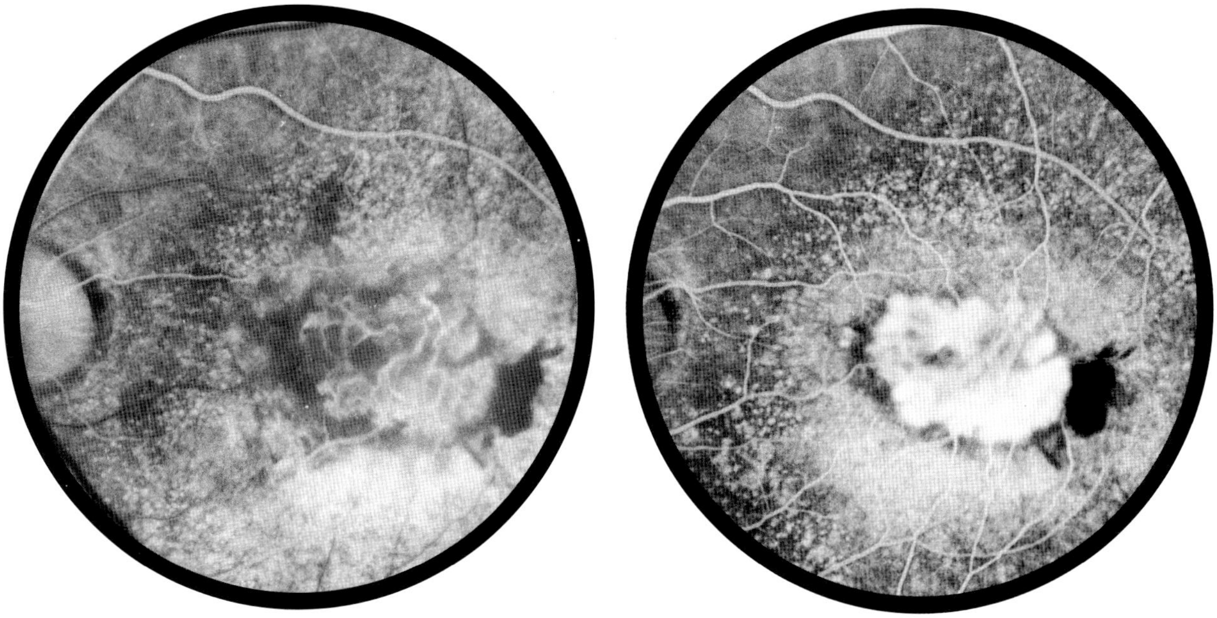

B

Figure 4.27. *A*, arterial phase angiogram. Note the hyperfluorescence in the center of the macula. It is a form of early hyperfluorescence and it is irregular and lacy in character, indicating that the fluorescence is due to abnormal vessels, partially obscured by turbid subretinal fluid. *B*, late venous phase angiogram. There is late hyperfluorescence originating from the abnormal vessels. Early lacy hyperfluorescence secondary to abnormal vessels, followed subsequently by late hyperfluorescence or leak is characteristic of neovascularization. In this case, the neovascularization has developed from the choroidal circulation forming a subretinal neovascularized membrane in involutional macular degeneration. The fluorescing dots elsewhere in the macular region are due to transmitted fluorescence at the site of drusen.

In the next patient there is an area of hyperfluorescence in the macula indicating either transmitted fluorescence, abnormal vessels, or leak (Fig. 4.28*A*). Note that the lesion reveals early hyperfluorescence even before there is fluorescence in some of the large retinal vessels. In Figure 4.28*B*, in the late venous phase of the angiogram, there is a diffuse hyperfluorescence well established in the lesion itself. This early hyperfluorescence is due to abnormal vessels. Since the retinal vessels can be observed overlying the lesion, the *abnormal vessels* are located subretinally and are choroidal in origin. This lesion was studied histopathologically and proved to be a malignant melanoma of the choroid. The early hyperfluorescence was produced by filling of the abnormal tumor vessels.

A

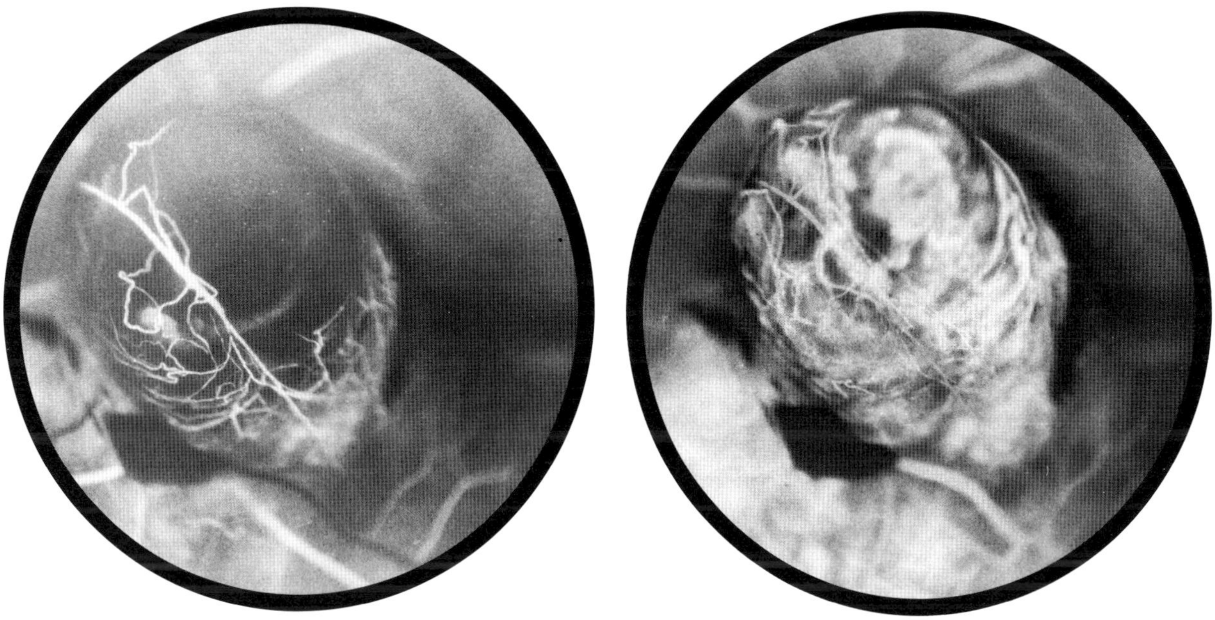

B

Figure 4.28. *A*, arteriovenous phase angiogram. Note the early hyperfluorescence at the site of an elevated lesion in the macular region. There is a lacy-like hyperfluorescence prior to perfusion of some of the larger retinal vessels. This early hyperfluorescence is due to abnormal vessels. *B*, late venous phase angiogram. Note the late hyperfluorescence well established within the lesion itself. Late hyperfluorescence is always due to leak, and in this case, it originated from the abnormal vessels present within a choroidal malignant melanoma retinal erosion.

Note the area of hyperfluorescence on this angiogram (Fig. 4.29, *A–C*). Is it due to choroidal transmission, abnormal vessels, or leak? A simple indicator of leak is the presence of late hyperfluorescence. Late hyperfluorescence is always due to leak. Since there is late hyperfluorescence in the macula of this patient (Fig. 4.29*C*) it must be due to leak. When leak is present, the next step is to determine its location. In Figure 4.29*C*, note that the fluorescein leakage is independent of any retinal vessels. The hyperfluorescence originates at the level of the pigment epithelium and extends into the space created by a sensory retinal detachment. The area of hyperfluorescence is initially barely evident and focal (Fig. 4.29*A*); it gradually increases in size in the midstage of the angiogram (Fig. 4.29*B*); and it has fuzzy margins late in the angiogram (Fig. 4.29*C*). This patient has central serous chorioretinopathy or idiopathic detachment of the sensory retina. Note that all of the fluid under the sensory retina does not completely fluoresce in the late stage of the angiogram (Fig. 4.29*C*).

Late hyperfluorescence or leak may occur into tissue and this is defined as staining or it may accumulate into an anatomic space which is defined as pooling. In the fundus there are four potential spaces for fluorescein to pool: (1) the vitreous cavity; (2) the intraretinal spaces (cystoid); (3) the subsensory retinal space; and (4) the subpigment epithelial space.

A

B

C

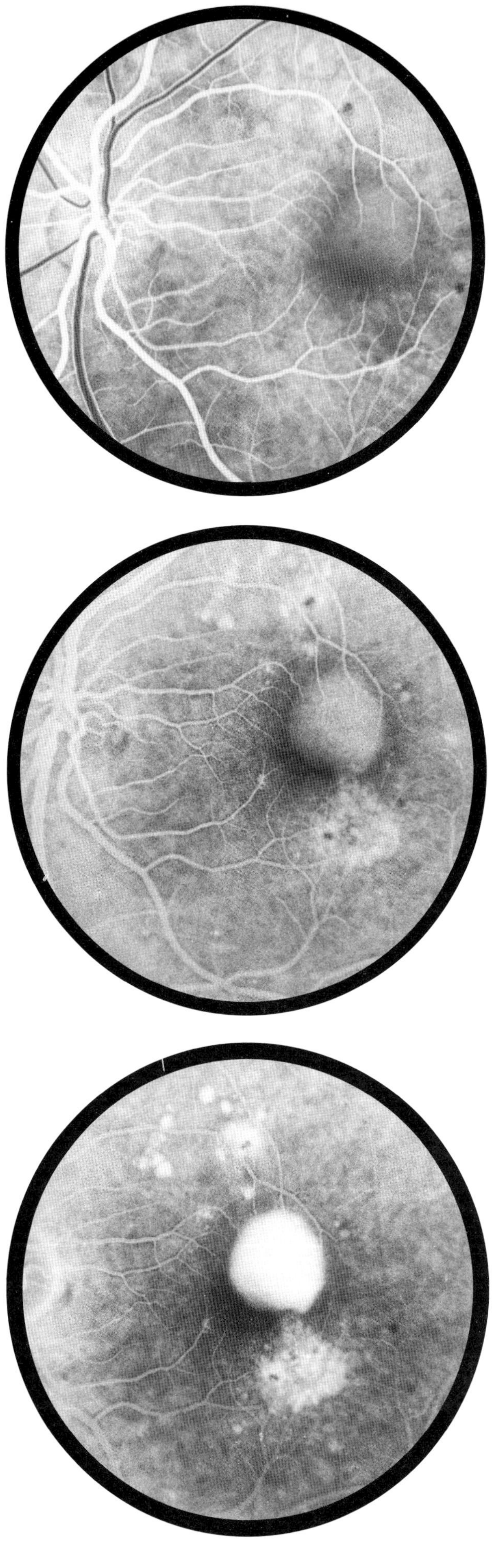

Figure 4.29. *A*, arteriovenous phase angiogram. Note the early hyperfluorescence at the site of a circumscribed macular detachment. *B*, early venous phase angiogram. Note that the area of hyperfluorescence has increased in intensity but not in size. *C*, late venous phase angiogram. The circumscribed area of hyperfluorescence has continued to increase in intensity although not in size completely filling the detachment with well demarcated margins. The late hyperfluorescence present in this patient is due to pooling beneath a detachment of the retinal pigment epithelium.

The macula in the next case, also reveals an area of hyperfluorescence (Fig. 4.30 *A–C*). The hyperfluorescence is again late which indicates a leak. When leak is present the next decision is to determine its location. The hyperfluorescence originates subretinally with no evidence of abnormal leakage from the retinal vessels. Note that the full extent of the late hyperfluorescence is evident on the early angiogram (Fig. 4.30*A*) and it increases in its intensity but not in its size in the later stages of the angiogram (Fig. 4.30, *B* and *C*). This is typical of the well demarcated, complete late hyperfluorescence that develops from pooling beneath a serous pigment epithelial detachment.

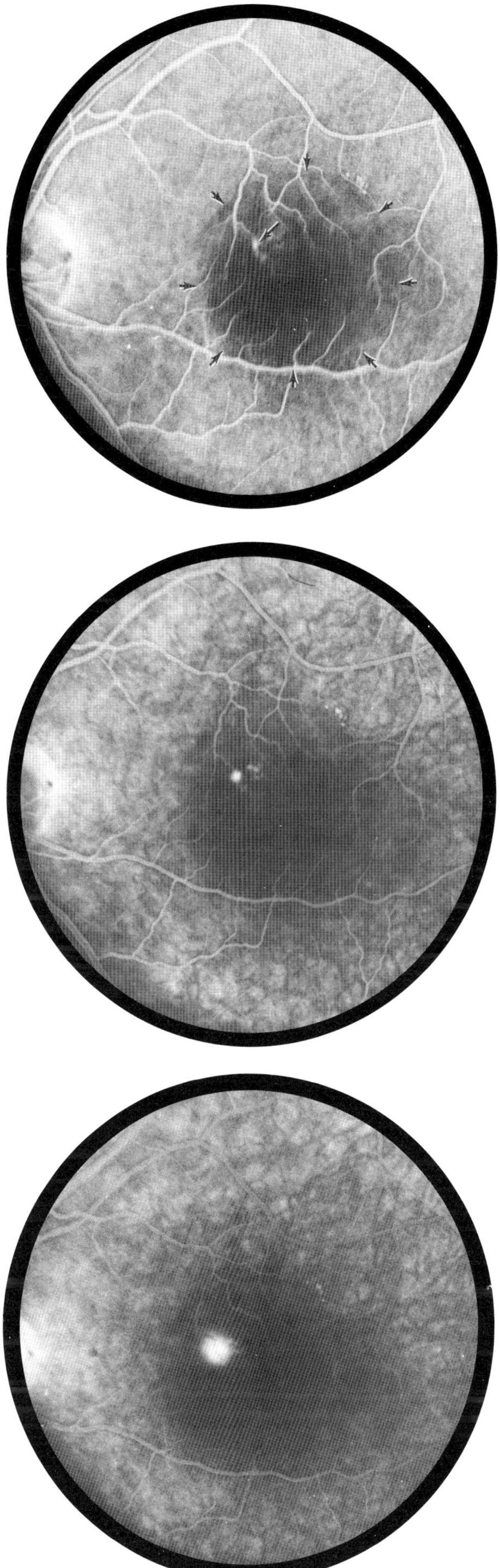

A

B

C

Figure 4.30. *A*, arteriovenous phase angiogram. Note the pinpoint area of hyperfluorescence just beneath a retinal vessel in the macula (*large arrow*). The retinal vasculature is out of focus because of a localized macular detachment (*small arrows*). *B*, early venous phase angiogram. Note that the focal area of hyperfluorescence has increased in size and intensity. Adjacent to the focal area of hyperfluorescence there is patchy hyperfluorescence which has not changed since the earlier stage of the angiogram. *C*, late venous phase angiogram. Note that the focal subretinal hyperfluorescence has continued to expand in size with fuzzy margins, but not enough to fill the macular detachment. The early hyperfluorescence adjacent to the focal leak has gradually faded indicating that it was due to pigment epithelial atrophic changes or choroidal transmission. The late hyperfluorescence in this patient is due to a focal leak in the pigment epithelium with pooling beneath an overlying sensory retinal detachment.

Examine the next case and note the late hyperfluorescence in the macula (Fig. 4.31, *A* and *B*). The presence of late hyperfluorescence always means leak. The next question suggested by the schematic guide is to determine what tissue is involved. Figure 4.31*A* indicates that there are small pockets or pools of late hyperfluorescence which on stereoscopic analysis were localized to the deep retinal layers. Fluorescein here has accumulated within the sensory retina showing the typical pattern of cystoid macular edema originating from the deep retinal capillaries in the macula evident in the early stages of the angiogram (Fig. 4.31*B*). This patient demonstrates intraretinal cystoid macular edema following surgery, the so-called Irvine-Gass syndrome. The angiogram revealed abnormal retinal capillaries in the macula which leaked resulting in marked cystoid macular edema.

Study the late phase fluorescein angiogram in the next case (Fig. 4.32) and note the late hyperfluorescence at the disc and along the course of adjacent retinal vessels. The presence of late hyperfluorescence indicates leak. As suggested by the schematic guide, the next question relates to the site of the leak. In this case the leak develops at the nerve head and within the sensory retina in a noncystoid area, the perivascular region. This form of leak which has occurred within tissue, is referred to as staining. Thus, in this case of optic neuritis there is staining of the optic nerve and adjacent retinal vessels. The fuzzy margins of the intraretinal staining contrasts with the discrete area of hyperfluorescence seen in pooling into the deeper intraretinal cystoid spaces.

Note the area of hyperfluorescence in the macula in the next case (Fig. 4.33, *A* and *B*). Since the hyperfluorescence is late, this is a leak. The normal retinal vessels are seen to overlie the lesion serving to localize the leak to the subretinal area. Also, the pattern is vascular in nature, indicating that the leak comes from abnormal choroidal vessels. The late hyperfluorescence due to leak corresponds to a yellowish subretinal lesion seen on the ophthalmoscopic view (Fig. 4.33*B*). This is a subretinal scar which typically tends to retain fluorescein and stains quite brightly in the later phases of the angiogram. The margins of the scar will usually stain in a well demarcated fashion unless there is an associated sensory retinal detachment. When an overlying detachment is present, fluorescein will pool into the subsensory retinal space from the scar and the margins of the scar will be fuzzy in the late phase angiogram.

A

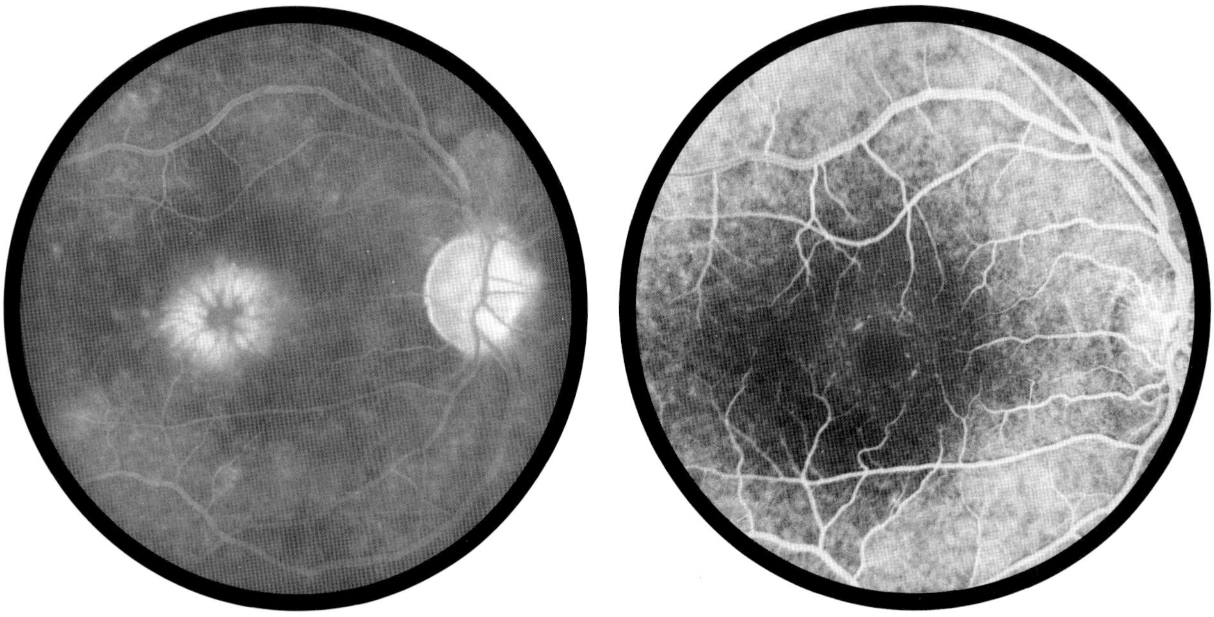

B

Figure 4.31. *A*, late venous phase angiogram. Note the late hyperfluorescence in the angiogram. These represent pockets of fluid accumulated within the sensory retina showing the typical pattern of cystoid macular edema. *B*, early venous phase angiogram. Note that the deep retinal capillaries in the macula are abnormally prominent and show evidence of early leakage. The cystoid macular edema in this patient originated from the deep capillaries of the retinal circulation.

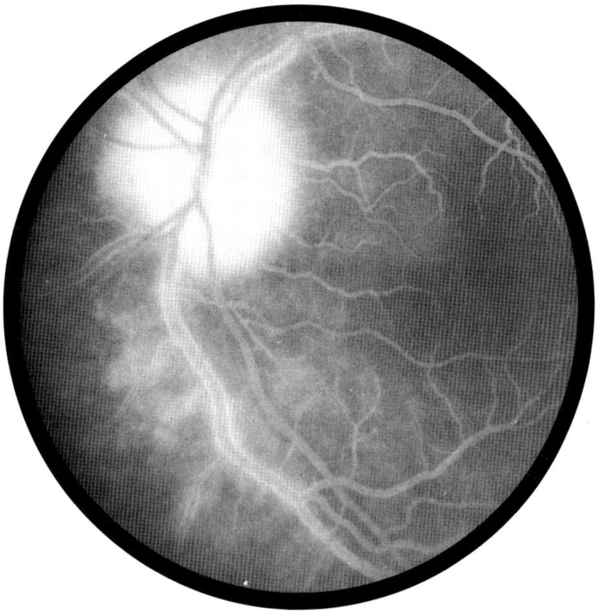

Figure 4.32. Late phase angiogram. Note the late hyperfluorescence or leak at the disc and along the course of adjacent retinal vessels. In this case the leak is due to staining of the optic nerve head as well as into the noncystoid perivascular areas of the retina.

A

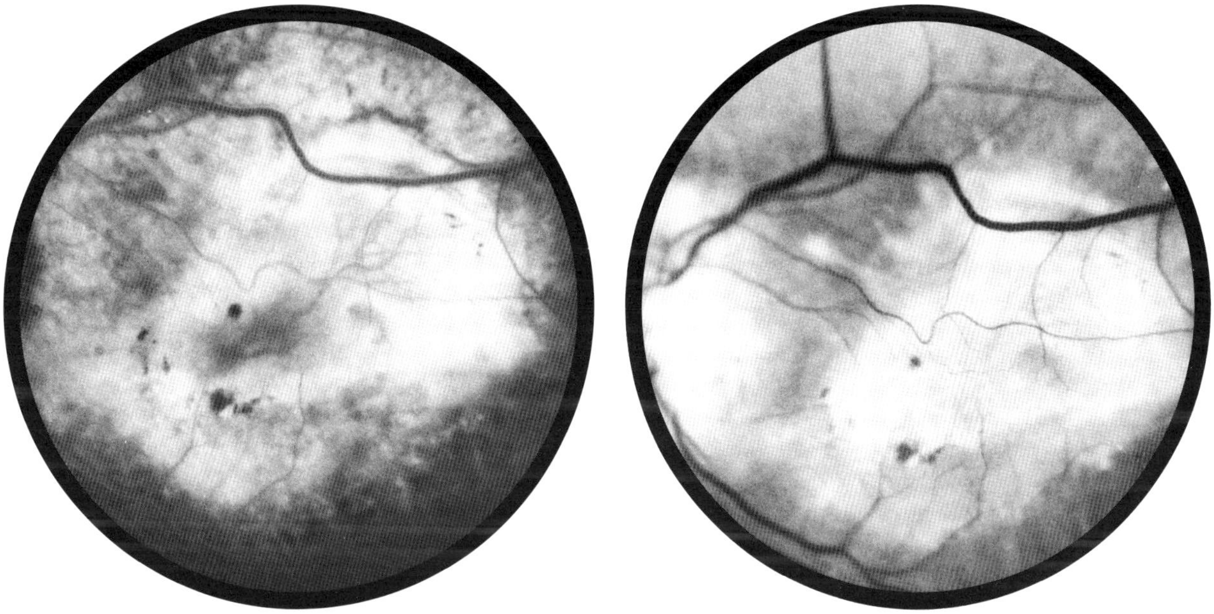

B

Figure 4.33. *A*, late phase angiogram. Note the late hyperfluorescence in the subretinal area associated with abnormal vessels which silhouette against the fluorescing background. *B*, ophthalmoscopic photograph. The subretinal late hyperfluorescence corresponds to a white disciform scar. Subretinal scars typically retain fluorescein and stain brightly in the late phase of the angiogram.

Examine the last case for areas of hypo- or hyperfluorescence (Fig. 4.34, *A–C*). Note that there is an area of hypofluorescence along the course of the retinal vessels in the early stages of the angiogram (Fig. 4.34*A*). It is due to blocked fluorescence or a vascular filling defect. A comparison with the color photographs (Fig. 4.34*B*) reveals no corresponding tissue or fluid barrier to account for the hypofluorescence. Therefore, the hypofluorescence is due to a vascular filling defect. Does the vascular filling defect involve the retinal or choroidal circulation? In Figure 4.34, *A–C*, the retinal vessels are perfusing normally. However, only the larger choroidal vessels are evident in the early stages of the angiogram and the typical "ground glass" appearance of the choriocapillaris doesn't become evident even in the late stages of the angiogram. Therefore, the vascular filling defect involves the choriocapillaris and it is complete in nature as these vessels failed to perfuse. The larger chroidal vessels are visible on the angiogram because there is atrophy of the retinal pigment epithelium. In spite of the atrophy of the pigment epithelial layer there is no early hyperfluorescence from transmitted fluorescence which requires an intact choriocapillaris. There is, however, a late hyperfluorescence or leak evident at first along the margins of the chorioretinal atrophy and gradually extending centrally beneath the normal overlying retinal vessels (Fig. 4.34*D*). This late hyperfluorescence or leak is a result of staining of the sclera which takes place anywhere in the fundus where it is visible. In this case of idiopathic perivascular helicoid chorioretinopathy, the scleral staining begins at the margins of the involved areas where there is normal choriocapillaris. A schematic representation of fluorescein leakage from the normal choriocapillaris into the extravascular choroidal spaces and sclera in an eye with absent choriocapillaris and pigment epithelium is illustrated (Fig. 4.34*B*).

Figure 4.34. *A,* arteriovenous phase angiogram. Note the hypofluorescence along the course of the retinal arcades and the nasal juxtapapillary region. *B,* color photograph on the same patient. Note that there is no corresponding tissue or fluid density to account for the hypofluorescence in this area. Therefore, the hypofluorescence is due to a vascular filling defect. *C,* late venous phase angiogram. The retinal vessels have filled normally. There is, however, an absence of the typical "ground glass" fluorescence of normal choriocapillaris along the area of hypofluorescence. The vascular filling defect producing the hypofluorescence is due to absence of the choriocapillaris. The larger choroidal vessels are seen through an atrophic retinal pigment epithelium. This is, therefore, a case of idiopathic helicoid paravenous chorioretinal atrophy. Note also that there is hyperfluorescence most evident at the margins of the chorioretinal atrophy. (From H. Schatz, T. Burton, L. Yannuzzi, and M. Rabb: Interpretation of Fundus Fluorescein Angiography, 1978, © C. V. Mosby Co., St. Louis; reprinted with permission.) *D,* late phase angiogram. Note the diffuse late hyperfluorescence in the region of the chorioretinal atrophy. Large choroidal vessels are seen as dark silhouettes overlying the late hyperfluorescence. The presence of the late hyperfluorescence indicates leak. In this case, the leak can be localized external to the large choroidal vessels at the level of the sclera. This form of late hyperfluorescence or leak is due to staining of the sclera where it is visible through areas of chorioretinal atrophy. *E,* schematic representation of the same case. There is an absence of the retinal pigment epithelium and choriocapillaris centrally. Intact choriocapillaris leaks at the margins of the lesion into the extrachoroidal space and stains the sclera centrally. *Decreasing arrows* suggest that the hyperfluorescence is most evident first at the margins of the chorioretinal atrophy adjacent to the leaking choriocapillaris.

A C

B D

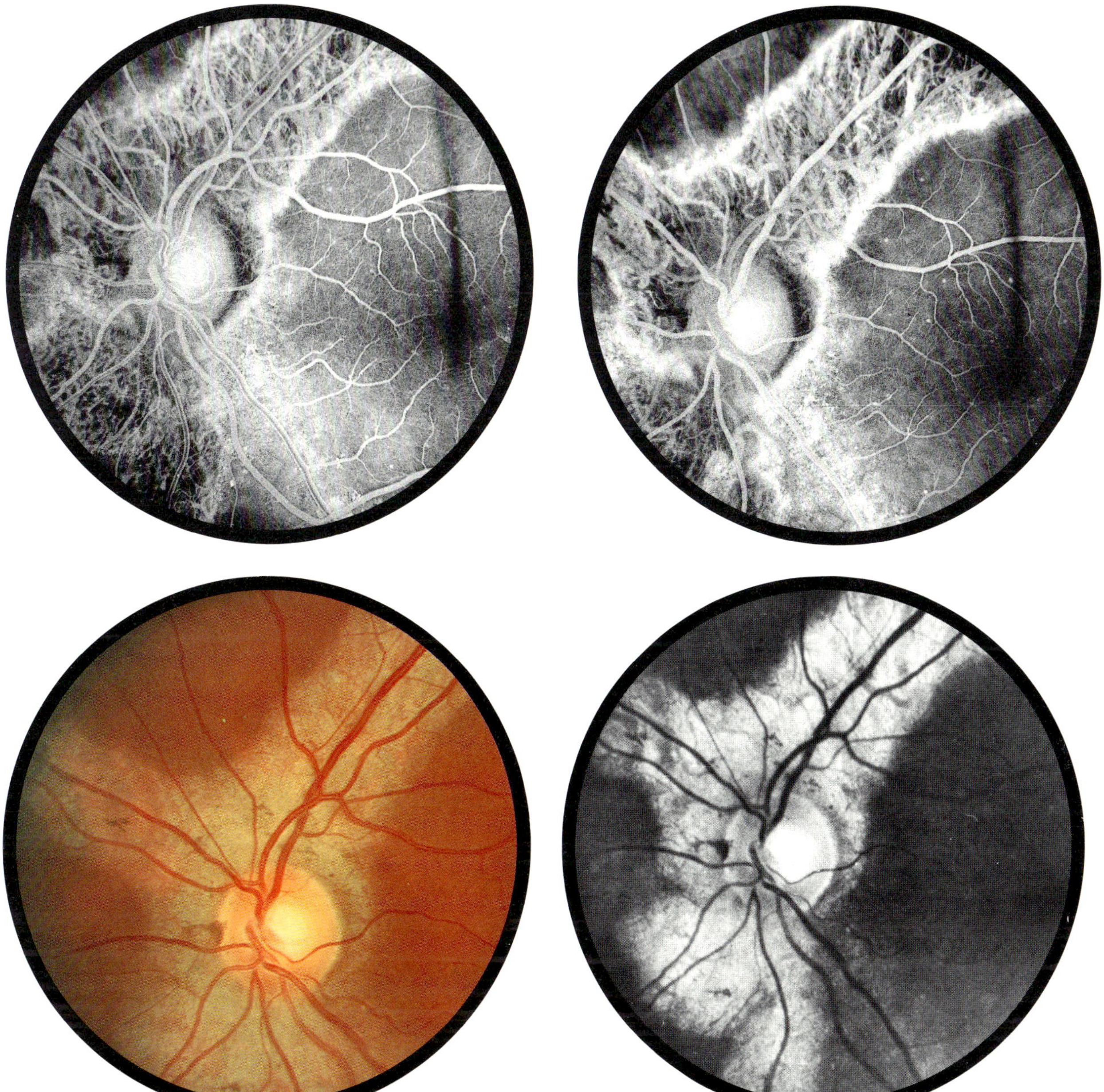

E

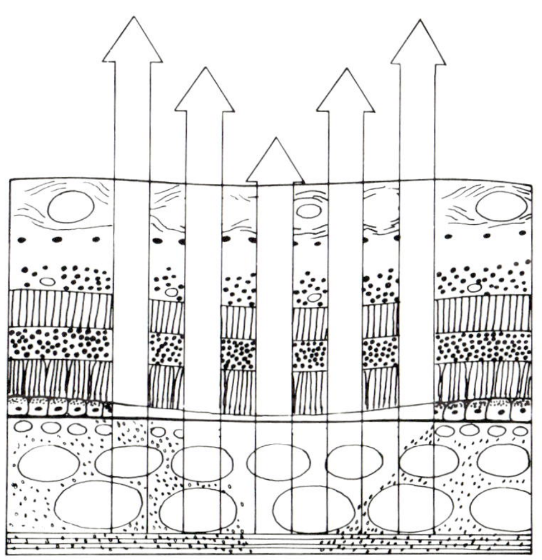

Absence of Chorio-Capillaris and Retinal Pigment Epithelium

SCLERAL STAINING

PREINJECTION FLUORESCENCE

Two other types of hyperfluorescence known as autofluorescence and pseudofluorescence, occur in the preinjection stage of the angiogram. That is, they are seen before the injection of the dye on the control photo. Pseudofluorescence is produced by a poor filter combination employed in the fluorescein angiographic technique. The excitatory blue filter overlaps in its transmission characteristics with the yellow barrier filter (Fig. 4.35). Thus, some green or "fluorescing light" is introduced into the fundus by the excitatory filter, and/or some blue excitatory light passes through the barrier filter to the film plane. Pseudofluorescence occurs at the site of any area of high surface reflectivity in the fundus such as exudate, myelinated nerve fibers, or even the optic nerve. Note in Figure 4.36, *A–C*, that exudate evident on the color photograph (Fig. 4.36*A*) appears to fluoresce on the preinjection photograph (Fig. 4.36*B*) because of the poor filters employed. When ideal filters are used in the same case, the pseudofluorescence disappears (Fig. 4.36*C*).

Autofluorescence occurs when ideal filters are employed. Ideal filters are, so-called mutually exclusive. That is, the excitatory and barrier filters have sharply cut off transmission spectra with no overlap (Fig. 4.37). Certain lesions of

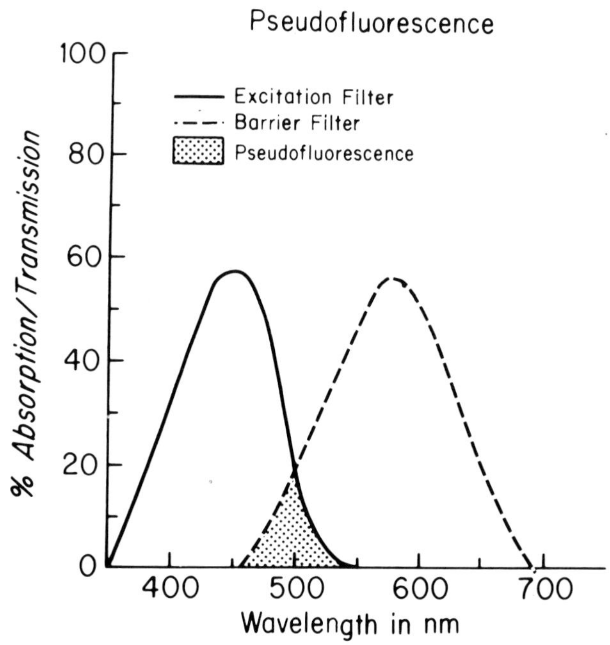

Figure 4.35. Transmission curves of a poor filter combination employed in fluorescein angiography. The triangular shape of overlap (*dots*) is the zone responsible for pseudofluorescence. Excitatory blue light overlaps in its transmission characteristics with the yellow barrier filter. Thus, some green or fluorescing light is introduced into the fundus by the excitatory filter and/or some blue excitatory light passes through the barrier filter to the film plane. (From H. Schatz, T. Burton, L. Yannuzzi, and M. Rabb: Interpretation of Fundus Fluorescein Angiography, 1978, © C. V. Mosby Co., St. Louis; reprinted with permission.)

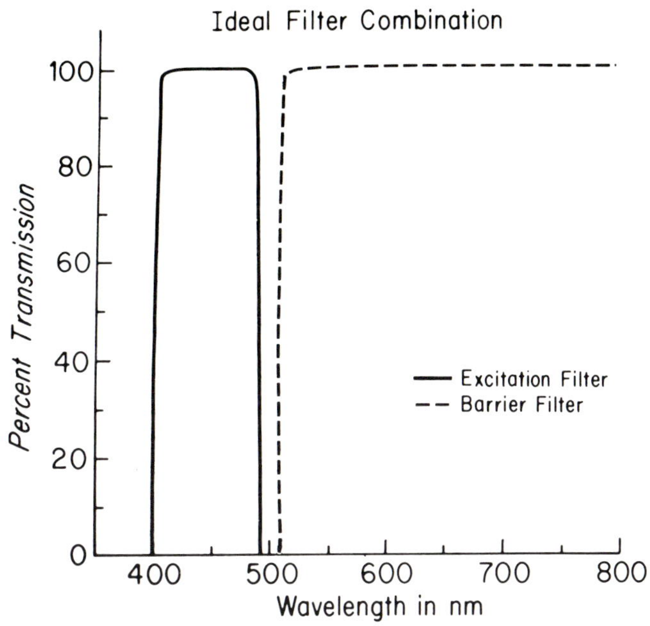

Figure 4.37. Transmission spectra of an ideal filter combination for fluorescein angiography. Note that there is no overlap between the transmission curve of the excitation filter and the barrier filter. (From H. Schatz, T. Burton, L. Yannuzzi, and M. Rabb: Interpretation of Fundus Fluorescein Angiography, 1978, © C. V. Mosby Co., St. Louis; reprinted with permission.)

A

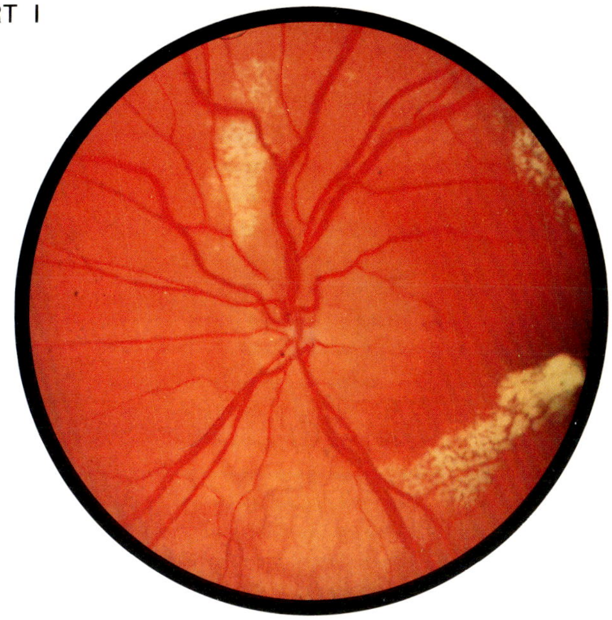

B

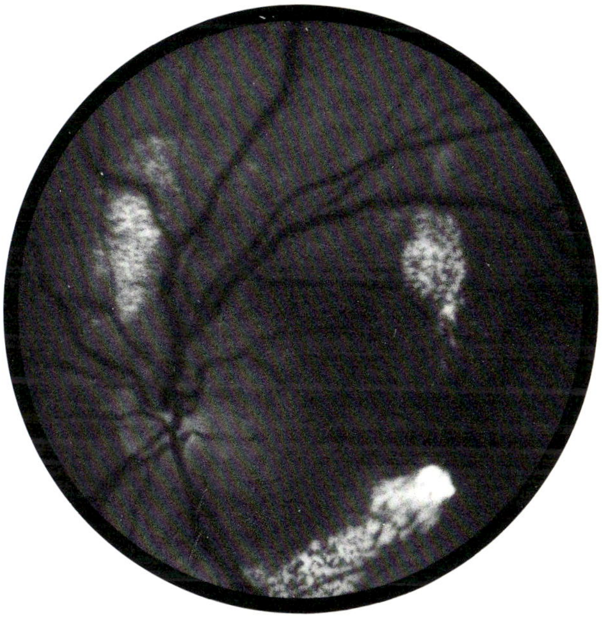

C

Figure 4.36. *A,* color photograph of a patient with a juxtapapillary exophytic hemangioma and exudate in the macula and above the disc. *B,* preinjection photograph on the same patient, employing a poor filter combination. Pseudofluorescence is evident at the site of the exudates. The less, highly reflective nerve head also has a small degree of pseudofluorescence. *C,* preinjection photograph taken on the same patient employing ideal filters, indicating the absence of any pseudofluorescence.

A B

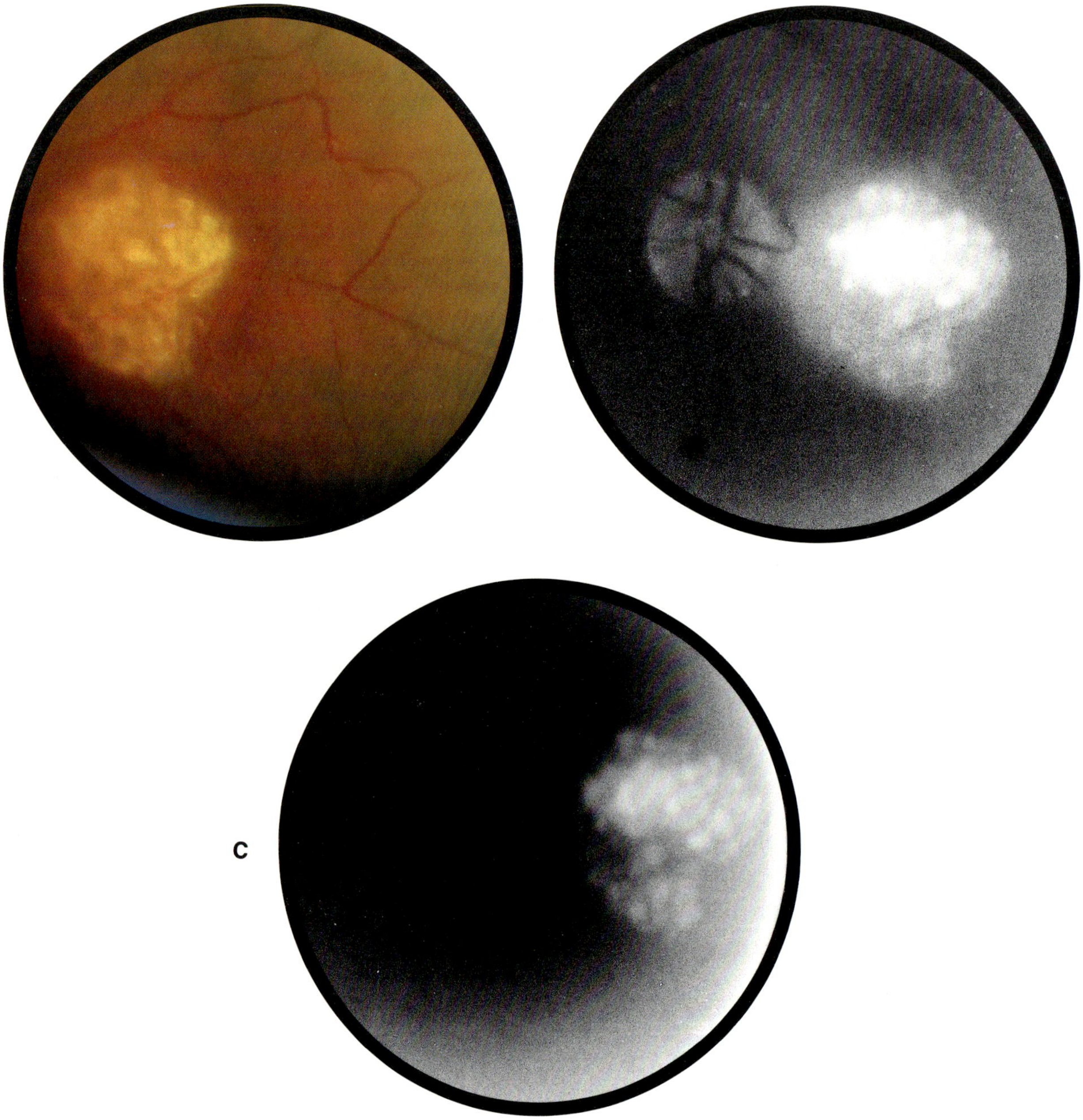

C

Figure 4.38. *A*, color photograph of a patient with an astrocytic hamartoma in the nasal retina. *B*, preinjection photograph on the same patient, employing a poor filter combination. Note the pseudofluorescence at the site of the astrocytic hamartoma as well as at the less reflective nerve head. *C*, preinjection photograph on the same patient employing ideal filters shows the presence of autofluorescence at the site of the astrocytic hamartoma. Pseudofluorescence has been eliminated by the use of the ideal filter combination.

the fundus, such as astrocytic hamartomas and some optic nerve head drusen, produce autofluorescence (Figs. 4.38, *A–C*). Note the astrocytic hamartoma nasal to the disc in the color photograph (Fig. 4.38*A*). The preinjection photograph employing poor filters can be seen in Figure 4.38*B*. This preinjection form of hyperfluorescence is a combined pseudofluorescence and autofluorescence because when ideal filters are used (Fig. 4.38*C*) only part of the preinjection fluorescence disappears (the pseudofluorescence) while the autofluorescence persists. Similarly a few optic nerve head drusen also show autofluorescence. Astrocytic hamartomas and optic nerve head drusen are the only lesions in the fundus to demonstrate autofluorescence (Fig. 4.39). These lesions that autofluoresce naturally emit light of the fluorescing green wavelength when exposed to blue excitatory light. They change blue light to green light much in the same way as a molecule of fluorescein. It is important to keep in mind that pseudofluorescence occurs only with a poor filter combination and that autofluorescence occurs, by definition, with an ideal filter combination. Both of these forms of hyperfluorescence are seen in the preinjection stage of the angiogram on the control photo. Fortunately, both are of little clinical significance today since most fluorescein angiographic systems employ ideal filter combinations in their technique.

In learning to interpret fluorescein angiograms, it is essential to review the histopathology of the fundus, to learn the photographic technique, to utilize fluorescein angiography, and to study the normal fluorescein angiogram. Once familiarized with these suggested prerequisites, a basic approach to interpretation can follow the schematic guide to the interpretation of fluorescein angiograms (Fig. 4.13) which states that there are only two major types of abnormal fluorescence, hypofluorescence and hyperfluorescence. Once the basic differentiation of hypo- or hyperfluorescence is made, it suggests a systematic series of decisions designed to arrive at the proper diagnosis. If hypofluorescence is present, there are only two possible explanations, blocked fluorescence or vascular filling defects. A comparison of the ophthalmoscopic view and the study of the filling characteristics of the retinal and choroidal circulations differentiates the two. When hyperfluorescence is present, there are three major possibilities. One is that there is an increase in the transmission of the choroidal fluorescence due to defects in the pigment epithelium. This is transmitted fluorescence or so-called pigment epithelial window defect. A second type is due to abnormal vessels, and the third is due to alterations in the permeability barriers in the fundus called leak. Transmitted fluorescence and abnormal vessels are seen as forms of early hyperfluorescence, and leak is always late hyperfluorescence. Minor forms of preinjection hyperfluorescence, known as autofluorescence and pseudofluorescence, are of little clinical importance today.

After the basic differentiation between the forms of hypo- and hyperfluorescence is made, the schematic guide follows a logical, stepwise progression through a series of sequential decisions, which lead to a better appreciation of the histopathologic manifestations involved, and ultimately to a more accurate diagnosis.

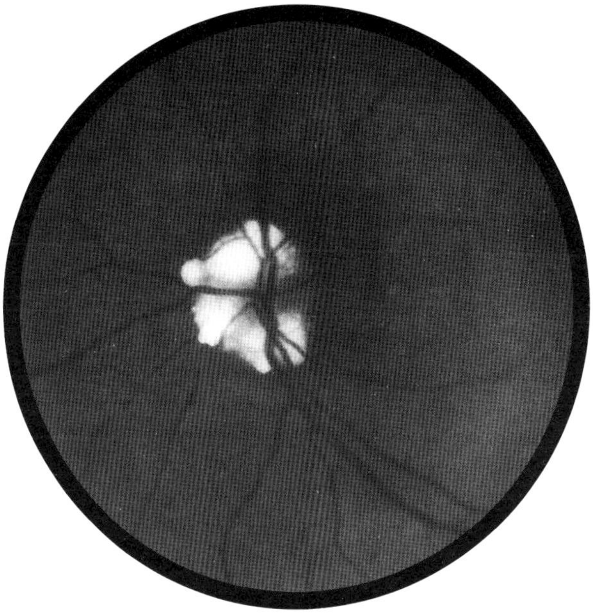

Figure 4.39. Preinjection fluorescence employing ideal filters. Note the autofluorescence at the site of an optic nerve head drusen. Astrocytic hamartomas tend to uniformly show a variable degree of autofluorescence, whereas optic nerve head drusen infrequently reveal this phenomenon.

Suggested Readings

Gass, J.D.M.: Stereoscopic Atlas of Macular Diseases: A Funduscopic and Angiographic Presentation, 2nd ed., C.V. Mosby, St. Louis, 1977.

Justice, J., Jr.: Ocular fundus photography. *Int Ophthalmol Clin, 16* (2): 23, 1976.

Rosen, E.S.: Fluorescence Photography of the Eye: A Manual of Dynamic Clinical Ocular Fundus Pathology, Butterworths, Woburn, Mass, 1969.

Schatz, H., Burton, T.C., Yannuzzi, L.A., and Rabb, M.F.: Fundus Fluorescein Angiography: A Comprehensive Text and Atlas, C.V. Mosby, St. Louis, 1978.

Shimizu, K.: Fluorescein Microangiography of the Ocular Fundus. Igaku Shoin Ltd., Tokyo, 1973.

Wessing A.: Fluorescein Angiography of the Retina. C.V. Mosby, St. Louis, 1969.

Wise, G.N., Dollery, C.T., and Henkind, P.: The Retinal Circulation, Harper & Row, New York, 1971.

Yanoff, M., and Fine, B.S.: Ocular Pathology: A Text and Atlas, Harper & Row, New York, 1975.

CHAPTER 5

Ultrasonography of the Macula

Yale L. Fisher, M.D.

Diagnostic ophthalmic ultrasonography can be of great aid in the evaluation of the macular region in situations of opaque as well as clear ocular media. When the media is opaque, it represents the only method of determining intraocular architecture. The Bronson-Turner B-Scan Ultrasonoscope, which has been well described in the literature [1], is an excellent apparatus for this purpose (Fig. 5.1). While precise localization is not possible, the experienced and careful technician can scan the general macular region very effectively [2]. To avoid ultrasonic artifacts induced by the lens, the posterior pole of the globe must be scanned from the scleral probe positions posterior to the limbus (Fig. 5.2). The optic nerve is utilized as a reference point. From this known reference, the probe is directed toward the macular region by scanning temporally. Similar scanning techniques are used to investigate the posterior pole from probe positions that parallel the upper and lower lids, always using the optic nerve shadow as a reference point. In utilizing this technique, the examiner must develop his ability in three-dimensional thinking, carefully collating the different cross-sectional images into a whole material picture of the posterior pole.

In situations of clear media, ultrasound provides information about tissue density and texture. Elevations and outlines of intraocular lesions are often more easily appreciated when seen in cross-section on the ultrasonic display screen. This is especially true of intraocular tumors hidden by secondary retinal detachments (Fig. 5.3, *A* and *B*).

To interpret reflections in relation to tissue density, the examiner must be familiar with the concept of acoustic impedance, which is an arithmetic product of the speed of sound transmission through any substance multiplied by the density of the substance. When adjacent tissues have large differences in acoustic impedance, a strong echo is returned to the ultrasonic probe and, after electronic processing, displayed as a strong white image. In contrast, when there are small differences in acoustic impedance between adjacent tissues, weaker echoes are returned and displayed as weaker signals (a shade of gray). When there is no difference, there is no echo (anechoic). With this simplified explanation, we can begin to interpret tissue density on the basis of images seen on the display screen. While ultrasonic interpretation should not be regarded as pathognomonic, it is helpful as an adjunct to the total diagnostic work-up of patients with tumors and distortions of global architecture [3].

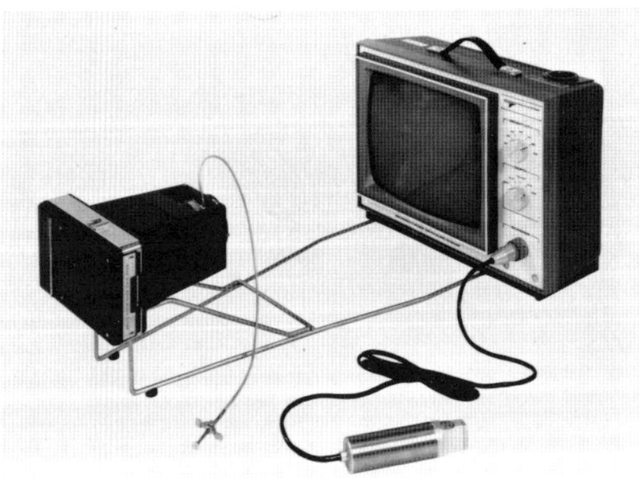

Figure 5.1. Bronson-Turner B-scan Ultrasonoscope with polaroid camera.

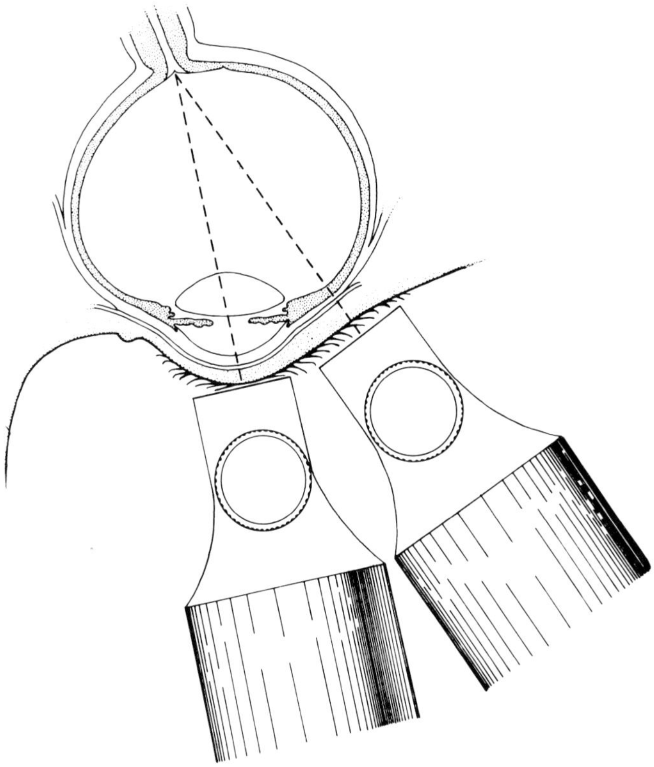

Figure 5.2. The examining probe is positioned behind the limbus. (From N. R. Bronson, Y.L. Fisher, *et al:* Ophthalmic Contact B-scan Ultrasonography for the Clinician, Intercontinental Publications, 1976; reprinted with permission.)

A

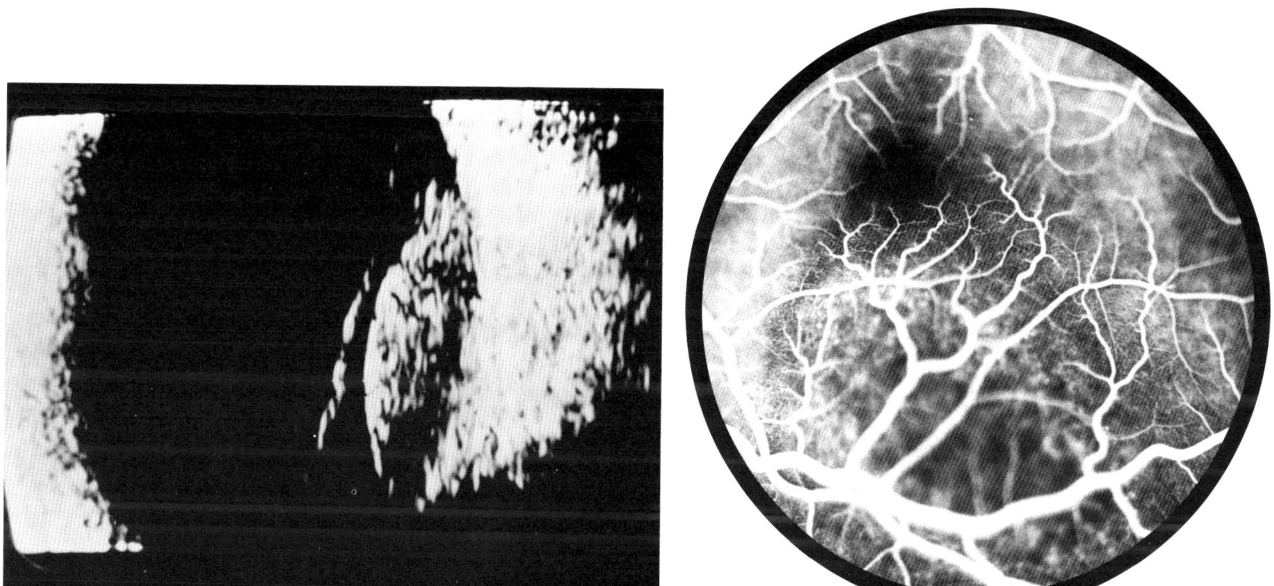

B

Figure 5.3. *A*, tumor hidden by retinal detachment on B-scan. *B*, fluorescein angiogram showing detached sensory retina overlying choroidal tumor.

Tumors of the Posterior Pole

MALIGNANT MELANOMA

Malignant melanomas of the choroid may be located anywhere within the globe. In most instances, the ultrasonic picture is remarkably similar. The tumor is classically dome-shaped, being well outlined against the sonically clear vitreous (Fig. 5.4). If Bruch's membrane is ruptured by the expanding mass, a mushroom configuration is common (Fig. 5.5*A*). Ultrasonic characteristics include strong border echoes and weaker internal reflections. The internal echoes are seen as a lighter shade of gray when compared to the strong white border echoes. Reduction in sensitivity from 80–70 dbs. accentuates this difference (Fig. 5.5*B*). The border echoes are still easily visible while almost all of the internal echoes disappear, giving the lesion a hollow appearance. The reason for this apparent hollowing of a known solid object is based on the relative acoustic homogeneity found within these masses especially at their base, where the homogeneous cells are packed tightly together giving little difference of acoustic impedance from area to area and, therefore, little echo production.

Careful observation of the orbital fat pattern behind the lesion demonstrates that the signal has been attenuated by the solid mass. This attenuation of orbital fat pattern echoes is called shadowing. It can be seen in many situations in which structures overlying the orbital fat pattern attenuate the exploring signal. One further comment should be made: interpretation of internal echoes involving small lesions below 1.5 mm is really not possible. With careful and thorough scanning, however, small lesions can be detected by their border echoes down to the limits of resolution which, for all practical purposes, is 1 mm.

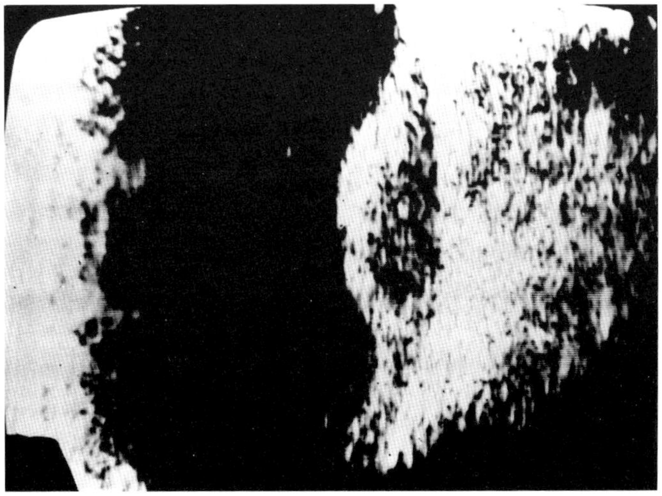

Figure 5.4. Dome-shaped malignant melanoma with strong border echoes. Note the well outlined contour as well as the internal hollowing deep in the mass. The orbital fat directly behind the tumor demonstrates shadowing, a result of signal attenuation of the mass lesion.

CHOROIDAL HEMANGIOMA

The choroidal hemangioma is a low-profile dome-shaped lesion usually located near the posterior pole and often associated with secondary retinal detachment (Fig. 5.6*A*). The lesion is well outlined and regular. Border echoes are strong, demonstrating a great difference between the acoustic impedance of the vitreous and this solid lesion. Internal reflections are of near equal intensity when compared to the border echoes producing a display image which is "white" throughout (Fig. 5.6*B*). The anatomic composition of this spongy vascular tumor accounts for the marked change in the acoustic impedance at all levels of the lesion. Reduction of the sensitivity setting demonstrates the persistence of the relatively strong internal echoes at 70 db (Fig. 5.6*C*).

These lesions are often difficult to visualize with indirect ophthalmoscopy because of their low profile and subtle coloring. The cross-sectional B-scan image, however, demonstrates the presence and internal acoustic texture extremely well.

A 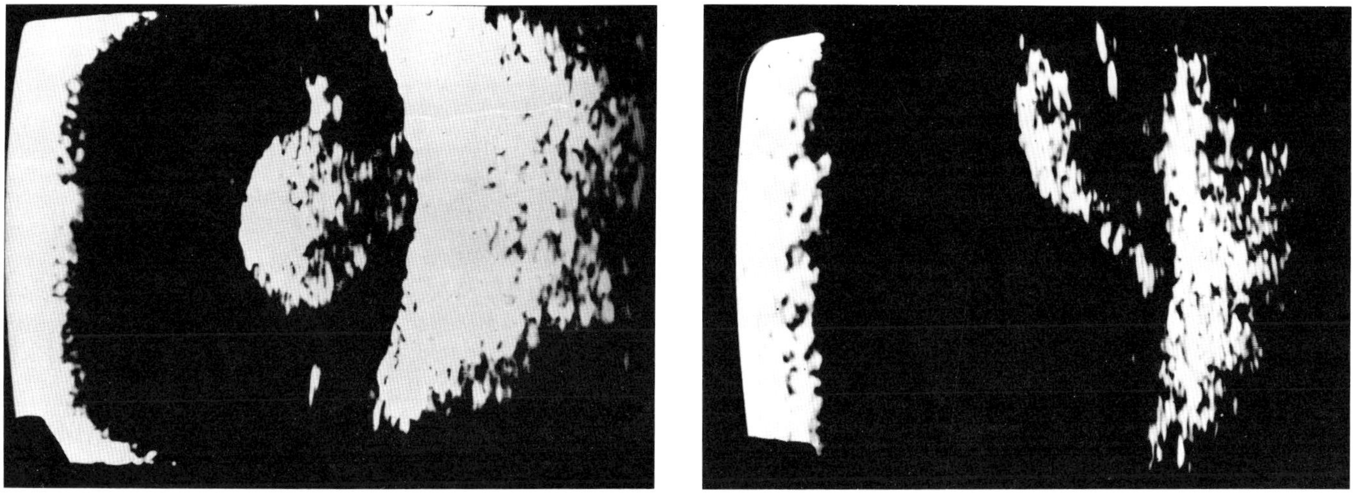 B

Figure 5.5. *A*, mushroom-shaped malignant melanoma with an associated secondary retinal detachment. *B*, reduction in sensitivity from 80–70 db (in same eye) accentuating the hollowing effect deep within the malignant melanoma. This is a consequence of low amplitude echoes seen in ultrasonically homogeneous tissue.

A 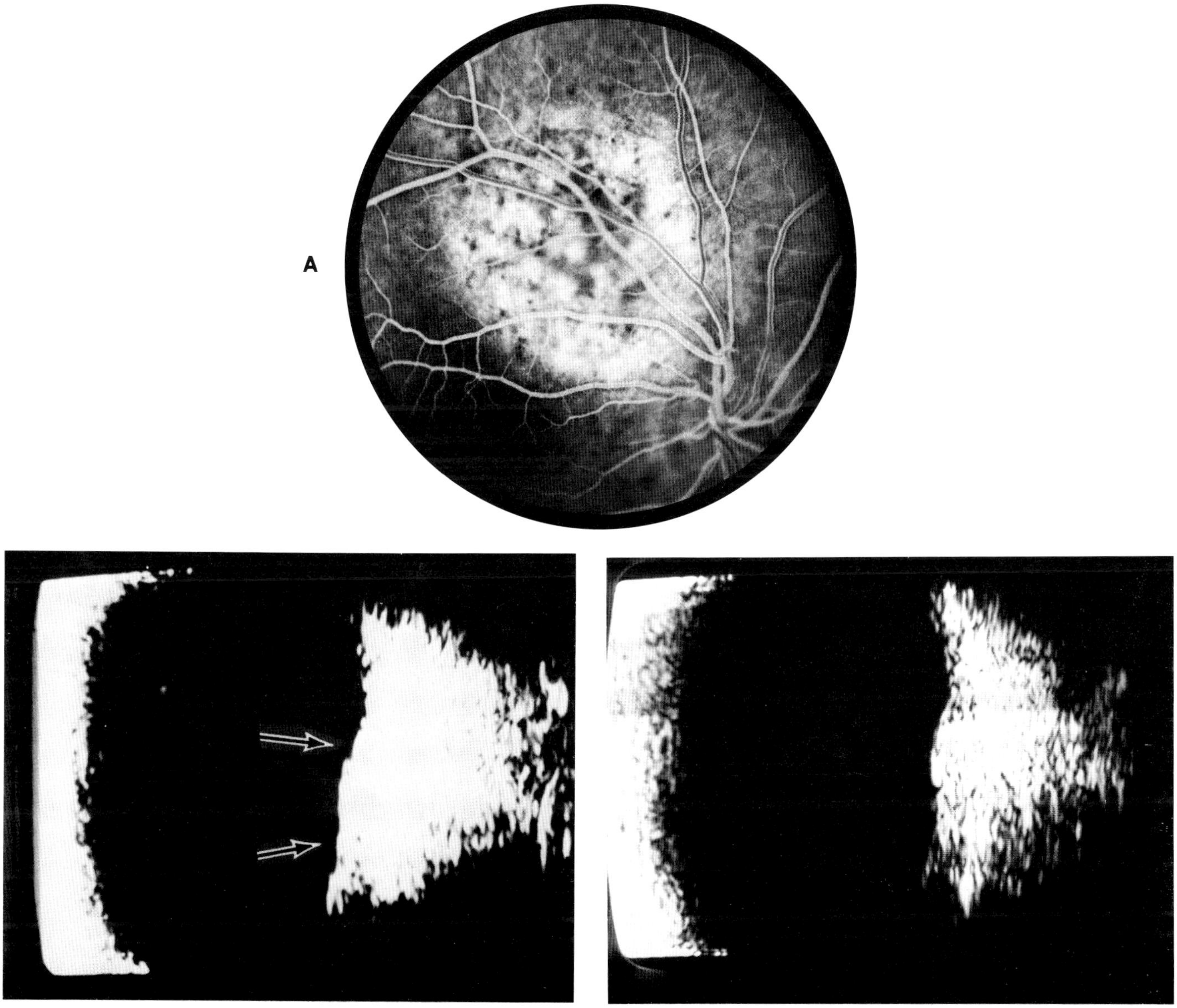 B C

Figure 5.6. *A*, fluorescein angiogram showing diffuse hyperfluorescence of choroidal hemangioma. *B*, choroidal hemangioma demonstrating strong border echoes and high reflectivity and a white image throughout the lesion. *C*, same eye with reduced sensitivity showing persistence of strong internal echoes without hollowing.

DISCIFORM DEGENERATION

Interpretation of disciform lesions on the basis of ultrasound alone is extremely difficult. In situations of clear media, a solid-appearing, elevated mass lesion often associated with subretinal pigment epithelial or subretinal blood located in the macular region is much more diagnostic than ultrasound. Sonically, these fibrovascular plaques have an irregular low profile with strong internal reflectivity, demonstrating the acoustic heterogeneity of the connective tissue components (Fig. 5.7). When the lesions are not classic in appearance and especially when eccentrically placed with no hemorrhagic component, concern over the possibility of a metastatic lesion is often raised. Ultrasound, unfortunately, is not very helpful in this differentiation since metastatic tumors often appear the same ultrasonically as disciform lesions, at least in the early stages of their growth (Fig. 5.8, *A–C*). When metastatic lesions are present, the growth and secondary changes often seen with these lesions can be appreciated and documented by ultrasound.

When the media is cloudy or opaque, careful scanning can definitely discern an elevated lesion in the posterior pole temporal to the optic nerve shadow, once the elevation exceeds the limits of resolution of the apparatus. Often it is possible to dynamically move vitreous debris away from the wall of the globe by asking the patient to move his eye back and forth while carefully observing the area in question (Fig. 5.9, *A* and *B*). This dynamic technique becomes more important in the preoperative evaluation of the patient being considered for vitreous surgery.

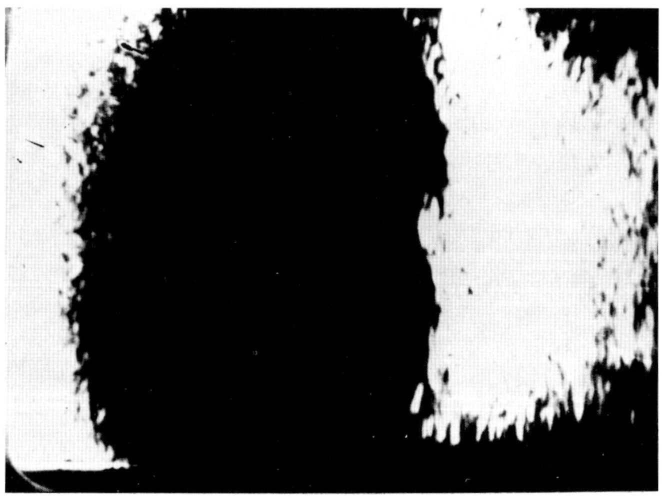

Figure 5.7. Disciform degeneration. Note the low profile, strong internal echoes, and irregular shape characteristic of these lesions.

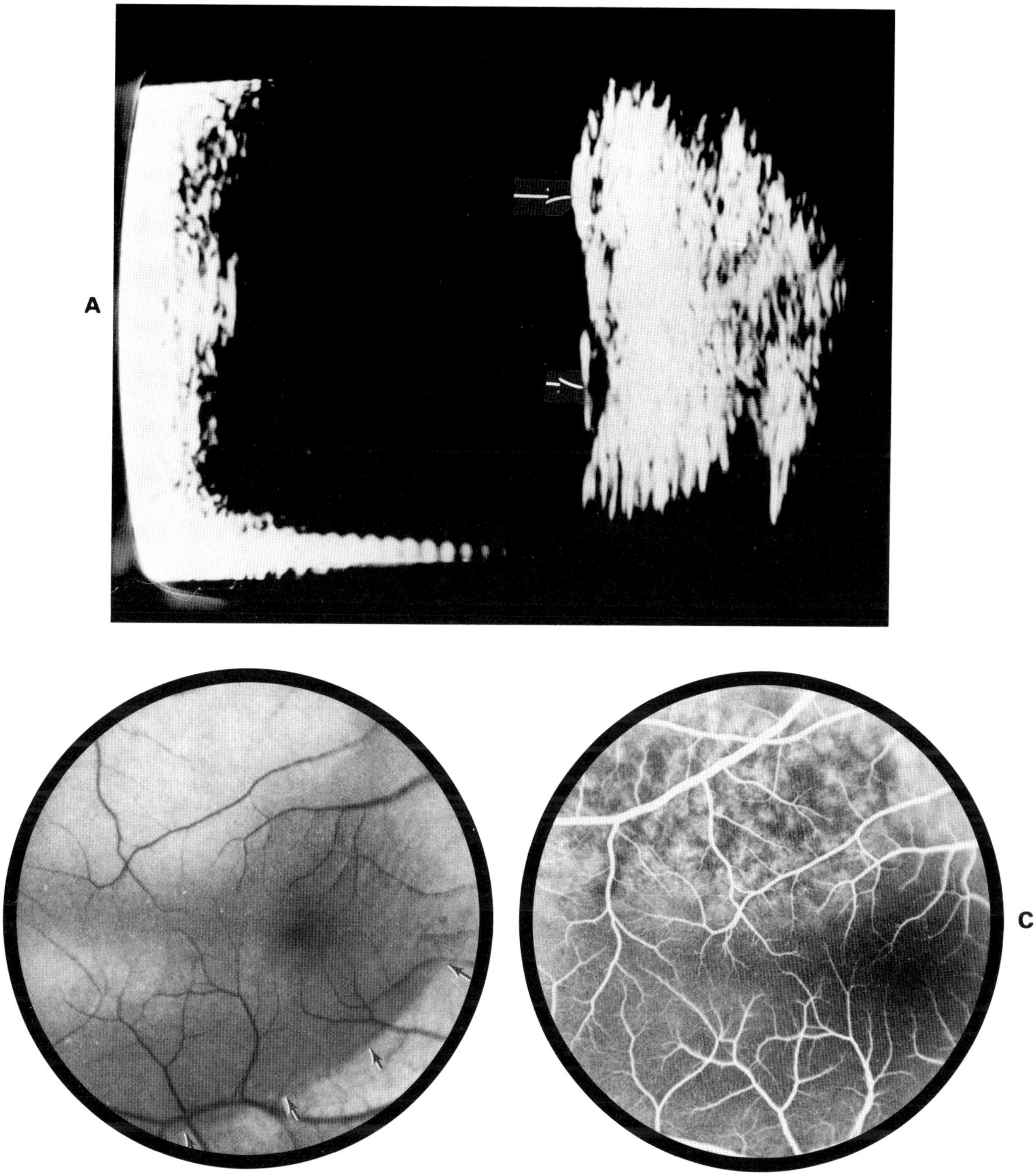

Figure 5.8. *A*, breast carcinoma metastatic to the choroid in the macula (*large arrow)* with an associated secondary retinal detachment (*small arrow*) seen at the inferior portion of the lesion. Note the similarity in acoustical appearance of this lesion when compared to that of a disciform degeneration (Fig. 5.7). *B*, ophthalmoscopic photograph of the sensory retinal detachment (*small arrows*) overlying the metastatic tumor in the superotemporal macula. *C*, arteriovenous phase angiogram, same eye showing patchy hypo- and hyperfluorescence of this tumor.

A 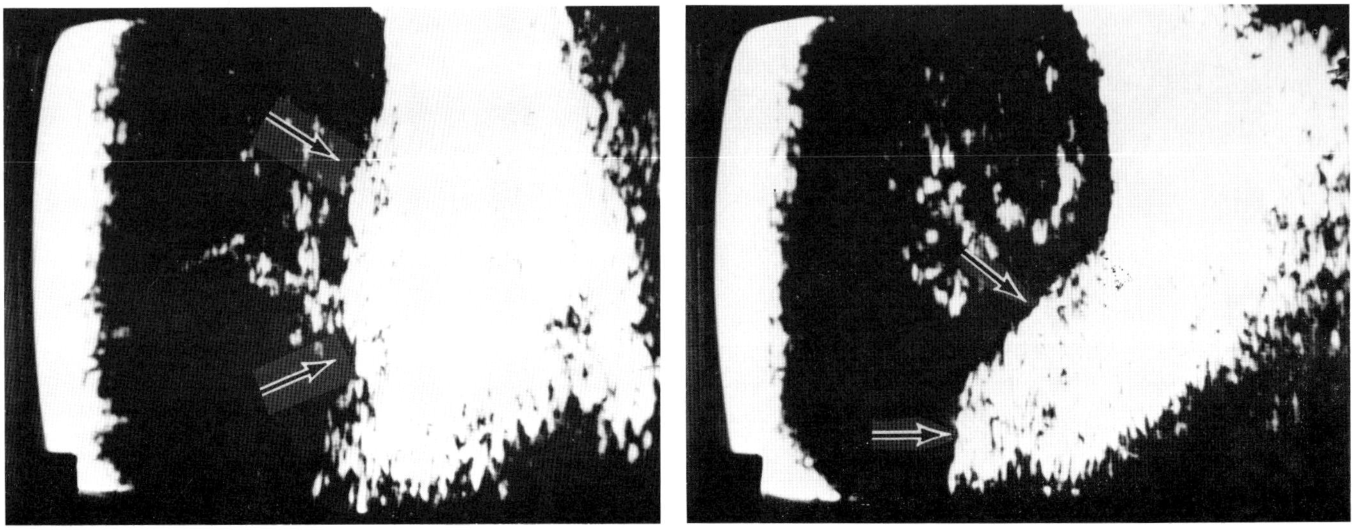 B

Figure 5.9. *A*, marked vitreous hemorrhage with associated posterior pole mass (*arrows*) which is difficult to visualize in this photograph. *B*, rapid command voluntary movement of the patient's eye accentuates the lesion as the vitreous debris separates from the surface of the mass.

A 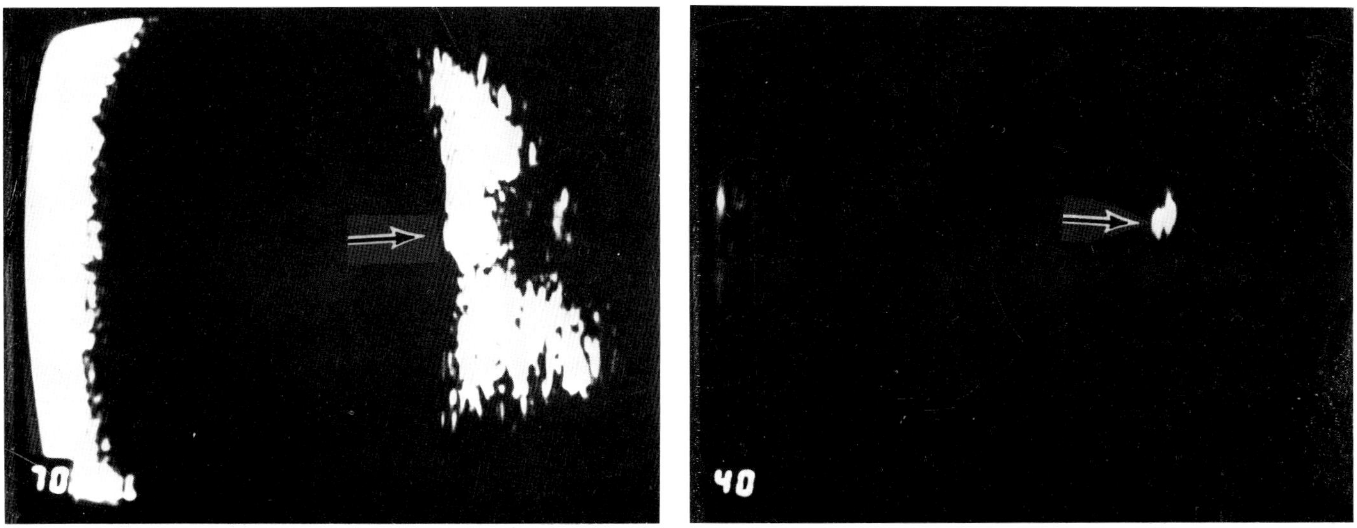

Figure 5.10. *A*, drusen of the optic nerve head at 70 db. *B*, drusen of the optic nerve head at 40 db. Note the persistent high reflectivity of this abnormality.

Miscellaneous Ultrasonic Abnormalities of the Posterior Pole

DRUSEN OF THE OPTIC NERVE HEAD

Primary disorders of the optic nerve, with secondary manifestations in the macular region, can be evaluated ultrasonographically even in clear media. Drusen of the optic nerve head can be detected by ultrasonography. Ultrasonically, the lesions appear as strongly reflective, small granular opacities situated on the head of the optic nerve (Fig. 5.10*A*). The strength of the echoes is demonstrated by reduction of the sensitivity setting to 40 db (Fig. 5.10*B*), at which level only the echoes from the drusen can be seen on the display screen. Presumably the calcium content of the drusen explains the marked difference of acoustic impedance between the drusen and the surrounding tissue, accounting for the strong echoes seen. Only an intraocular foreign body, an astrocytic hamartoma, or a choroidal osteoma has been noted to produce similar echoes.

In most patients ultrasonography is a confirmatory test since ophthalmoscopy and fluorescein angiography will usually substantiate the presence of optic nerve head drusen. In situations in which drusen are deeply buried in the nerve head, ultrasound has proven to be the only method of detection.

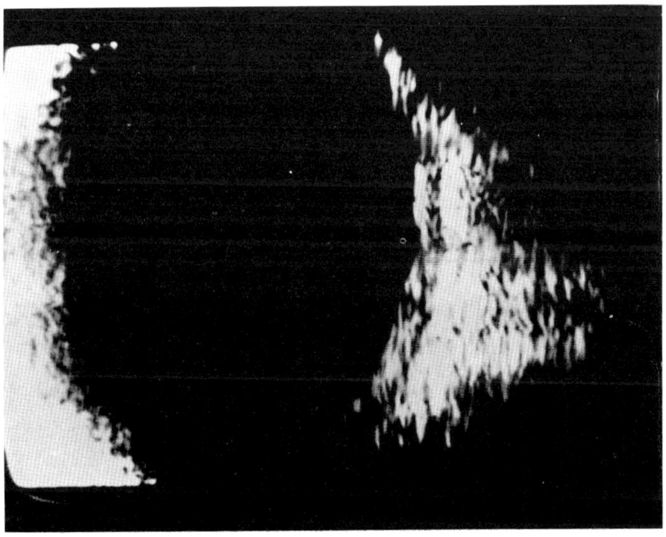

Figure 5.11. Thickening of the choroid is demonstrated in an eye with hypotony. Choroidal thickening may be seen in hypotony, Harada's disease, uveal effusion, hemangioma of Sturge-Weber disease, sympathetic uveitis, neurofibromatosis, uveoscleritis and any diffuse infiltrative process such as reactive lymphoid hyperplasia.

CHOROIDAL THICKENING

The normal choroidal pattern can usually be detected as a thin layer just inside the scleral echo during routine ultrasonographic examination. This highly vascular tissue is well outlined by the clear vitreous and the strongly reflective scleral shell. The thickness of this layer varies, and at times it is almost imperceptible on the display screen. In a number of disease processes, however, the choroidal pattern thickens and can be easily demonstrated by contact B-scan ultrasonography. Perhaps the most common one is hypotony (Fig. 5.11). Thickening may also be seen in situations that are not the result of a hypotonous state such as those of uveomeningeal-type syndromes such as Harada's disease, sympathetic ophthalmia, uveal effusion, neurofibromatosis, hemangioma of Sturge-Weber disease, uveosclerosis, or a diffuse infiltrative process such as reactive lymphoid hyperplasia.

Ultrasonography has proven to be a valuable adjunct to the examination of the globe with clear media when information concerning tissue density is desired. It is invaluable when the media is opaque [4–7]. While the information obtained is not pathognomonic, an experienced examiner can gain clinically useful information from a thorough study of ultrasonically resolvable intraocular lesions involving the macula.

References

1. Bronson, N.R.: Development of a simple B-scan ultrasonoscope. *Trans Am Ophthalmol Soc, 70*: 365, 1972.
2. Bronson, N.R., Fisher, Y.L., Pickering, N., and Trayner, E.: Ophthalmic Contact B-Scan Ultrasonography for the Clinician. Intercontinental Publications, Westport, Conn., 1976.
3. Fisher, Y.L., Bronson, N.R., Schutz, J.S., and Llovera, I.N.: Contact B-scan ultrasonography: clinicopathological correlations. *Ann Ophthalmol, 7*: 779, 1975.
4. Fisher, Y.L.: The current status of ophthalmic B-scan ultrasonography. *J Clin Ultrasound, 3*: 219, 1975.
5. Coleman, D.J.: Reliability of ocular and orbital diagnosis with B-scan ultrasound. I: Ocular diagnosis. *Am J Ophthalmol, 73*: 501, 1972.
6. Coleman, D.J., Abramson, D.H., Jack, R.L., and Franzen, L.A.: Ultrasonic diagnosis of tumors of the choroid. *Arch Ophthalmol, 91*: 344, 1974.
7. Purnell, E.W.: Ultrasound in ophthalmological diagnosis. *In* Diagnostic Ultrasound, *In* Proceedings of the First International Conference, University of Pittsburgh, 1965, ed. by C.C. Grossman, J.H. Homes, C. Joyner, *et al.*, Plenum Press, New York, 1966, p. 95.

CHAPTER 6

Low Vision Correction in Macular Disease

Alan H. Barnert, M.D., and Eleanor E. Faye, M.D.

In view of the sophisticated modalities now employed in the diagnosis and treatment of macular diseases and the advances in knowledge of their pathogenesis, one might suppose that there is little need for optical treatment of disability. However, anyone familiar with macular disease will be only too aware that even with the best management, there are some patients whose final visual function is sufficiently impaired to be disabling. They will be interested in obtaining maximum use of their visual capabilities.

The old maxim, "Treat the patient and not the disease," leads to an effective approach along three lines: (1) informing the patient about his disease so that he understands it and is able to accept it; (2) considering how he will cope with his social and occupational problems; and (3) doing a low vision evaluation.

This chapter describes some pitfalls the doctor should avoid and the goals he should keep in mind in communicating with patients with macular disease. It then defines and describes low vision evaluation and sets forth the therapeutic categories into which macular patients fall, together with the aids most appropriate for each group.

Communication with the Patient

Ophthalmologists do not always realize what special meanings patients attach to certain words and concepts. In explaining to a patient that he has macular disease, it is important to emphasize (as applicable, of course) that it happens to people in good health; that it usually remains confined to a very small area of the retina; that it is *not* associated with poor circulation outside the macula; and that it rarely leads to "complete blindness," or even to such poor vision that the patient cannot function independently. Many patients get the impression, from the physician's explanations, that they are losing their sight altogether, or that macular degeneration is a sign of impending cerebral or peripheral arteriosclerosis or a stroke, or that they will soon be walking with a cane or a seeing-eye dog or not at all.

Of course, one must not gloss over the fact that the disease often progresses to about 20/200 or even worse, that unilateral disease often becomes bilateral, and that treatment seldom improves the vision. One can emphasize, however, how much a patient *can* do rather than dwell on possible limitations and such words as "senile" or "degeneration." These words, as well as many others (some prime examples are: blind, old, circulation, and arteriosclerosis), have strong emotional overtones. It is important to recognize this and to avoid them, lest their significance be misunderstood. Also, a patient can be told that there is often a disparity between the aging eye and other tissues or organs which may show no degenerative changes, and that macular disease can be independent of age.

Similarly, many patients equate any visual handicap, even moderate difficulty in reading, with blindness. Explaining the prognosis and ways to adjust to the condition often relieves anxiety. When told that they will never lose "side vision" and will, thus, always be able to get around independently, they will no longer fear becoming helpless and dependent upon a traveling companion or dog. Most patients with macular disease can adjust to their poor distance vision much as the moderate myope does when he elects not to use his glasses. What bothers macular patients most, in addition to the fear of going blind or becoming senile, is the inability to perform *near* tasks.

The physician is usually primarily concerned with the diagnosis and treatment of the local lesion. But he should realize that the patient's main concern is not the etiology or anatomic cure of his condition but the end result in terms of function. Function means not only his visual acuity, but also how his acuity loss will affect his whole life situation. Macular dysfunction can lead to problems in all sorts of areas. The patient may worry about his job, or his future: about his daily living, his ability to get around town, or to care for himself. He may worry about his hobbies, recreation, friends, social life, and other activities. He may have adapted to his level of function either well or poorly; he may have a clear idea about his status or be badly misinformed about important aspects of it. He may continue to fear going blind and need continual reassurance or, on the other hand, he may exhibit denial and have unrealistic plans that require discussion.

The ophthalmologist is well prepared for the discussion of treatment and prognosis. A patient's social, emotional, or vocational problems, should be recognized and the patient referred for appropriate counseling; this may be to a social worker, an employment counselor, a rehabilitation service, a psychiatrist, or to several of these. Each case must be handled in an individual way. Even with the same acuity, fields, and general situation, patients will vary tremendously in their attitudes, adaptation, and general ability to cope.

Low Vision Evaluation

Stated simply, a low vision evaluation involves an analysis for the purpose of obtaining the best function out of whatever visual acuity a patient may have. *Distant* vision is helped by the best available refraction: glasses, contact lenses, telescopes, sunglasses; or by such nonoptical measures as having him move closer to the blackboard or TV set.

Near vision is usually helped by strong plus reading glasses, hand or stand magnifiers, or occasionally by telescopic reading devices or a closed-circuit reading apparatus (CCTV). Accessory aids for near vision include large-print books, broad point (felt) pens, check writing guides, and telephone dial attachments with large numerals.

Intermediate vision is corrected in special cases by the use of telescopic lenses.

Many patients with macular disease will already have experimented with some type of visual aid, often successfully. Sometimes they consult an ophthalmologist only when the almost universally available plus 5 to plus 11 hand magnifier is no longer helpful. Others with residual vision will be in search of instruction to achieve additional mobility or help in areas of personal management.

Macular disease in general involves a central scotoma with good peripheral field. Because of this, travel vision and capability are good, and patients are able to adapt to using gross vision for most ordinary tasks. It is only in discrimination of fine detail that patients are handicapped and it is here that low vision aids offer the most promise.

Almost all cases of macular disease should be considered for possible low vision aids, regardless of whether they are suitable for any form of active treatment. It may also be wise to evaluate some cases before treatment; often rehabilitation with low vision aids is so effective that heroic treatment becomes unnecessary*. Among the many macular diseases considered untreatable by ophthalmologists but which can benefit from low vision aids, are: involutional nonexudative (dry) degeneration; holes; cysts; central scars from any cause including iatrogenic, end-stage disciform disease, and central chorioretinitis.

The range of visual acuity amenable to low vision help is extremely wide, varying from 4/200 to 20/40. Better acuity than this will respond to normal refractive methods and correction; worse acuity than this is only rarely responsive because the requirement of high adds, close reading distance, and strong illumination make adaption difficult.

It is important to measure the visual acuity of all patients accurately. Do not use "count fingers" technique; use a 200-foot Snellen letter at 10, 8, 5, or 3 feet. If the "E" can be read at almost any distance, it is probably worth trying a low vision examination.

When evaluating a patient for treatment of macular disease, sophisticated studies are needed to determine the etiology, pathology, histopathology, proximity to the fovea, or the papillomacular bundle, and probable response of various tissues to treatment. In contrast, when considering correction in low vision, treatment factors are important only in relation to their effect on the retinal area that the patient will be using. In reading, for example, it is vital that there be no scotoma immediately to the right of fixation; otherwise, it is impossible to follow a line of print. If the left eye is the better one, and the area just temporal to the macula is treated by photocoagulation (as is done when a "C" or onside "U" pattern is made around the macula, sparing the papillomacular bundle), a very disabling iatrogenic defect can be produced.

IMPORTANT FACTORS

For all patients with macular disease the following factors in the care and evaluation of low vision are significant:

(1) Central Visual Acuity

(2) Scotoma Size, Steepness, and Location

A small localized central scotoma is far less disabling than one extending into the paracentral or peripheral fields; it does not reduce the visual acuity below that of the immediately surrounding retina, which means fairly good vision. A larger scotoma can reduce vision to any level. In addition, the surrounding retina is used when employing a low vision aid; a central scotoma does not interfere with this unless the scotoma is large enough to interfere with the scanning of lines of print.

(3) The Patient's Motivation

(4) The Patient's Adaptability

An older patient with sudden visual loss does less well than a younger patient with stationary or slowly progressive diminution of vision.

(5) The Patient's Needs

A typical loss in a child with macular disease is inability to see a baseball or the blackboard. In older children and young adults the loss is inability to drive, read, and succeed in occupational plans. Older persons miss leisure reading and independence in pursuing personal interests. All three instances require different types of low vision appliances.

(6) The Nature of the Disease (Stationary or Progressive)

Progressive disease is discouraging to the physician and more so to the patient, but some cases can be handled

* Faye and Yannuzzi (unpublished data, 1976) began a study of low vision evaluation before and after laser photocoagulation. The study was discontinued as an evaluation of laser treatment because all the patients demonstrated improvement of visual function with simple low vision devices. The emphasis had to be changed, since the philosophy of treating the macula had undergone a change at the time. The exception was localized macular edema with diabetic retinopathy originating from extramacular sites; this condition responded well to photocoagulation, after which the use of low vision aids was more suitable or no longer necessary. About 90% of the patients in the study received and used low vision aids.

satisfactorily by means of extra help and training to enable the patient to remain independent.

(7) Special Factors

Aphakia, amount of available accommodation, presence of other ocular complications such as opacities of the media, field defects or extraocular muscle problems, or systemic complications such as diabetes, tremors, low intelligence, or neurologic disease, further complicate a patient's potential response to low vision correction.

LOW VISION CORRECTION

On the basis of the above factors most patients with macular disease fall into the following five natural groups that suggest the means for correcting their low vision:

Group A: Older Patients with Macular Degeneration and Favorable Factors

This group includes such diseases as well localized involutional macular degeneration (IMD), cysts, or holes. In this group the surrounding retina is healthy and the patient is well motivated, adaptable, and has no other significant associated factors.

This is the group which furnishes the large bulk of low vision practice. Their main complaint is inability to read letters, bills, newspapers, and bibles, in approximately that order. They cannot recognize people or see street signs and bus and house numbers.

Low vision evaluation usually leads to one or more of the following aids: high-plus spectacles for reading, a small hand-held magnifier for near tasks, a low-power monocular hand-held telescope for spotting distant numbers. Most patients do not do well either with the complicated CCTV for reading or with high-power telescopes for distance, because of difficulty in their use. Nonoptical aids, such as large-print books, telephone dials, and check writing guides are helpful; felt pens are useful to both patient and his correspondents.

Group B: Older Patients with Less Favorable Factors

This group includes IMD with extensive involvement beyond the immediate macular area; widespread permanent macular damage from diabetes; any rapidly progressive disease; and patients with poor adaptation or motivation.

These patients constitute a smaller but (unfortunately) not negligible group. Although their needs are the same as those in group A, the optical results are discouraging—anything from inability to complete the examination because of poor cooperation, to a patient owning but not using his devices because of extensive pathology. Counseling may help the patient adjust to his more severe disability.

Group C: IMD with Aphakia

This group is separated from group B because the problem for these patients is principally optical. Since aphakic spectacles cause diminution of and distortion in the peripheral field, patients are hampered in the use of that part of the retina that functions best for them. A spectacle-induced ring scotoma is an added disability, also interfering with an important part of their total field. For near vision, the high-plus add required because of low vision, combined with the high-plus distance correction, results in very thick glasses with their accompanying optical disadvantages. (None of this applies, of course, to high myopic aphakes or to patients who have had cataract extractions with intraocular lens implantations.) Contact lenses, when usable, are often a solution for this group. When contact lenses cannot be used, aspheric aphakic glasses offer better correction than spherical ones. They are available with high-add bifocal segments of plus 6, plus 9, plus 12, and plus 18 diopters (American Optical Corporation, Bedford, Mass.). In patients with macular degeneration and a cataract, cataract extraction combined with pseudoaphakic implantation may ultimately prove to be the most beneficial form of management.

Group D: Young Adults with Localized Lesions

These can be solar burns, central chorioretinal scars from any cause, such as toxoplasmosis, presumed ocular histoplasmosis, pars planitis with macular edema, degenerative myopia, certain hereditary maculopathies, and trauma.

Patients in this group vary in age, needs, progression of their disease, and degree of associated systemic disorders. The ingenuity of the low vision practitioner is often taxed in meeting their requirements, which may be occupational, scholastic, social, the pursuit of hobbies or sports, or any of the myriad activities of normal, active young people. Fortunately, many of their requirements can be met.

These patients are very adaptable, highly motivated, and often ingenious themselves. Many find no inconvenience in having a large number of aids, such as telescopes or binoculars of varying strengths; magnifiers of different sizes and strengths, with and without self-illumination; several different spectacles including bifocals for differing tasks; and if needed in cases of very poor vision or special vocational situations, CCTV. As accommodation gradually decreases with age, thus decreasing the focal range of each of their devices, they may require additional aids. Unless theirs is a rapidly progressing disease they continue to do well with aids.

Group E: Children

This fairly large group of patients differs from the others in many respects. Having large accommodation, they supply their own built-in "high-plus," so that they usually need no additional aid for reading. They are very adaptable, particularly since they have either congenital eye diseases, or a disease which developed in early childhood and, thus, they do not miss the vision that they never had.

Visual acuity, even in normal very young children, is not 20/20, hence a mild reduction in macular function is not as disabling in this group. Also, preschool children are not significantly handicapped by even fairly poor vision, since they have no need for reading, driving, recognition of distance, small objects, or other tasks requiring critical cone function. It is not until about the age of 7 that a child's 20/200 may present any sort of problem, or even become noticeable to him or his family.

What is usually needed after this age is a monocular telescope for reading blackboards. It is important to tell the family and teachers that the child is not functionally blind and should not be treated as blind, whether legally blind or not; that the child can and should use his eyes, remain in regular class, and read regular print and not Braille. Also, he should participate in sports and gym with other children. Exceptions include children with associated mental deficiency or a learning disability; for them the situation is less favorable. Aphakia is of special concern because of the inability to accommodate. As a rule, however, children with stationary defects and no complicating factors are easy to treat successfully.

Accommodation decreases as children grow older, whereas the need to read small print and meet other fine discrimination requirements increases. They may then begin to need a near correction; often best prescribed as a bifocal. Hand magnifiers can be used for such occasional extra tasks as reading exponents, fractions, or the dictionary. Children also appreciate and easily learn (better than adults can) to use devices for distance magnification, such as handheld 2.5–8× telescopes and spectacle-mounted telescopes up to about 4×.

In summary, patients with macular disease, after completion of whatever active treatment is possible, often have a visual disability. Attention to this, including low vision evaluation, proper communication with the patient about his condition, and counseling in specific areas when indicated, may be of great benefit to the patient.

In evaluating and correcting low vision there are several factors to consider. Patients can be divided into five therapeutic categories on the basis of these factors. These categories provide a guide both for evaluation and for choosing corrective aids that will give individual patients the maximum use of their actual vision. The response varies according to the category; the overall response rate is high.

What the patient is told, and the language and manner in which he is told, affect the patient's ability to cope with his social and occupational problems. Consequently, the physician should take care to explain the patient's condition in a language he can understand, emphasizing whatever positive aspects pertain, and describing clearly the adjustments that will help him make full use of his visual acuity. Guidance by other professionals or paraprofessionals may be indicated.

Suggested Readings

American Foundation for the Blind, Office of Low Vision Projects, 15 East 16th Street, New York, 10011.

Faye, E.: The Low Vision Patient, Grune & Stratton, New York, 1970.

Faye, E., and Hood, C.M.: Low Vision: A Symposium Marking the 20th Anniversary of the Lighthouse Low Vision Service. Charles C Thomas, Springfield, Ill., 1975.

Fonda, G.: Management of the Patient with Subnormal Vision, 2nd ed, C.V. Mosby, St. Louis, 1970.

Freid, A.N., and Mehr, E.B.: Low Vision Care. The Professional Press, Chicago, 1974.

Hood, C.M.: Low Vision Clinical Society, 121 East 60th Street, New York, 10021.

Lighthouse Catalogue of Optical Aids, 4th ed, New York Association for the Blind, New York, 1976.

PART II

Retinal Vascular Disease

CHAPTER 7

Diabetic Retinopathy

Kurt A. Gitter, M.D., Howard Schatz, M.D., and Lawrence A. Yannuzzi, M.D.

Diabetic retinopathy is one of the most difficult and discouraging diseases which confronts ophthalmologists today. Diabetes mellitus presently affects 1.5% of the population in the Western World with wide geographic and ethnic differences. The retinopathy occurs in slightly less than one-half of all diabetics and represents a major cause of blindness in these countries.

An increase in the life expectancy of the diabetic patient promises to potentiate the problem of diabetic retinopathy in the future. Because of its serious nature and high frequency of occurrence, it is extremely important for ophthalmologists to understand and recognize the pathophysiology, clinical manifestations, and treatment of diabetic retinopathy. This chapter discusses the classification, incidence and natural history, pathogenesis and clinical findings, related systemic and ocular factors, fluorescein angiographic characteristics, and treatment of diabetic retinopathy.

Classification

For the purposes of understanding and recognizing specific clinical features and determining therapy, diabetic retinopathy is best classified into two types: nonproliferative or background diabetic retinopathy and proliferative diabetic retinopathy.

The clinical findings in nonproliferative diabetic retinopathy include retinal venous beading, microaneurysms, cotton wool infarcts, hard waxy exudates, superficial and deep intraretinal hemorrhages, preretinal membrane formation, intraretinal edema, retinal vascular ischemia and occlusion, and intraretinal microvascular abnormalities (IRMA). The diabetic retinopathy is classified as proliferative when, in addition to these other findings, neovascularization develops from the disc and/or retinal vessels. This form of diabetic retinopathy invariably becomes associated with preretinal hemorrhage, fibrosis, posterior retinal breaks, anterior-posterior vitreous traction with secondary retinoschisis, and detachment.

Incidence and Natural History

In the United States, diabetes mellitus occurs in 1 to 2% of the population, and diabetic retinopathy affects 40% of all diabetics. It is this country's leading cause of blindness today. The retinopathy is reported to be directly related to the duration of the disease [1]. For juvenile diabetics, about 10% will have retinopathy after 5 years, 25% after 10 years, 50% after 15 years, and 90% after 25 years. In adult onset diabetics, diabetic retinopathy develops earlier in relationship to the onset of diabetes. It is not rare for diabetic retinopathy to be the first clinical sign of adult onset diabetes. Approximately 30% of adult onset diabetics have diabetic retinopathy after 5 years and about 50% after 10 years.

More than 90% of patients with diabetic retinopathy have the nonproliferative form. This retinopathy is frequently minimal and demonstrates mild ophthalmoscopic changes with no visual loss. Often the changes are fluctuant with periods of spontaneous improvement as well as stabilization and progression. Severe forms of nonproliferative diabetic retinopathy may occur, each of which may result in marked and irreversible reduction in vision. One form is associated with diffuse leakage of the perifoveal retinal capillaries. This usually leads to circumpapillary cystoid macular edema with confluent macular cyst formation and a gradual but progressive reduction in central vision. This form of diabetic maculopathy is not benefitted by photocoagulation therapy. Other manifestations in nonproliferative diabetic retinopathy leading to profound irreversible reduction in central vision include preretinal membrane formation with macular cyst or hole, subfoveal hemorrhage, and perifoveal capillary nonperfusion from occluded capillaries. Since only 6% of the diabetic retinopathy cases are of the proliferative variety, the macular dysfunction induced by nonproliferative manifestations is highly significant, representing the major cause of visual decline in diabetics.

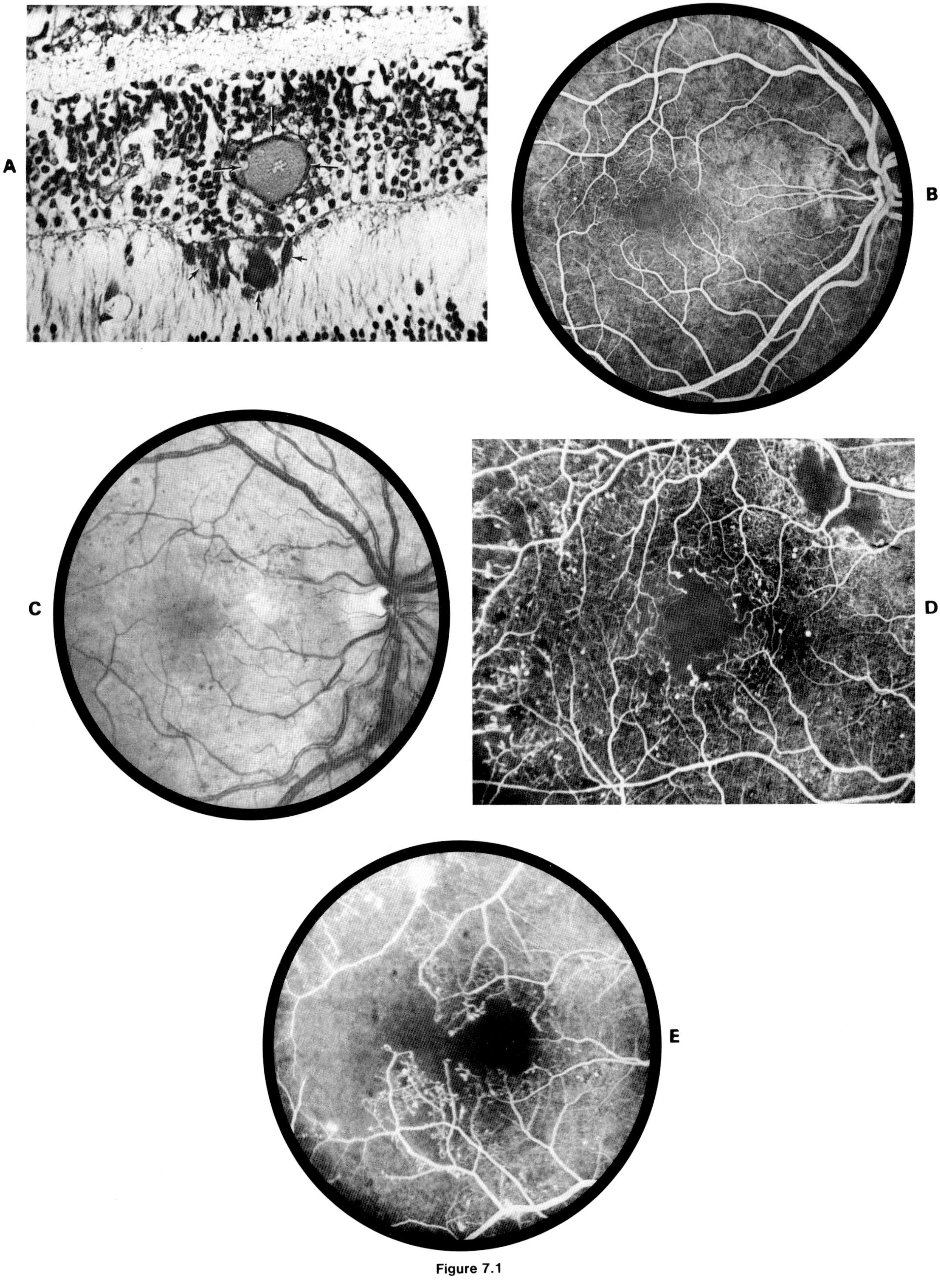

Figure 7.1

The visual prognosis in proliferative diabetic retinopathy is generally extremely poor [2]. The average duration of diabetes before its development is 17 years in juvenile diabetics and approximately 10 years in adult onset diabetes. After vision declines in one eye to 20/200 or worse, a significant number of patients become bilaterally blind in less than a year, and approximately 9 out of 10 of the fellow eyes deteriorate to the same vision in 5 years or less. It has been found that diabetics blinded by proliferative diabetic retinopathy have an average life expectancy of less than 6 years after the onset of blindness.

Neovascularization of the disc leads to blindness in 4 out of 5 (80%) untreated eyes within 5 years. When neovascularization is away from the disc, blindness occurs in 1 out of 5 (20%) untreated eyes over this period [3].

In general, however, diabetic retinopathy and its implications are highly variable and extremely unpredictable, and this alone may be its most distinctive feature.

Pathogenesis and Clinical Findings

Although the pathogenesis of diabetic retinopathy is not fully clear, in large part it is associated with arteriolar compromise and obliterated capillaries [4]. The earliest visible retinal vascular changes are usually prominence or engorgement of the venous system or capillary microaneurysms.

Capillary microaneurysms are tiny out-pouchings of the capillary bed which may be hypercellular or acellular, as seen by trypsin digestion. They appear as tiny red dots scattered in the posterior pole of the fundus, with their greatest predilection for the temporal macula. They may be difficult to distinguish from small intraretinal hemorrhages, but they can be identified by fluorescein angiography because they usually perfuse while small hemorrhages appear as hypofluorescent spots.

Small superficial flame-shaped hemorrhages, deep dot and blot-like hemorrhages, patches of waxy edudation, intraretinal edema, capillary occlusion, and IRMA are other early findings (Fig. 7.1). IRMA are irregularly dilated (telangiectatic) capillaries, usually associated with, and located adjacent to, areas of capillary nonperfusion. These capillaries tend to leak and also contain microaneurysms along their course. They are frequently the only vascular channels connecting arterioles and venules and thus, function as arteriovenous collaterals. Some have suggested that IRMA represent early endothelial proliferation or shunts, but most probably they are simply dilated capillaries compensating for adjacent vascular occlusions.

IRMA and associated capillary occlusion can lead to two major problems. One is abnormal retinal vascular permeability which results in serous leakage from the affected and remaining patent retinal capillaries as well as from microaneurysms. This produces intraretinal edema and deposits of lipid exudation. Massive intraretinal edema may seep beneath the sensory retina to produce a shallow macular detachment. When the macula becomes edematous or exudate deposition occurs in the fovea, central vision is reduced.

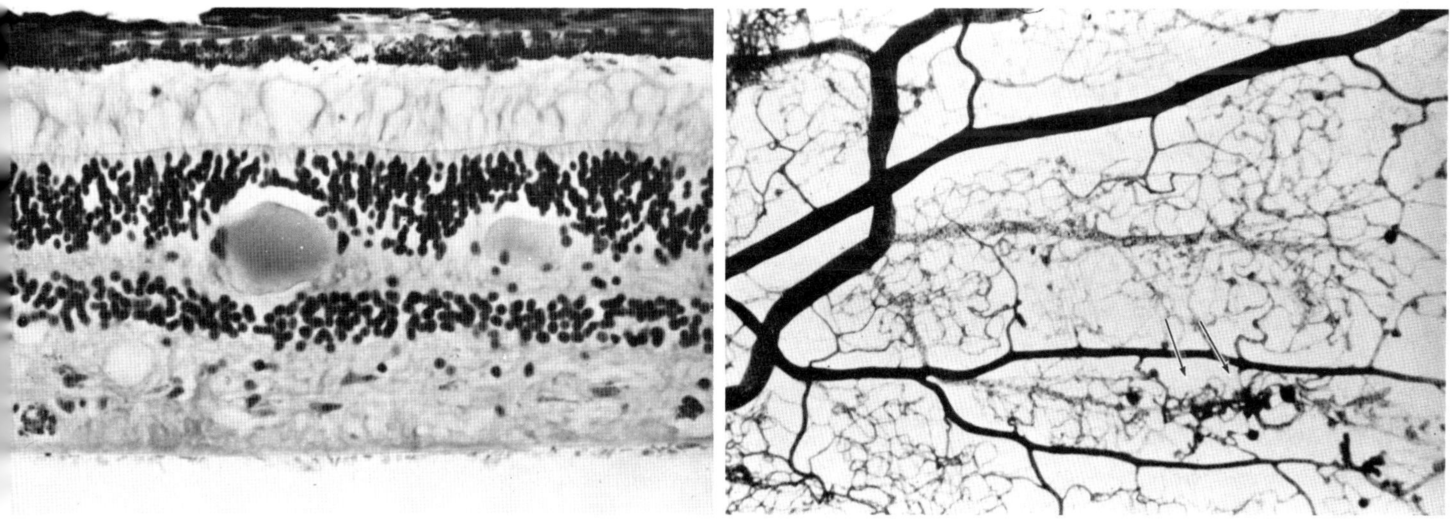

G

Figure 7.1— *continued*

Figure 7.1. *A*, histopathologic cross-section of retina showing microaneurysm (*large arrows*) from deep capillary plexus leaking exudate (*small arrows*) into outer plexiform layer. ×25. (Courtesy of Martin H. Vogel, M.D.). *B*, fluorescein angiogram of early nonproliferative diabetic retinopathy showing microaneurysms at their usual site of predilection in the temporal macula. The retinal capillary bed is still intact. *C*, ophthalmoscopic photograph of patient with nonproliferative diabetic retinopathy with hemorrhages, microaneurysms, and marked venous irregularities. *D*, fluorescein angiogram of the perifoveal circulation in diabetic retinopathy. Note the capillary irregularities and microaneurysms. *E*, fluorescein angiogram of the macula in diabetic retinopathy. Note the capillary nonperfusion which begins in the perifoveal area and includes the temporal macula. *F*, histopathologic cross-section of the retina showing intraretinal exudation in diabetic retinopathy (Courtesy of Myron Yanoff, MD). *G*, retinal digest preparation in diabetic retinopathy showing intraretinal microangiopathy (IRMA), including capillary dilatation, capillary acellularity, and capillary microaneurysms. There are also areas of dilated, hypercellular capillaries (arrows) adjacent to nonperfused vessels. These abnormal capillaries probably represent early proliferative changes or compensatory collaterals adjacent to ischemic areas. (Courtesy of Myron Yanoff, MD).

A second major problem is retinal vascular endothelial proliferation in response to the retinal ischemia caused by the capillary nonperfusion. This leads to neovascularization which usually occurs first at the disc or on the retinal surface along the course of the large vascular arcades. The vascular complexes break through the internal limiting membrane, proliferate on the surface of the retina, and eventually attach to the posterior hyaloid. When the posterior hyaloid detaches from the internal limiting membrane, the new vessels are lifted off the surface of the retina with it. Vitreous contraction may cause traction on the new blood vessels and subhyaloid and/or vitreous hemorrhage. Fibrosis and organization of the vitreous may evolve, and this can lead to retinal traction detachment and total loss of vision. The exact mechanism or etiology predisposing to vitreous contraction and its sequelae is not known [5].

Whether the major problem is one of increased vascular permeability with macular edema, preretinal membrane formation, macular capillary nonperfusion, fibrovascular proliferation, vitreous hemorrhage or retinal traction detachment, diabetic retinopathy tends to result in progressive loss of vision, making any clinical evidence of its presence a serious finding.

Systemic and Ocular Factors

Various systemic and ocular factors can have an adverse effect on diabetic retinopathy and others appear to inhibit its formation.

Pregnancy is known to aggravate the retinopathy of a juvenile diabetic [6]. Neovascularization, hemorrhage, edema of the optic nervehead, and retinal edema may increase markedly during pregnancy. Termination of the pregnancy by abortion (therapeutic or spontaneous) may cause immediate and marked regression. There are some, however, who argue that there is no definite relationship between pregnancy and worsening of diabetic retinopathy.

Hypertension and renal decompensation may also increase the severity of the diabetic retinopathy. These conditions tend to increase vascular occlusion and lead to further hypoxia. Increased retinal vascular permeability may occur and result in a greater serous outpouring into as well as beneath the sensory retina. Some reports have suggested that abnormal blood coagulability, increased capillary fragility, and increased platelet aggregation may worsen proliferative diabetic retinopathy.

There is some evidence that poor diabetic control can aggravate retinopathy and that high serum lipids may cause increased deposition of hard exudate in the retina. Since many systemic factors are important in diabetes, especially when retinopathy is present, it is essential for the ophthalmologist to work closely with the diabetic patient and his/her internist to manage these factors.

Certain ocular factors seem to decrease the incidence of retinopathy or reduce its severity. Axial myopia, greater than 5 diopters, seems to have a beneficial effect. This is also true with increased intraocular pressure, optic atrophy, severe chorioretinal scarring, reduced central retinal artery diastolic pressure, and central retinal artery occlusion. Each of these ocular disorders should be considered if diabetic retinopathy is monocular or markedly asymmetric in severity. It has been theorized that in each of these conditions, fewer retinal elements are viable, thereby reducing the production of the unknown, abnormal biochemical factor which may stimulate or potentiate the development of the retinopathy.

Fluorescein Angiographic Characteristics

As with other retinal vascular diseases, the fluorescein angiogram is indispensible in the evaluation, treatment, and management of diabetic retinopathy. In the early (or vascular) phase of the angiogram, the IRMA findings are most clearly seen. The fluorescein angiogram demonstrates that these are irregularly dilated capillaries adjacent to areas of capillary nonperfusion. They appear to be arteriovenous collaterals, compensating for adjacent capillary occlusions.

Microaneurysms, areas of capillary nonperfusion, retinal neovascularization, dilation, tortuosity, and telangiectasia of the involved capillary bed are well defined by fluorescein angiography in an eye with relatively clear media. The late (or extravascular) phase of the angiogram shows the effect of these changes on the macula with intraretinal leakage (cystoid and noncystoid) and vitreous leakage from new blood vessels.

The extent of the capillary nonperfusion can be carefully assessed with a panoramic type of angiogram in which fluorescein angiophotographs are taken of the entire posterior pole and midperiphery. The specific areas and extent of involvement can be readily assessed with this technique. If a diabetic's vision is reduced and the reason is not evident on clinical examination, the angiogram may show capillary nonperfusion of the perifoveal capillary net, thus explaining the visual loss (Fig. 7.2).

Fluorescein angiography is especially useful in helping to determine the management and specific treatment of the

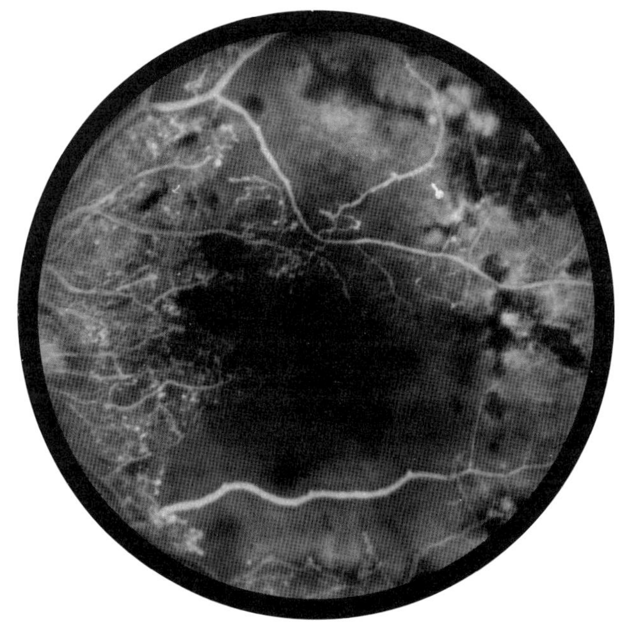

Figure 7.2. Fluorescein angiogram of a juvenile diabetic with marked areas of hypofluorescence due to capillary nonperfusion of the macula. This degree of foveal and macular capillary ischemia carries a very poor visual prognosis with or without treatment.

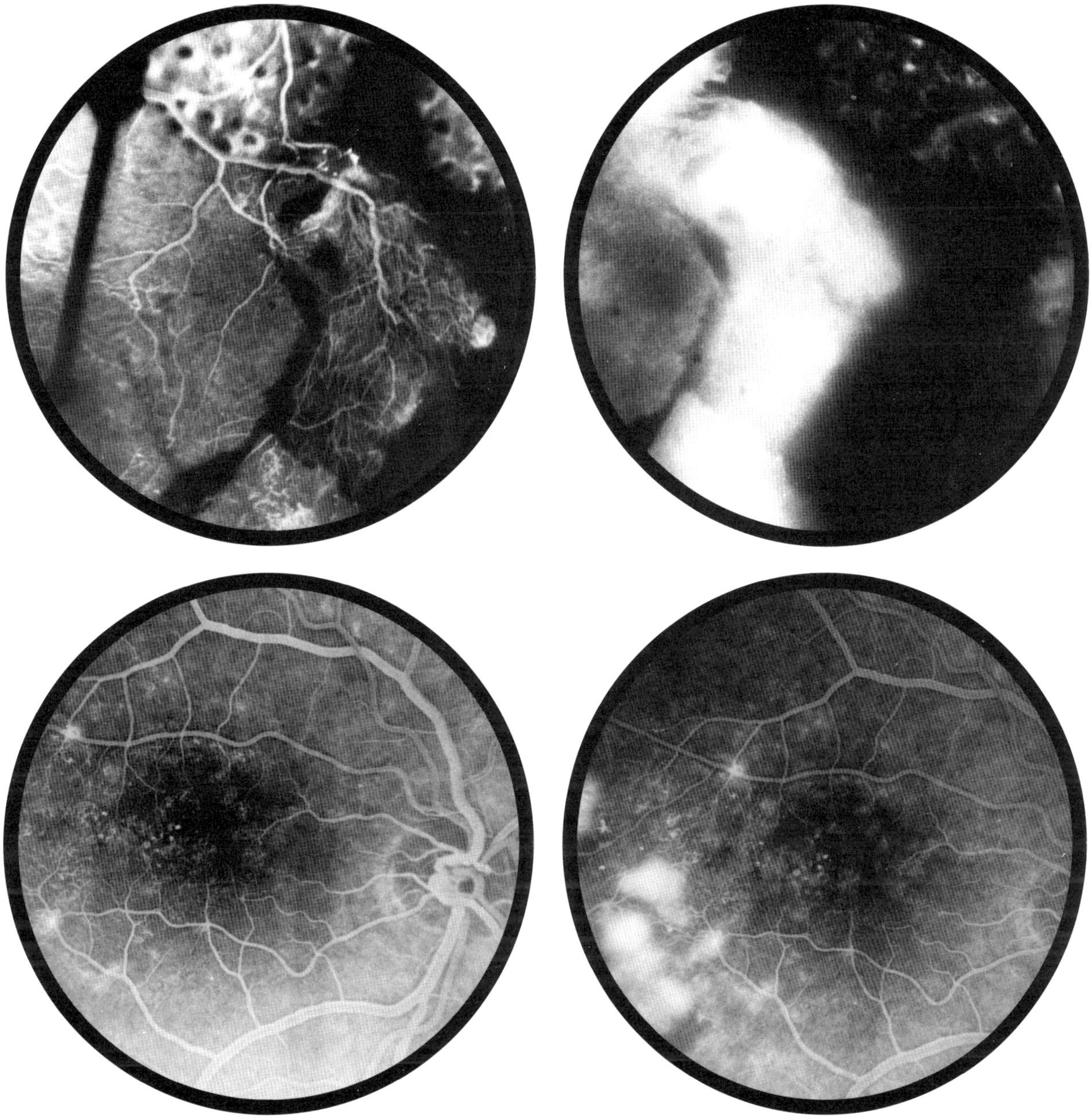

A B C D

Figure 7.3. Retinal neovascularization in diabetic retinopathy. *A,* early venous phase fluorescein angiogram. Note the lacy configuration of preretinal neovascularization. *B,* late phase angiogram, same patient. Note marked pooling of dye into the vitreous. *C,* early venous phase angiogram. Note abnormally dilated and tortuous capillaries in the macula of this patient with proliferative diabetic retinopathy. *D,* late phase angiogram, same patient. "Cottonball" hyperfluorescence is now evident in the vitreous. Late hyperfluorescence of this type is always indicative of retinal or disc neovascularization. When neovascularization is close to the retinal surface, fluorescein angiography is helpful in documenting its presence.

diabetic retinopathy. If the intraretinal vascular leakage is focal, the angiogram can be used to localize each specific leaking area so that argon laser photocoagulation can be exact and minimal. If the angiogram demonstrates diffuse fluorescein leakage in the macula, the prognosis is usually poor and photocoagulation is not helpful.

In proliferative diabetic retinopathy, there is no better way to demonstrate and confirm the exact extent and location of neovascularization than with fluorescein angiography (Fig. 7.3). Early lacy hyperfluorescence precedes late hyperfluorescence produced by leakage into the vitreous. Often the leaking neovascularization appears as a "cottonball" suspended in the posterior vitreous overlying the retinal vessels.

Finally, angiography is helpful in assessing the state of the postphotocoagulated eye. A panoramic type of angiogram taken in an eye that has been photocoagulated for neovascularization will clearly show the presence, regression, or absence of retinal neovascularization. Similarly, the angiogram performed in a patient who has had photocoagulation for nonproliferative diabetic retinopathy with retinal vascular leakage will clearly show resolution of leakage areas, continued leakage from areas in which treatment was attempted, or new leakage.

The angiogram is not generally utilized to diagnose diabetic retinopathy, but rather to help manage the diabetic patient by explaining obscure reductions in vision, by establishing a prognosis, and by serving as a guide to therapy.

Treatment

Diabetic retinopathy is difficult to manage; therefore, a variety of treatments have been proposed. These treatments include medical and diet, photocoagulation, pituitary ablation, vitrectomy, and scleral buckling procedures.

Medical forms of treatment including diets, Atromid-S, salicylates, and other drugs have all been advocated, but to date, none has been proven effective. Strict control of diabetes, although significant to the general health of the diabetic, does not appear to retard definitely the incidence or severity of the retinopathy.

Pituitary ablation, although possibly effective in some few instances, is no longer employed in the majority of centers because of inconclusive evidence of its usefulness and because of major problems in postoperative care.

Photocoagulation treatment for diabetic retinopathy is presently the most widely employed modality and provides the best choice available for halting the progression of the disease and stabilizing visual acuity.

The major rationale for photocoagulation therapy is based on the observation that eyes with widespread chorioretinal degeneration are spared from the development of retinopathic changes.

Photocoagulation was first employed in the 1950's by Meyer-Schwickerath [7] with xenon arc photocoagulation. Others [8, 9] promoted this modality in the early 1960's, and Aiello and coworkers [10] in 1968 advocated panretinal ablation with ruby laser for proliferative diabetic retinopathy. Later, argon laser photocoagulation was introduced [11, 12].

Although results of photocoagulation (by all modalities) have been encouraging, many early reports did not include adequate control subjects and, thus, accumulated statistics were often of questionable significance. Nevertheless, in those studies in which control subjects were available [13, 14], the effect on vision in eyes with nonproliferative diabetic retinopathy treated by photocoagulation appeared to be encouraging.

For nonproliferative diabetic retinopathy in which focal areas of retinal vascular leakage result in macular edema and lipid exudate which reduce vision, laser photocoagulation is used to treat the leakage to resorb the retinal edema and exudates. Often, treatment of the retinal area surrounded by a circinate exudate which cuts through the fovea and reduces vision will result in greatly improved vision as the exudate resolves (Fig. 7.4).

However, when these hard exudates become long-standing in the fovea with development of cholesterol crystals, vision is markedly disturbed and the prognosis for visual improvement is dim, regardless of therapy, because of retinal fibrotic reaction and pigment epithelial scar formation. Photocoagulation in these eyes can sometimes show disappearance of the exudate, but vision most often is unimproved.

There are specific manifestations in nonproliferative diabetic retinopathy which imply a poor visual prognosis when photocoagulation is employed. These include perifov-

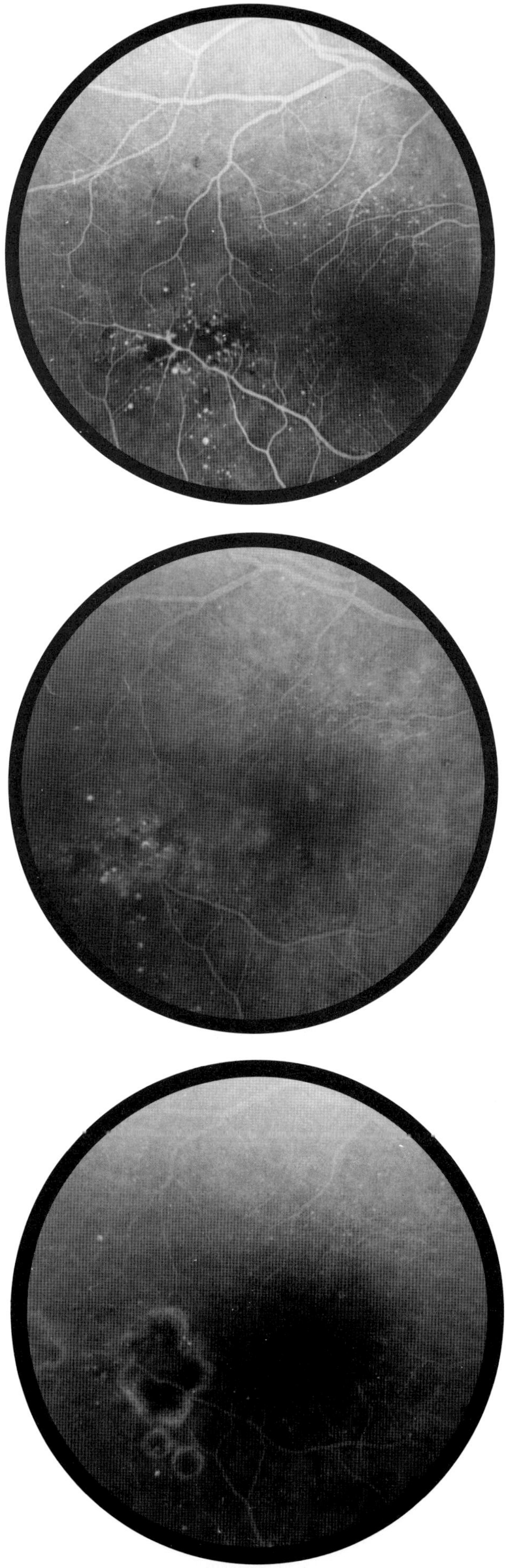

A

B

C

Figure 7.4. Nonproliferative diabetic retinopathy. *A,* intraretinal microangiopathy (IRMA) with capillary nonperfusion, capillary microaneurysms, capillary telangiectasia, and capillary leakage within a ring of circinate exudation. *B,* late phase angiogram showing dye leakage extending into the macula. *C,* postphotocoagulation late phase angiogram, same eye. Note the obliteration of abnormal capillaries and the resolution of macular edema.

eal capillary nonperfusion [15, 16], circumfoveal cystoid macular edema with confluent cyst formation [17], preretinal membrane formation with macular cyst or hole, long-standing heavy lipid deposition in the fovea, subfoveal hemorrhage, other submacular pathology, severe renal disease, or systemic hypertension. While there have been no prospective, controlled studies of the use of focal laser treatment for nonproliferative diabetic retinopathy, many feel this modality is promising if not highly useful.

Panretinal photocoagulation is used throughout the world to treat proliferative diabetic retinopathy. Recently, the National Institutes of Health Diabetic Retinopathy Study concluded that eyes with proliferative diabetic retinopathy and disc neovascularization fared better with xenon and/or argon laser photocoagulation than control eyes [18]. This study and others indicate that photocoagulation of eyes with moderate or severe neovascularization within one disc diameter of the disc, or eyes with neovascularization elsewhere and vitreous hemorrhage should be treated with the panretinal photocoagulation technique. The current working theory is that one or more biochemical products of ischemic or hypoxic retina stimulate endothelial proliferation and cause neovascularization. Destruction of the hypoxic retina eliminates the toxic stimulus and neovascularization regresses.

The specific method of treatment is to place combinations of 200, 500, and 1000 μ spot sizes of argon laser photocoagulation, or comparable spots of xenon arc photocoagulation, in a scattered method over the entire fundus from the posterior pole to the equator, avoiding the macular area (Fig. 7.5). Laser burns are placed approximately 1/4 to 1/2 a spot size apart from each other, and the burns are of low to medium intensity rather than "hot" white. The treatment may be divided into three or four sessions to reduce complications.

The beneficial effects of this type of photocoagulation include regression and disappearance of neovascular fronds and the establishment of a temporary state of quiescence of the abnormal retinal vascular changes. Complications include a slight reduction in acuity and field, iritis, increased retinal vascular leakage and macular edema with reduced vision, secondary retinal detachment, increased fibrotic preretinal traction and traction detachment, inadvertent photocoagulation of the fovea or a large retinal vessel with vitreous hemorrhage, and puncture of the pigment epithelium resulting in hemorrhage from the choriocapillaris under the sensory retina, and subsequent choroidal-retinal-vitreal neovascularization. Despite these numerous potential complications, panretinal photocoagulation, if used properly, is a fairly safe and effective method of therapy.

Unfortunately, photocoagulation cannot be considered as a cure for diabetic retinopathy, as retinal and retinal pigment epithelial destruction by photocoagulation only acts as a stopgap to prevent further visual decline. Further basic research is necessary to determine the pathogenic mechanisms of this disorder which will ultimately provide better answers.

The advent and development of pars plana microsurgical vitrectomy for eyes with long-standing organized vitreous hemorrhage secondary to diabetic retinopathy or other pathologic states is a significant surgical advance in ophthalmology. It is estimated by an analysis of over 500 cases [19] that 50% or more eyes were salvaged with resultant visual improvement following vitrectomy. In almost all cases, vitrectomy represents the last hope for visual improvement and, when successful, means the difference between blindness and travel vision, or better.

Eyes with vitreous hemorrhage obscuring retinal clarity should be considered for vitrectomy after a duration of 1 year, providing there is a potential for visual recovery as determined by preoperative evaluation of visual function, including ultrasonography and bright-flash electroretinography. The major complications of surgery are the development of retinal detachment, vitreous hemorrhage, and postoperative rubeosis iridis; the latter is particularly disconcerting. Notwithstanding, this new surgical technique represents a major surgical breakthrough.

Other surgical techniques, particularly scleral buckling and/or scleral resection, often combined with vitrectomy, have been advocated in eyes with both traction and rhegmatogenous retinal detachments secondary to diabetic retinopathy in an effort to retain minimal levels of visual acuity. These are, in general, final efforts at retaining minimal vision in eyes with otherwise clear ocular media.

Finally, ophthalmic surgeons must be prepared to deal with the real and psychologic difficulties associated with the onset of blindness in an adult. They must be able to offer advice and direction regarding rehabilitation programs and be familiar with local, state, and national agencies capable of aiding these individuals. The ophthalmologist must always be available for consultation, discussion, and advice to his patient and family.

In summary, diabetic retinopathy is one of the most severe, challenging, chronic, and perplexing problems for the ophthalmologist to manage. Great attention to detail including a careful history and ocular examination, along with an understanding of the natural history and pathogenesis of the disease, will lead to the proper management of such patients.

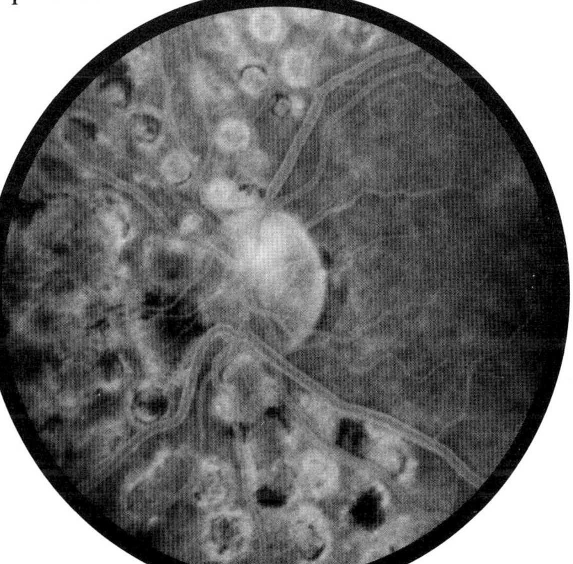

Figure 7.5. Postphotocoagulation of eye with proliferative diabetic retinopathy showing involution of disc neovascularization and burn placement in the ablation technique.

References

1. Caird, F.I.: Diabetic retinopathy as a cause of visual impairment. *In* Symposium on the Treatment of Diabetic Retinopathy, ed. by M. Goldberg and S. Fine, U.S. Department of Health, Education and Welfare, Washington, D.C., 1968.
2. Patz, A., and Berkow, J.W.: Visual prognosis in advanced diabetic retinopathy. *In* Symposium on the Treatment of Diabetic Retinopathy, ed. by M. Goldberg and S. Fine, U.S. Department of Health, Education and Welfare, Washington, D.C., 1968.
3. Berkow, J.W., Shugarman, R.G., Maumenee, A.E., and Patz, A.: A retrospective study of blind diabetic patients. *JAMA, 193:* 867, 1965.
4. Davis, M.D., and Myers, F.L.: Clinical observations concerning the pathogenesis of diabetic retinopathy. *In* Symposium on the Treatment of Diabetic Retinopathy, U.S. Department of Health, Education and Welfare, Washington, D.C., 1968.
5. Davis, M.: Symposium on Retinal Diseases, NOA Ophthalmol, 1977, C. V. Mosby, St. Louis.
6. Okun, E., *et al.:* Management of Diabetic Retinopathy: A Stereoscopic Presentation, C.V. Mosby, St. Louis, 1971.
7. Meyer-Schwickerath, G.: Light Coagulation, C.V. Mosby, St. Louis, 1960.
8. Wetzig, P.C., and Worlton, J. T.: Treatment of diabetic retinopathy by light coagulation: a preliminary study. *Brit J Ophthalmol, 47:* 539, 1963.
9. Okun, E., and Cibis, P.A.: The role of photocoagulation in the therapy of proliferative diabetic retinopathy. *Arch Ophthalmol, 75:* 337, 1966.
10. Aiello, L.M., Beetham, W.P., *et al.:* Ruby laser photocoagulation in treatment of diabetic proliferative retinopathy. *In* Symposium on the Treatment of Diabetic Retinopathy, ed. by M. Goldberg and S. Fine, U.S. Department of Health, Education and Welfare, Washington, D.C., 1968.
11. L'Esperance, F.A., Jr.: The treatment of ophthalmic vascular disease by argon laser photocoagulation. *Trans Am Acad Ophthalmol Otolaryngol, 73:* 1077, 1969.
12. Little, H.L., Zweng, H.C., and Peabody, R.R.: Argon laser slit-lamp retinal photocoagulation. *Trans Am Acad Ophthalmol Otolaryngol, 74:* 85, 1970.
13. Rubinstein, K., and Myska, V.: Treatment of diabetic maculopathy with photocoagulation: limitation and prospects for retinal surgery, *Mod Prob Ophthalmol, 12:* 272, 1974.
14. Patz, A., Schatz, H., Ryan, S.J., Berkow, J.W., and Lazarus, M.G.: Argon laser photocoagulation for treatment of advanced diabetic retinopathy. *Trans Am Acad Ophthalmol Otolaryngol, 76:* 984, 1972.
15. Patz, A., Schatz, H., Berkow, J.W., Gittlesohn, A.M., and Ticho, U.: Macular edema: an overlooked complication of diabetic retinopathy. *Trans Am Acad Ophthalmol Otolaryngol, 77:* 34, 1973.
16. Bresnick, G.H., DeVenecia, G., Myers, F.L., Harris, J.A., and Davis, M.D.: Retinal ischemia in diabetic retinopathy. *Arch Ophthalmol, 93:* 1300, 1975.
17. Schatz, H., and Patz, A.: Cystoid maculopathy in diabetics. *Arch Ophthalmol, 94:* 761, 1976.
18. Diabetic Retinopathy Study Research Group: Preliminary report on effects of photocoagulation therapy. *Am J Ophthalmol, 81:* 383, 1976.
19. Gitter, K.A. (ed.): Current Concepts of the Vitreous Including Vitrectomy, C.V. Mosby, St. Louis, 1976.

CHAPTER 8

Retinal Occlusive Disease

Arnall Patz, M.D. and Ronald L. Radius, M.D.

Arterial Occlusion

As early as 1859, von Graefe [1] described the familiar picture of an acute occlusion of the central retinal artery. The typical patient complains of a sudden and dramatic loss of vision. Fundus examination reveals attenuated arterioles and blood segmentation within the retinal veins (Table 8.1). The retina rapidly loses its transparency, assuming a milky white appearance reflecting cloudy swelling and coagulative necrosis within the ganglion cell and nerve fiber layers [2–4]. The absence of inner retinal layers at the fovea allows visualization of the normal choroidal pattern producing the characteristic red spot. Branch retinal artery or cilioretinal artery occlusions produce essentially identical fundus pathology limited to the involved retinal quadrant or sector. Fluorescein angiography reveals an absence or delay in the perfusion of the obstructed vessels (Fig. 8.1).

The pathogenesis of these occlusions can be grouped into three major categories including angiospastic, embolic, and thromboangiitic etiologies [5] (Table 8.2). It remains a controversial question what role vascular spasm may play in retinal arterial occlusion, but in patients with angiospastic symptomatology including migraine and Raynaud's disease, vascular occlusion secondary to arterial spasm has been described [6–9].

Embolic phenomena appear to be of greater significance in producing arterial obstruction. Various sources of emboli have been implicated in arterial occlusion, especially in cases of tributary obstruction which is characteristically an embolic event. Most frequently emboli are atheromatous debris including cholesterol, platelets, and fibrin as well as other blood products [10–14]. Numerous vascular lesions including carotid atheromatous plaques, rheumatic vegetations, valvular disease, mural thrombi, valve prostheses, and even septic endocarditis have been implicated as the source of these arterial emboli [4, 15–19]. Other embolic phenomena have included atrial myxomata, fat, air, and various iatrogenically introduced materials [5, 20–24] (Table 8.3).

The most frequent cause of arterial occlusion, however, is thrombosis which may account for as much as 80% of all obstructions [5]. Carotid and ophthalmic artery disease contributes to the incidence of retinal artery occlusion by reducing vascular perfusion [25]. Other disease states associated with retinal thrombosis include Buerger's disease, dissecting aneurysm of the ophthalmic artery, cranial arteritis, local orbital disease, polyarteritis nodosa, sickle cell disease, and elevated intraocular pressure [26–35] (Table 8.4).

In an effort to identify the correct etiology in a given occlusion, various clinical parameters should be investigated. Medical consultation may be requested, especially to evaluate the possibility of embolic disease from cardiac as well as vascular pathology. A complete blood count, collagen vascular disease screen, hemoglobin electrophoresis, and lipid screen are indicated (Table 8.5). An erythrocyte sedimentation rate is certainly important, but if the clinical presentation is suggestive of cranial arteritis, steroid therapy must be instituted without delay. Finally, the suggestion that retinal vascular occlusion portends more extensive embolic disease remains unanswered. Nevertheless, in younger patients, or in any patient with symptomatology suggestive of embolic disease, cardiac angiography should be considered [36–38].

Whatever the etiology, an arterial occlusion represents a true ocular emergency. Various modes of therapeutic intervention have been suggested [5, 34] (Table 8.6). Massage to reduce intraocular pressure as well as propel an embolus into more peripheral vessels appears to be beneficial. Rapid decompression of ocular tension is most effectively accomplished by anterior chamber paracentesis [39]. Subsequently, medications such as carbonic anhydrase inhibitors may be utilized to maintain a state of relative ocular hypotension. Efforts at vasodilatation including ganglionic blockade, retrobulbar aminophylline and tolazoline have met with success in isolated cases [34, 40]. High oxygen tension (95%) with carbon dioxide (5%) to relieve vasoconstriction is advocated, but great care must be exercised to recognize early signs of toxicity especially in patients with cardiopulmonary disease [34, 41]. The effectiveness of anticoagulant and thrombolytic agents has not been conclusively demonstrated, and both medications have a high risk potential. Although these efforts may often seem heroic, experimental and clinical experience suggest that if adequate perfusion can be restored within from 1–2 hours, return of good visual function can be expected [33, 39, 43–46].

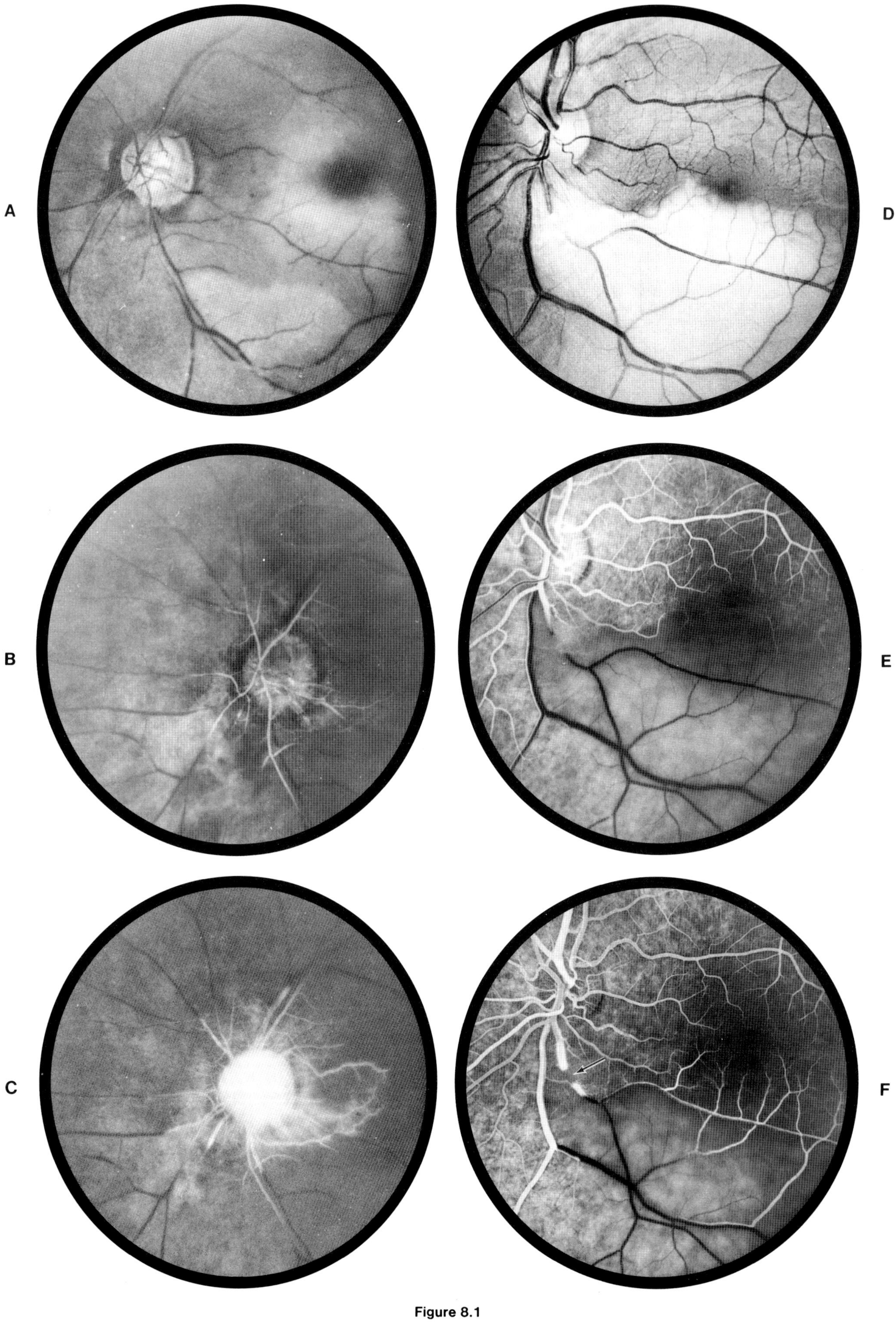

Figure 8.1

G

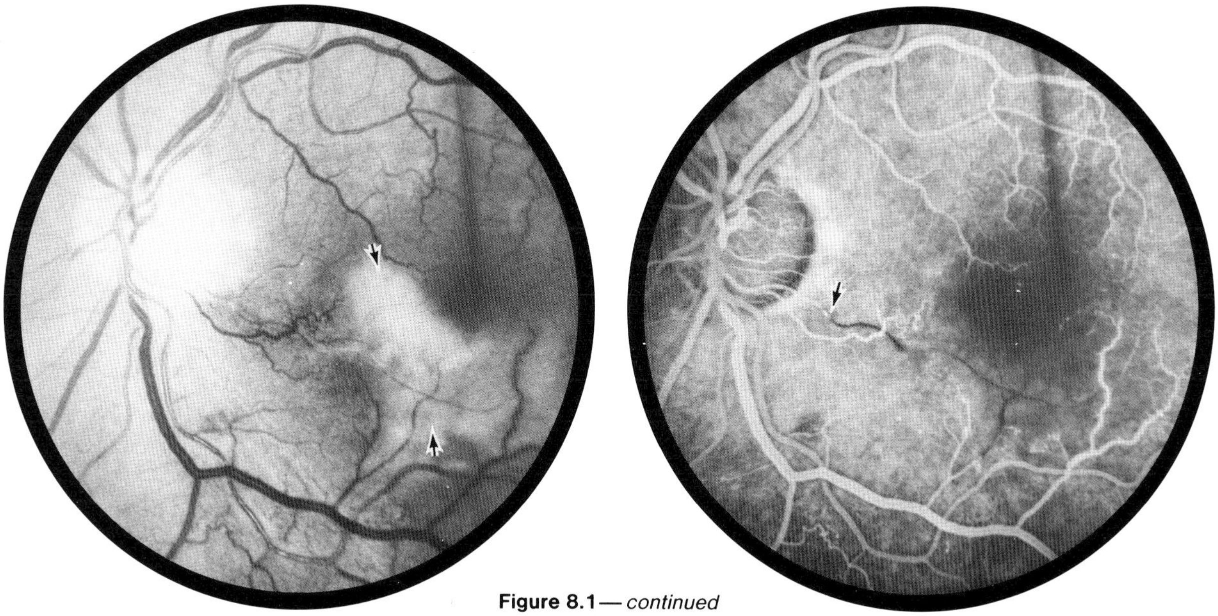

H

Figure 8.1—*continued*

Figure 8.1. Arterial occlusions. *A,* ophthalmoscopic photograph of central retinal artery occlusion. Note the generalized retinal vascular attenuation, the cloudy swelling of the retina, and the cherry red spot. *B,* early phase angiogram, same patient. Note the incomplete filling of the central retinal artery and its branches. *C,* late phase angiogram, same patient. Note that the occlusion is complete and only corresponding segments of veins show hyperfluorescence. *D,* ophthalmoscopic photograph of a branch artery occlusion. Note the cloudy swelling along the inferotemporal arcade. *E,* arterial phase angiogram, same patient. Note the nonperfusion of the inferotemporal artery and its branches. *F,* arteriovenous phase angiogram, same patient. Note that the site of occlusion is still hypofluorescent (*arrow*). Distal to the occlusion, the involved artery is being perfused in a retrograde fashion. *G,* ophthalmoscopic photograph of branch arteriolar occlusion. Note the cloudy swelling of the retina in the inferior and nasal macular (*arrows*). *H,* late venous phase angiogram, same patient. Note the obstructed branch retinal artery in the juxtapapillary area (*arrow*). There is delayed filling of the corresponding venules and widespread compensatory capillary dilatation. (Courtesy of Thomas C. Burton, M.D.)

Table 8.1 Clinical picture in arterial occlusion

Marked fall in visual acuity
Afferent pupillary defect
Thinned arterioles
Segmentation in veins
Necrosis of ganglion cell layer
Cherry red spot
Decrease in b-wave of ERG

Table 8.2. Etiology of arterial occlusion

Angiospasm
Migraine
Raynaud's disease
Embolism
Thrombo-angiitis

Table 8.3. Embolus

Cholesterol-platelets-fibrin
Carotid disease
Mural thrombus
Rheumatic disease
Endocarditis
Atrial myxoma
Valvular disease
Fat embolus
Air embolus
Iatrogenically induced materials

Table 8.4. Thrombosis

Retinal arterial atheroma
Carotid atheroma
Ophthalmic artery aneurysm
Orbital disease
Beurger's disease
Cranial arteritis
Polyarteritis nodosa
Sickle cell disease
Ocular hypertension

Table 8.5. Patient evaluation

Medical consultation
Hematology profile
Hemoglobin electrophoresis
Erythrocyte sedimentation
Lipid screen
Collagen vascular screen
Cardiovascular angiography

Table 8.6. Treatment of arterial occlusion

Anterior chamber paracentesis
Ocular massage
Carbonic anhydrase inhibitor
95% oxygen, 5% carbon dioxide
Amyl nitrate
Retrobulbar aminophylline
Ganglionic blockade
Anticoagulation
Thrombolytic agents
Surgical decompression of optic nerve

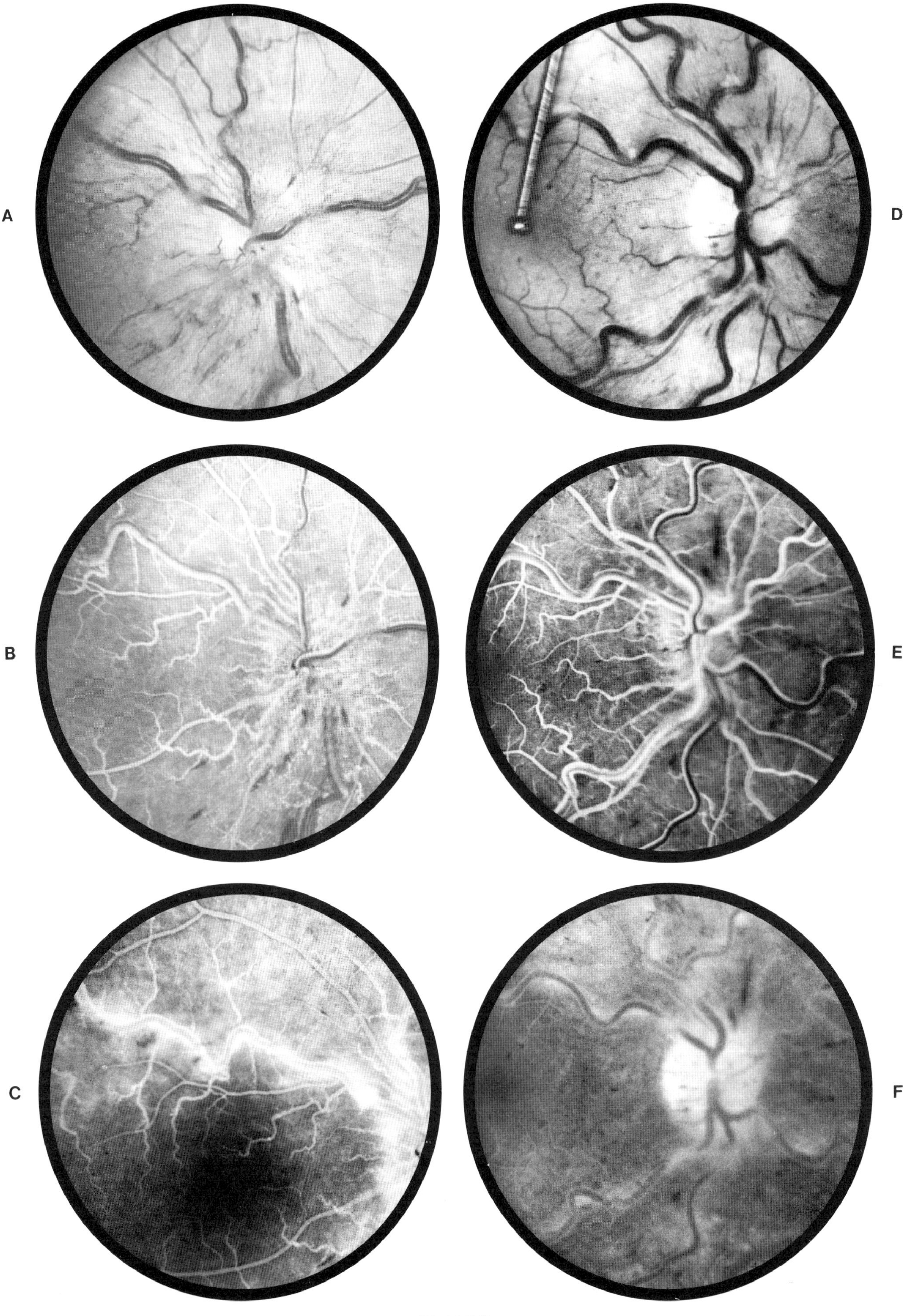

Figure 8.2

Venous Occlusion

Central retinal vein thrombosis presents an equally dramatic fundus appearance (Table 8.7). Dilated, engorged tortuous retinal vessels, superficial and deep retinal vessels, superficial and deep retinal hemorrhages scattered widely throughout the fundus, and variable degrees of retinal edema, collateralization, and ischemia are apparent. Hayreh [47] has suggested that central retinal vein occlusion represents two distinct clinical entities: venous stasis retinopathy and hemorrhagic retinopathy (Figs. 8.2 and 8.3).

Venous stasis retinopathy is the more common form of representation, involving a complete occlusion of the central retinal vein without significant hypoxia or ischemia. It has been associated erroneously with such terms as "partial," "incipient," or "impending" central retinal vein occlusion. It is a relatively benign, self-limiting condition. The ultimate visual recovery potential depends on the severity and duration of the induced macular edema and possibly the site of the occlusion; i.e., the deeper the site of the occlusion within the optic nerve, the greater the potential for compensatory collateralization available, the less severe the retinopathy, and the better the prognosis.

Hayreh has further divided venous stasis retinopathy into two groups. The condition in young patients appears to be on the basis of a phlebitis of the central retinal vein, which produces venous thrombosis. In older patients the thrombosis appears to be related to atherosclerosis of the adjacent central retinal artery. Fluorescein angiography in both instances shows an accentuation of the engorged vessels, venous filling defects, and variable degrees of disc, macular and perivascular leakage. (Fig. 8.2). The phlebitis in younger patients is also evident angiographically as late perivascular leakage.

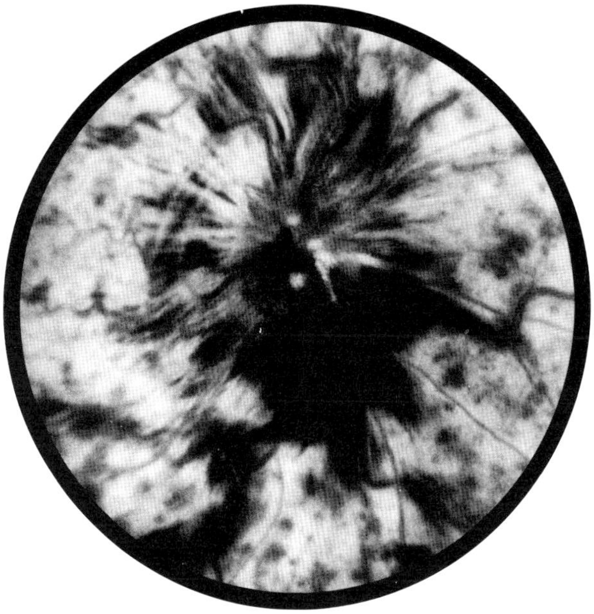

G

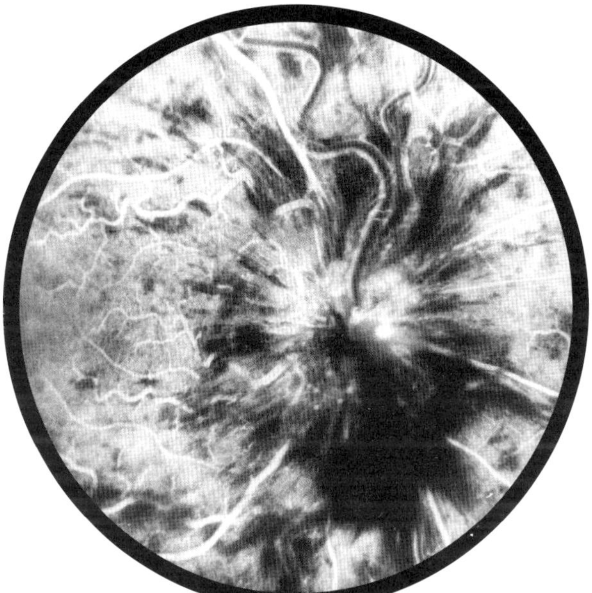

H

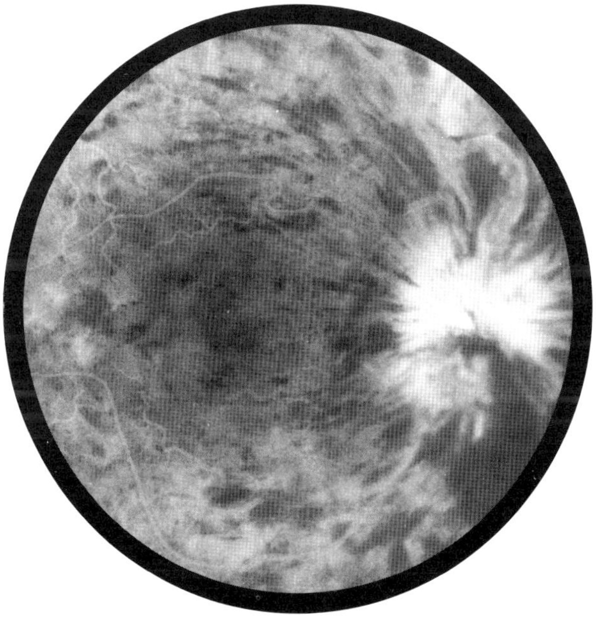

I

Figure 8.2. Central retinal vein thrombosis (venous stasis retinopathy). *A*, ophthalmoscopic photograph of a 20-year-old female with 20/20 vision. Note the dilated tortuous retinal veins, disc edema, and scattered hemorrhages in this case of papillophlebitis. *B*, arteriovenous phase angiogram. Note the markedly dilated superficial papillary and deep papillary capillaries and the multifocal areas of hyperfluorescence along the course of numerous veins. *C*, late venous phase angiogram. Note the disc edema and the segmental perivascular late hyperfluorescence of the veins, indicative of phlebitis. *D*, ophthalmoscopic photograph of a mild case of venous stasis retinopathy. Note the marked venous engorgement and dilatation and the scattered hemorrhages in four quadrants. A fixation target is centered at the macula. *E*, arteriovenous phase angiogram, same patient. Note the scattered hemorrhages produced by superficial and deep intraretinal hemorrhages. The retinovascular perfusion is delayed. *F*, late phase angiogram, same patient. Note the disc and perivascular staining. Some dye leakage into the posterior vitreous obscures some of the fundus details. There is minimal edema in the macula of this patient with 20/20 visual acuity. *G*, ophthalmoscopic photograph of a severe case of venous stasis retinopathy in a middle-aged patient. Note the widespread retinal hemorrhages and massive hemorrhage at the disc. *H*, arteriovenous phase angiogram, same patient. There is blocked hypofluorescence from hemorrhages and marked vascular tortuosity. There is good arteriolar perfusion with no evidence of ischemia. *I*, late phase angiogram. Note the marked disc and perivascular staining. There is a moderate degree of cystoid edema present in this patient with 20/50 visual acuity.

Figure 8.2—*continued*

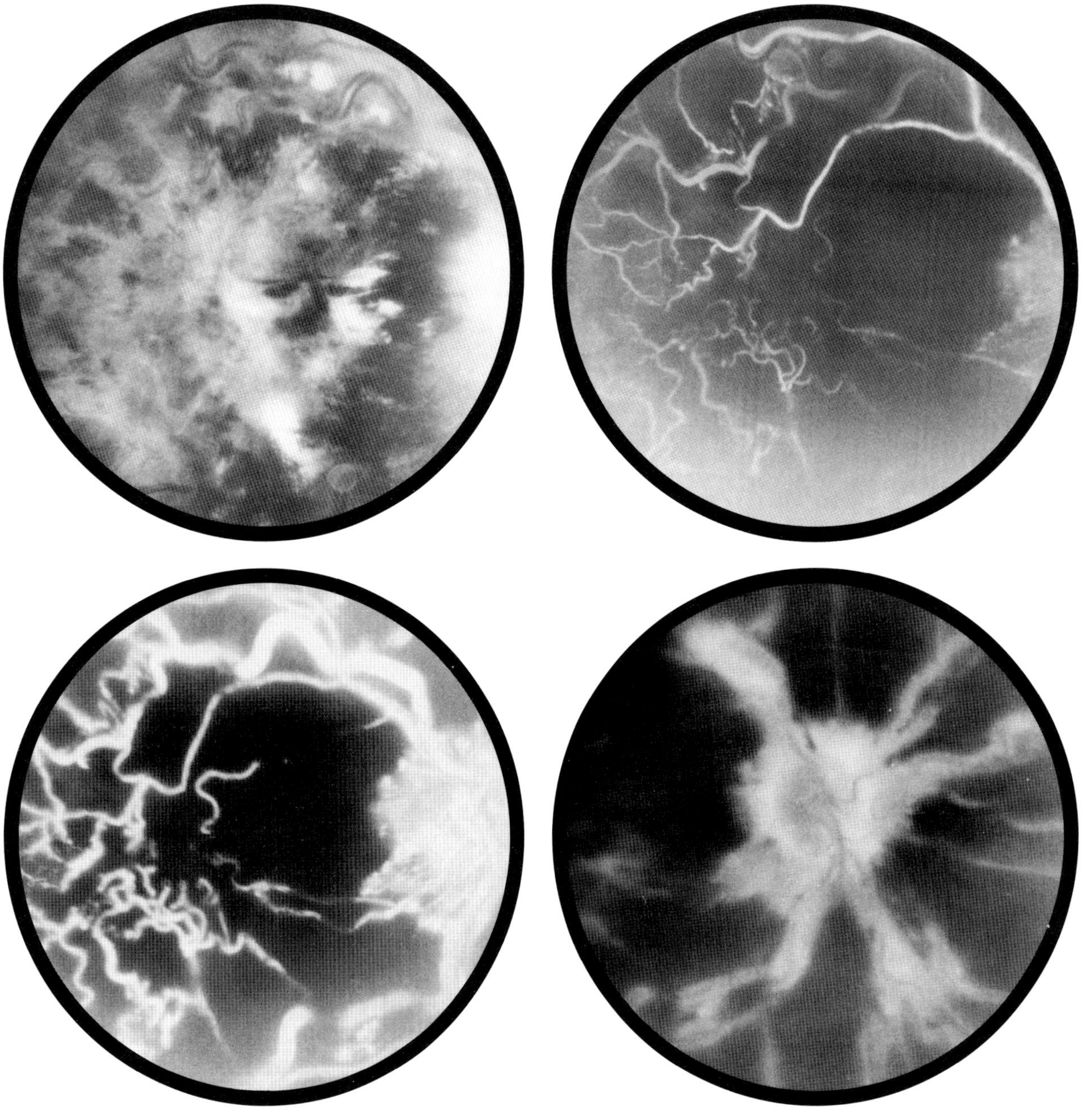

A B C D

Figure 8.3. Central retinal vein thrombosis (hemorrhagic retinopathy). *A,* ophthalmoscopic photograph. Note the massive hemorrhage and exudation in the macula associated with dilated and tortuous retinal veins and disc swelling. *B,* arterial phase angiogram. Note the extensive hypofluorescence from blockage caused by hemorrhage and exudation, but also by a severe degree of arteriolar ischemia and capillary nonperfusion throughout the macula. *C,* late venous phase angiogram. Widespread hypofluorescence persists, and there is early staining at the nerve and along the larger venules. *D,* late phase angiogram. Note the extensive leakage along the course of the retinal vessels in four quadrants and at the nerve head.

Hemorrhagic retinopathy occurs much less frequently than venous stasis retinopathy. Unlike venous stasis retinopathy which occurs in young or middle-aged patients, hemorrhagic retinopathy is seen most often in patients past middle age. The occlusion of the central retinal vein in this condition is associated with marked retinal ischemia. The visual acuity and field are more significantly depressed in this disorder. Larger hemorrhages, cotton-wool spots, more pronounced disc edema, and more extensive atherosclerosis of the arterioles are seen in this form of central vein occlusion.

The fluorescein angiogram in hemorrhagic retinopathy reveals all of the changes seen in venous stasis retinopathy but, in addition, delayed or incomplete arteriolar filling and capillary nonperfusion predominate (Fig. 8.3).

A poor visual prognosis from capillary obliteration of the macula, cystic macular degeneration, vitreous hemorrhage, and thrombotic glaucoma are more common in this variety.

The etiology of venous occlusion remains unclear (Table 8.8). Hayreh [47] has suggested that the characteristic central vein occlusion cannot occur without significant arterial disease. In many instances, primary arterial disease is the dominant factor in producing venous pathology and obstruction [42, 44, 48–51]. Sclerotic arterial disease, encroaching upon an adjacent vein, produces a reactive endothelial proliferation and ultimate thrombosis. The observation that tributary venous occlusions occur uniformly at arteriovenous crossings supports this hypothesis. Similarly, frequent association with hypertensive vascular disease is incriminating [42, 50]. Other investigators have indicated, however, that primary venous disease may occur in certain instances of clinical occlusion. Stagnation of blood flow within the venous channels almost certainly shares a significant role in producing these occlusions. Central retinal vein obstruction has been described in a variety of conditions which indict this common mechanism. These states include severe carotid disease, various hyperviscosity syndromes, glaucoma, and phlebitis [5, 34, 42, 48, 49, 51–53].

Management of central venous occlusion has been generally unrewarding [5, 34]. Several authors have noted a beneficial response to systemic anticoagulant therapy although this therapy has not been conclusively documented [42, 50–51, 54]. Fibrinolytic agents have not been adequately evaluated [50]. Management of secondary complications including hemorrhagic glaucoma and retinal neovascularization has been similarly discouraging. Probably the most beneficial intervention the clinician can make is to institute a general systemic examination to investigate the various possible etiologies of a given venous occlusion. Nevertheless, continued investigation of anticoagulation, enzymatic fibrinolysis, and photocoagulation may yield effective modes of therapeutic intervention. The role of photocoagulation deserves special consideration in view of its widespread usage for branch vein occlusion. There is a significant priority for branch vein occlusion, as next to diabetic retinopathy it is the most frequent retinal vascular disorder encountered by the ophthalmologist. The most common cause of visual impairment in patients with branch vein occlusion is macular edema.

It is convenient to classify the branch vein occlusions according to the locus of the occlusion (Fig. 8.4). In the vast majority of patients, the site of obstruction is at an arteriolar venous crossing. The occlusion can be near the disc margin, involving a major branch vein, between the disc margin and the macular area, or involving a small macular tributary branch vein (Fig. 8.5). Occasional occlusions may be temporal to the macula. Patients suffering nasal branch vein occlusions may have the obstruction anywhere along the distribution of the nasal vessels; however, nasal branch vein occlusions do not cause visual impairment from macular edema.

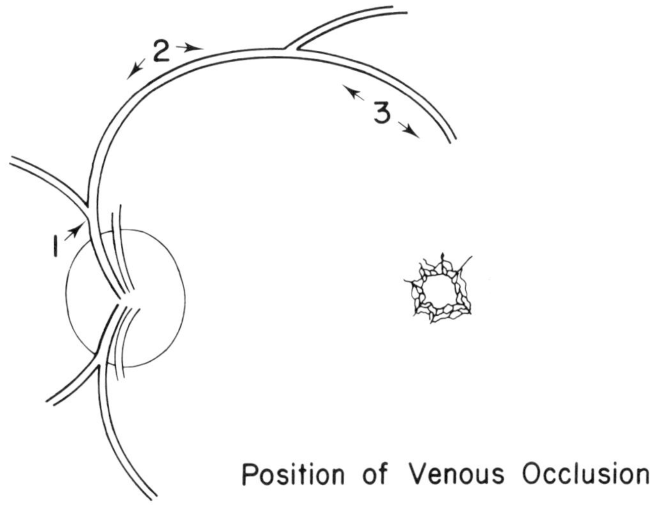

Figure 8.4. Diagrammatic representation of most common sites of branch vein occlusion: (1) near the disc margin, (2) between the disc margin and macula, and (3) at the small macular tributary branch vein.

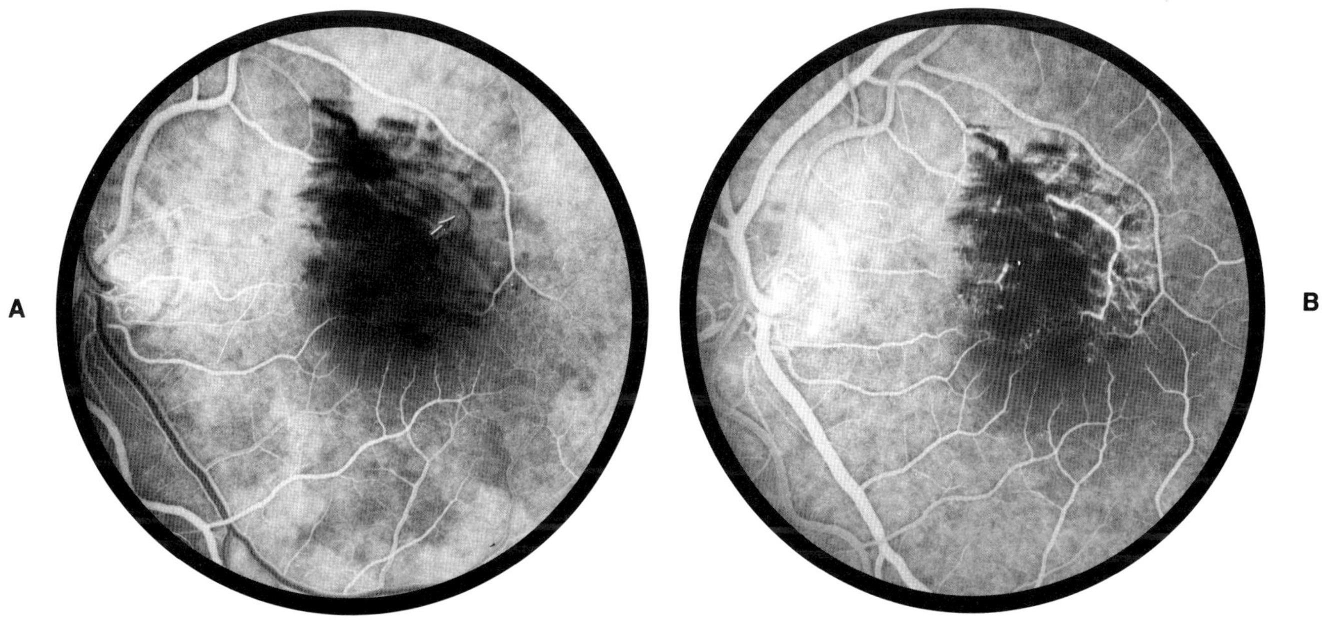

Figure 8.5. Arteriovenous phase fluorescein angiogram of branch vein occlusion. *A*, note the delayed filling of superotemporal branch vein occlusion (*arrow*) and associated intraretinal hemorrhage. *B*, venous phase angiogram showing late staining of the involved vein and mild dilation and tortuosity of the surrounding capillary bed.

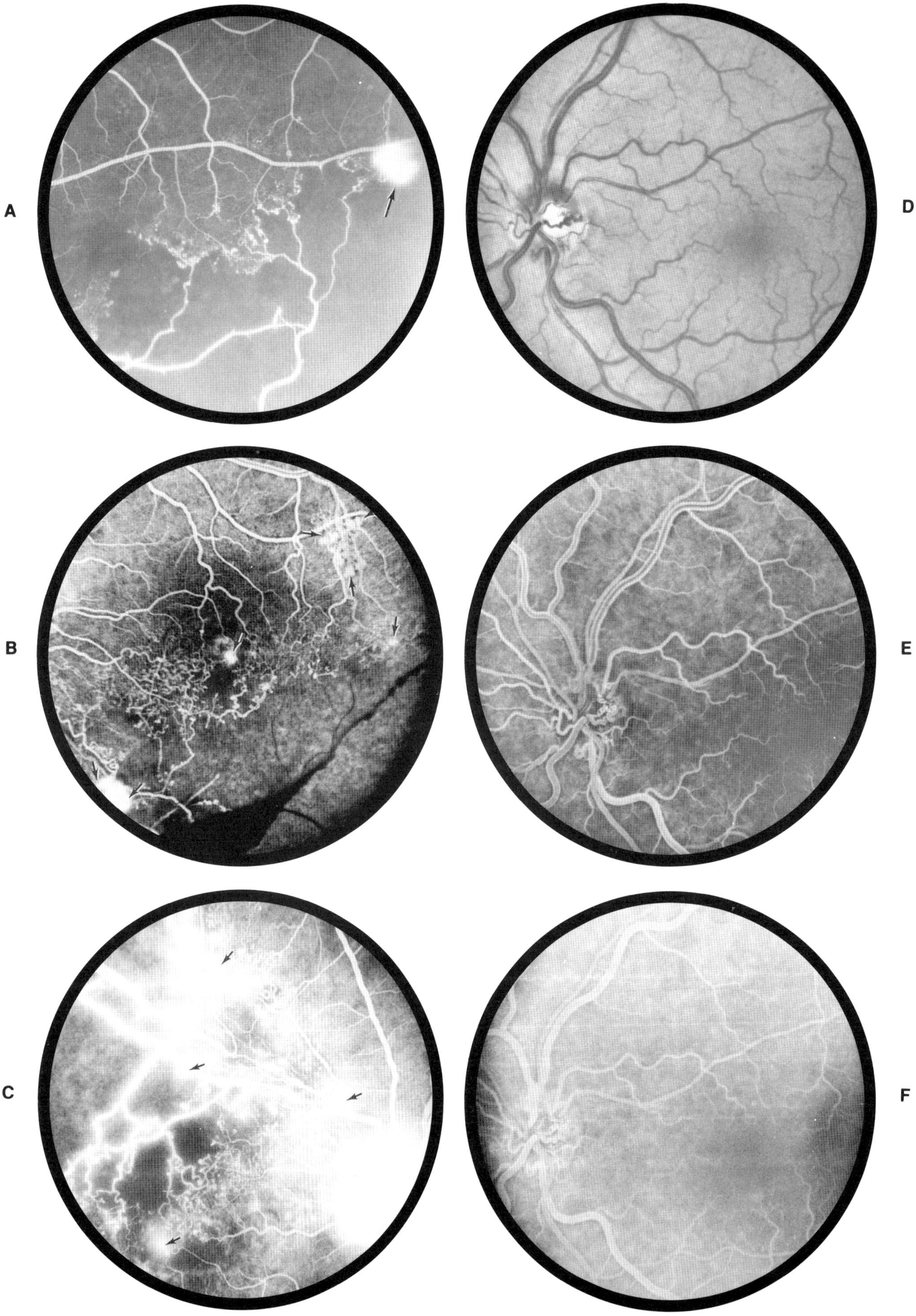

Figure 8.6

In addition to the common problem of macular edema in these patients, not infrequently, patients with long-standing major branch vein occlusion will develop neovascularization at the disc or in the area immediately adjacent to the area of nonperfusion in the quadrant involved by the occlusion (Fig. 8.6, *A–C*). Abnormal disc vessels following central retinal vein thromboses are invariably retinal ciliary collaterals except in hemorrhagic retinopathy when disc neovascularization may rarely occur (Fig. 8.6, *D–F*). Frequently, collateral vessels in branch vein occlusion develop immediately around the area of venous obstruction, and collateralization across the horizontal raphe into the vascular bed in the opposite vertical portion of the fundus takes place (Fig. 8.7). Long-standing branch vein occlusion may result in internal limiting membrane contracture and disturbance of the underlying retinal pigment epithelium. It is important to recognize that small macular tributary branch vein occlusions near the center of the macula may present no visible signs on routine fundus examination.

Table 8.7. Clinical picture in venous occlusion

Dilated tortuous veins
Deep punctate hemorrhage
Diffuse deep and superficial hemorrhage
Rarely, soft exudate and ischemic infarct
Disc edema
Retinal edema
Vitreous hemorrhage

Table 8.8. Factors in venous occlusion

Arterial disease
Hypertension
Diabetes
Dysproteinemias
Polycythemia
Hemoglobinopathies
Lymphocytoses
Glaucoma
Phlebitis

A

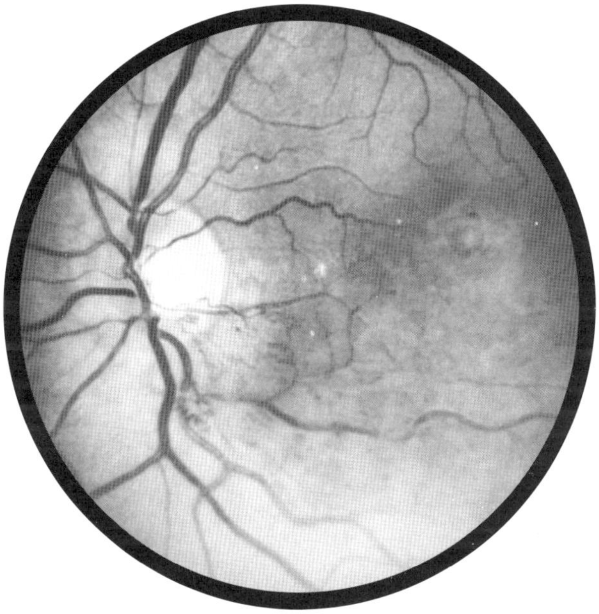

B

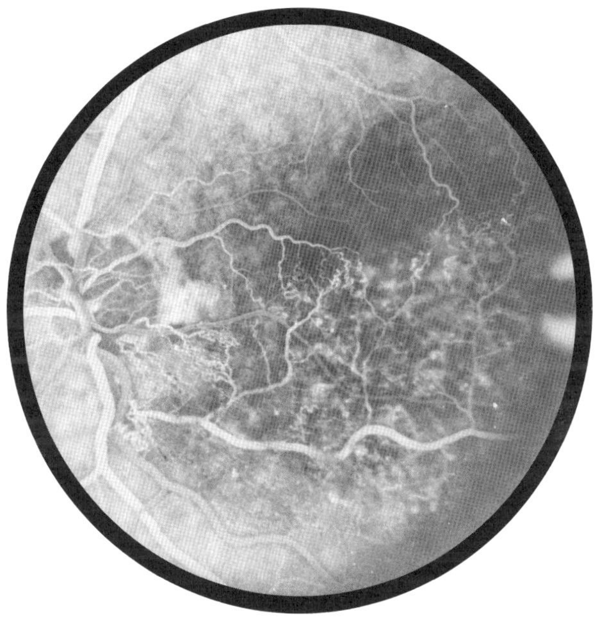

Figure 8.7. *A*, ophthalmoscopic photograph of an inferior temporal branch vein occlusion showing three typical locations of dilated collateral vessels: between the area of obstruction and disc, near the area of obstruction, and across the horizontal raphe. *B*, early venous phase fluorescein angiogram of same patient demonstrating collateral blood flow as described.

Figure 8.6. *A*, arteriovenous phase angiogram of long-standing branch vein occlusion showing large zones of capillary nonperfusion, intraretinal microangiography, and an adjacent patch of neovascularization (*arrow*). *B*, arteriovenous phase angiogram of a patient with an inferotemporal branch vein occlusion. Note the capillary nonperfusion, the irregular band of hypofluorescence from vitreous hemorrhage, the compensatory collaterals crossing the horizontal raphe, and multiple areas of neovascularization (*arrows*). *C*, late venous phase anglogram showing disc neovascularization secondary to branch vein occlusion. Note the "cotton-like" hyperfluorescence at the optic nerve head secondary to neovascularization. Compensatory venous/venous collaterolization is evident along the horizontal and from retinal neovascularization adjacent to ischemic areas (*arrows*). (Courtesy of Dr. Hong-Zen Lin and Mr. Michael Feldman.) *D*, ophthalmoscopic photograph of retinociliary disc collateralization following central vein thrombosis. Note the dilated and irregular vessels at the nerve head. There is widespread retinal vascular prominence but no other gross fundus abnormality in this eye with antecedent central retinal vein thrombosis. *E*, arteriovenous phase angiogram, same patient. Note the filling of the retinal venous ciliary venous collaterals at the nerve head. *F*, late venous phase angiogram, same patient. These collaterals reveal no evidence of leakage differentiating them from neovascularization. The retinal vascular transient time was normal, and the macula was free of edema. Thus, the only evidence of previous central vein thrombosis in this eye is the presence of the retinal-ciliary collaterals at the nerve head. These collaterals are often mistaken for disc neovascularization, which is rare following central retinal venous occusion.

A B C

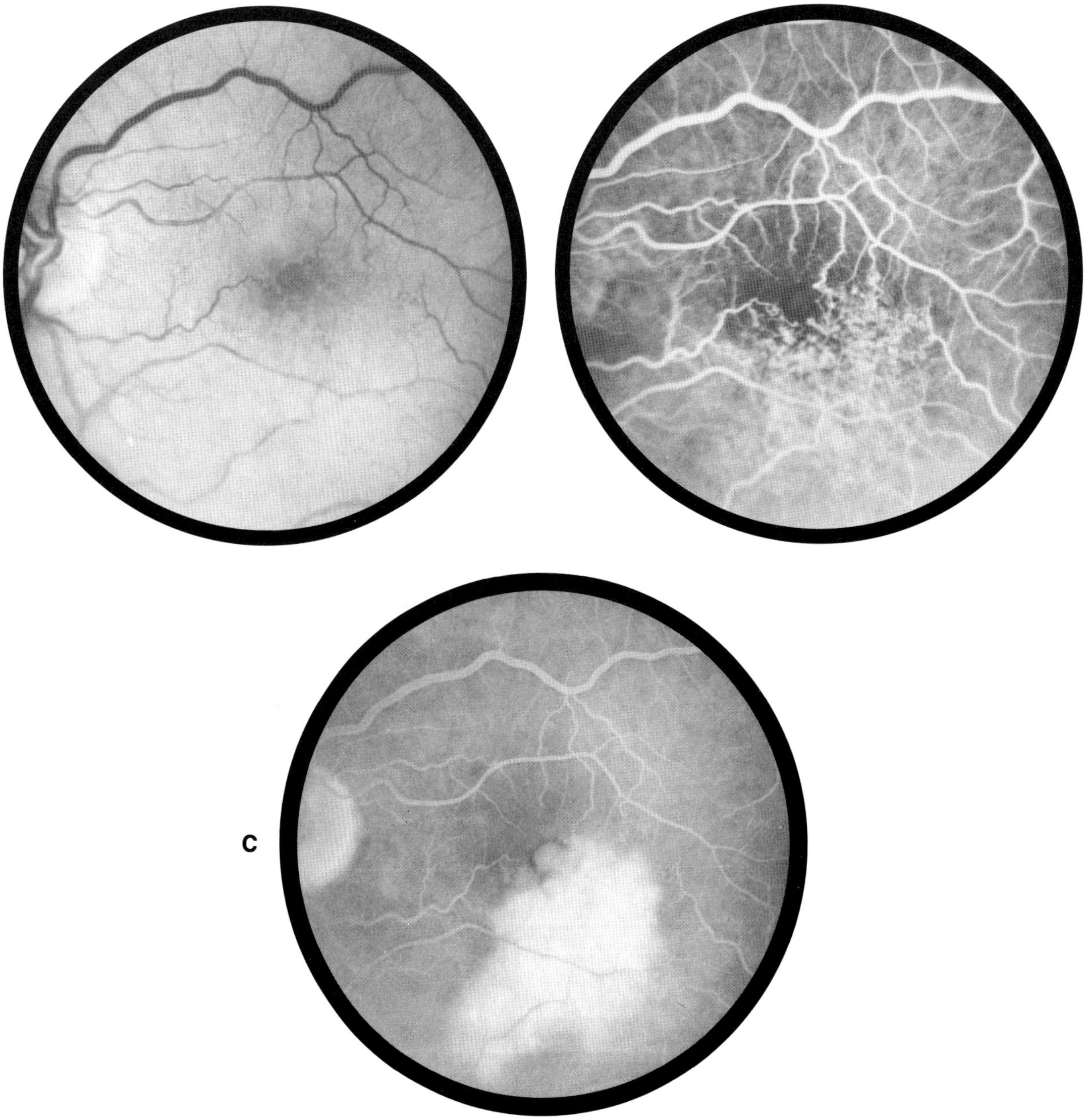

Figure 8.8. *A*, ophthalmoscopic photograph of a patient with small inferior macular tributary branch vein obstruction with a surprisingly normal fundus. *B*, early venous phase fluorescein angiogram of the same patient dramatically demonstrates microvascular abnormalities and collateral vessels crossing the mid-line raphe characteristic of venous obstruction. *C*, late phase angiogram, showing retinal staining with leakage of fluorescein and cystoid macular edema, responsible for decreased visual acuity.

A

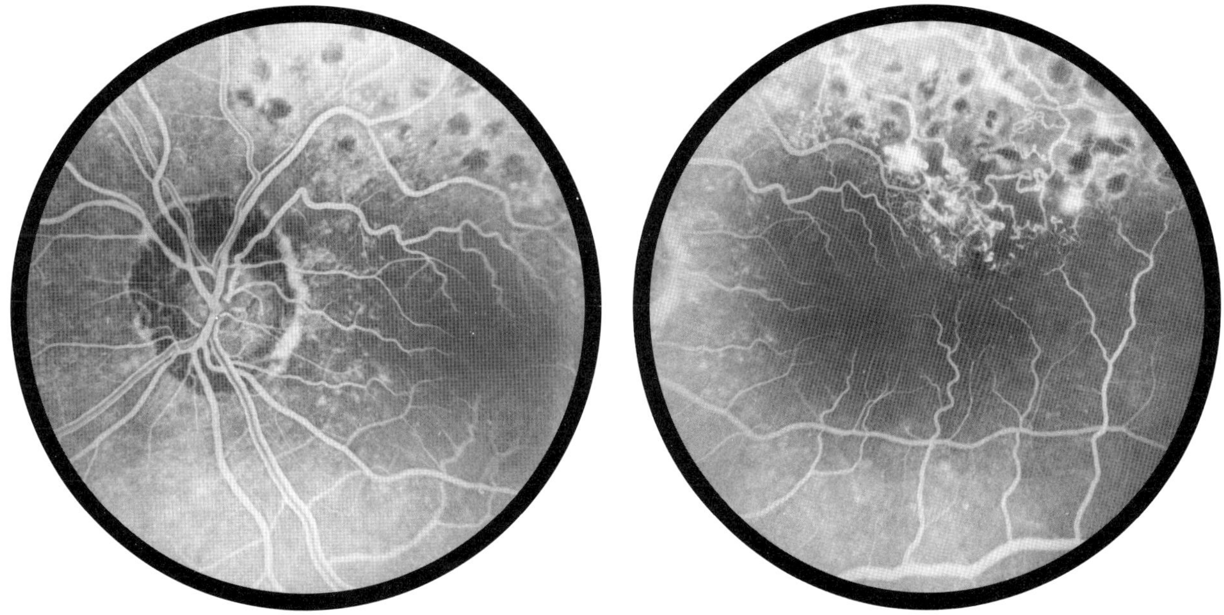

B

Figure 8.9. *A*, arteriovenous phase fluorescein angiogram, postphotocoagulation, showing typical distribution and size of therapy for a superior branch retinal vein occlusion. *B*, late venous phase angiogram, same patient, showing focal dye leakage in macular area.

Even with the slit-lamp and contact lens examination, no obvious residual of the branch vein occlusion may be detected, unless there is some cystoid macular edema. Only with fluorescein angiography will the retinal vascular abnormalities be detected as illustrated in Fig. 8.8.

The treatment of branch vein obstruction is highly controversial. Since the results of anticoagulant therapy are inconclusive, we do not recommend their usage. In recent years, photocoagulation has been advocated by many investigators. Unfortunately, these studies have not been conducted on the basis of a randomized controlled clinical trial. Furthermore, the natural history studies of Michels and Gass [55] and of Gutman and Zegarra [56] have shown that about 50% of patients with branch vein occlusion maintain fairly good vision (20/50 or better) during a significant period of follow-up. Since the remaining patients in these series and approximately 50% of our own cases [57] will lose a significant degree of visual acuity, we have instituted and are presently participating in a randomized controlled clinical trial to test, as objectively as feasible, the role of photocoagulation for patients with branch vein occlusion.

Our management of patients in the controlled study that is now under way consists of: first, categorizing the patient according to the locus of the obstruction; and, second, considering the patient in terms of presence or absence of neovascularization either at the disc or elsewhere in the general area of the obstruction. No patient is considered for photocoagulation until a minimum of 6 months lapse following the initial symptoms to be certain that sufficient time has elapsed for the development of collateral vessels and to permit whatever compensation will occur spontaneously to develop. It is recognized that even after 6 months an occasional patient will develop further collateralization and compensation of his obstruction. After this interval, patients who have visual impairment down to the level of 20/40 as a result of macular edema are then randomly assigned to treatment (or no treatment) based on a computer-generated table of random numbers. Since the mean follow-up period is only 1½ years at the time of this writing, it is much too early to present any data concerning therapy.

Since the ophthalmologist, when faced with a patient with branch vein occlusion, may not be in a position to enroll that patient in a controlled clinical study, some practical guidelines can be made for the management of these patients. First, photocoagulation should not be considered, in our opinion, for a minimum of 6 months following the initial vascular obstruction. Second, unless the visual acuity has been compromised to at least the level of 20/40, we do not recommend therapy. In these cases with 20/40 or worse vision, we recommend photocoagulation therapy and we prefer the argon laser modality as the energy of choice. For those not having argon laser photocoagulation capability, the xenon arc can be used with special care in treating within 1 disc diameter of the center of the fovea. The distribution of treatment is shown in Fig. 8.9. In placement of the photocoagulation lesions we try to cover the entire area of nonperfusion involved in the venous obstruction. We deliberately avoid coming closer than 1 disc diameter to the center of the fovea with scatter-type of treatment.

We recommend treatment of all patients showing obvious neovascularization, either from the disc or in the area of obstruction away from the disc, using a scatter-type of distribution covering the entire area of nonperfusion up to 1½ disc diameters from the center of the fovea. If the patient had sustained a vitreal hemorrhage from the neovascularization, we recommend that treatment be deferred until the media is sufficiently clear to provide good visualization for the area to be treated.

References

1. von Graefe, A.: Über Embolie der Arteria centralis retinae als Ursache plötzlicher Erblindung. *Albrecht von Graefes Arch Ophthalmol, 5:* 136, 1859.
2. Kroll, A.J.: Experimental central retinal artery occlusion. *Arch Ophthalmol, 79:* 453, 1968.
3. Reinecke, R.D., Kuwabara, T., Cogan, D.G., and Weis, R.D.: Retinal vascular patterns. V. Experimental ischemia of the cat eye. *Arch Ophthalmol, 67:* 470, 1962.
4. Zimmerman, L.E.: Embolism of central retinal artery secondary to myocardial infarction with mural thrombosis. *Arch Ophthalmol, 73:* 822, 1965.
5. Duke-Elder, S. (ed.): System of Ophthalmology, vol. 10: Diseases of the Retina, C.V. Mosby, St. Louis, 1967.
6. Wagener, H.P. and Gipner, J.F.: Arterial spasm in production of occlusion of branches of central artery of the retina. *Am J Ophthalmol, 10:* 650, 1927.
7. Krapin, D.: Occlusion of the central retinal artery in migraine. *N Engl J Med, 270:* 359, 1964.
8. Anderson, R.G., and Gray, E.B.: Spasm of the central retinal artery in Raynaud's disease: report of a case. *Arch Ophthalmol, 17:* 662, 1937.
9. Dunphy, E.B.: Ocular manifestations of Raynaud's disease. *Trans Am Ophthalmol Soc, 30:* 420, 1932.
10. Hollenhorst, R.W., Lensink, E.R., and Whisnant, J.P.: Experimental embolization of retinal arterioles. *Trans Am Ophthalmol Soc, 60:* 316, 1962.
11. Ball, C.J.: Atheromatous embolism to the brain, retina and choroid. *Arch Ophthalmol, 76:* 690, 1966.
12. Honour, A.J., and Russell, R.R.: Intra-arterial embolism in response to injury. *Trans Ophthalmol Soc U K, 81:* 451, 1961.
13. Russell, R.W.R.: Atheromatous retinal embolism. *Lancet, 2:* 1354, 1963.
14. Denny-Brown, D.: Reccurent cerebrovascular episodes. *Arch Neurol, 2:* 194, 1960.
15. Hollenhorst, R.W.: Carotid and vertebral-basilar arterial stenosis and occlusion: neuro-ophthalmologic considerations. *Trans Am Acad Ophthalmol Otolaryngol, 66:* 166, 1962.
16. Hollenhorst, R.W.: Significance of bright plaques in the retinal arterioles. *Trans Am Ophthalmol Soc, 59:* 252, 1961.
17. Penner, R., and Font, R.L.: Retinal embolism from calcified vegetations of aortic valve: a spontaneous complication of rheumatic heart disease. *Arch Ophthalmol, 81:* 565, 1969.
18. Woldoff, H.S., Gerber, M., Desser, K.B., and Benchimol, A.: Retinal vascular lesions in two patients with prolapsed mitral valve leaflets. *Am J Ophthalmol, 79:* 382, 1975.
19. Ide, C.H., Almond, C.H., Hart, W.M., Simmons, E.M., and Wilson, R.J.: Hematogenous dissemination of microemboli: eye findings in a patient with Starr-Edwards aortic prosthesis. *Arch Ophthalmol, 76:* 769, 1973.
20. Anderson, J.D., and Lubow, M.: Atrial myxoma as a source of retinal embolism. *Am J Ophthalmol, 76:* 769, 1973.
21. Jampol, L.M., Wong, A.S., and Albert, D.L.: Atrial myxoma and central retinal artery occlusion. *Am J Ophthalmol, 75:* 242, 1973.
22. Inkeles, D.M., and Walsh, J.B.: Retinal fat emboli as a sequela to acute pancreatitis. *Am J Ophthalmol, 80:* 935, 1975.
23. Landolt, E.: Ein Fall von Fettembolie der Augen. *Klin Monatsbl Augenheilkd, 131:* 538, 1957.
24. Sachsenweger, R.: Luftembolie und Auge. *Klin Monatsbl Augenheilkd, 130:* 813, 1957.
25. David, N.J., Norton, E.W.C., Gass, J.D.M., and Sexton, R.: Fluorescein retinal angiography in carotid occlusion. *Arch Neurol, 14:* 281, 1966.
26. Gresser, E.B.: Partial occlusion of retinal vessels in a case of thromboangitis obliterans. *Am J Ophthalmol, 15:* 235, 1932.
27. Lisch, K.: Embolie der Zentralarterie bei der Buergerschen Krankheit. *Klin Monatsbl Augenheilkd, 99:* 812, 1937.
28. Wagener, H.P., and Hollenhorst, R.W.: The ocular lesions of temporal arteritis. *Trans Am Ophthalmol Soc, 55:* 249, 1957.
29. Godfrey, R.C.: Occlusion of the retinal artery in two cases of orbital granuloma. *Brit J Ophthalmol, 53:* 703, 1969.
30. Boeck, J.: Ocular changes in periarteritis nodosa. *Am J Ophthalmol, 42:* 567, 1956.
31. Bernstein, A.: Periarteritis nodosa without peripheral nodules diagnosed antemortem. *Am J Med Sci, 190:* 317, 1935.
32. Michelson, P.E., and Pfaffenbach, D.: Retinal artery occlusion following ocular trauma in youths with sickle-trait hemoglobinopathy. *Am J Ophthalmol, 74:* 494, 1972.
33. Radius, R.L., and Finkelstein, D.: Central retinal artery occlusion (reversible) in sickle trait with glaucoma. *Brit J Ophthalmol, 60:* 428, 1976.
34. Wise, G.N., Dollery, C.T., and Henkind, P.: The Retinal Circulation, Harper & Row, New York, 1971.
35. Givner, E., and Jaffee, N.: Occlusion of the central retinal artery following anesthesia. *Arch Ophthalmol, 43:* 197, 1950.
36. Appen, R.E., Wray, S.H., and Cogan, D.G.: Central retinal artery occlusion. *Am J Ophthalmol, 79:* 374, 1975.
37. Kollarits, C.R., Lubow, M., and Hissong, S.L.: Retinal strokes. *JAMA, 222:* 1273, 1972.
38. Liversedge, L.A., and Smith, V.H.: Neuromedical and ophthalmic aspects of central retinal artery occlusion. *Trans Ophthalmol Soc U K, 82:* 571, 1962.
39. Simmonds, N.T.: Embolus of central retinal artery: successfully treated by paracentesis. *Am J Ophthalmol, 54:* 1129, 1962.
40. Leffertstra, L.J.: Results of early treatment in a case of spasm of the central retinal artery. *Ophthalmologica, 144:* 433, 1962.
41. Patz, A.: Oxygen inhalation in retinal arterial occlusion: a preliminary report. *Am J Ophthalmol, 40:* 789, 1955.
42. Anderson, B., and Vallotton, W.: Etiology and therapy of retinal vascular occulsions. *Arch Ophthalmol, 54:* 6, 1955.
43. Arden, G.B., and Greaves, D.P.: The reversible alterations of the electroretinogram of the rabbit after occlusion of the retinal circulation. *J Physiol, 133:* 266, 1956.
44. Hamasaki, D.I., and Kroll, A.J.: Experimental central retinal artery occlusion: an electrophysiological study. *Arch Ophthalmol, 80:* 243, 1968.
45. Wegner, W.: Die Funktion der menschlichen Netzaut bei experimenteller Ischaemia retinae. *Arch Augenheilkd, 98:* 514, 1928.
46. Böck, J., Bornschein, H., and Hommer, K.: Die Erholungslatenz der Helligkeitsempfindung und des Elektroretinogramms nach retinaler Ischämie. *Albrecht von Graefes Arch Ophthalmol, 167:* 276, 1964.
47. Hayreh, S.S.: An experimental study of the central retinal vein occlusion. *Trans Ophthalmol Soc U K, 84:* 586, 1964.
48. Lubow, M.: Carotid-cavernous fistula. *Am J Ophthalmol, 53:* 121, 1962.
49. Weiss, DI., Shaffer, R.N., and Nehrenberg, T.R.: Neovascular glaucoma complicating carotid-cavernous fistula. *Arch Ophthalmol, 69:* 304, 1963.
50. Paton, A., Rubinstein, K., and Smith, H.V.: Arterial insufficiency in retinal venous occlusion. *Trans Ophthalmol Soc U K, 84:* 559, 1964.
51. Klien, B.A., and Olwin, J.H.: A survey of the pathogenesis of retinal venous occlusion. *Arch Ophthalmol, 56:* 207, 1956.
52. Rothstein, T.: Bilateral, central retinal vein closure as the initial manifestation of polycythemia. *Am J Ophthalmol, 74:* 256, 1972.
53. Bertelsen, T.I.: The relationship between thrombosis in the retinal veins and primary glaucoma. *Acta Ophthalmol, 39:* 603, 1961.
54. Vannas, S., and Raitta, C.: Anticoagulant treatment of retinal venous occlusion. *Am J Ophthalmol, 62:* 874, 1966.
55. Michels, R.G., and Gass, J.D.M.: The natural course of retinal branch vein obstruction. *Trans Am Acad Ophthalmol Otolaryngol, 78:* 166, 1974.
56. Gutman, F.A., and Zegarra, H.: Natural course of temporal retinal branch vein occlusion. *Trans Am Acad Ophthalmol Otolaryngol, 78:* 178, 1974.
57. Kelley, J.S., Patz, A., and Schatz, H.: Management of retinal branch vein occlusion: the role of argon laser photocoagulation. *Ann Ophthalmol, 6:* 1123, 1974.

CHAPTER 9

Peripheral Retinal Occlusive Disease

Lee Jampol, M.D. and Maurice F. Rabb, M.D.

The retinal manifestations of many occlusive vascular diseases (e.g., diabetes mellitus and hypertension) are usually most prominent in the posterior pole, particularly the macula. However, the major changes in other retinal diseases are noted at or anterior to the equator. These diseases show occlusion of peripheral retinal vessels with the development of peripheral proliferative retinopathy. The prototype for this class of diseases is sickle cell retinopathy. This chapter will describe the retinal manifestations of sickle cell disease and other peripheral proliferative retinopathies and, when applicable, their associated features in the macula.

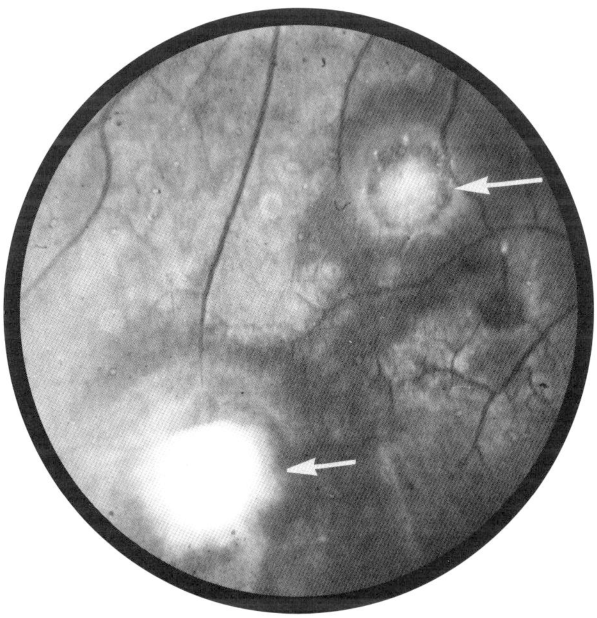

Figure 9.1. Ophthalmoscopic photograph of relatively recent salmon patches with surrounding hemorrhage in hemoglobin S-C disease (*arrows*).

Sickle Cell Retinopathy

Cook [1], in 1930, first described peripheral retinal changes in sickle cell anemia. In 1971, Goldberg [2] introduced a five-stage classification of proliferative sickle cell retinopathy which described the various retinal changes in their natural sequence. The two forms of retinopathy in sickle cell diseases are: (1) nonproliferative retinopathy and (2) proliferative retinopathy. Proliferative retinopathy is usually progressive and leads to reduced visual acuity; nonproliferative retinopathy is nonprogressive and rarely leads to reduced visual acuity.

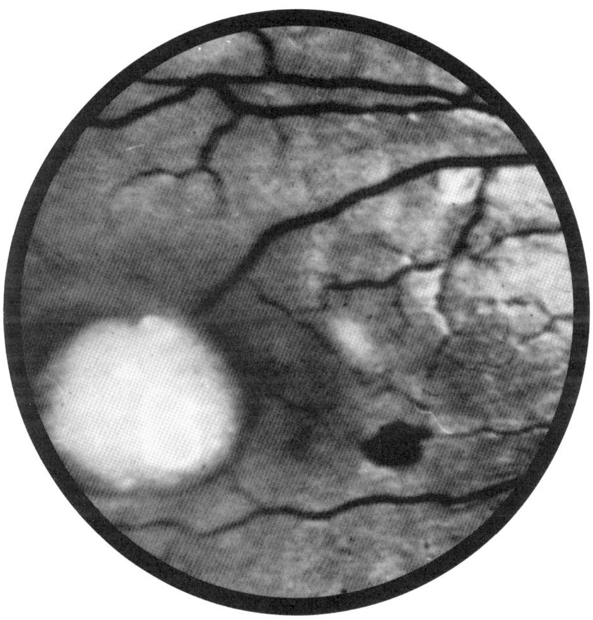

Figure 9.2. Ophthalmoscopic photograph of ovoid pink-orange collection of blood (salmon patch) apparently located between internal limiting membrane and remainder of retina. (From Duane's Textbook of Ophthalmology, volume 3, chapter 17; reprinted with permission.)

NONPROLIFERATIVE RETINOPATHY

Nonproliferative retinopathy is characterized by salmon-colored patches, schisis cavities, iridescent spots, black sunbursts, white without pressure, mottled brown areas, and venous tortuosity.

Salmon Patches

In 1956, Hannon [3] first described the typical salmon color of retinal hemorrhages, which are flat or elevated, and

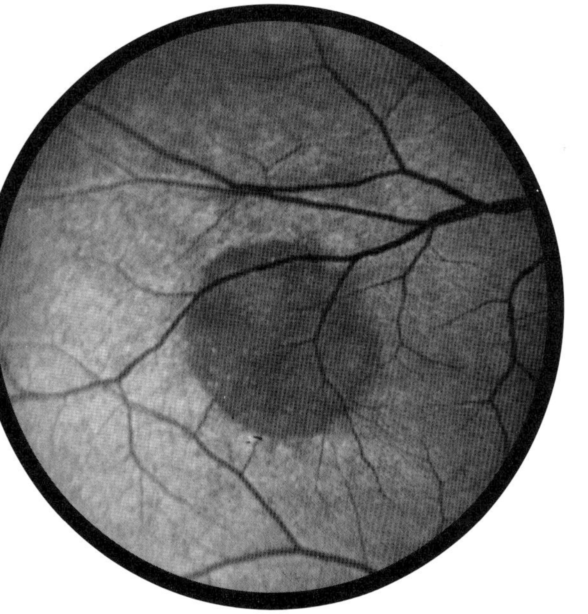

Figure 9.3. Ophthalmoscopic photograph of schisis cavity in S-thalassemia thought to follow an intraretinal hemorrhage.

may be found in the various types of sickle cell diseases (i.e., SS, SC, and S-thalassemia). Salmon patches may be homogeneous with well defined borders and vary in color from a bright red to a yellowish white, depending upon the age of the lesion. The acute lesions are bright red; the older lesions turn white in a matter of months (Fig. 9.1). Most salmon patches are seen in the mid- or far-periphery of the retina; they rarely occur at the posterior pole. They are usually adjacent to a retinal arteriole; an occlusive process very likely leads to infarction of the arteriole resulting in a hemorrhage (Fig. 9.2). Salmon patches range size from ½ to 1 disc diameter, and their shape depends on location of the lesions in the superficial or deeper layers of the retina. Some salmon patches extend into the preretinal space and, therefore, have linear borders, whereas intraretinal hemorrhages have round borders. The hemorrhage may break through the internal limiting membrane of the retina, producing diffuse vitreous hemorrhages, or it may extend in the opposite direction, elevating the retina or pigment epithelium.

Salmon patches are almost pathognomonic of sickle cell disease; they are rarely seen in other occlusive retinal diseases. The cause of their peculiar coloration is unknown.

Schisis Cavities and Iridescent Spots

In some instances, the salmon patch is absorbed, leaving only an area of atrophic retina or a schisis cavity. Schisis cavities are usually bordered anteriorly by the internal limiting membrane and posteriorly by the sensory retina (Fig. 9.3). They contain small pockets of red blood cells, which are broken down to hemosiderin which is then ingested by macrophages. This process results in the iridescent or copper-colored refractile bodies known as iridescent

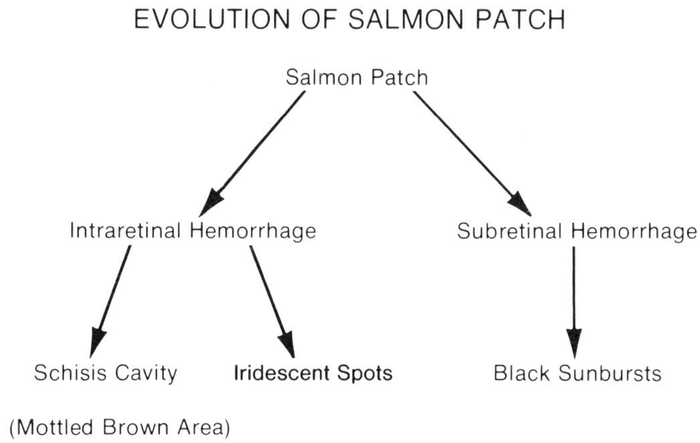

Figure 9.4. Evolution of salmon patch.

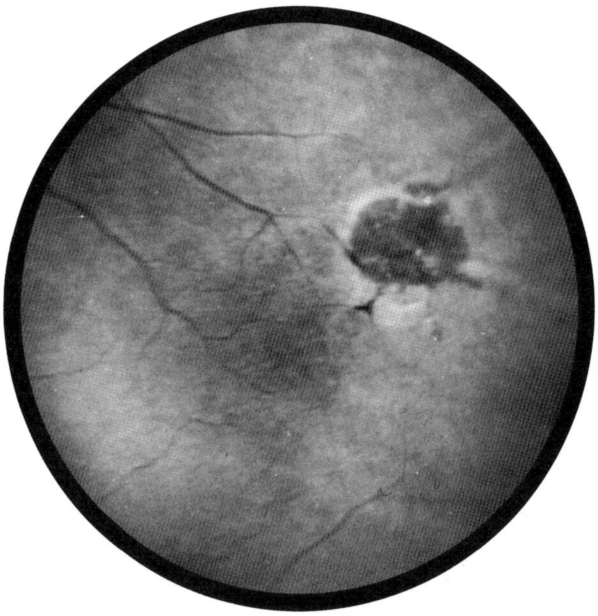

Figure 9.5. Ophthalmoscopic photograph of black sunburst in S-thalassemia. Note pigment deposition and ovoid shape.

spots (Fig. 9.4). They may be found in hemoglobin SC disease, S-thalassemia, and sickle cell anemia.

Black Sunbursts

As described above, intraretinal salmon patches may remain stationary or may change in color with time. For example, they may evolve into black chorioretinal scars called black sunbursts (Fig. 9.5). The term black sunburst was first used by Welch and Goldberg [4] in 1966. These lesions develop most often in the peripheral retina, usually near arterioles (Fig. 9.6). They are found in 35% of patients with hemoglobin SS (sickle cell anemia), 20% of those with S-thalassemia, and 41% of those with hemoglobin SC disease. Asdourian, *et al.* [5] demonstrated that deep retinal hemorrhages (salmon patches) are precursors of black sunbursts. The patient's subretinal blood irritates the retinal

A

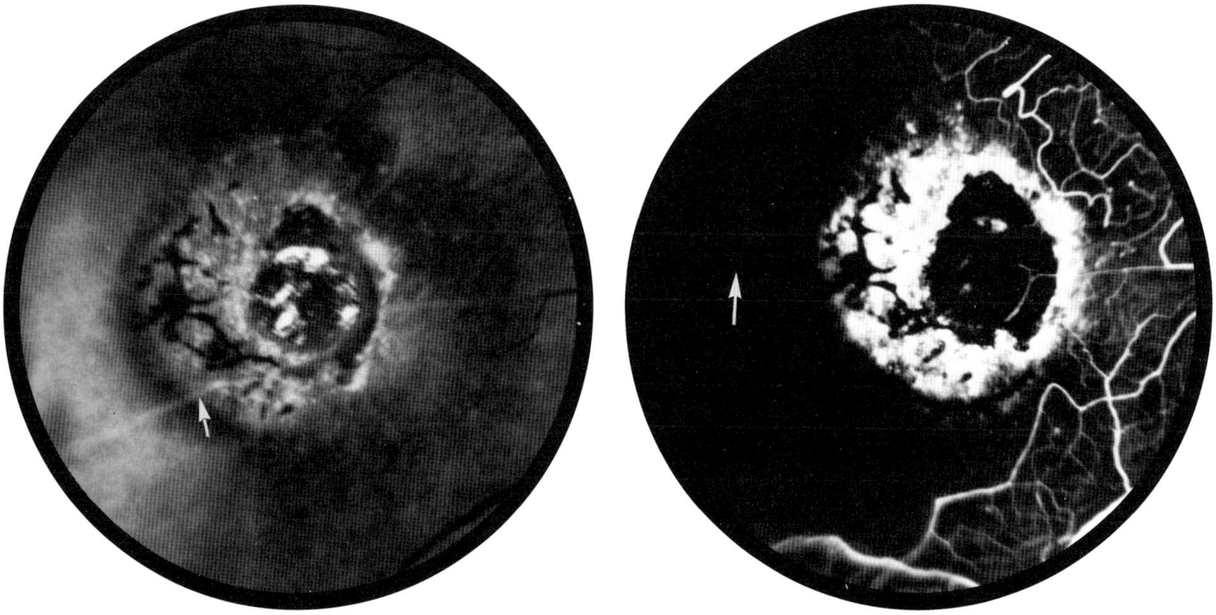

B

Figure 9.6. *A*, ophthalmoscopic photograph of large black sunburst adjacent to apparently occluded arteriole (*arrow*). *B*, early venous phase fluorescein angiogram demonstrating hyper- and hypofluorescence of the sunburst. *Arrow* indicates large zone of avascularity anterior to the sunburst.

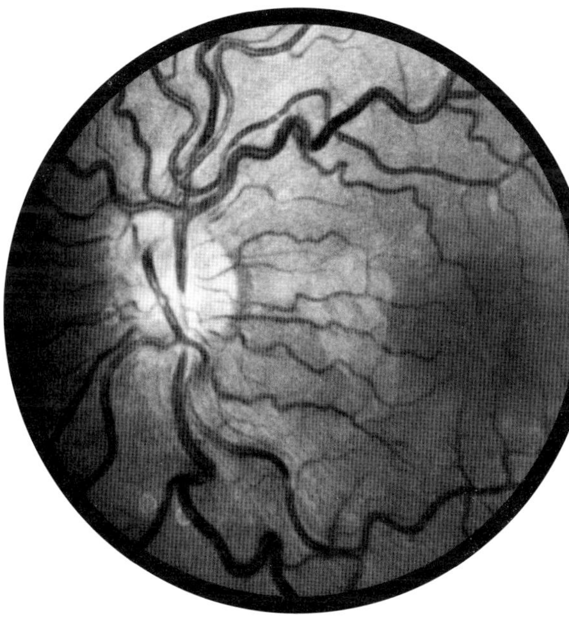

Figure 9.7. Ophthalmoscopic photograph of vascular tortuosity in sickle hemoglobin SC disease.

pigment epithelium resulting in pigment epithelial hypertrophy and hyperplasia, processes leading to a black sunburst (Fig. 9.4).

White Without Pressure and Mottled Brown Areas

Whitening of the peripheral retina, a common finding in patients with sickle cell disease [6–9], may simply represent the condition called white without pressure, normally seen in the general population, not specifically in individuals with sickle cell disease [10]. Mottled brown areas also may be only an intermediate stage of a subretinal hemorrhage that eventually becomes a black sunburst [6] (Fig. 9.6).

Retinal Tortuosity

Tortuosity of the retinal blood vessels, particularly the venules, is common in patients with sickle hemoglobin [4] (Fig. 9.7), but this condition may be noted in patients with hypertension, polycythemia vera, and hyperviscosity syndrome, and, rarely in normal individuals. It is still uncertain whether vascular tortuosity is more common in sickle hemoglobinopathy than in normal persons.

PROLIFERATIVE SICKLE RETINOPATHY

Proliferative sickle retinopathy (PSR), the most severe ocular complication of sickle cell disease, is more prevalent in patients with hemoglobin SC and S-thalassemia than in those with homozygous SS disease [4, 6–8]. This condition is characterized by neovascularization, better known as sea fans. According to Goldberg [2], PSR evolves in five stages (Fig. 9.8):

(1) peripheral arteriolar occlusions
(2) arteriolar-venular anastomoses
(3) neovascular proliferation (sea fans)
(4) vitreous hemorrhage
(5) retinal detachment

The most important stage in the long-term follow-up of PSR is stage 2, arteriolar-venular anastomosis (Fig. 9.9). Although vision is not affected, areas of neovascularization often originate from these arteriolar-venular anastomoses. Neovascular proliferation, which develops in stage 3, can lead to vitreous hemorrhage and retinal detachment. Close evaluation and follow-up are necessary to determine

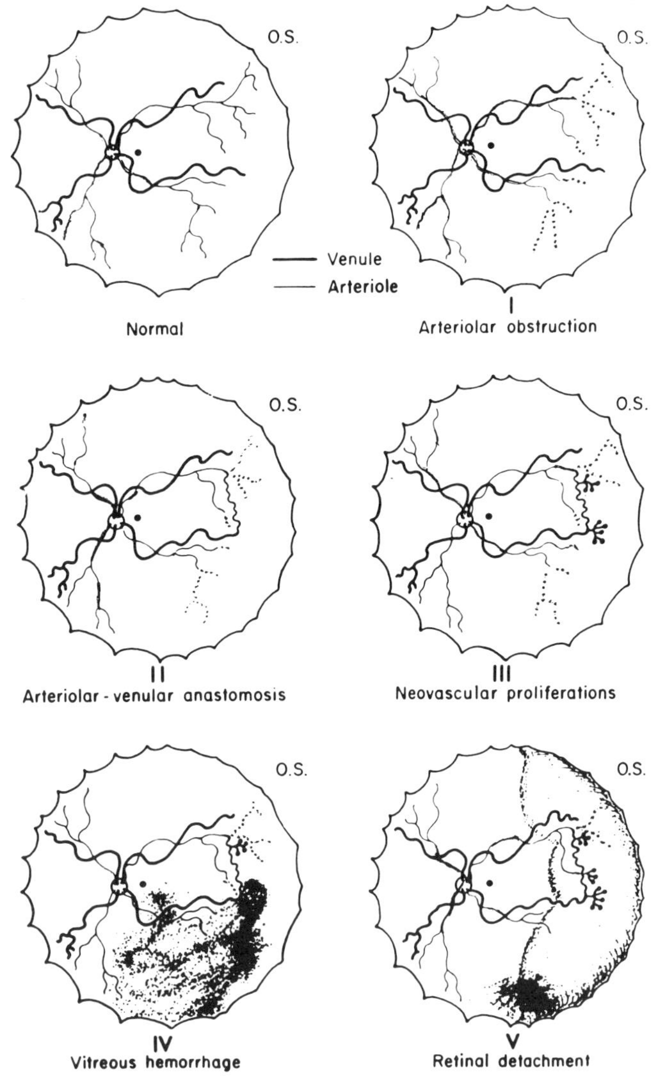

Figure 9.8. Classification of PSR. Note peripheral location. The series of events begins with arteriolar obstructions followed by arteriolar-venular anastomosis, neovascular proliferation, vitreous hemorrhage, and finally retinal detachment. (From Goldberg, M.F.: *Am J Ophthalmol, 71:* 649, 1971; reprinted with permission.)

whether these neovascular lesions are proliferating and should be treated. Photocoagulation before they increase in size seems to reduce the risk of future vitreous hemorrhage and retinal detachment, although this has not been proven.

The sea fans of sickle cell disease are neovascular abnormalities, most often seen in the peripheral superotemporal quadrant of the retina. They are commonly found in patients with hemoglobin SC disease and S-thalassemia (Fig. 9.10). The incidence of proliferative changes in sickle cell anemia, or homozygous SS disease, is much lower in young patients (less than 3%), but can be as high as 29% in patients over 50 years of age [11]. It may be difficult to visualize the actual neovascularization in the peripheral retina without the use of fluorescein angiography. The areas of neovascularization, or vascular fronds, are frequently indistinct, particularly with white light. With fluorescein angiography, single or multiple areas of PSR throughout the peripheral retina can be visualized and photographed (Fig. 9.11). They slowly perfuse, revealing one or more filling arterioles and venules. The sea fans typically are at the avascular-vascular interface in the peripheral retina with a convex margin facing the peripheral avascular zone. These patches of neovascularization (sea fans) become particularly hazardous if they break through the retinal surface and extend into the vitreous. Thirty seconds after fluorescein injection, the areas of proliferative growth may be seen; however, in the later stages of the angiogram, the vitreous may be filled with dye since these abnormal vessels leak heavily (Fig. 9.11).

Nagpal *et al.* [12] reported spontaneous regression of sea fans; e.g., in 8 of 45 patients with proliferative sickle retinopathy. Similar regression of neovascularization has been noted in patients with diabetes and retrolental fibroplasia.

Although neovascularization in sickle disease was formerly thought to develop only in the third or fourth decade of life, or even later, proliferative retinopathy has been seen in 5- and 6-year-old children of both sexes. Why the condition is manifested at an early age in some cases and in the middle years in others is not yet clear. The time needed for PSR to progress from stage to stage is still not well established. However, it has been suggested that prolifera-

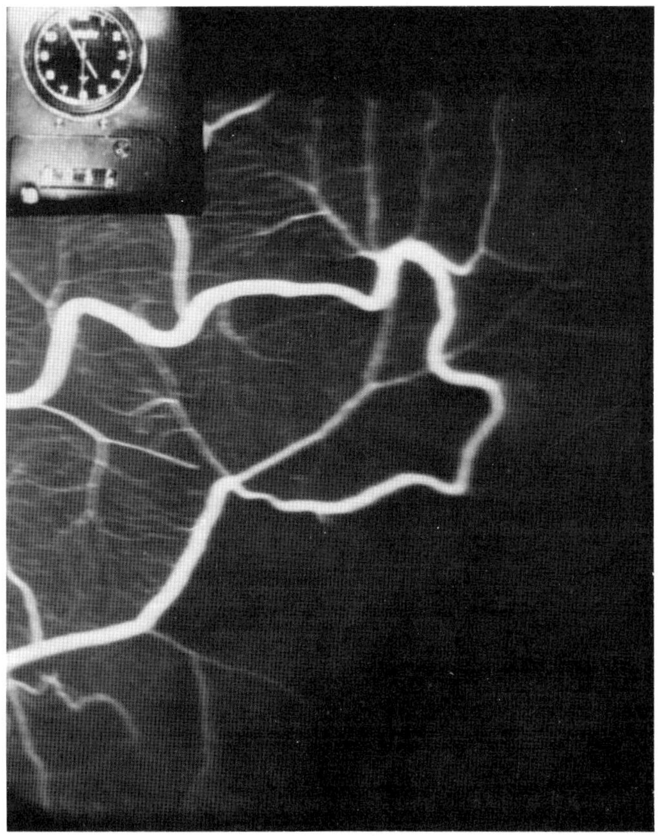

Figure 9.9. Stage 2 PSR. Fluorescein angiogram of peripheral arteriolar-venular anastomosis in SC hemoglobin angiogram. The wider and more tortuous vessel is the arteriole. (From Goldberg, M.F.: *Am J Ophthalmol, 71:* 649, 1971; reprinted with permission.)

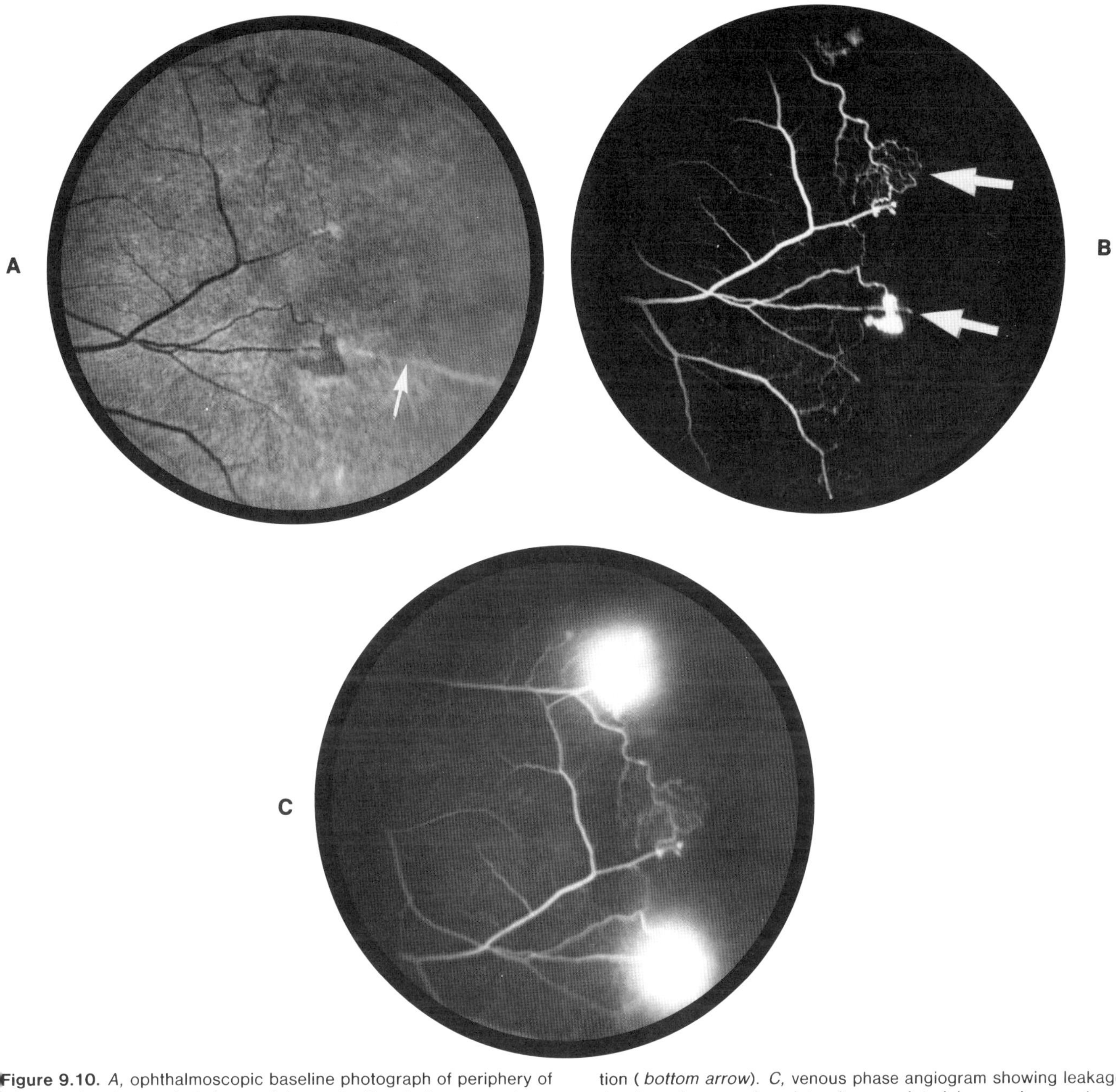

Figure 9.10. *A*, ophthalmoscopic baseline photograph of periphery of left eye showing occluded vessel (*arrow*). *B*, arteriovenous phase fluorescein angiogram of temporal periphery, demonstrating stage 2 (arteriolar-venular anastomosis) (*top arrow*) and early neovascularization (*bottom arrow*). *C*, venous phase angiogram showing leakage of dye from two sea fans into vitreous. Arteriolar-venular anastomosis does not leak.

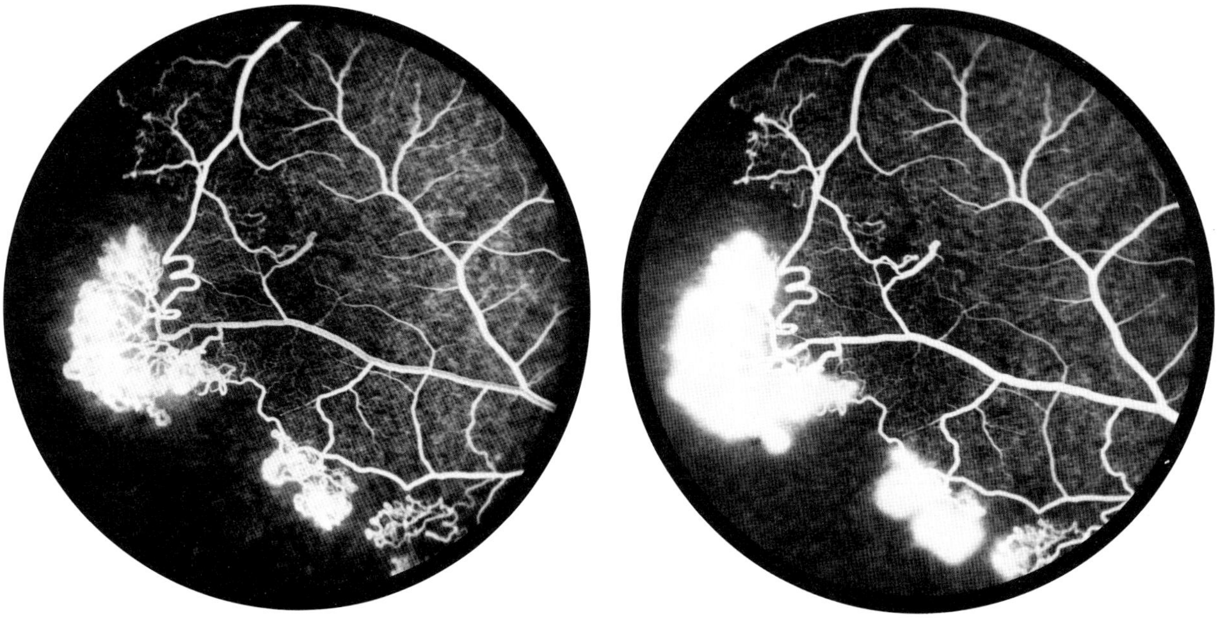

A B

Figure 9.11. *A,* fluorescein angiogram of multiple sea fans in hemoglobin S-thalassemia. *B,* leakage of dye from sea fans into vitreous in the venous phase.

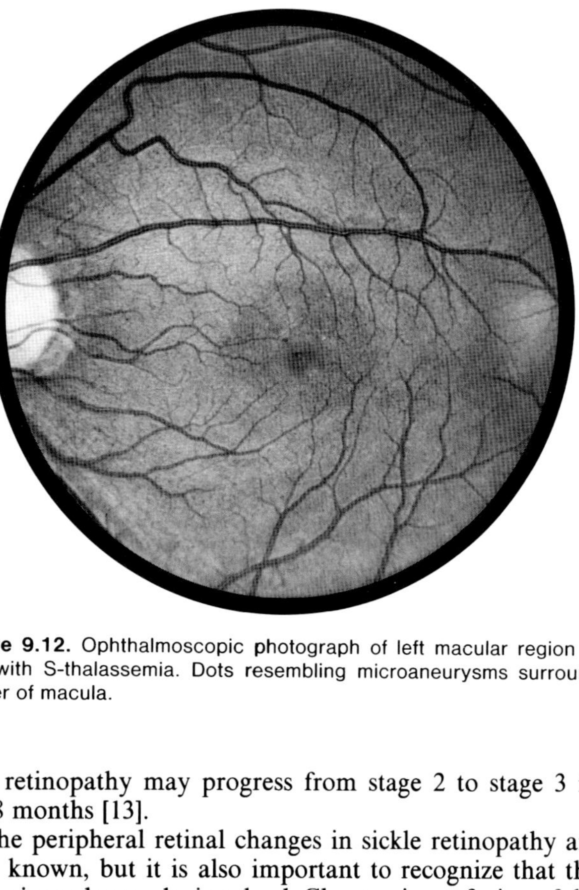

Figure 9.12. Ophthalmoscopic photograph of left macular region in eye with S-thalassemia. Dots resembling microaneurysms surround center of macula.

tive retinopathy may progress from stage 2 to stage 3 in 4–18 months [13].

The peripheral retinal changes in sickle retinopathy are well known, but it is also important to recognize that the posterior pole may be involved. Changes in perfusion of the fine vasculature in the macular and perimacular areas are evident [14], which may or may not diminish visual acuity. Asdourian and associates [15] reported a series of 100 patients of whom 22% had abnormalities in and around the macula (Fig. 9.12). Pathologic changes in the macular area were believed basically to involve the single layer of capillary network surrounding the foveal avascular zone (Fig. 9.13). There was poor correlation between the angioscopic appearance of the capillaries around the foveal avascular zone and the visual acuity. Some eyes have a loss of capillaries adjacent to the foveal avascular zone, yet retain normal macular function (Fig. 9.14). Field defects were sometimes demonstrated corresponding to areas of capillary nonperfusion. Macular fibrosis, arteriolar occlusions, and neovascularization from the arcades in the posterior pole may be seen, but macular lipid exudation and cystoid edema are *not* manifestations in the macula in sickle retinopathy.

Optic Nerve

Optic disc involvement in sickle cell disease has received little attention. Comma-shaped vascular segments which have been noted on the disc are often detected only with fluorescein angiography and do not result in reduced visual acuity [6, 16]. In rare instances there is actual neovascularization of the disc (Fig. 9.15).

TREATMENT OF SICKLE RETINOPATHY

Proliferative sickle cell retinopathy may be treated by: (1) diathermy, (2) xenon arc photocoagulation, (3) argon laser photocoagulation, or (4) cryocoagulation. Although penetrating diathermy seals abnormal feeder vessels in areas of neovascularization, it is rarely used now that effective photocoagulation techniques have been developed. Goldbaum [17] has treated PSR with the Zeiss xenon arc photocoagulation system with a slit-lamp delivery system. The

A
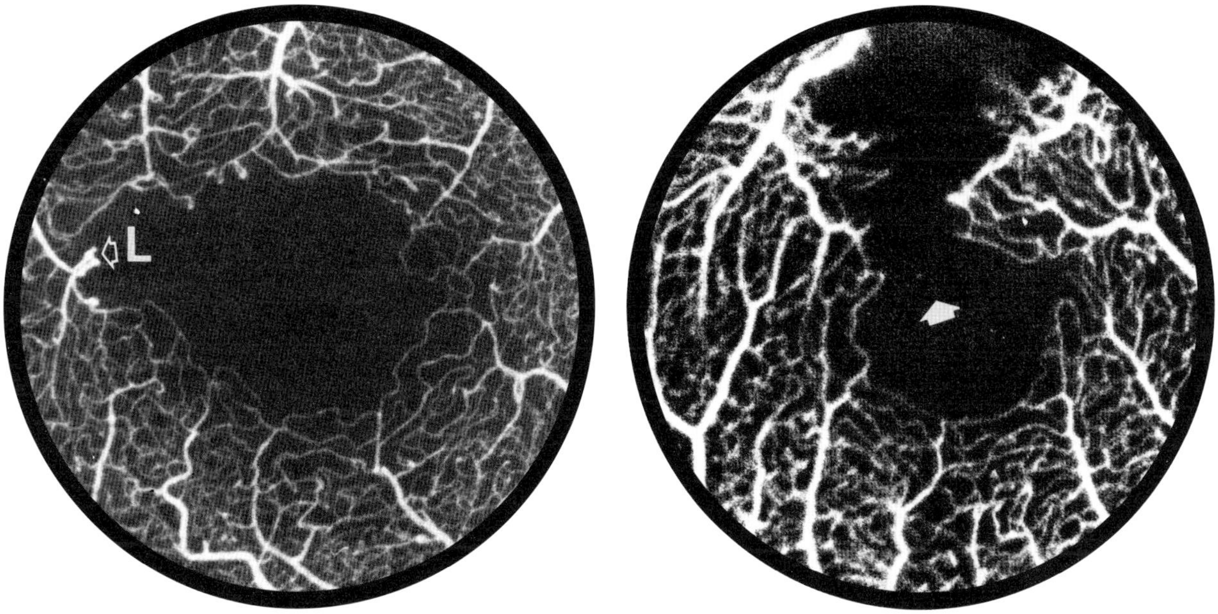
B

Figure 9.13. *A,* late venous phase fluorescein angiogram of right posterior pole showing abnormally shaped foveal avascular zone with loss of vascular arcades at 9 to 10 o'clock meridian; Venular loop (*L*) directed into avascular zone. (From G.K. Asdourian *et al.*: *Brit J Ophthalmol, 60:* 431, 1976; reprinted with permission.) *B,* fluorescein angiogram of right posterior pole 48 hours after an acute episode of infarction. Enlarged view showing nonperfusion of single capillary bridging superior border of foveal avascular zone (*arrow*). (From G.K. Asdourian *et al.*: *Brit. J Ophthalmol, 60:* 431, 1976; reprinted with permission.)

A
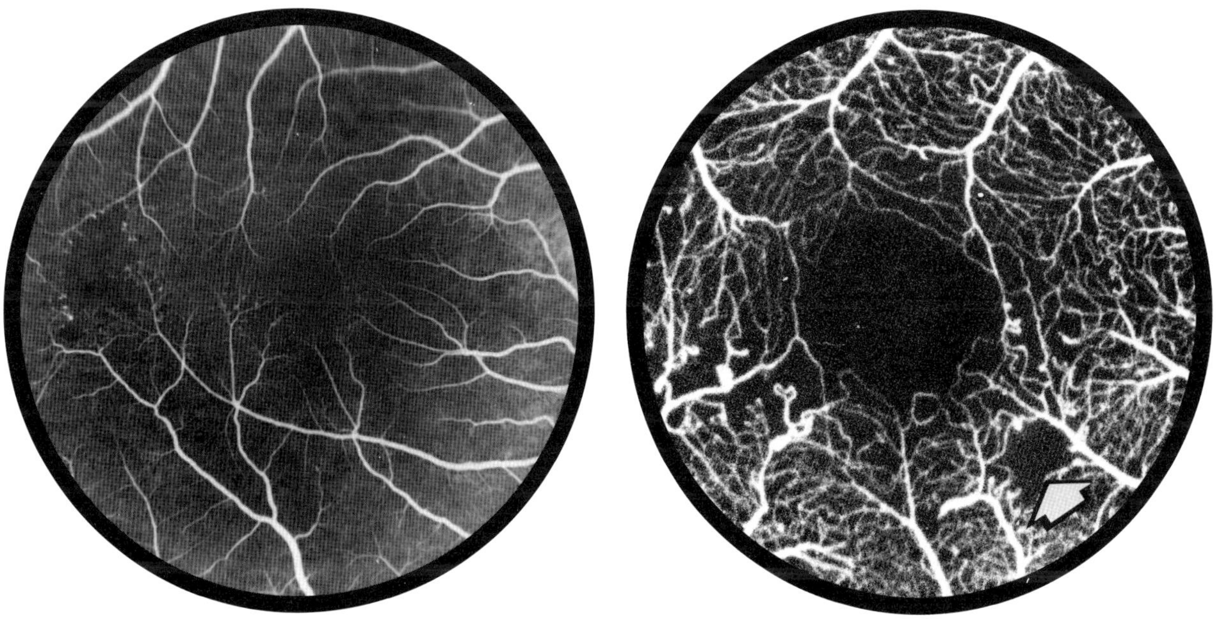
B

Figure 9.14. Fluorescein angiogram in sickle retinopathy. *A,* beads of fluorescein are apparent in the capillaries surrounding the foveal avascular zone. Temporal to the zone is a pathologic avascular zone. *B,* in enlarged view of the foveal avascular zone, spaces of the surrounding capillary meshwork show abnormal variation in size. *Arrow* shows where capillary loss occurred. Capillary nonperfusion in the macula may or may not have associated defects in visual function. (From G.K. Asdourian *et al.*: *Brit J Ophthalmol, 60:* 431, 1976; reprinted with permission.)

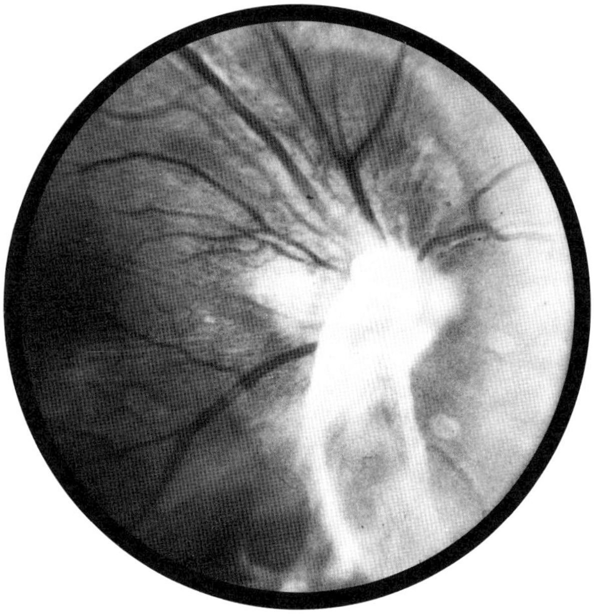

Figure 9.15. Ophthalmoscopic photograph of fibrotic tuft secondary to neovascularization superimposed on right disc in sickle cell disease.

usual settings are 1.5°C with a 0.2- to 0.5-second exposure time. Flat sea fans on the retinal surface may be treated directly but for elevated proliferative retinal lesions, the feeder arterioles, and, later, the draining venules should be occluded. The feeder vessels are treated on the retina just proximal to the elevated sea fans—first the arterioles, then the venules. The treatment is stopped when there is obvious segmentation of the blood column in the vessel. Angiography is performed immediately to determine that the neovascular bed has been closed.

Proliferative sickle retinopathy has also been treated with argon laser photocoagulation [18–21] with large, intense spots of long duration (Fig. 9.16). The feeder vessels are treated with at least 2½ times the baseline power (the power required to produce an intermediate intensity white spot next to the area to be treated).

Among the complications of light photocoagulation are vitreous hemorrhage, choroidal ischemia, and choroidoretinovitreal neovascular membranes that appear after treatment [18, 23]. Use of small spot sizes with the argon laser can produce holes in Bruch's membrane, through which choroidal vessels may grow resulting in choroidovitreal vascularization. This devastating complication has not been seen following xenon arc photocoagulation, or with use of the 500-μm spot size of the argon laser. However, Condon and Serjeant [22] reported choroidovitreal neovascularization with 1500 μ xenon spot sizes.

Cryotherapy is employed in cases in which vitreous hemorrhage partially or completely obscures the neovascular sea fans, precluding photocoagulation. The area of suspected neovascularization, including the feeder vessels, is frozen. The treatment is carried out if possible under direct observation with the indirect ophthalmoscope. Single or triple freeze-thaw techniques at −60 to −80°C have been used [24, 25], but the latter is no longer recommended. Hemorrhage and retinal detachment have been reported following cryotherapy of PSR.

EALES' DISEASE (IDIOPATHIC PERIPHERAL NEOVASCULARIZATION)

In 1880, Eales [26]) described a disease in young men characterized by retinal hemorrhages associated with epistaxis and constipation. Many investigators [27–32] since that time have reported cases of vitreous hemorrhage and peripheral retinal neovascularization associated with peripheral retinal vascular occlusions. Constipation and epistaxis have not proven to be important features of the disease. Eales' disease, or idiopathic periphlebitis retinae, is a "wastebasket" category. Patients originally thought to have Eales' disease after careful diagnostic evaluation were found to have such disorders as sickle cell retinopathy, chronic leukemia, sarcoidosis, systemic vasculitis, multiple sclerosis, branch or central retinal vein occlusion, or dysproteinemia. Increased diagnostic acumen will certainly lead to the elimination of other cases from this category. Until then the designation of idiopathic peripheral neovascularization seems appropriate.

Clinical Appearance

Eales' disease is much less common in the United States than in Europe, India, and other areas of the world. It usually affects young men 20- to 45-years old, although men in other age groups and women may be affected. The disease is bilateral in 90% of the cases. The patient consults an ophthalmologist because of visual loss related to vitreous hemorrhage.

Eales' disease, like most other ischemic retinopathies, affects the temporal peripheral retina more frequently than the nasal periphery [32]. Early cases are characterized by areas of peripheral capillary dropout, and by arteriovenous communications. Fluorescein angiography reveals small arterioles and venules that appear opacified and nonperfused. Chorioretinal scars, microaneurysms, capillary dilatation, and perivascular (usually perivenous) sheathing are observed (Fig. 9.17). Peripheral fluorescein angiography [32–34] is helpful in verifying capillary dropout, vascular obstruction, and neovascularization (Fig. 9.18). Signs of vasculitis or perivasculitis (especially periphlebitis) suggest an inflammatory cause for the vascular changes. There may be concomitant uveitis with anterior chamber reaction or, more commonly, vitreous cellular reaction. Neovascular tissue develops at the border between vascular and avascular retina (Fig. 9.19), which appears identical with sickle cell sea fans. These new vessels proliferate from the surface of the retina and frequently develop a prominent fibrous matrix. Possible complications include retinal and vitreous hemorrhage and tractional or rhegmatogenous retinal detachment. Severe cases show rubesosis iridis, cataract, and glaucoma. The disease remains active for months to years, but in time usually becomes quiescent. As it progresses, there may be a centripetal contraction of the margin of perfused retina, similar to sickle cell disease and Takayasu's disease.

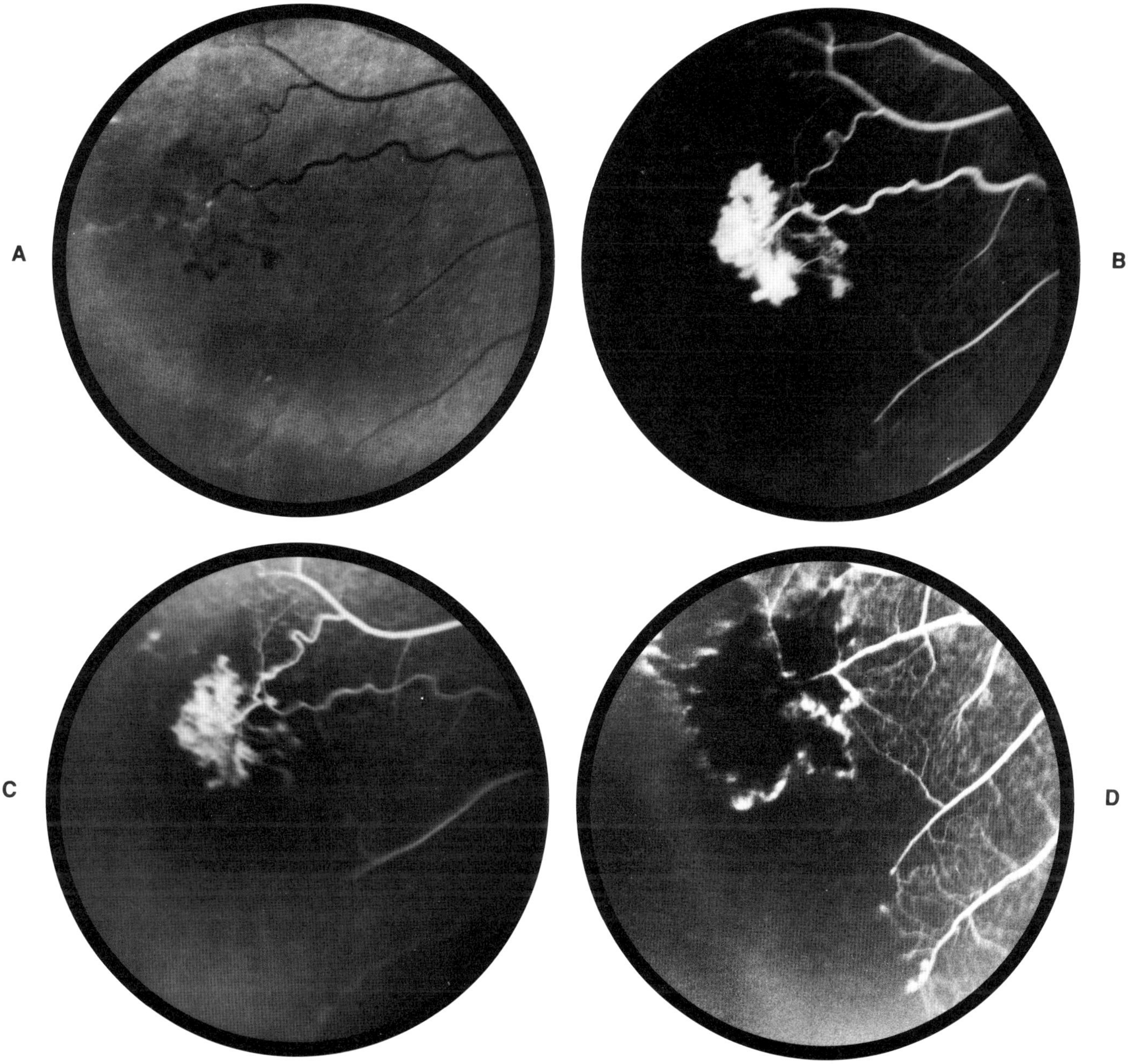

Figure 9.16. *A,* ophthalmoscopic photograph of sea fan. *B,* prior to laser photocoagulation, fluorescein angiogram shows perfused neovascular sea fans at 9:30 o'clock position. Note typical zone of ischemia peripheral to neovascular tissue. *C,* persistent perfusion 1 day after initial photocoagulation directly to sea fan (early venous phase), indicates need for retreatment. *D,* thirty-nine days after second argon laser photocoagulation, fluorescein angiogram shows no further perfusion of sea fan. (From M.F. Goldberg, and I. Acacio.: *Arch Ophthalmol, 90:* 35, 1973; reprinted with permission.)

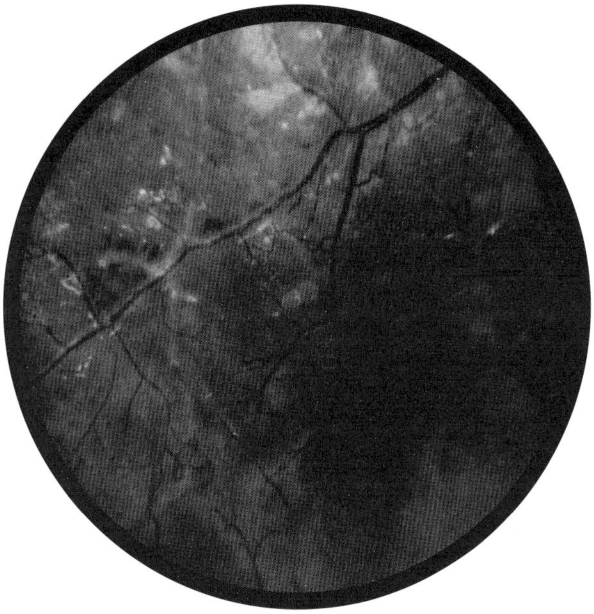

Figure 9.17. Ophthalmoscopic photograph of extensive perivenous sheathing with abnormal venous-venous anastomoses in a patient with Eales' disease.

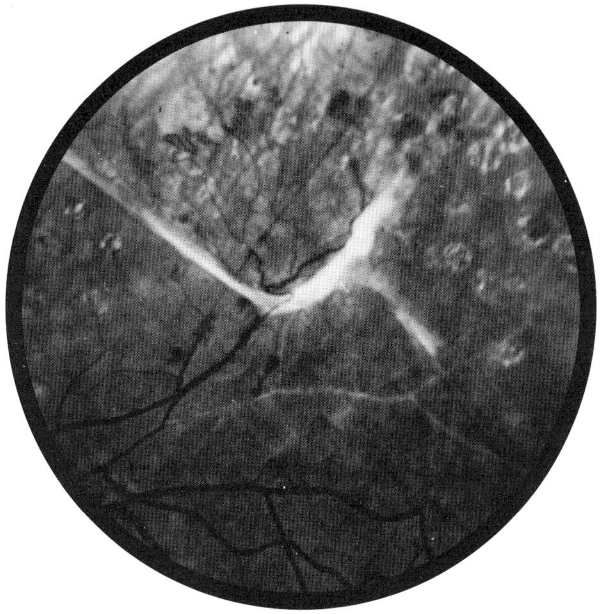

Figure 9.19. Ophthalmoscopic photograph of fibrovascular proliferation in the midperiphery of patient with Eales' disease. Argon laser photocoagulation spots surround neovascularization.

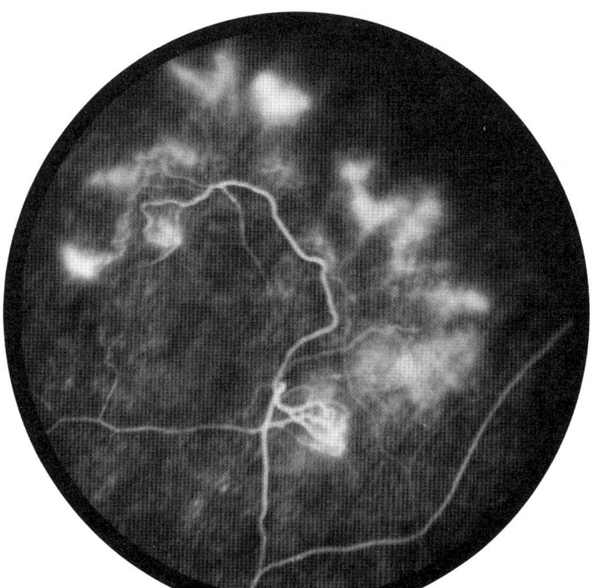

Figure 9.18. Fluorescein angiogram of "sickle like" sea fan in Eales' disease. (Courtesy of Department of Ophthalmology, Yale University School of Medicine.)

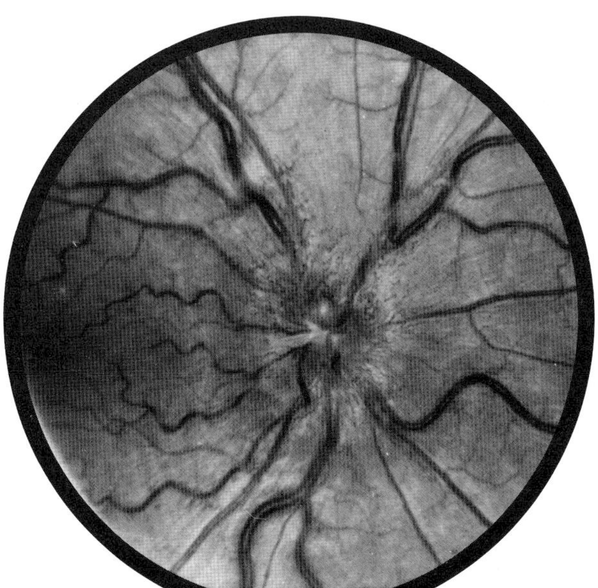

Figure 9.20. Ophthalmoscopic photograph of disc edema and venous congestion in a patient with papillophlebitis. (Courtesy of the Ophthalmology Clinic, Walter Reed Hospital.)

Although most reports of Eales' disease have focused on peripheral retinal involvement, inflammation of the central retinal vein—so-called papillophlebitis or optic disc vasculitis—has also been described [35–37]. This syndrome, usually unilateral, is characterized by disc edema, venous congestion, and some retinal hemorrhage in younger patients who are apparently otherwise healthy (Fig. 9.20). The clinical picture resembles impending central retinal vein obstruction, but the central vision is spared unless cystoid macular edema develops. The disease usually runs a course of 3–12 months, and the visual prognosis is good in most cases. Some patients show signs of peripheral vasculitis (Eales' disease) and papillophlebitis [35].

The macula is rarely involved in Eales' disease, although if the process is extensive it may lead to cystoid macular edema or perimacular hemorrhages. In rare cases, retinal vasculitis involves blood vessels in the posterior pole and macula [38] (Fig. 9.21).

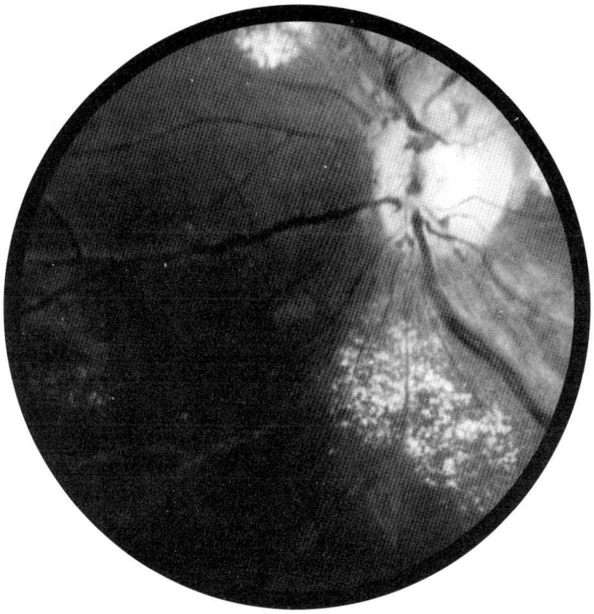

Figure 9.21. Ophthalmoscopic photograph of perivascular sheathing and lipid exudation in a patient with retinal vasculitis.

Etiology

There are two major theories of the cause of the peripheral retinal changes in Eales' disease [39]. Most investigators have felt that it represents a perivasculitis or vasculitis predominantly with venous involvement. The term "periphlebitis retinae" has, thus, become a synonym for Eales' disease. In fact, many of the pathologic specimens from patients with Eales' disease show perivascular or intramural infiltration of lymphocytes in the retina and, occasionally, giant cells or a granulomatous reaction. The process affects mainly the venules. The inflammation has been attributed to active tuberculosis, allergy to tuberculoprotein, syphilis, viral infections, collagen vascular disease, multiple sclerosis, thromboangiitis obliterans, and other systemic diseases—so far, without substantiation. Similarity of the clinical findings of retinal vasculitis to an intraocular Arthus reaction indicates the possibility of an immune complex (antigen-antibody-complement) disease involving the retinal circulation. The antigen(s) involved is, as yet, unknown.

Other investigators favor the theory of a noninflammatory disease of peripheral retinal blood vessels [32]. Changes in the vessel wall corresponding to hyaline thickening or intramural deposition of some material lead to opacification and obstruction of the vessels. The cause of this process is unknown. The absence of vasculitis in some histopathologic specimens [40] certainly does not rule out prior vasculitis as the source.

Differential Diagnosis

Patients with the clinical picture of Eales' disease must be evaluated for evidence of other diseases associated with peripheral retinopathies. The work-up should include: (1) hemoglobin electrophoresis to rule out sickle cell disease; (2) evaluation for sarcoidosis; (3) a complete blood cell count to rule out leukemia or polycythemia; (4) serum protein electrophoresis to rule out dysproteinemias; (5) neurologic evaluation to rule out demyelinating disease; (6) vascular evaluation to rule out aortic arch syndromes, hypertension, diabetes mellitus, collagen diseases and other vascular diseases.

Prognosis

Since the term Eales' disease probably covers a variety of conditions, it is difficult to arrive at a sound prognosis. The outcome is generally good, with bilateral blindness a rarity [31]. Nevertheless, some eyes do develop intractable vitreous hemorrhages, tractional or rhegmatogenous retinal detachment, or rubeotic glaucoma. As noted above, since the disease is, in general, peripheral, the macula is usually not involved. The prognosis in most cases of optic nerve vasculitis is favorable.

Therapy

Treatment of Eales' disease includes diathermy, cryopexy, photocoagulation, and corticosteroids. To date, corticosteroids have demonstrated no proven efficacy. Direct light coagulation of the vascular abnormalities is the therapy of choice in most centers [41]. No large controlled series has been reported, but the response to light coagulation has been excellent. Remarkably low energy levels are needed for successful closure of the neovascularization [41], although some sea fans are markedly resistant to treatment. In one series, 91% of the eyes were morphologically unchanged over a mean observation period of 5 years after the completion of treatment [41]. Since the natural history of the untreated disease is unclear, controlled studies are needed to substantiate claims of improved prognosis for patients undergoing photocoagulation. On the other hand, repeat vitreous hemorrhage or expansion of the neovascularized complex necessitates a more aggressive approach until definitive studies are available because of dreaded sequela such as retinal detachment with vitreous contraction.

Complications of photocoagulation include bleeding, preretinal membrane formation, and rarely, chorioretinal or choriovitreal vascular anastomosis [42].

In addition to direct treatment of vascular abnormalities (neovascularization, microaneurysms), it may be efficacious to employ retinal ablative therapy in the involved area to destroy hypoxic retina and thereby prevent neovascularization. Successful ablation in a diabetic retinopathy [43] certainly would suggest the value of this type of therapy.

SARCOIDOSIS

Patients with sarcoidosis may show retinopathy. Features of the disease include chorioretinitis, periphlebitis, perivenous candle-way drippings, macular edema, optic disc edema, optic atrophy, vitreous and preretinal opacities, and disc, retinal, and choroidal granulomas. Periphlebitis may lead to branch vein occlusions with retinal hemorrhages. Peripheral retinal neovascularization has been noted in at least four patients with sarcoidosis, in whom there was evidence of peripheral vascular venous occlusions, perivenous sheathing, and capillary dropout [44, 45]. As in sickle cell disease, sea fan-like neovascularization was present at the border between anterior avascular retina and posterior perfused retina. However, a perfused vessel did pass anterior to the sea fan into avascular retina (Fig. 9.22), as occurs in most cases of proliferative sickle retinopathy. Since sarcoid retinopathy is usually characterized by perivenous inflammation, the peripheral neovascularization seems likely to result from venous compromise with sluggish blood flow, and from capillary nonperfusion. The ensuing hypoxia then stimulates neovascular growth.

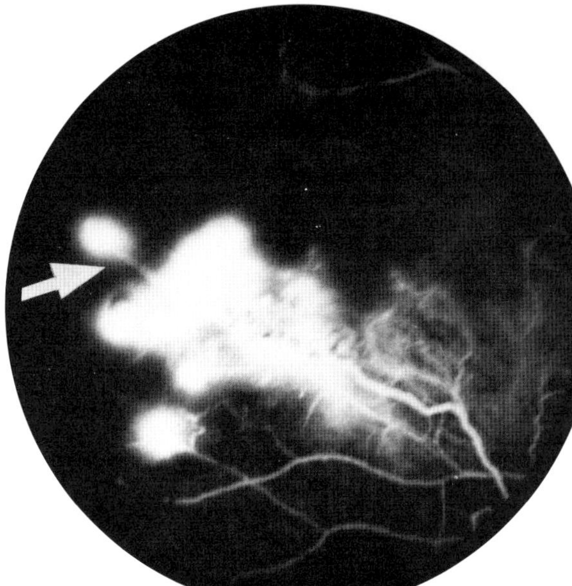

Figure 9.22. Late phase fluorescein angiogram of sea fan neovascularization in right fundus, due to sarcoidosis, shows profuse leakage of dye and single vessel (*arrow*) passing through neovascularization into area of avascular retina, as well as small leaking sea fan at tip of protruding vessel. (Courtesy of Department of Ophthalmology, Yale University School of Medicine.)

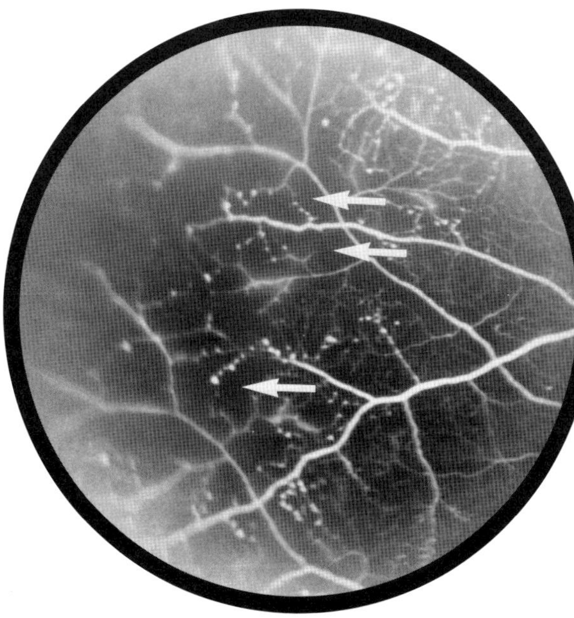

Figure 9.23. Early venous phase fluorescein angiogram of peripheral retinal microaneurysms in patient with chronic granulocytic leukemia. *Arrows* indicate areas of capillary nonperfusion. (From L. Jampol *et al.*: *Am J Ophthalmol, 80:* 242, 1975; reprinted with permission.)

LEUKEMIA

Retinopathy can be considered a manifestation of acute or chronic leukemia. Findings may include dilated, tortuous veins; retinal, preretinal, or vitreous hemorrhages; cotton-wool spots; Roth's spots; and retinal lipid exudation; as well as disc edema, pigment epithelial changes, and nonrhegmatogenous retinal detachment. Hyperviscosity retinopathy may also be seen in association with chronic granulocytic or, less frequently, chronic lymphocytic leukemia [46]. Prolonged leukocytosis in some cases of chronic leukemia can lead to increased whole blood viscosity, and, perhaps, in turn to comma-like changes in the conjunctiva similar to those noted in sickle cell disease [47]. The leukocytosis may also result in peripheral retinal-capillary nonperfusion, vascular stagnation, perivenous sheathing, and microaneurysm formation (Fig. 9.23). Peripheral retinal microaneurysms were seen clinically in 2 of 8 patients with chronic lymphocytic leukemia and 6 of 17 patients with chronic granulocytic leukemia [46]. Microaneurysms have also been demonstrated histopathologically [48]. Two reported patients with chronic granulocytic leukemia demonstrated sea fan-like neovascularization at the margin of perfused and nonperfused retina [49, 50]. This retinopathy was virtually identical with that in sickle cell disease, sarcoidosis, and Eales' disease. Fluorescein angiograms from a patient with chronic granulocytic leukemia revealed central macular capillary dropout, again very similar to that in sickle cell maculopathy (Fig. 9.24).

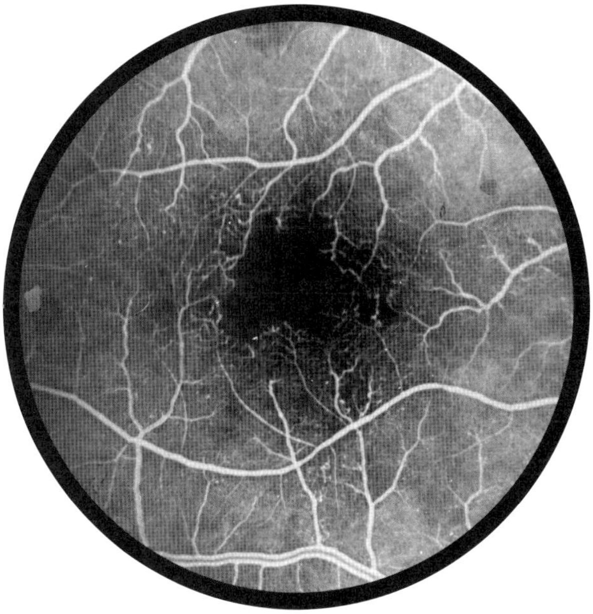

Figure 9.24. Fluorescein angiogram of macular capillary nonperfusion in a patient with chronic granulocytic leukemia. Multiple irregularities are evident at the margins of the photograph from darkroom artifacts.

RETROLENTAL FIBROPLASIA

Although the pathogenesis of retrolental fibroplasia (oxygen toxicity) differs from that of the other retinopathies, the clinical picture is somewhat similar. The initial manifestation is peripheral arteriolar occlusion(s) leading to retinal ischemia. The temporal aspect of the retina is more likely to be affected than other portions. Neovascular proliferations resemble those seen in proliferative sickle retinopathy, i.e., into the peripheral avascular retina and then into the vitreous (Fig. 9.25). Subsequent hemorrhage and fibrous proliferation result in dragging of the disc and retina, membrane formation, retinal detachment, and the development of intravitreal fibrous sheets and bands.

Ophthalmoscopy and fluorescein angiography demonstrate many similarities between retrolental fibroplasia and proliferative sickle retinopathy, among which are temporal ischemia and a proliferative edge of granulation tissue growing on the surface of the retina. Fluorescein angiography reveals an abrupt interface, with active growth of neovascular tissue, between the anterior nonperfused retina and the posterior perfused retina [51].

A

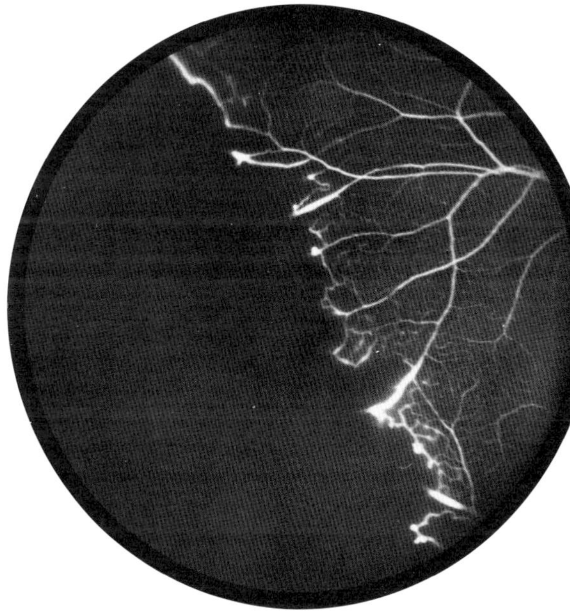

Figure 9.25. Fluorescein angiogram of a patient with retrolental fibroplasia. Note the distinct vascular-avascular zone in the peripheral temporal retina, resembling the changes seen in the proliferative sickle retinopathy.

A

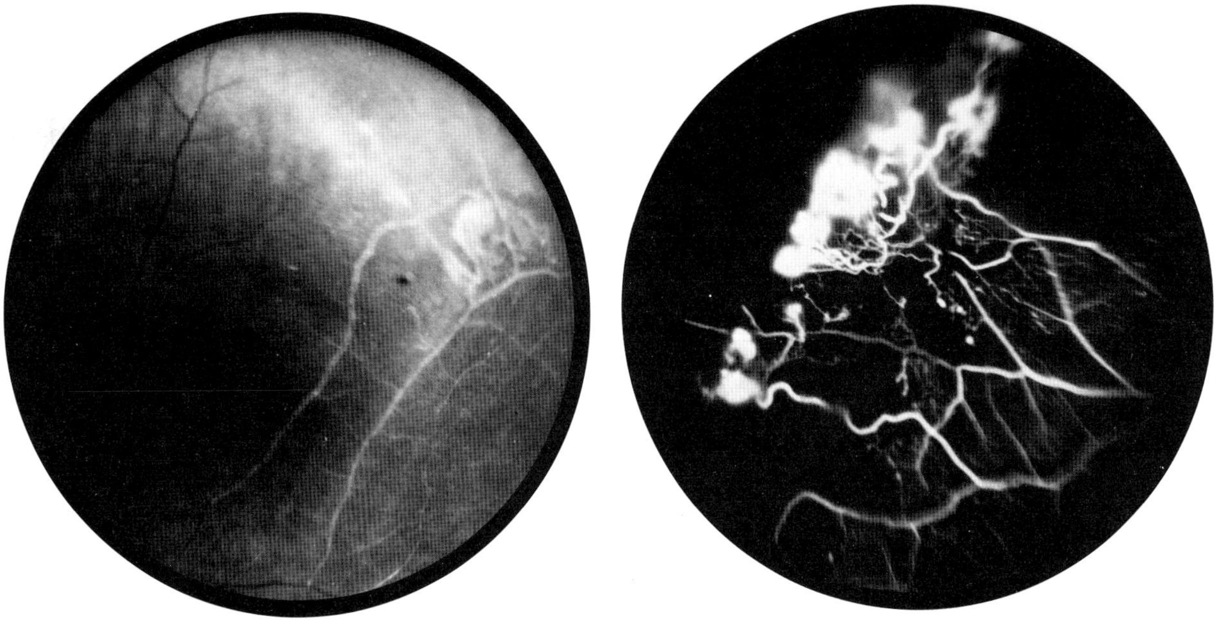

B

Figure 9.26. Peripheral neovascularization in systemic hypertension. *A*, ophthalmoscopic photograph of multiple opacified (sclerotic) vessels supplying superotemporal quadrant with sea fan neovascularization in right eye of patient with hypertension. *B*, fluorescein angiogram of same patient showing capillary nonperfusion, microaneurysms, and neovascular sea fans. (Courtesy of Tom Stevens, M.D., University of Wisconsin.)

HYPERTENSION AND OTHER DISEASES

Retinal neovascularization is a common manifestation of branch retinal vein occlusions. Branch occlusions, which usually occur in the posterior pole, are frequently associated with hypertension. In a 75-year-old black man with longstanding hypertension, the fundus demonstrated multiple old branch vein occlusions bilaterally (Fig. 9.26). An unusual feature was opacification of multiple peripheral venules and arterioles. Sea fan-like neovascularization was visible at the junction of anterior avascular retina and posterior perfused retina, and the patient also had multiple microaneurysms.

A young woman with bilateral occlusive retinal arteriolitis (compare Eales' disease with its periphlebitis) had a sea fan neovascular lesion in one eye (Fig. 9.27) [52].

Sea fan-like neovascularization has also been noted in patients with AC hemoglobin [53], sickle cell trait (rare), incontinentia pigmenti [54], aortic arch syndromes (e.g., Takayasu's disease) retinal detachment and in some families as a dominantly inherited proliferative vascular disorder. In other patients peripheral neovascularization may have been related to syphilis, trauma (boxing), or intravenously administered drugs. The cause may still remain obscure in some patients despite extensive ophthalmic and medical evaluations.

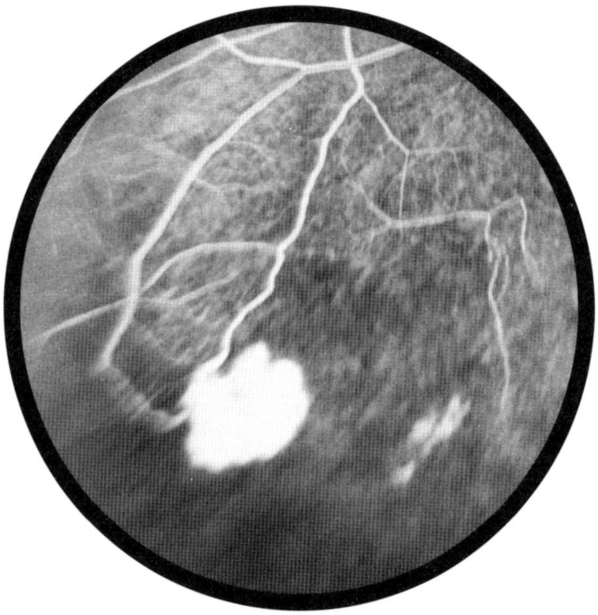

Figure 9.27. Fluorescein angiogram of sea fan lesion with occlusive arteriolitis in patient with extensive capillary nonperfusion. (From L. Jampol *et al.*, *Am J Ophthalmol, 81:* 583, 1976; reprinted with permission.)

References

1. Cook, W.C.: A case of sickle cell anemia with associated subarachnoid hemorrhage. *J Med, 11:* 541, 1930.
2. Goldberg, M.F.: Classification and pathogenesis of proliferative sickle retinopathy. *Am J Ophthalmol, 71:* 649, 1971.
3. Hannon, J.F.: Vitreous hemorrhages associated with sickle-cell hemoglobin C disease. *Am J Ophthalmol, 42:* 707, 1956.
4. Welch, R.B., and Goldberg, M.F.: Sickle-cell hemoglobin and its relation to fundus abnormality. *Arch Ophthalmol, 75:* 353, 1966.
5. Asdourian, G., Nagpal, K.C., Goldbaum, M., Patrianakos, D., Goldberg, M.F., and Rabb, M.: Evolution of the retinal black sunburst in sickling haemoglobinopathies. *Brit J Ophthalmol, 59:* 710, 1975.
6. Condon, P.I., and Serjeant, G.R.: Ocular findings in homozygous sickle cell anemia in Jamaica. *Am J Ophthalmol, 73:* 533, 1972.
7. Condon, P.I., and Serjeant, G.R.: Ocular findings in hemoglobin SC disease in Jamaica. *Am J Ophthalmol, 74:* 921, 1972.
8. Condon, P.I., and Serjeant, G.R.: Ocular findings in sickle cell thalassemia in Jamaica. *Am J Ophthalmol, 74:* 1105, 1972.
9. Condon, P.I., and Serjeant, G.R.: The progression of sickle cell eye disease in Jamaica. *Doc Ophthalmol, 39:* 203, 1975.
10. Nagpal, K.C., Huamonte, F., Constantaras, A., Asdourian, G., Goldberg, M.F., and Busso, B.: Migratory white-without-pressure retinal lesions. *Arch Ophthalmol, 94:* 576, 1976.
11. Condon, P.I., and Serjeant, G.R.: Ocular findings in elderly cases of homozygous sickle-cell disease in Jamaica. *Brit J Ophthalmol, 60:* 361, 1976.
12. Nagpal, K.C., Patrianakos, D., Asdourian, G.K., Goldberg, M.F., Rabb, M., and Jampol, L.: Spontaneous regression (autoinfarction) of proliferative sickle retinopathy. *Am J Ophthalmol, 80:* 885, 1975.
13. Raichand, M., Goldberg, M.F., Nagpal, K.C., Goldbaum, M.H., and Asdourian, G.K.: Evolution of neovascularization in sickle cell retinopathy: a prospective fluorescein angiographic study. *Arch Ophthalmol, 95:*1543, 1977.
14. Stevens, T.S., Busse, B., Lee, C.-B., Woolf, M.B., Galinos, S.O., and Goldberg, M.F.: Sickling hemoglobinopathies: macular and perimacular vascular abnormalities. *Arch Ophthalmol, 92:* 455, 1974.
15. Asdourian, G.K., Nagpal, K.C., Busse, B., Goldbaum, M., Patrianakos, D., Rabb, M.F., and Goldberg, M.F.: Macular and perimacular vascular remodelling in sickling haemoglobinopathies. *Brit J Ophthalmol, 60:* 431, 1976.
16. Goldberg, M.F.: Retinal vaso-occlusion in sickling hemoglobinopathies. *Birth Defects, 12* (3): 475, 1976.
17. Goldbaum, M.H., Goldberg, M.F., Nagpal, K.C., *et al.:* Quantitative photocoagulation and the treatment of proliferative sickle retinopathy. *In* Current Diagnosis and Management of Chorioretinal Disease, ed. by F. L'Esperance, C.V. Mosby, St. Louis, 1977.
18. L'Esperance, F.A.: The treatment of ophthalmic vascular disease by argon laser photocoagulation. *Trans Am Acad Ophthalmol Otolaryngol, 73:* 1077, 1969.
19. Little, H.L., Zweng, H.C., and Peabody, R.R.: Argon laser slit-lamp photocoagulation. *Trans Am Acad Ophthalmol Otolaryngol, 74:* 85, 1970.
20. Goldberg, M.F.: Treatment of proliferative sickle retinopathy. *Trans Am Acad Ophthalmol Otolaryngol, 75:* 532, 1971.
21. Goldberg, M.F., and Acacio, I.: Argon laser photocoagulation of proliferative sickle retinopathy. *Arch Ophthalmol, 90:* 35, 1973.
22. Condon, P.I., and Serjeant, G.R.: Photocoagulation and diathermy in the treatment of proliferative sickle retinopathy. *Brit J Ophthalmol, 58:* 650, 1974.
23. Galinos, S.O., Asdourian, G.K., Woolf, M.B., Goldberg, M.F., and Busse, B.J.: Choroido-vitreal neovascularization after argon laser photocoagulation. *Arch Ophthalmol, 93:* 524, 1975.
24. Lee, C.-B., Woolf, M.B., Galinos, S.O., Goldbaum, M.H., Stevens, T.S., and Goldberg, M.F.: Cryotherapy of proliferative sickle retinopathy. Part I. Single freeze-thaw cycle. *Ann Ophthalmol, 7:* 1299, 1975.
25. Goldbaum, M.H., Asdourian, G.K., Nagpal, K.C., *et al.:* Cryotherapy of proliferative sickle retinopathy. Read before Meeting of the Association for Research in Vision and Ophthalmology, Sarasota, Florida, April 1975.
26. Eales, H.: Cases of retinal haemorrhage associated with epistaxis and constipation. *Birmingham Med Rev, 9:* 262, 1880.
27. Donders, P.C.: Eales's disease. *Doc Ophthalmol, 12:* 1, 1958.
28. Cross, A.G.: Vasculitis retinae. *Trans Ophthalmol Soc U K, 83:* 133, 1963.
29. Cross, A.G.: Vasculitis retinae: prognosis and treatment. *Trans Ophthalmol Soc U K, 85:* 11, 1965.
30. Elliot, A.J., and Harris, G.S.: The present status of the diagnosis and treatment of periphlebitis retinae (Eales' disease). *Can J Ophthalmol, 4:* 117, 1969.
31. Elliot, A.J.: Thirty-year observation of patients with Eales's disease. *Am J Ophthalmol, 80:* 404, 1975.
32. Spitznas, M., Meyer-Schwickerath, G., and Stephan, B.: The clinical picture of Eales' disease. *Albrecht von Graefe's Arch Klin Ophthalmol, 194:* 73, 1975.
33. Theodossiadis, G.: Fluorescein angiography in Eales' disease. *Am J Ophthalmol, 69:* 271, 1970.
34. Wessing, A., and Meyer-Schwickerath, G.: Fluorescein studies in Eales' disease and related lesions of the retina. *In* Proceedings of the International Symposium on Fluorescein Angiography, Karger, Basel, 1971, p. 608.
35. Lyle, T.K., and Wybar, K.: Retinal vasculitis. *Brit J Ophthalmol, 45:* 778, 1961.
36. Hayreh, S.S.: Optic disc vasculitis. *Brit J Ophthalmol, 56:* 652, 1972.
37. Hunter, C.P., and Thompson, H.S.: Papillophlebitis. *In* Current Concepts in Ophthalmology, vol. 4, ed. by F.C. Blodi, C.V. Mosby, St. Louis, 1974, p. 353.
38. Karel, I., Votocková, J., and Peleška, M.: Fluorescence angiography in unusual forms of idiopathic retinal vasculitis. *Ophthalmologica, 168:* 446, 1974.
39. Ashton, N.: Pathogenesis and aetiology of Eales' disease. *In* XIX Concillium Ophthalmologicum, vol. II, ed. by Y.K. Pandit, Times of India Press, Bombay, 1962, p. 828.
40. Elliot, A.J.: Recurrent intraocular hemorrhage in young adults (Eales's disease): a report of 31 cases. *Trans Am Ophthalmol Soc, 52:* 811, 1954.
41. Spitznas, M., Meyer-Schwickerath, G., and Stephan, B.: Treatment of Eales' disease with photocoagulation. *Albrecht von Graefe's Arch Klin Ophthalmol, 194:* 193, 1975.
42. Theodossiadis, G., and Velissaropoulos, P.: Choroidal vascular involvement in Eales' disease. *Ophthalmologica, 166:* 1, 1973.
43. Diabetic Retinopathy Study Research Group: Preliminary report on effects of photocoagulation therapy. *Am J Ophthalmol, 81:* 383, 1976.
44. Algvere, P.: Fluorescein studies of retinal vasculitis in sarcoidosis: report of a case. *Acta Ophthalmol, 48:* 1129, 1970.
45. Asdourian, G.K., Goldberg, M.F., and Busse, B.J.: Peripheral retinal neovascularization in sarcoidosis. *Arch Ophthalmol, 93:* 787, 1975.
46. Jampol, L.M., Goldberg, M.F., and Busse, B.: Peripheral retinal microaneurysms in chronic leukemia. *Am J Ophthalmol, 80:* 242, 1975.
47. Swartz, M., and Jampol, L.M.: Comma-shaped venular segments of conjunctiva in chronic granulocytic leukemia. *Can J Ophthalmol, 10:* 458, 1975.
48. Duke, J.R., Wilkinson, C.P., and Sigelman, S.: Retinal microaneurysms in leukemia. *Brit J Ophthalmol, 52:* 368, 1968.
49. Morse, P.H., and McCready, J.L.: Peripheral retinal neovascularization in chronic myelocytic leukemia. *Am J Ophthalmol, 72:* 975, 1971.
50. Frank, R.N., and Ryan, S.J., Jr.: Peripheral retinal neovascularization with chronic myelogenous leukemia. *Arch Ophthalmol, 87:* 585, 1972.
51. Patz, A.: Retrolental fibroplasia. *Surv Ophthalmol, 14:* 1, 1969.
52. Jampol, L.M., Isenberg, S.J., and Goldberg, M.F.: Occlusive retinal arteriolitis with neovascularization. *Am J Ophthalmol, 81:* 583, 1976.
53. Moschandreou, M., Galinos, S., Valenzuela, R., Constantaras, A.A., Goldberg, M.F., and Adams, J., III: Retinopathy in hemoglobin C trait (AC hemoglobinopathy). *Am J Ophthalmol, 77:* 465, 1974.
54. Watzke, R.C., Stevens, T.S., and Carney, R.G., Jr.: Retinal vascular changes of incontinentia pigmenti. *Arch Ophthalmol, 94:* 743, 1976.

CHAPTER 10

Retinal Telangiectasia

Kurt A. Gitter, M.D., Lawrence A. Yannuzzi, M.D., and Howard Schatz, M.D.

Retinal telangiectasia is a congenital retinal vascular anomaly of unknown etiology with a broad spectrum of clinical presentation including Coats' disease, Leber's miliary aneurysms and macular and paramacular telangiectasia. It may present with one, all, or a combination of these clinically recognizable anatomic patterns.

In 1908 [1] and 1912 [2], Coats described an "exudative retinitis" in childhood associated with congenital retinal telangiectasia. He classified this disorder into three types based on their apparent histopathologic causes and clinical appearance: type I, external exudate retinopathy; type II, external hemorrhagic retinopathy; and type III, angiomatosis and arteriovenous communications.

Later, type III became regarded as von Hippel-Lindau's angiomatosis [3], and Coats' type I and II were combined to form a single exudative retinopathy in children and young adults.

Leber [4], in 1912 described a unilateral retinal capillary disorder characterized by aneurysmal dilations and exudations primarily affecting males, which produced visual loss. He termed this condition "miliary aneurysms."

Many authors subsequently noted the similarity between Coats' retinal telangiectasia and Leber's miliary aneurysms.

In 1956, Reese [6] coined the term retinal telangiectasia to include all of these conditions.

Pathology

The histopathology was first described by Coats [1, 2] and, subsequently, by Leber [4] and many others [5–12]. Leber believed these lesions were inflammatory in nature, whereas Reese [6] felt that the primary problem was the development of abnormal retinal vessels. Manschot and deBruijn [10] in 1967 and Tripathi and Ashton [12] in 1971 clarified the pathology of this disorder and demonstrated that the primary lesion is retinal telangiectasia, which is probably congenital. Tripathi and Ashton studied the histopathology of Coats' by electron microscopy and concluded that the essential abnormality involved the retinal vascular endothelium (Fig. 10.1). They postulated that an abnormality of permeability of the capillary or vein endothelium led to the deposition of plasma in the vessel wall. Gradual disruption of the vascular tissue enables blood components to pass through the wall with serum and lipid exudation.

Congenital retinal telangiectasia with abnormal arteriovenous communications and defective capillary endothelium account for the leakage of serum and blood cells. When intraretinal fluid accumulation is prolonged, cystoid macular edema may result. Likewise, degeneration of retinal elements results in lipid deposits mimicking exudate throughout the retina. The propensity for this lipid to migrate toward the macula (even when the telangiectasia is peripheral) is not fully understood. Nevertheless, longstanding macular lipid results in permanent visual decline secondary to scar formation. Subretinal exudate also causes secondary retinal detachment and proliferation of retinal pigment epithelium cells.

Clinical Characteristics

The clinical characteristics depend on the degree and severity of the retinal vascular involvement (Table 10.1). The most widespread involvement, defined as Coats' disease, usually is monocular and affects young males in the first decade of life. In these eyes, large zones of retina (one quadrant or more) are involved with telangiectasia, aneurysmal dilation, arteriovenous communications, and intraretinal and subretinal exudation. The macula is frequently involved with lipid deposition (Figs. 10.2, and 10.3) and zones of capillary nonperfusion can be seen.

This full blown manifestation of retinal telangiectasia, (called Coats' disease) can result in secondary retinal detachment and leukokoria and can simulate retinoblastoma. Ultimately, the eye may become phthisical.

A more moderate form of retinal telangiectasia occurring in the second and third decades of life is Leber's miliary aneurysms. This degree of telangiectasia presents with hemorrhage, exudate, aneurysmal dilation, and the vascular involvement is usually less widespread occupying a smaller zone of retinal tissue several disc diameters in size. These eyes may be asymptomatic until cystoid edema, circinate retinopathy, localized detachment, or hemorrhage occur.

The least severe form of retinal telangiectasia consists of isolated small zones of macular or paramacular telangiectasia (Fig. 10.4). This form is usually asymptomatic until

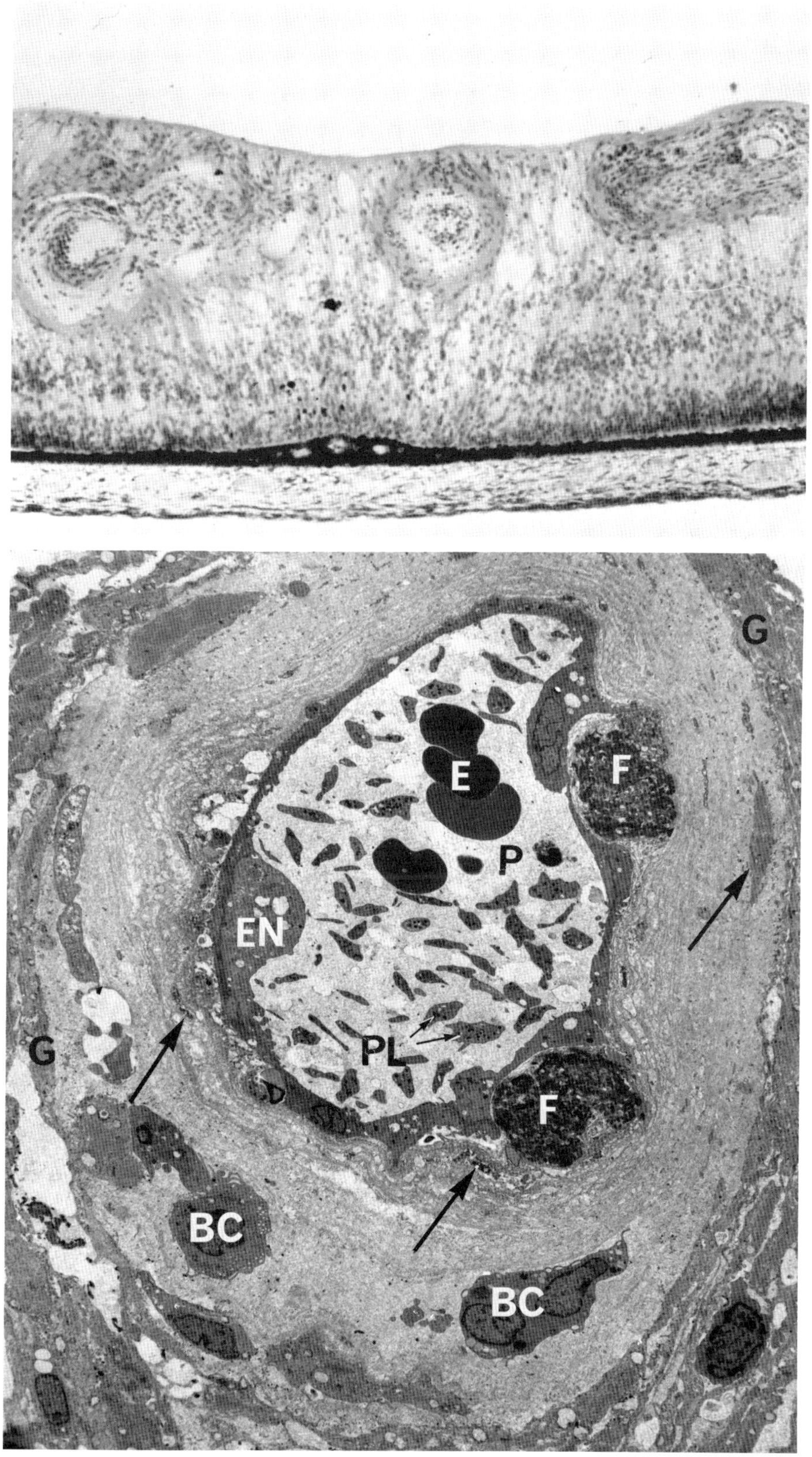

Figure 10.1. *A,* histopathology of Coats' disease showing swollen retina, with exudate foam cells and glial proliferation. Hematoxylin and eosin. ×100. (From Tripathi and Ashton, *Brit J Ophthalmol, 55:* 289, 1971; reprinted with permission.) *B,* electron microscopic photograph of blood vessel with Coats' disease showing a lumen containing plasma (*P*), platelets (*PL*), and erythrocytes (*E*). The vessel wall is infiltrated with plasma, blood corpuscles (*BC*), and cellular debris (*arrows*). The endothelium (*EN*) is still continuous with collection of fibrin (*F*) in the subendothelial space. ×3650. (From Tripathi and Ashton, *Brit J Ophthalmol, 55:* 289, 1971; reprinted with permission.)

Table 10.1. Retinal telangiectasia

Type	Age group	Degree, location	Severity	Vision
I:Coats	1st–2nd decade	1 or more quadrants	Severe and progressive	Often compromised with lipid in macula; may progress to 2° detachment
II:Leber's	2nd–3rd decade	Usually less than 1 quadrant several disc diameters	Moderate	VA decreases only when lipid or edema in macula
III:Isolated	2nd–5th decade	Often 1–2 disc diameters or less	Mild	Usually asymptomatic until late edema or lipid accumulation in macula

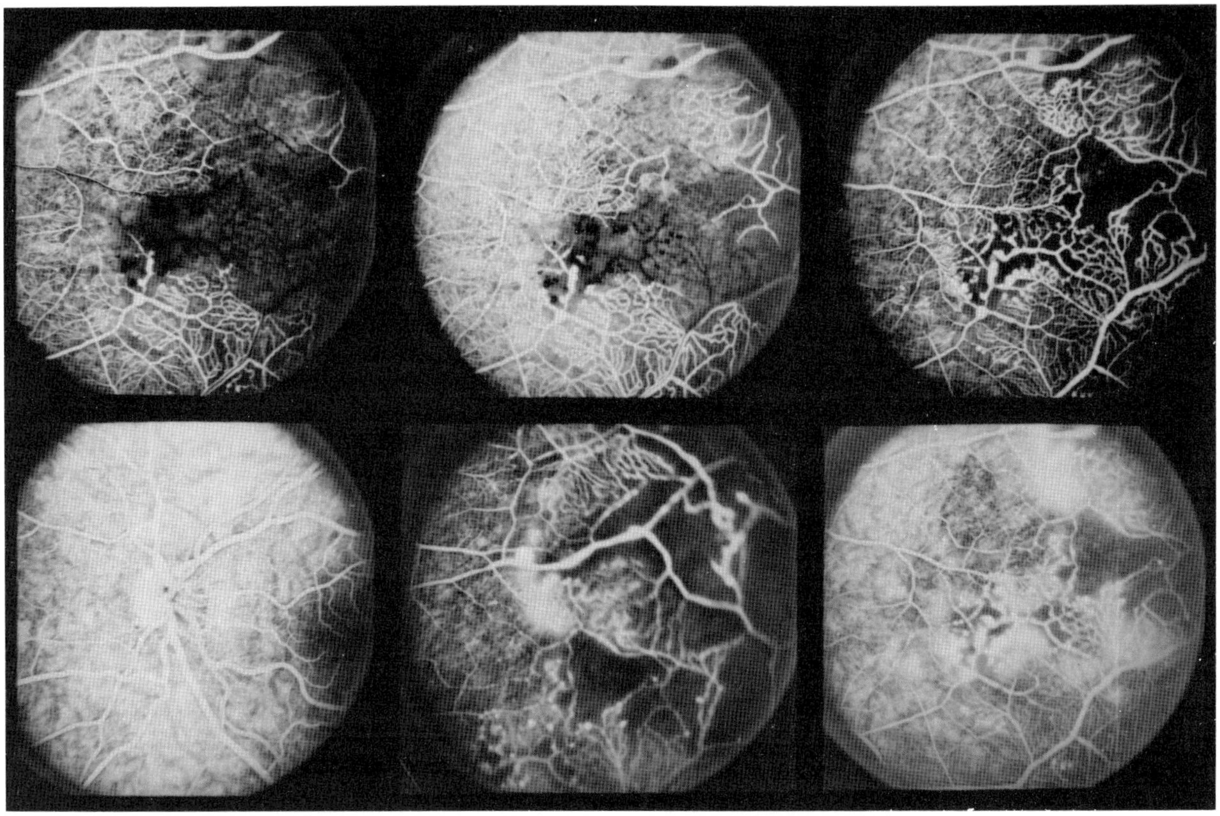

Figure 10.2. Fluorescein composite of eye with Coats' disease showing areas of capillary nonperfusion, arteriovenous communications, dilation and tortuosity of retinal vessels, aneurysms, and dye leakage.

A

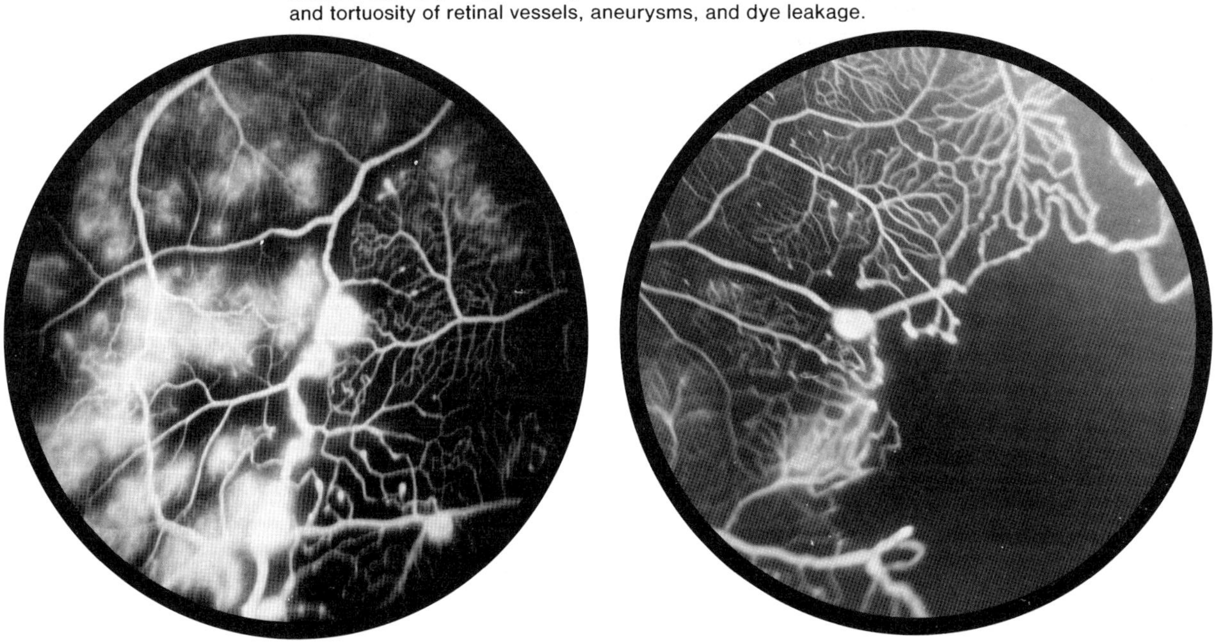

B

Figure 10.3. *A*, venous phase fluorescein angiogram of a 16-year-old male with Coats' disease showing leaking retinal telangiectatic vessels, and sacular aneurysm. *B*, venous phase angiogram in a 38-year-old black male with Coats' disease isolated to the superior temporal quadrant. Note the widespread area of capillary nonperfusion.

the second to fourth decade of life at which time edema or lipid deposition in the fovea may cause visual decline. Slow progression is the rule with increasing amounts of fluid and lipid deposition causing visual reduction when the macula is affected.

FLUORESCEIN ANGIOGRAPHY

The diagnosis and understanding of the wide spectrum of retinal telangiectasia is more fully appreciated with the aid of fluorescein angiography. The fluorescein angiogram shows the location, extent, and severity of the vascular involvement. The specific observable retinal vascular changes include micro- and macroaneurysmal dilation, dilation of existing capillary bed, arteriovenous communications, and areas of capillary nonperfusion (Figs. 10.2 through 10.5).

The permeability of all telangiectatic vessels is increased with staining and leakage of dye. Zones of capillary nonperfusion can be seen both within the telangiectatic areas and the peripheral retina anterior to the zones of involvement. Significantly, there is an absence of true new vessel formation (retinal or preretinal neovascularization) as is frequently found in other peripheral vaso-occlusive disorders such as Eales', retrolental fibroplasia, sarcoid, and sickle cell retinopathies. These angiographic findings are pathognomonic of retinal telangiectasia.

DIFFERENTIAL DIAGNOSIS

The differential diagnosis of retinal telangiectasia is shown in Table 10.2.

One must exclude certain disorders such as retinal angiomatosis, a dominantly inherited phacoma which affects the central nervous system as well in 25% of cases.

Retinal cavernous hemangioma may simulate isolated telangiectasia, but angiographically differs in that the early phases block fluorescein and show delayed filling and late stages show filling of the aneurysmal dilation without leakage. This condition is usually nonprogressive and benign.

Radiation retinopathy can produce a clinical picture identical with isolated retinal telangiectasia and can be seen up to 20 years after treatment.

Retinal arterial macroaneurysm can appear as retinal telangiectasia, but is differentiated by the angiographic findings of arterial bulb-like fluorescence and the older age group.

Other vaso-occlusive diseases, including diabetic retinopathy, vein occlusion, and peripheral occlusive diseases, may simulate retinal telangiectasia, but are differentiated on the basis of the absence of true neovascularization in telangiectasia and the more usual widespread involvement of the later condition.

Tributary vein occlusion geographically occurs along the involved vein and the associated telangiectasia does not cross the horizontal raphe. This contrasts with macular telangiectasia, which has no respect for horizontal raphe and is often seen on both its sides. Accentuation of the site of occlusion, geographic distribution beginning at the occluded site (at an A/V crossing) and extending along the course of the involved tributary vein, late perivascular staining evident collaterals, and neovasculararization are fluorescein angiographic features that differentiate primary macular telangiectasia from telangiectasia secondary to branch vein occlusion. These two entities can otherwise be clinically indistinguishable (Fig. 10.6).

A

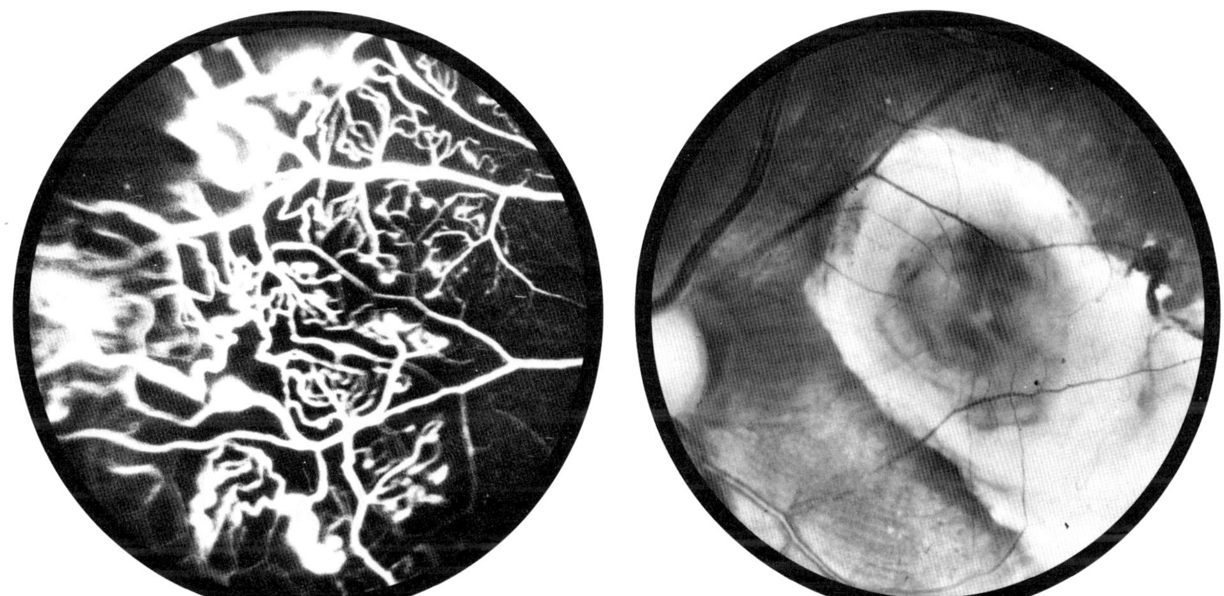

B

Figure 10.4. *A*, fluorescein angiogram of Coats' disease with involvement in the periphery and macula. The angiogram documents nonperfusion, arteriovenous communication, retinal telangiectasia, and marked dye leakage. *B*, ophthalmoscopic photograph of same eye with heavy lipid exudation in the macula.

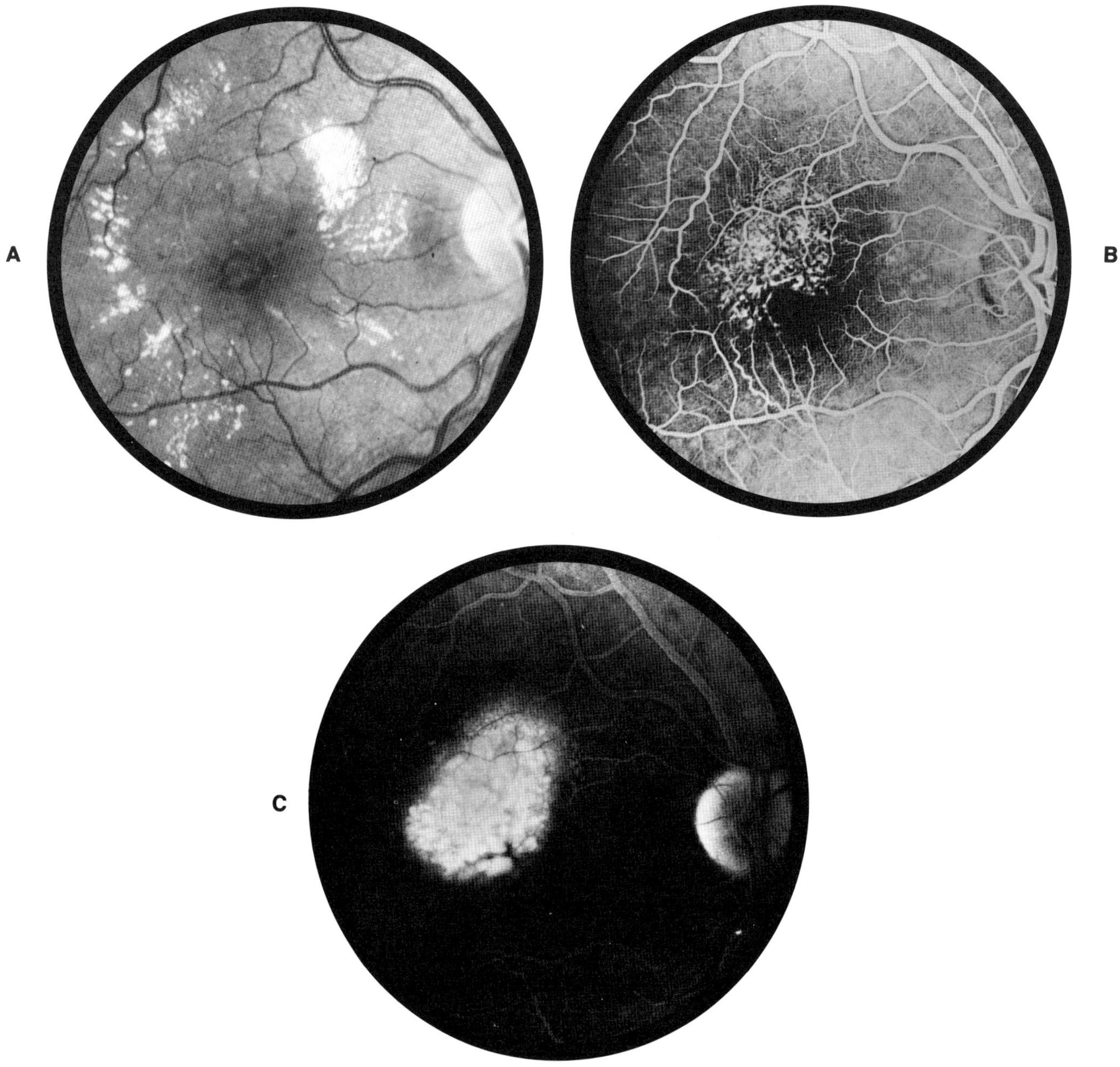

Figure 10.5. Macular telangiectasia. *A*, ophthalmoscopic photograph showing ring of circinate exudation in the macula. *B*, venous phase angiogram showing telangiectatic vessels, which cross the horizontal raphe. *C*, late phase angiogram showing heavy intraretinal, cystoid edema.

A

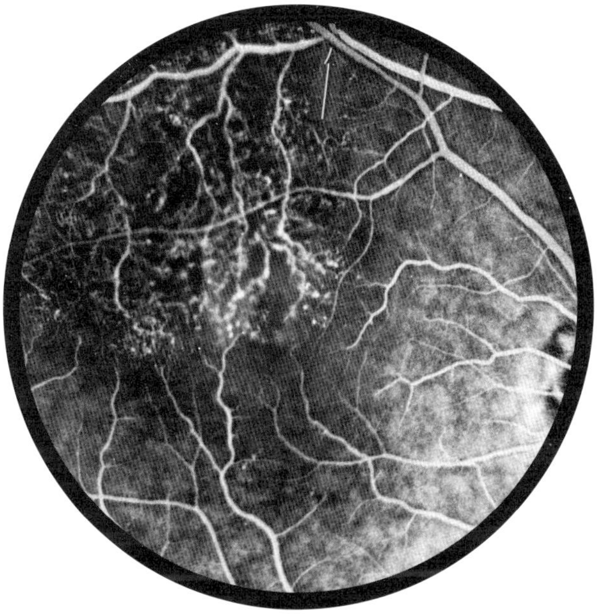

B

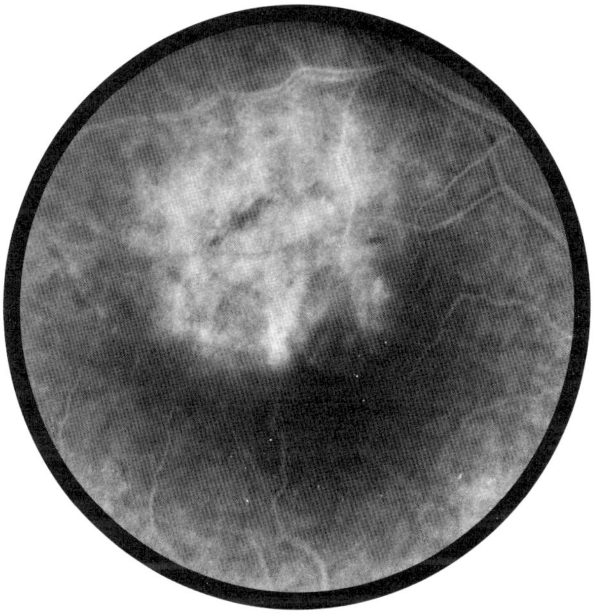

Figure 10.6. Macular telangiectasia following branch vein occlusion. *A*, venous phase angiogram. Note the capillary telangiectasia in the superior macula which does not cross the horizontal raphe. The site of occlusion is seen at an arteriovenous crossing (*arrow*). *B*, late phase angiogram with diffuse intraretinal edema and staining of the involved vessel wall. Unlike primary macular telangiectasia, branch vein occlusion is associated with telangiectatic changes which always respect the horizontal raphe and begins at an A/V crossing.

TREATMENT

The purpose of treatment of this condition is 2-fold. One is to improve vision by reducing lipid and fluid accumulation in the macula and the other to prevent exudative retinal detachment and phthisis bulbi.

These goals can be achieved by destroying the telangiectatic vessels. The methods advocated for treatment of these abnormal vessels include cryopexy, diathermy, and photocoagulation (Figs. 10.7 and 10.8).

Finally, destruction of peripheral abnormal vessels, even in those eyes where central vision has been compromised due to scar and long-standing lipid, may be justified in an attempt to reduce secondary retinal detachment.

A

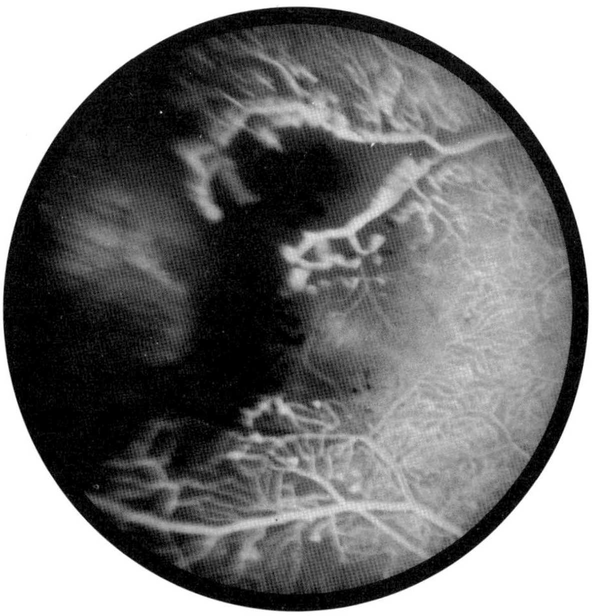

B

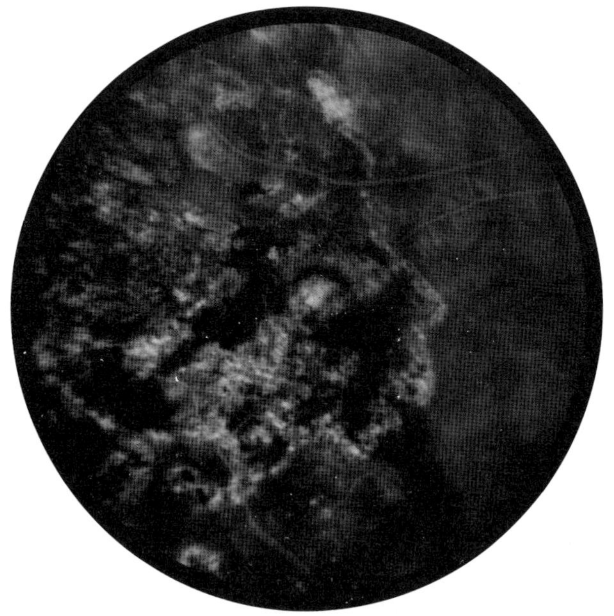

Figure 10.7. *A*, pretreatment fluorescein angiogram of Coats' disease showing capillary nonperfusion and retinal telangiectasia with dye leakage. *B*, fluorescein angiogram 2 years after intense photocoagulation, showing good scar formation and no evidence of telangiectasia leakage.

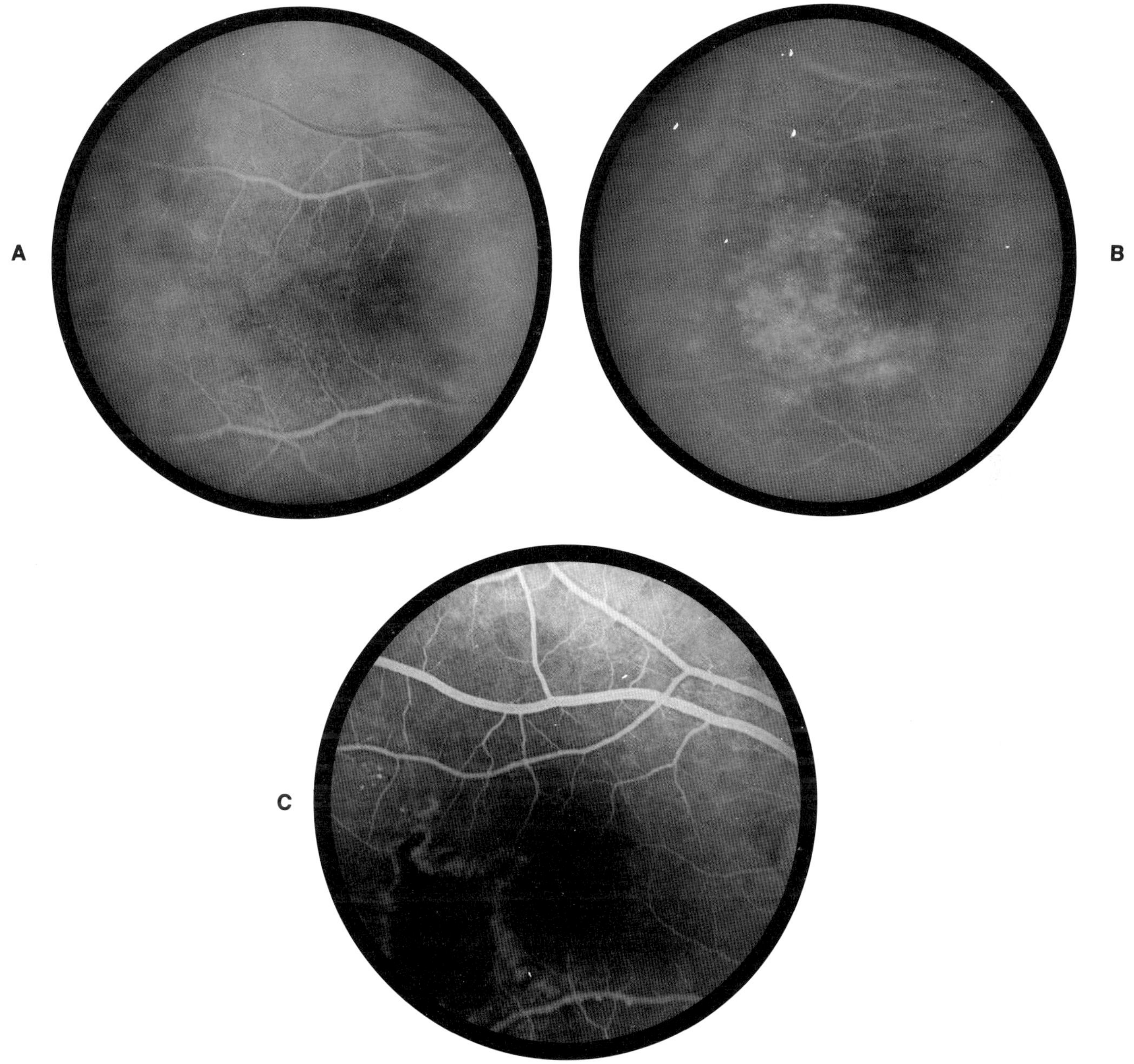

Figure 10.8. Isolated paramacular retinal telangiectasia. *A*, preoperative arteriovenous phase fluorescein angiogram of isolated paramacular telangiectasia in a 48-year-old male presenting with reduced vision secondary to macular edema. *B*, late phase angiogram showing leakage crossing the horizontal raphe. *C*, post-argon laser photocoagulation showing good burn treatment with no residual leakage. Vision improved from 20/60 to 20/30.

Table 10.2. Differential diagnosis of retinal telangiectasia

	Age group	Degree of involvement	Location	FA characteristic
Retinal telangiectasia	1–4th decade usually 1–3rd	Localized to widespread	Posterior pole or periphery	A-V* communications with leakage, aneurysmal dilation; no neovascularization; peripheral capillary nonperfusion
Retinal macroaneurysms	Usually 6th decade and higher	Localized	Posterior pole	Arterial bulb-like filling of macroaneurysm with staining and leakage; associated capillary tortuosity, leakage and A/A anastomoses. No neovascularization or nonperfusion
Retinal cavernous hemangioma	Adult	Localized	Mid-periphery or posterior pole	Early blockage, delayed filling and late accumulation of dye with saccules without leakage
Angiomatosis retinae	Usually 1st 4 decades	Localized to widespread	Peripheral occasionally on disc	Early arterial filling and leakage; widened tortuous feeding vessels, nonperfusion anterior to angiomas
Radiation retinopathy	Any age post-radiation	Localized	Usually posterior pole	Capillary nonperfusion retinal telangiectasia and neovascularization with leakage
Diabetes	Adult Variable	Widespread	Widespread	Nonperfusion, microaneurysms, neovascularization and leakage
Peripheral vaso-occlusive, SC, Sarcoid, RLF, Eales'	Variable	Localized to widespread	Peripheral	Capillary nonperfusion arteriolar attenuation, neovascular tufts (fans) dye leakage
Branch or tributary vein occlusion	Greater than 4th decade	Localized to area of involved vein	Involved vein doesn't cross horizontal raphe	Delayed filling of vein, capillary nonperfusion, collaterals, neovascularization, macular edema

* A-V, arteriovenous.

References

1. Coats, G.: Forms of retinal disease with massive exudation. *Royal London Ophthalmol Hosp Rep, 17:* 440, 1908.
2. Coats, G.: Über Retinitis exudativa. *Albrecht von Graefes Arch Ophthalmol, 18:* 275, 1912.
3. von Hippel, E.: Angiomatosis retinae und Retinitis Exudativa Coats. *Albrecht von Graefes Arch Ophthalmol, 127:* 27, 1931.
4. Leber, T.: Über eine durch Vorkommen multipler Miliaraneurysmen Charakteristik, Form von Retinaldegeneration. *Albrecht von Graefes Arch Ophthalmol, 18:* 1, 1912.
5. Maggi, C.: Leber's retinal degeneration with miliary aneurysms. *Am J Ophthalmol, 56:* 901, 1963.
6. Reese, A.B.: Telangiectasis of the retina and Coats' disease. *Am J Ophthalmol, 42:* 1, 1956.
7. Sugar, H.S.: Coats' disease: telangiectatic or multiple vascular origin? *Am J Ophthalmol, 45:* 508, 1958.
8. Tour, R.L: Miliary retinal aneurysms. *Am J Ophthalmol, 43:* 426, 1957.
9. Wise, G.N.: Coats' disease. *Arch Ophthalmol, 58:* 735, 1957.
10. Manschot, W.A., and deBruijn, W.C.: Coats' disease: definition and pathogenesis. *Brit J Ophthalmol, 51:* 145, 1967.
11. Archer, D., and Krill, A.E.: Leber's miliary aneurysms and optic atrophy. *Surg Ophthalmol, 15:* 384, 1971.
12. Tripathi, R., and Ashton, N.: Electron microscopical study of Coats's disease. *Brit J Ophthalmol, 55:* 289, 1971.

CHAPTER 11

Retinal Macroaneurysms

Kurt A. Gitter, M.D., Howard Schatz, M.D. and Lawrence A. Yannuzzi, M.D.

Retinal arterial macroaneurysm is a distinct clinical entity characterized by single or multiple aneurysmal outpouchings of the first three orders of retinal arterial bifurcation.

Several reports of isolated aneurysms of the retinal arteries appeared in the ophthalmic literature early in this century [1–3].

In 1973, Robertson [4] defined this entity and introduced the term retinal macroaneurysm. In his description of 13 patients, hemorrhage and exudates producing scotomas and impairment of macular vision were frequently present. He emphasized that the natural tendency of macroaneurysms was to heal spontaneously, resulting in good vision. He, therefore, advocated conservative management.

Later in 1973, Hudomel and Imre [5] reported a solitary aneurysm which produced progressive central visual loss over a 12-month period that resolved following photocoagulation treatment with subsequent visual improvement. Schults and Swan [6] reported on five cases of macroaneurysm, three of whom had spontaneous pulsation and hemorrhage.

In 1975 Cleary, *et al.* [7] studied the natural history of 20 patients with macroaneurysms of which 14 (70%) suffered visual loss. Of these 14, six (30% of total number of patients) had permanent visual loss of less than 20/80 due mostly to macular edema and/or exudates. The authors suggested that patients with macroaneurysms may benefit from a course of photocoagulation treatment to prevent permanent visual loss. Nadel and Gupta [8] in 1976 reported six cases and emphasized that recurrent vitreous hemorrhage can lead to visual decline. Most recently, Perry, Zimmerman and Benson [9] reported that two eyes with macroaneurysms and hemorrhage were enucleated because of a mistaken diagnosis of malignant melanoma.

We have had the opportunity to personally evaluate and manage 29 cases of retinal macroaneurysms over the past 7 years, with photocoagulation treatment performed in 16 cases and conservative management in 13 [10]. Our results confirm that eyes with edema and/or lipid in the macula may show considerable visual improvement after photocoagulation.

Etiology

The etiology of this condition is unknown. Aging, hypertension, and arteriosclerosis appear to be common denominators. Similar aneurysms have been described in cerebral arteries in similar type patients [11]. With aging and arteriosclerosis, retinal arteries lose their muscularis layer. The vessels become thin-walled and fibrotic and with increased intra-arterial pressure can be more easily dilated.

Other associated conditions include sarcoid, which was found in two of Bird's cases [7] and three of our cases.

Clinical Characteristics and Natural History

Acquired retinal arterial macroaneurysm is a distinct entity unassociated with evidence of widespread ocular disease. There is no evidence of retinal telangiectasia, although small areas of capillary dilation can often be seen adjacent to the arterial macroaneurysm.

The condition is usually unilateral (90% or more) and found in patients usually over 50 years of age who frequently have a history of hypertension. It is much more prevalent in females than males.

Vision may be reduced by a variety of mechanisms including hemorrhage, exudates, and/or edema. Most commonly, hemorrhage occurs in the retina, but may be subretinal, sub-retinal pigment epithelium, preretinal, or in the vitreous. Lipid and fluid exudation can involve the fovea, and when it does, it results in visual decline. Other causes of visual loss include neurosensory detachment of the macula, cystoid macular edema, and macular hole formation.

Examination reveals a red outpouching of a second or third order arteriole that may be surrounded by a ring of hard exudates or edema, or be partially obscured by overlying hemorrhage. The arterial aneurysm may be single and, occasionally, multiple and may be pulsatile.

The natural history of these macroaneurysms is variable. Spontaneous improvement occurs in the majority of eyes, particularly when vision is initially reduced because of a hemorrhage. Some eyes, however, may rebleed causing

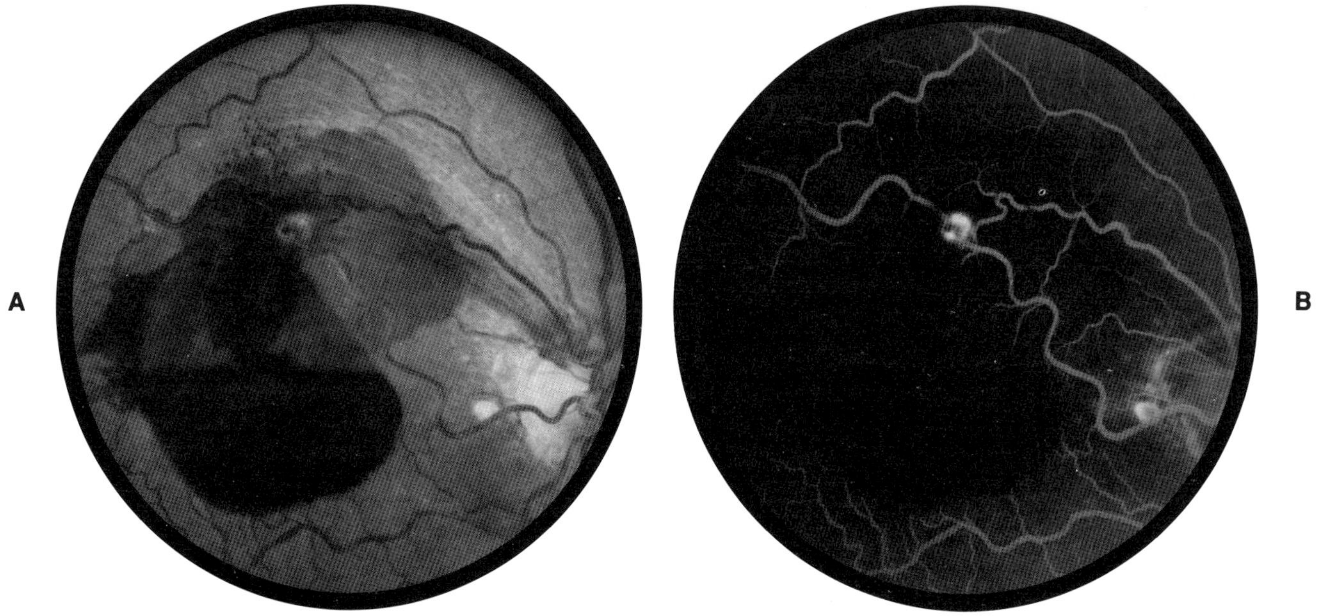

Figure 11.1. *A,* ophthalmoscopic photograph showing preretinal, retinal, and subretinal hemorrhage in the macula. *B,* early arteriovenous phase angiogram showing bright hyperfluorescence from arterial macroaneurysm superotemporal to macula. Another macroaneurysm is noted adjacent to the disc. (Courtesy of Maurice Rabb, M.D.)

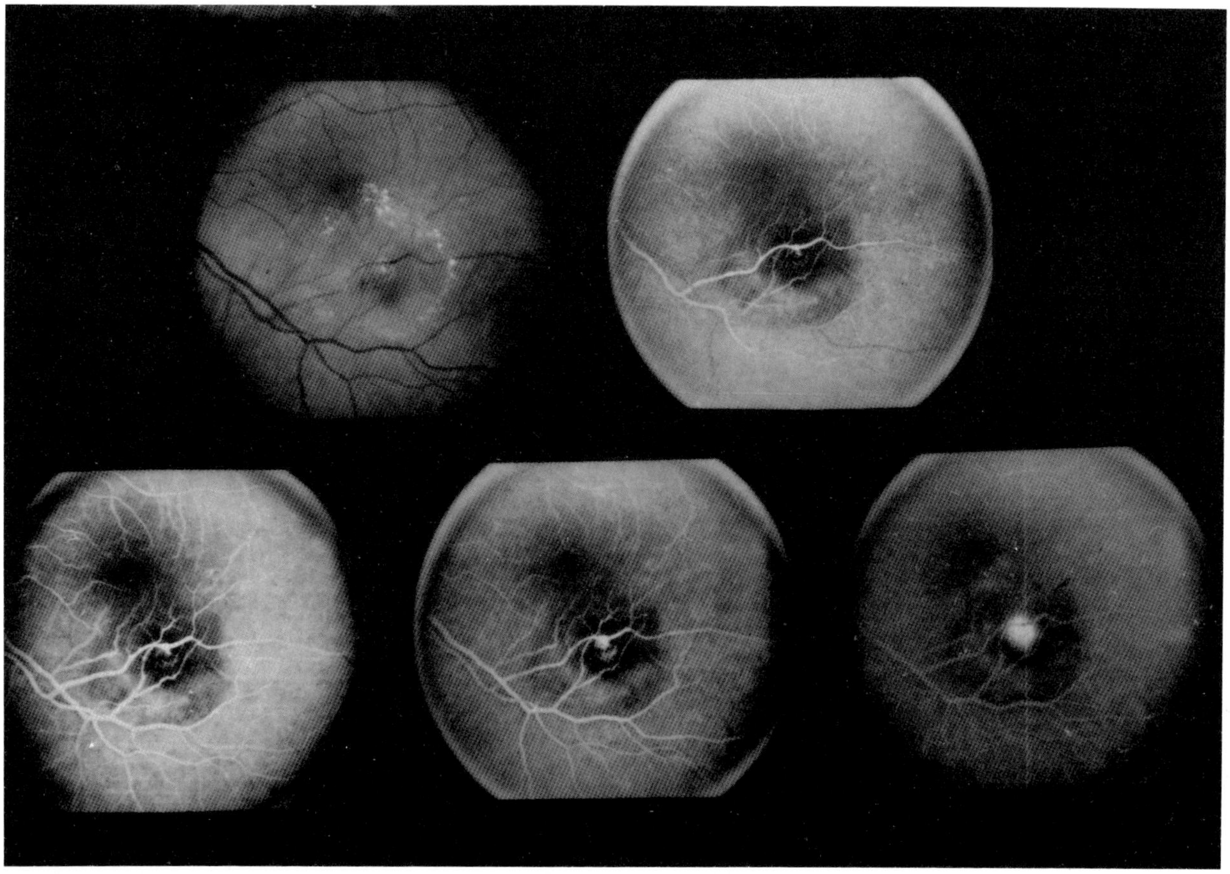

Figure 11.2. Composite fluorescein study of eye with reduced vision and lipid in macula as seen in ophthalmoscopic photograph (*upper left*). Angiogram shows early arterial hyperfluorescence and late "light bulb phenomenon" (*bottom right*) due to permeability changes in the wall of the aneurysm.

permanent visual loss. We have one eye in which a macular subretinal hemorrhage ruptured through into the vitreous causing a macular hole.

Cleary, *et al.* [7] documented that a significant percentage of untreated eyes (approximately 30%) suffer permanent reduction in vision. These eyes are usually those with lipid or fluid in the macula which, when untreated, lead to irreversible macular damage.

Fluorescein Angiography and Pathology

Fluorescein angiography (Figs. 11.1 and 11.2) demonstrates the nature of the lesion by documenting early fluorescence of the macroaneurysm simultaneous to filling of the retinal artery. In the later stages, staining and leaking of the aneurysm is noted, appearing like a bright light or "light bulb phenomenon." Often there is an associated dilated capillary bed which also leaks fluorescein. In addition, A-A collaterals are occasionally observed.

The fluorescein angiographic and clinical findings correlate with the known histopathology of arterial aneurysms as recently described by Gold *et al.* [12]. They demonstrated an arterial macroaneurysm surrounded by hemosiderin deposits and lipoidal and proteinaceous exudates (Fig. 11.3). These histopathologic findings confirm the angiographic findings of leakage of blood, serum, and fluid from the wall of the aneurysm to adjacent retinal tissue. The exudates, when seen, are for the most part located in normal retina and frequently migrate into the fovea even when the macroaneurysm is located several disc diameters from the fovea.

Treatment

The conservative management of retinal arterial macroaneurysm, as advocated by Robertson [4], is indicated when there is no visual compromise or when vision is reduced by acute hemorrhage only. However, when recurrent bleeding occurs or when lipid and fluid maculopathy predominates, we feel photocoagulation should be employed.

We used argon laser photocoagulation in 16 cases during the past 7 years without serious complications. Our criteria for treatment were the presence of fluid or exudate threatening or deposited in the fovea, and reduced vision. Our results were uniformly good. All eyes either remained unchanged or showed visual improvement in contrast to

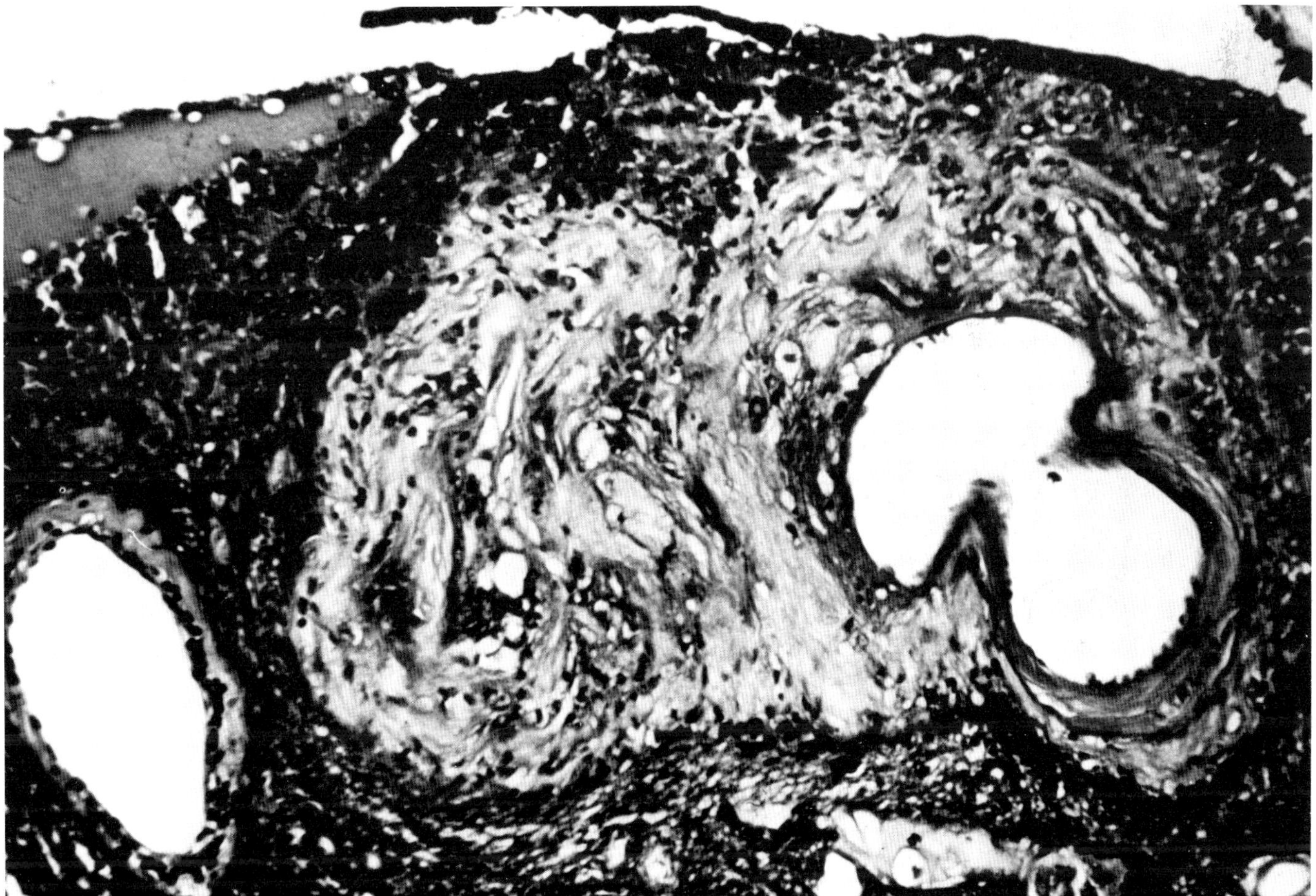

Figure 11.3. Note the retinal arterial macroaneurysm (*arrows*) with an extensive fibroglial reaction around it. Dilated retinal capillaries, hemosiderin deposits, and both lipoidal and proteinaceous exudates are also formed in the adjacent retina. Verhoeff-van Gieson's, ×95. (AFIP Neg. 73-9420; courtesy of Daniel H. Gold, M.D.)

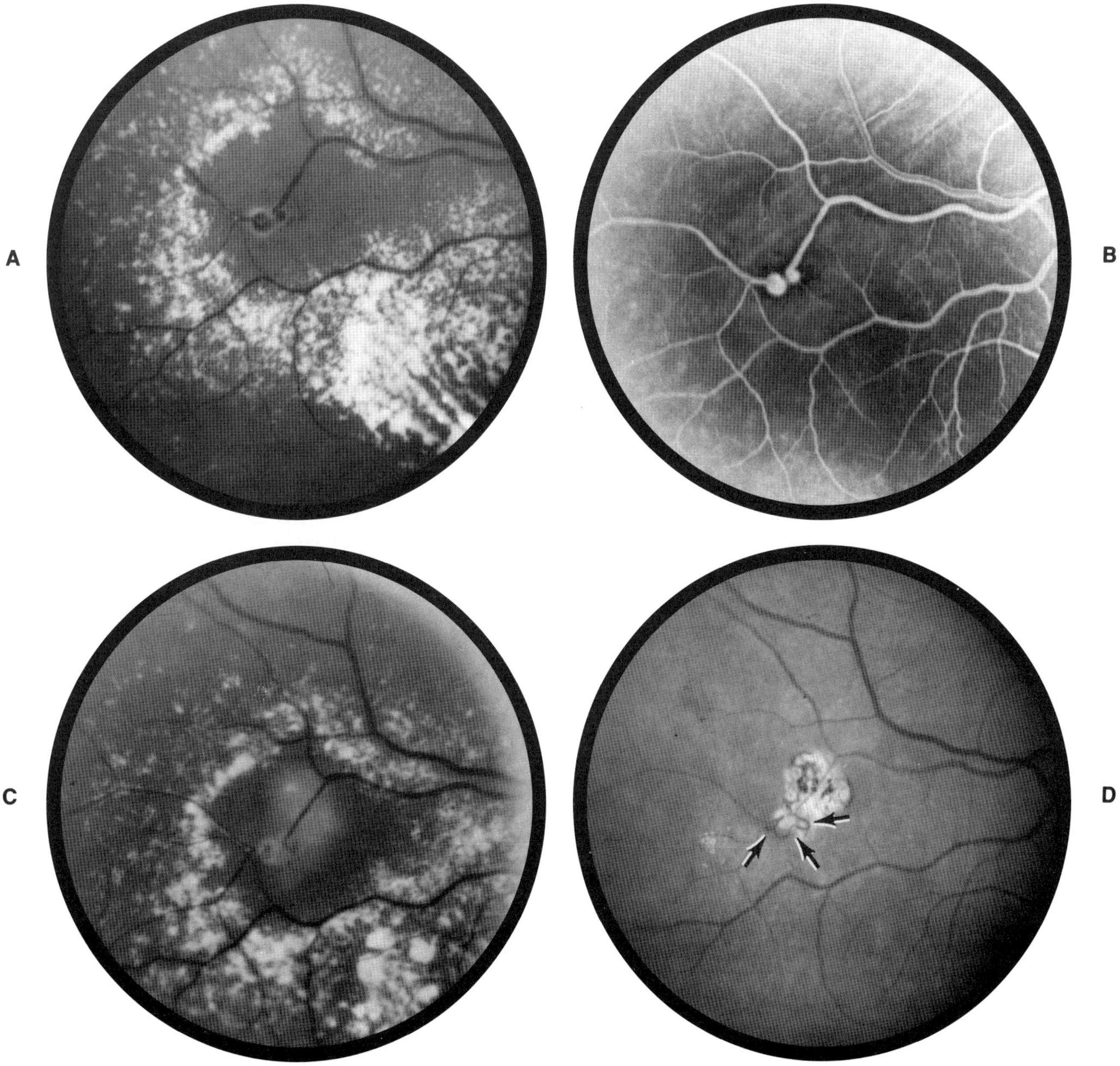

Figure 11.4. *A*, preoperative ophthalmoscopic photograph of macroaneurysm with surrounding lipid. *B*, angiogram of same eye showing two adjacent arterial macroaneurysms. *C*, ophthalmoscopic photograph immediately post-argon laser photocoagulation. *D*, ophthalmoscopic photograph one year post-argon laser photocoagulation showing good scar formation and absence of surrounding lipid. A small arteriole-arteriole collateral is present at the prior site of the macroaneurysms. (*arrows*)

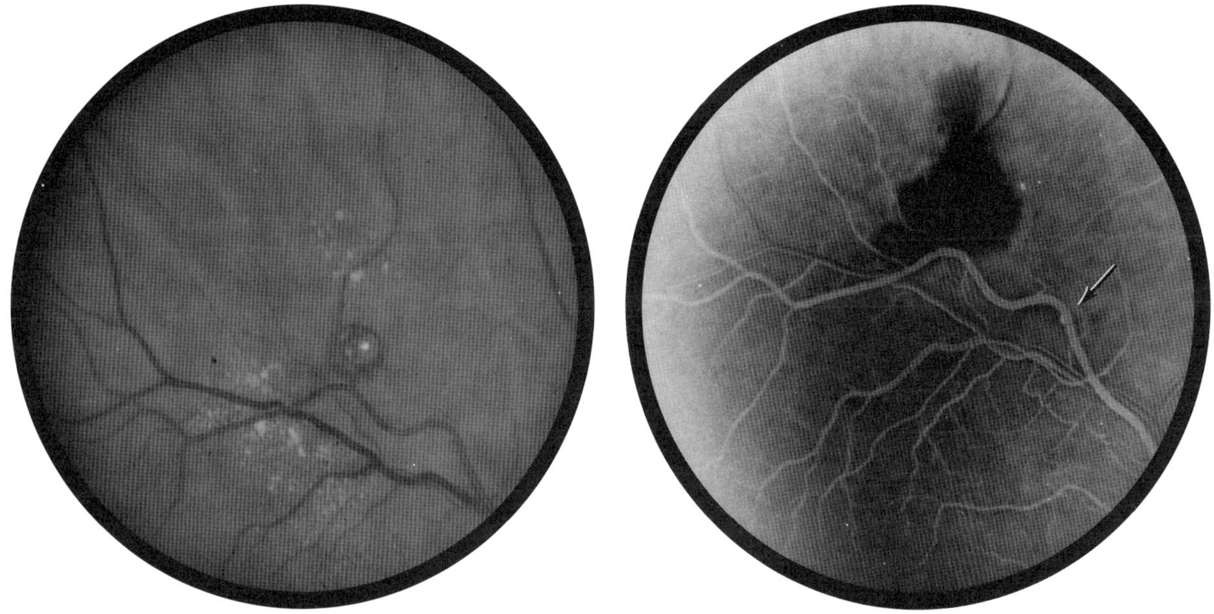

Figure 11.5. *A*, ophthalmoscopic photograph of preoperative macroaneurysm with surrounding exudate. *B*, immediately postphotocoagulation fluorescein angiogram showing destruction of macroaneurysm. Note another small aneurysm proximal to the treated area (*arrow*).

Cleary's group [7] which had 30% with permanent visual loss.

Photocoagulation must be performed with care and precision as complications can occur. These include hemorrhage, incomplete closure, and arterial or vein occlusion. Other possible complications include preretinal membrane formation (not seen yet) and recurrent macroaneurysms proximal to the treated site (not uncommon). Treatment by focal and direct closure is possible when the lesion is small (Fig. 11.4). With large macroaneurysms, multiple treatments may be necessary employing low thermal reactions to accelerate the fibrous response needed to seal the aneurysm with minimal risk of hemorrhage. The argon laser spot size should never be smaller than the caliber of the lesion so as not to puncture a hole through an already thinned aneurysmal wall. Initially, treatment should be with low energy to reduce flow in the vessel and allow maximal absorption with subsequent applications. Burns should be long (0.2 second or longer) to ensure adequate tissue uptake of the laser's thermal energy. Fluorescein angiography is used after laser photocoagulation to determine if therapy has been successful and if the lesion is impermeable or obliterated and the retinal artery patent (Figs. 11.5 and 11.6).

Differential Diagnosis

This condition must be differentiated from other retinal vascular disorders that produce localized vascular responses. Arterial macroaneurysms are rare, usually single, and unassociated with widespread retinal vascular disease.

Diagnostic possibilities include diabetic retinopathy, venous occlusive disease, retinal telangiectasia, retinal angiomatosis, and cavernous hemangioma of the retina.

Arterial macroaneurysms can occasionally simulate von Hippel-Lindau's disease, but the latter is seen in younger patients and is associated with dilated and tortuous vasculature and arteriovenous shunts. Furthermore, the angiomas are usually seen in the periphery in contrast to macroaneurysms which always occur in the posterior pole.

Retinal telangiectasia can appear clinically similar and may have aneurysmal outpouchings very similar to macroaneurysms. The associated arteriovenous communications, marked telangiectasia and capillary nonperfusion without neovascularization characterize this disorder, which generally affects younger patients. In particular, many published instances of Leber's miliary aneurysms are probably retinal arterial macroaneurysms.

Retinal cavernous hemangioma, a benign vascular tumor, also may resemble macroaneurysms. Fluorescein angiography is instrumental in differentiating this rare benign vascular tumor, which rarely affects vision. On angiography, outpouchings on the venous side are usually hypofluorescent in the early phase and show delayed filling. In the late phase, these aneurysms may fill with dye or show serum blood layers without leakage.

Finally, diabetic retinopathy and venous occlusive disease can mimic this condition. These conditions both have microaneurysms and not arterial macroaneurysms. The degree and areas of involvement are more widespread than in isolated macroaneurysms.

In summary, retinal arterial macroaneurysm is a distinct entity, mostly affecting elderly females with hypertension. Vision can be reduced by hemorrhage, fluid, and/or exudate which arise from the arterial macroaneurysm. Although the natural course of this disease frequently shows spontaneous improvement of vision, some eyes suffer permanent loss of vision and are potentially aided by photocoagulation. This disease must be differentiated from other simulating retinal vascular disorders.

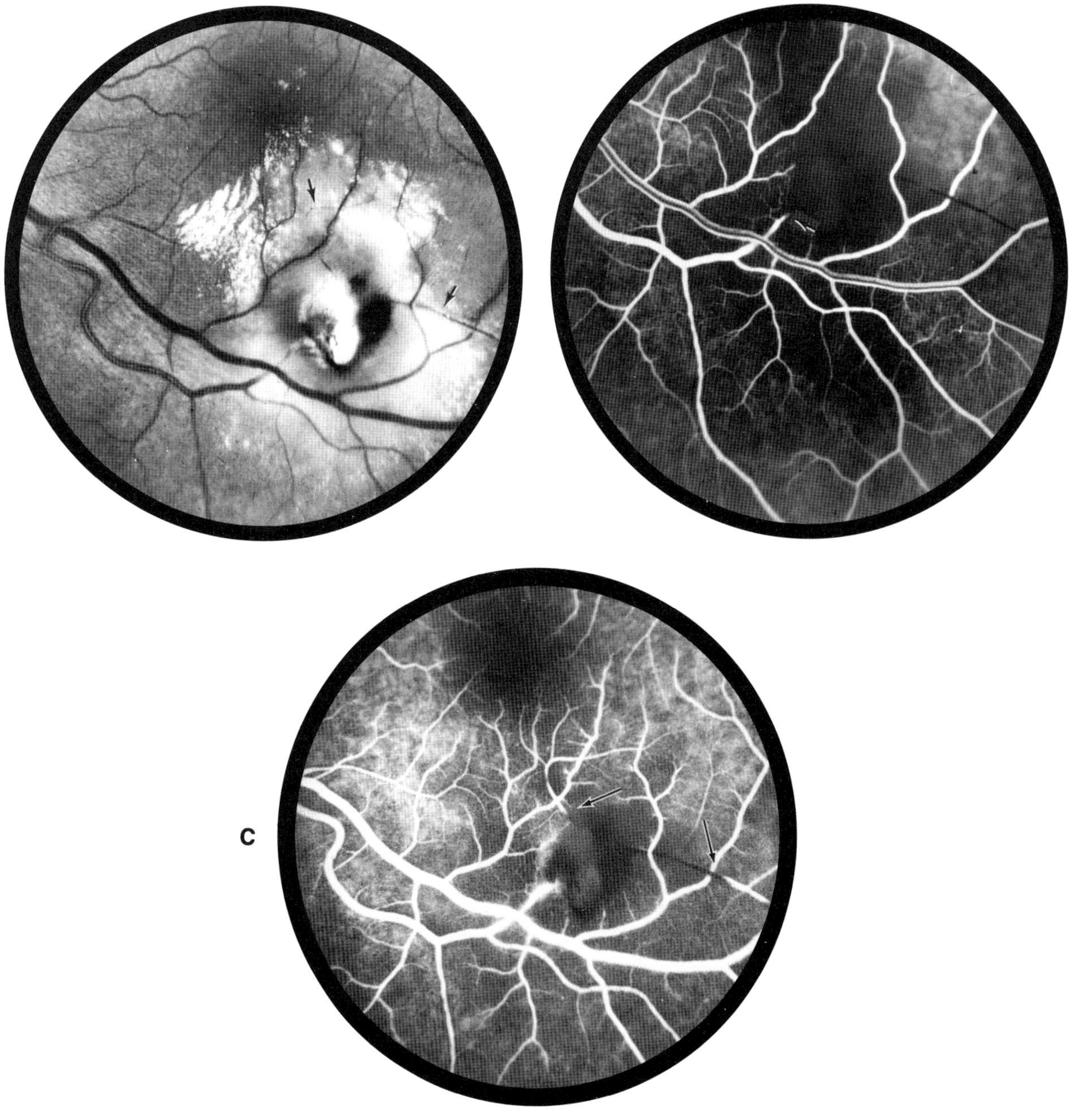

Figure 11.6. Postphotocoagulation of retinal arterial macroaneurysm. *A,* ophthalmoscopic photograph. Note the intense, white photocoagulation burn at the site of a macroaneurysm, which was located near a bifurcation. It is associated with hemorrhage, intraretinal edema, and heavy lipid exudation extending toward the macula. A "boxcar" phenomenon is present at the distal segments of the involved artery (*arrows*). *B,* arteriovenous phase angiogram (*arrow*). Note the delayed perfusion of the involved arteriole. Capillary nonperfusion distal to the aneurysm site is also evident. *C,* late venous phase angiogram. Note the retrograde filling of the distal branches of the involved artery (*arrows*), compatible with the "boxcar" phenomenon seen on the ophthalmoscopic view. Delayed and retrograde perfusion are commonly seen following photocoagulation of a retinal arterial macroaneurysm.

References

1. Pringle, J.A.: A case of multiple aneurysms of the retinal arteries. *Brit J Ophthalmol, 1:* 87, 1917.
2. Fernandez, F.M.: Multiple aneurysm of retinal arteries. *Am J Ophthalmol, 3:* 641, 1920.
3. Jennings, J.E.: Aneurysms of the retinal arteries. *Am J Ophthalmol, 1:* 12, 1918.
4. Robertson, D.M.: Macroaneurysms of the retinal arteries. *Trans Am Acad Ophthalmol Otolaryngol, 77:* 55, 1973.
5. Hudomel, J., and Imre, G.: Photocoagulation treatment of solitary aneurysm near the macula lutea: report of a case. *Acta Ophthalmol, 51:* 633, 1973.
6. Schults, W.T., and Swan, K.C.: Pulsatile aneurysms of the retinal arterial tree. *Am J Ophthalmol, 77:* 304, 1974.
7. Cleary, P.E., Kohner, E.M., Hamilton, A.M., and Bird, A.C.: Retinal macroaneurysms. *Brit J Ophthalmol, 59:* 355, 1975.
8. Nadel, A.J., and Gupta, K.K.: Macroaneurysms of the retinal arteries. *Arch Ophthalmol, 94:* 1092, 1976.
9. Perry, H.D., Zimmerman, L.E., and Benson, W.E.: Hemorrhage from isolated aneurysm of a retinal artery: report of two cases simulating malignant melanoma. *Arch Ophthalmol, 95:* 281, 1977.
10. Gitter, K.A., Schatz, H., and Yannuzzi, L.: Unpublished data.
11. Russell, R.W.R.: Observations on intracerebral aneurysms. *Brain, 86:* 425, 1963.
12. Gold, D.H., LaPiana, F.G., and Zimmerman, L.E.: Isolated retinal arterial aneurysms. *Am J Ophthalmol, 82:* 848, 1976.

CHAPTER 12

Retinal Vascular Anastomoses

Howard Schatz, M.D., Lawrence A. Yannuzzi, M.D., and Kurt A. Gitter, M.D.

Retinal vascular anastomoses are abnormal interconnections of retinal blood vessels that function as alternate pathways for normal blood flow. Two types of retinal vascular anastomoses known to occur are shunts and collaterals.

Retinal Shunts (Vascular Shortcuts)

A retinal shunt is an arteriovenous connection that either completely or partially circumvents the retinal capillary bed. It is a type of vascular shortcut in which an artery connects directly with a vein rather than flowing into a precapillary arteriole and capillary bed.

A shunt may involve a single pair of vessels (Fig. 12.1), a small focal section of the retina (Figs. 12.2 and 12.3), a quadrant or half of the retina (Fig. 12.4), or in some conditions, the entire fundus (Fig. 12.5).

In the Wyburn-Mason syndrome the vasculature of the entire fundus is incorporated into a mass of arteriovenous shunts (Fig. 12.5) which may also involve the orbit, cranium, or other parts of the body.

Arteriovenous shunts are often large, dilated channels (Fig. 12.4), although smaller vessels may also be involved. In some cases the shunt may bleed, although the hemorrhage is usually self-limiting. Auto-occlusion of an arteriovenous shunt may also occur.

The area of an arteriovenous shunt has either no interposed capillary bed, or else the capillary bed connecting the arterioles with the venules is a large dilated channel (Fig. 12.3). In some cases, the capillaries surrounding the shunt area are dilated.

In large shunts, the tortuous retinal vessels may lie parallel with the plane of the retina or be perpendicular, occupying the entire thickness of the retina from the internal limiting membrane down to the pigment epithelium.

Blood flows more rapidly through an arteriovenous shunt than through normal vessels. Consequently, on angiography, fluorescein reaches the venous side of the shunt before it reaches the normal venous channels elsewhere in the fundus. Leakage does not occur.

A type of retinal arteriovenous shunt occurs associated with a retinal hemangioma or angiomatosis, as in von Hippel's disease. Large arterial channels feed into the retinal vascular hamartoma and rapidly empty into large venous draining channels (Fig. 12.6). As in other retinal vascular arteriovenous shunts, flow is rapid. Retinal hemangiomas, unlike pure arteriovenous shunts, do leak fluorescein.

A B C D

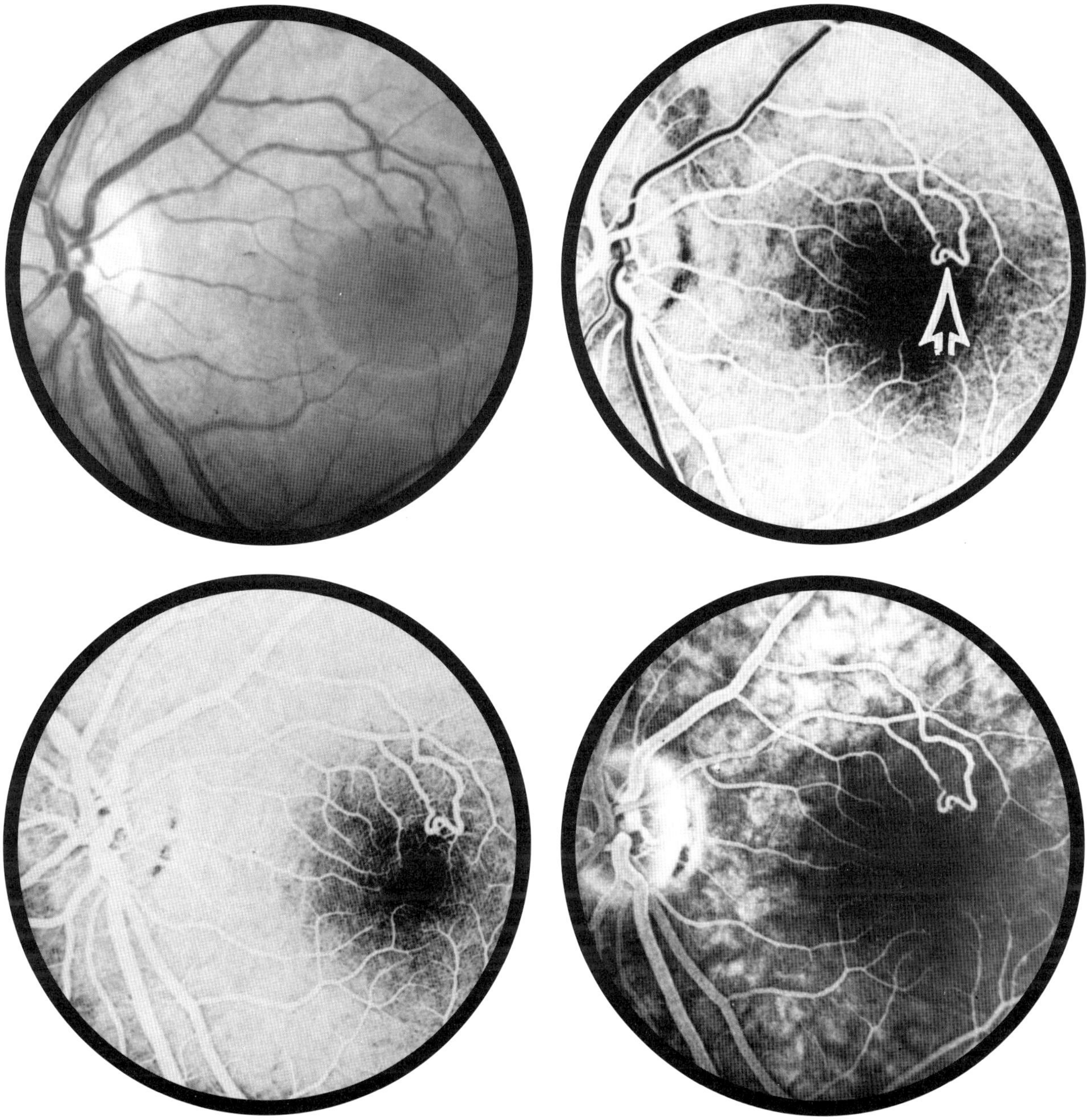

Figure 12.1. Retinal arteriovenous shunt (single pair of vessels). *A*, ophthalmoscopic photograph of the fovea shows a tortuous irregular vessel about the fovea. *B*, arteriovenous phase of the angiogram shows fast flow through a retinal artery connected to a retinal vein (*arrow*) bypassing the capillary bed. *C*, early venous phase angiogram shows that the other retinal vessels have filled normally. *D*, late phase angiogram showing that there is no leakage from the arteriovenous shunt. This patient had a small isolated arteriovenous shunt with a second order arteriole directly connected to a second order venule, avoiding the capillary bed and demonstrating no other retinal vascular abnormalities or leakage.

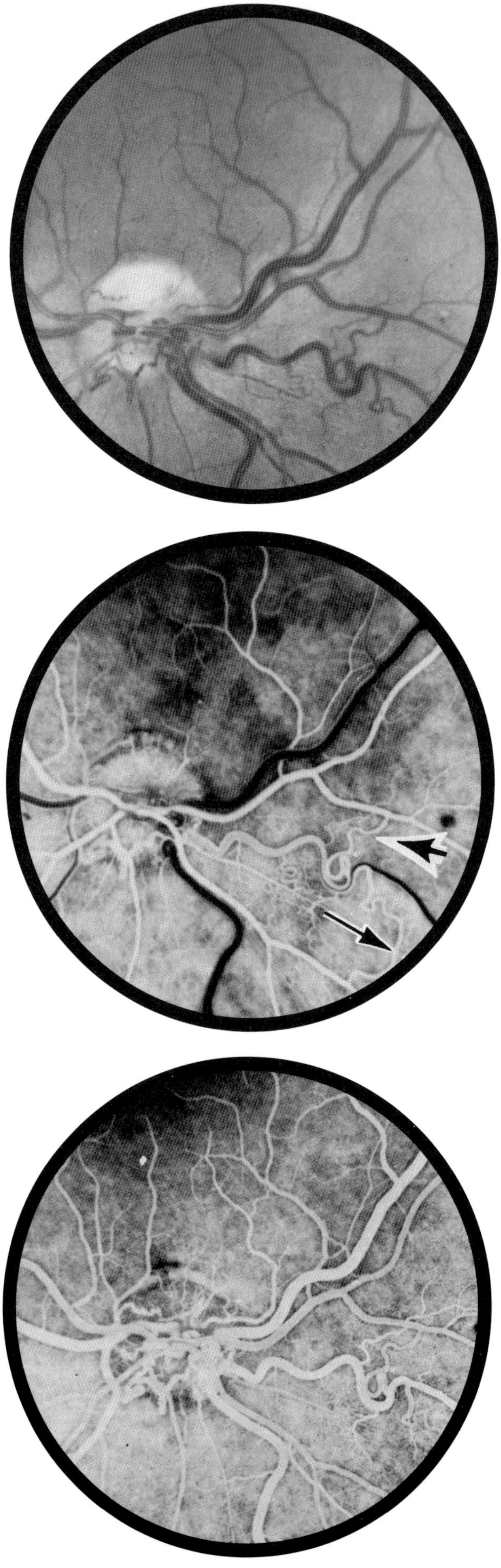

Figure 12.2. Arteriovenous shunt (focal section of retina). *A,* ophthalmoscopic photograph of the area above the right disc shows irregular, tortuous retinal vessels. *B,* arteriovenous phase angiogram shows retinal arteries connected to a retinal vein (*arrows*). The proximal segment of the involved vein is already filled with dye before the filling of comparable venule segments, indicative of fast flow through the shunt. *C,* early venous phase angiogram shows that the remainder of the retinal vasculature has filled and that there is no leakage. The vessels on the optic nerve head are also tortuous and represent small retinal vascular shunts. In this case multiple shunts empty into their connecting vein before the other retinal venous channels because of fast flow.

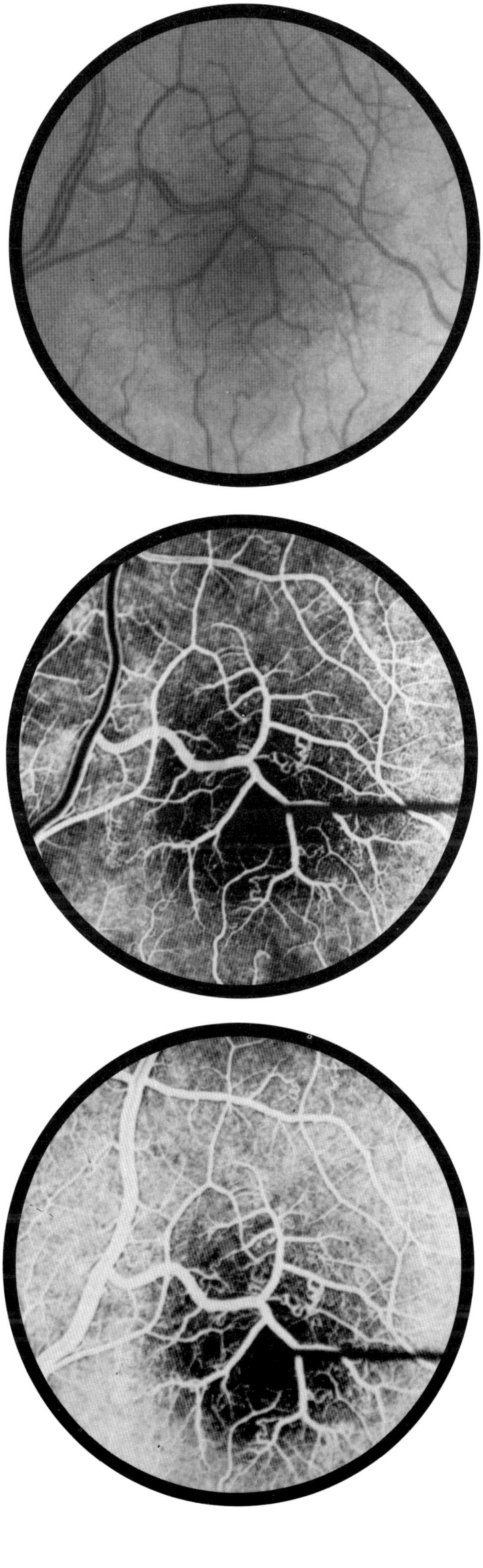

Figure 12.3. Multiple small arteriovenous shunts (focal section of retina). *A*, ophthalmoscopic photograph of right macula shows a large retinal vessel coursing through the center of the macular area. *B*, arteriovenous phase angiogram shows that the large retinal vessel is a vein with many small (capillary) connections which shunt blood from the arterial system. *C*, early venous phase, the remainder of the retinal vessels have filled. There is no fluorescein leakage. In this case, there are multiple arteriovenous connections composed of dilated channels at the level of the capillary bed shunting blood into a large retinal vein.

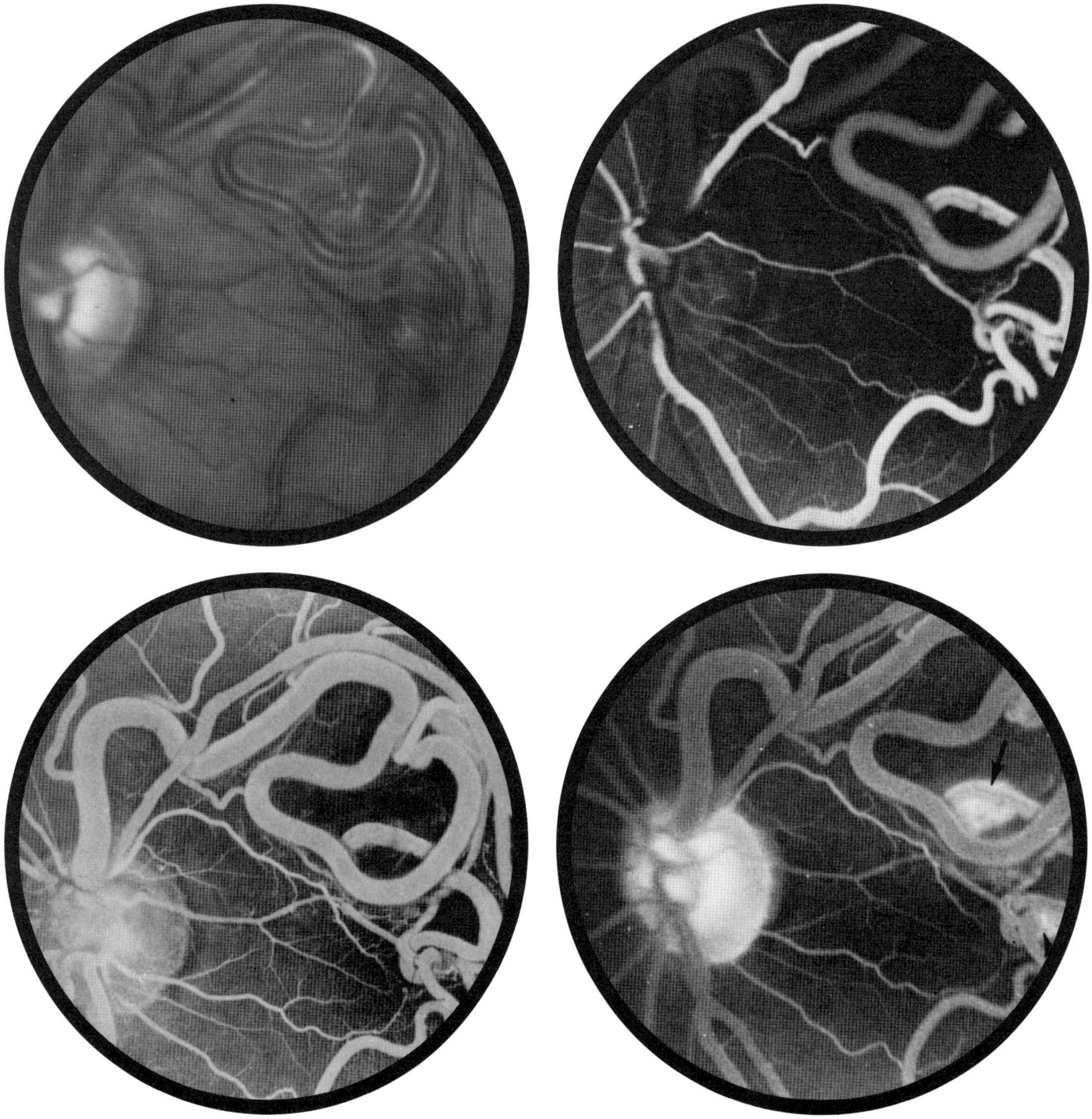

A B C D

Figure 12.4. Large arteriovenous shunts (posterior pole). *A*, ophthalmoscopic photograph of the left disc and macula demonstrates large tortuous retinal vessels. *B*, arteriovenous phase angiogram shows large retinal arterioles shunting flow into large tortuous veins in the macular area. *C*, early venous phase angiogram shows that the entire arteriovenous shunt and the remainder of the retinal vasculature have filled. Small dilated tortuous capillaries are also seen in the center of the macula associated with the shunt. *D*, late phase angiogram. A few sections of the shunt in the center of the macula show very faint perivascular leakage (*arrows*).

A

B

C

D

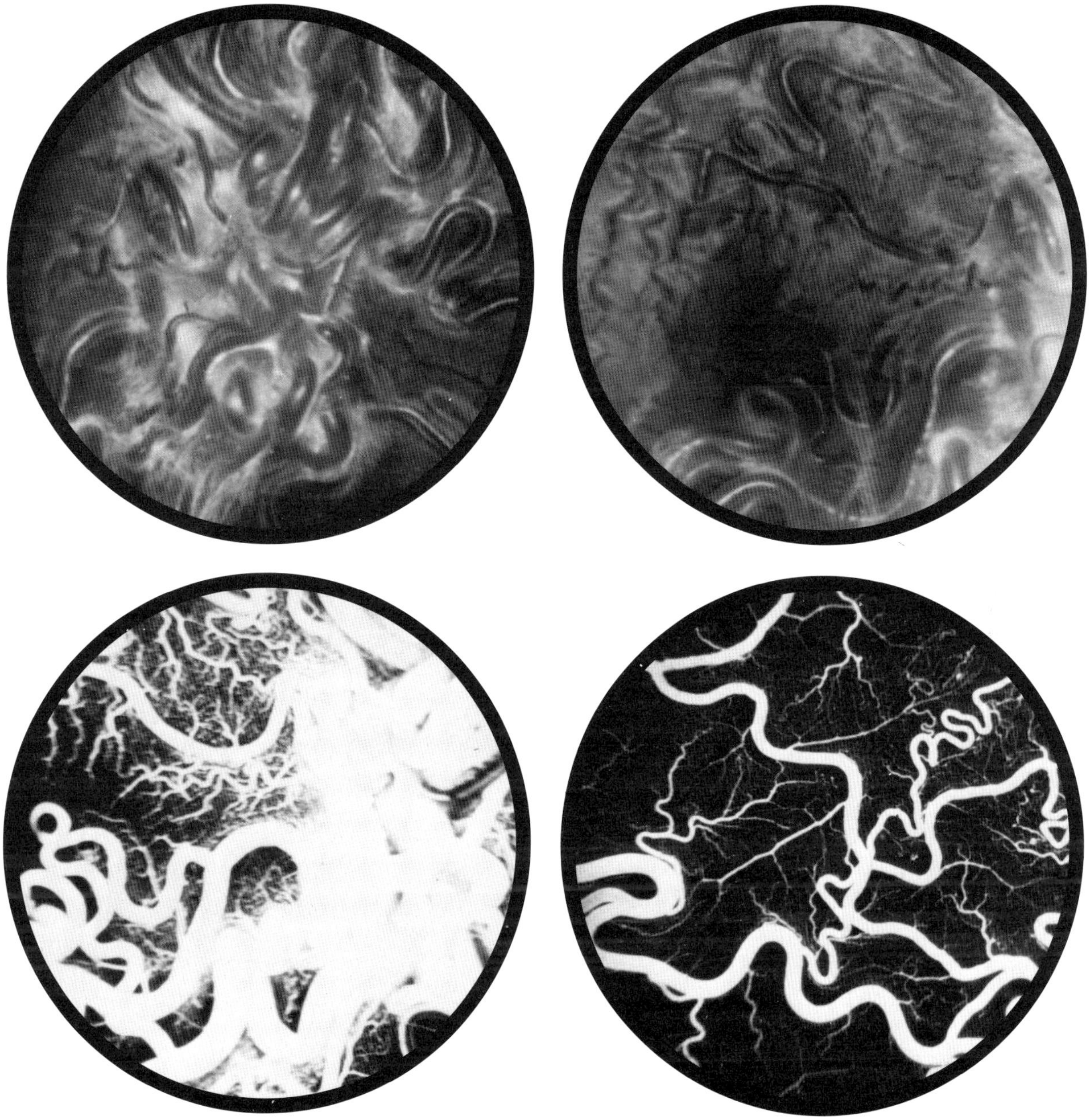

Figure 12.5. Multiple arteriovenous shunts of the entire fundus in Wyburn-Mason syndrome. *A* and *B*, ophthalmoscopic photographs of the right disc and macula showing racemose tortuous dilated blood vessels. *C*, arteriovenous phase angiogram showing rapid filling of the large blood vessels. *D*, multiple arteriovenous shunts of variable size are seen throughout the midperiphery. (Courtesy of Johnny Justice)

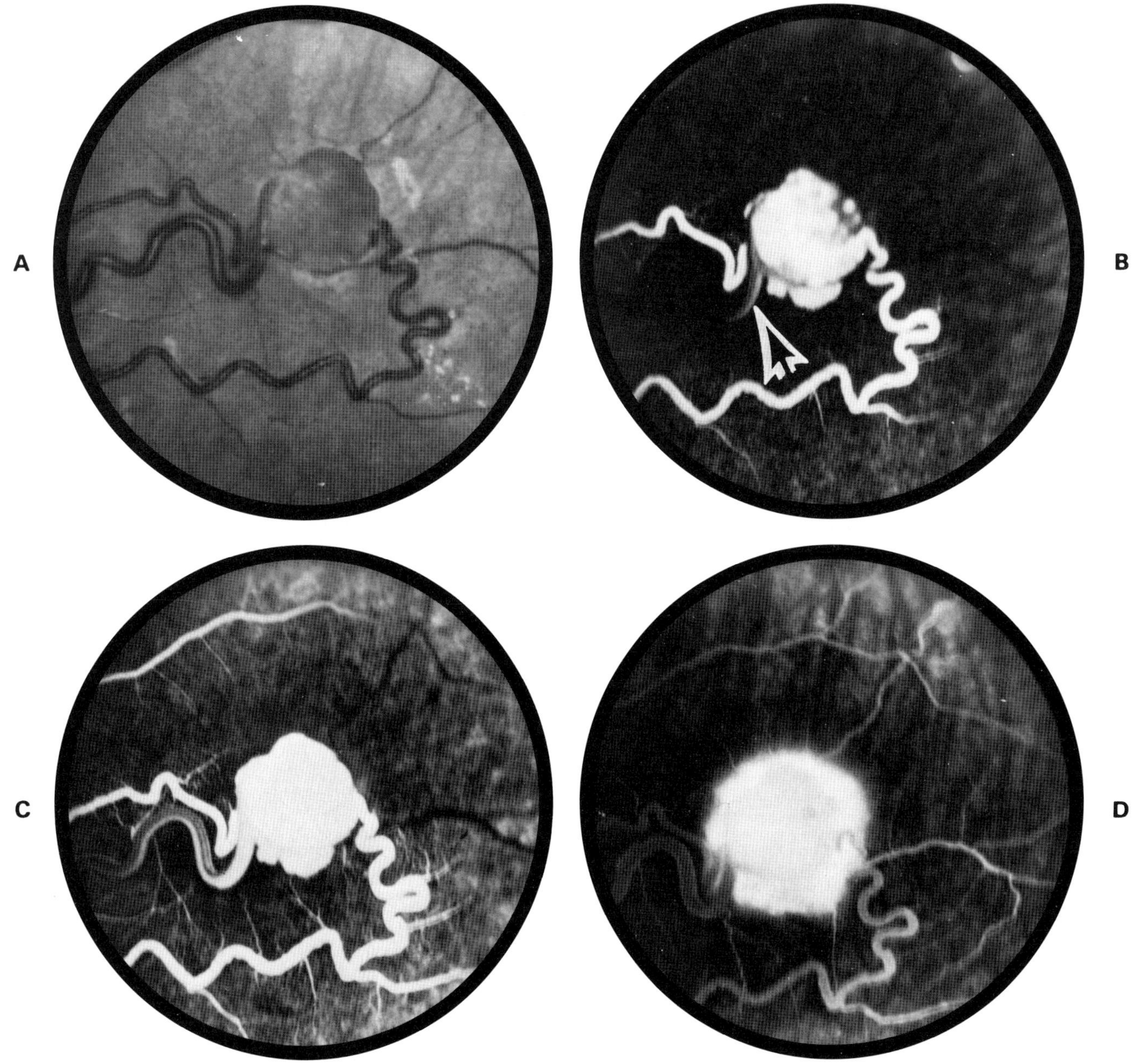

Figure 12.6. Retinal angioma (von Hippel's disease). *A*, ophthalmoscopic photograph demonstrates a red, disc-diameter sized retinal mass connected to three dilated tortuous retinal vessels in the superotemporal quadrant of the left midperiphery. *B*, arteriovenous phase angiogram showing two retinal arterioles feed into the mass; a venous emptying channel begins to fill (*arrow*). *C*, one second later, the mass fills completely with fluorescein and the venous emptying channel shows increased fluorescence. *D*, late phase angiogram demonstrating that the retinal angioma leaks fluorescein into its wall, the neighboring retina, and the overlying vitreous.

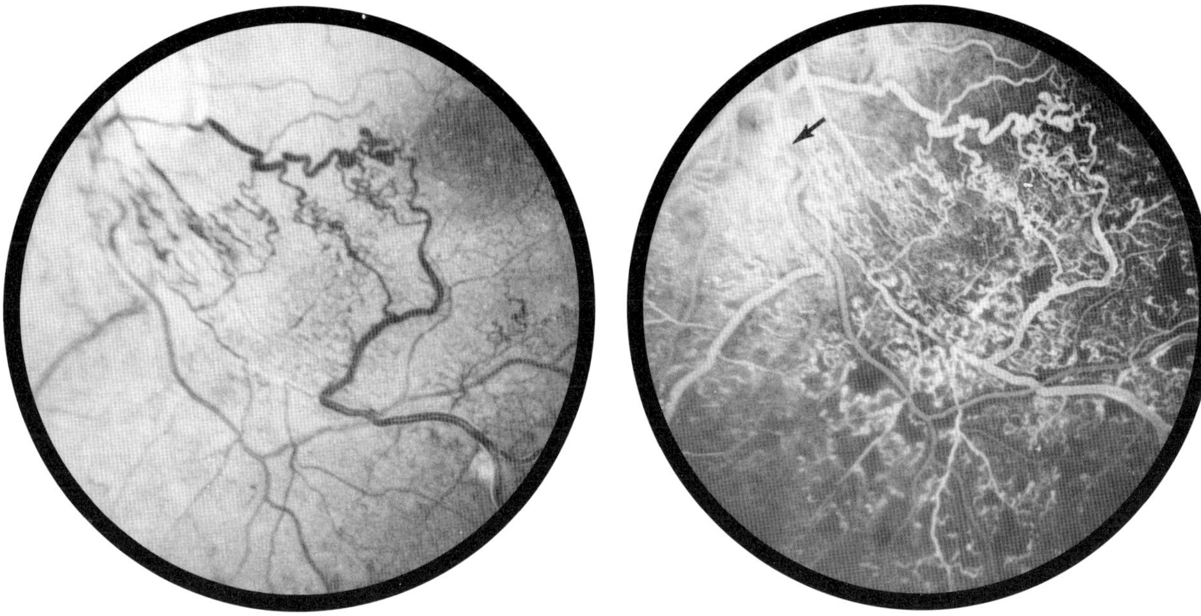

Figure 12.7. Venous-venous collaterals in branch vein occlusion. *A*, ophthalmoscopic photograph of left fundus. Dilated tortuous retinal vessels are present below the papillomacular bundle. *B*, arteriovenous phase angiogram. The abnormal vessels prove to be venous-venous collaterals, detouring venous blood flow around a large, old, branch vein occlusion located just inferotemporal to the optic nerve-head (*arrow*).

Retinal Collaterals (Vascular Detours)

Retinal collateral channels are anastomotic connections of vessels derived from the retinal capillary bed in response to a vascular occlusion in an adjacent area. Collaterals develop from and utilize a pre-existing retinal capillary bed. When a retinal vascular occlusion occurs, retinal blood flow is delayed or closed off completely. Intravascular pressure is increased by the greater volume of blood, causing the capillaries adjacent to the occluded area to take up the excess blood flow. These capillaries enlarge and develop into collaterals which then bypass the obstructed site, linking the patent portion of an occluded blood vessel with an adjacent patent vessel. In this manner, a vascular bypass or detour around the occlusion develops.

The capillaries functioning as collaterals become dilated and tortuous. The blood flow is often slow. When collaterals first develop, fluorescein angiography demonstrates that leakage is not uncommon, but after they have become well developed, leakage does not usually occur. Fluorescein angiography also demonstrates that the adjacent capillary bed is often abnormally dilated or nonperfused.

Specific types of collaterals develop in response to specific types of vascular occlusions. Collaterals that develop following a vein occlusion are venous. At the border of the area involving the occluded vein, capillaries drain blood from the involved area and empty into patent venous channels; thus, circumventing the occluded area. These collaterals are termed venous-venous (V/V) collaterals (Fig. 12.7.) Retinal-ciliary-venous collaterals develop at the optic nerve head in response to a central retinal vein occlusion and, occasionally, to a branch vein occlusion at the disc. Through these collaterals, the ciliary system drains blood flow from the retinal circulation, circumventing the retinal venous occlusion at the disc (Fig. 12.8). These collaterals can also occur with optic nerve sheath tumors, such as glioma or meningioma.

Arterial (A/A) collaterals occur in arterial occlusion and arteriovenous (A/V) collaterals develop following occlusion of the capillary bed. The classic example of arteriovenous collateralization is intraretinal microvascular abnormalities (IRMA), occurring in diabetic retinopathy adjacent to areas of capillary nonperfusion (occlusion). Also, a peripheral retinal arteriolar occlusion, such as in sickle retinopathy, evolves into an arteriovenous collateral.

The function of each type of collateral is readily apparent on fluorescein angiography as a detour of blood flow around an occlusion.

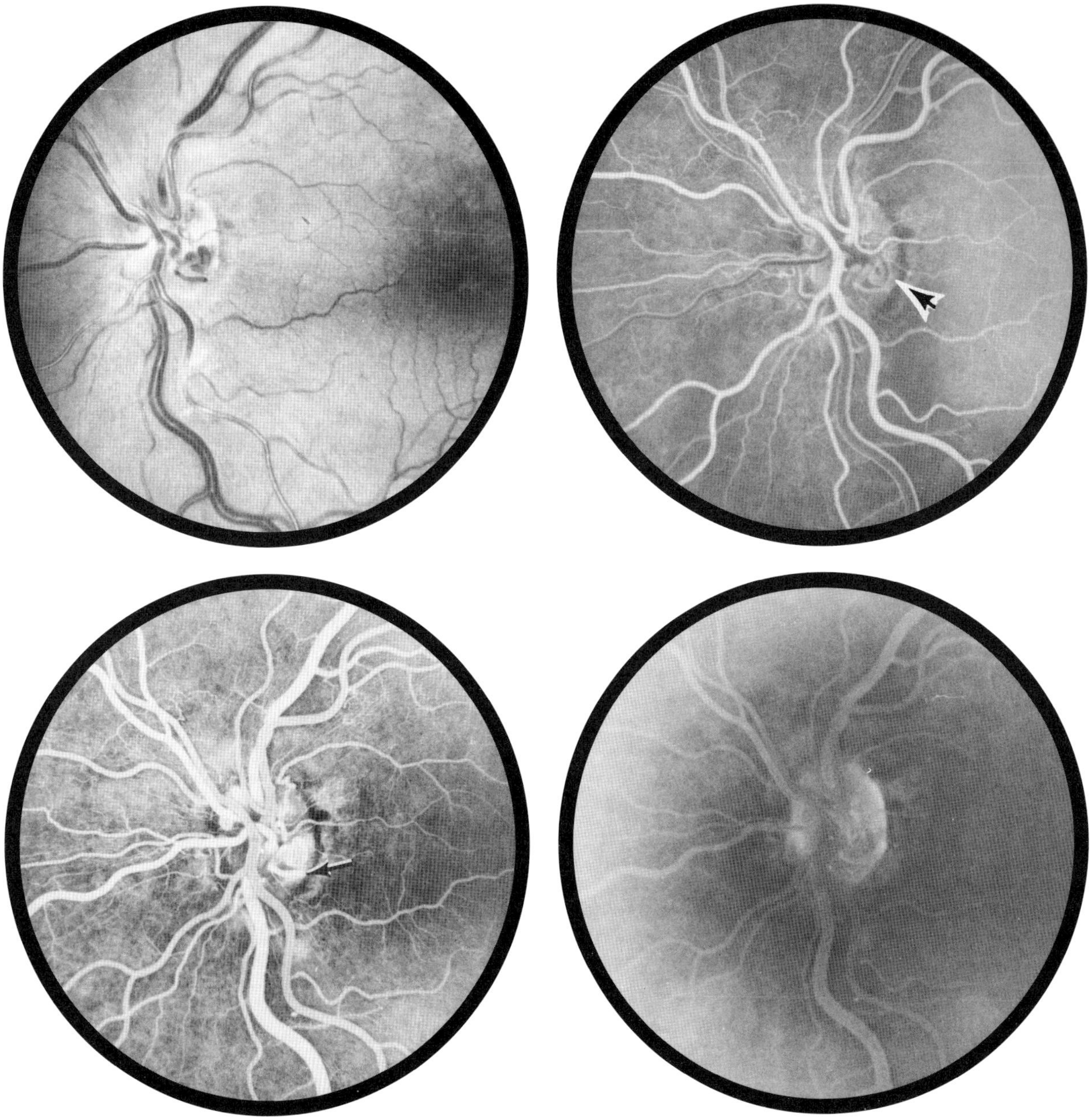

A B C D

Figure 12.8. Retinal venous-ciliary venous collaterals secondary to an old central retinal vein occlusion. *A,* ophthalmoscopic photograph showing dilated tortuous retinal vessels on the temporal margin of the disc. *B,* arteriovenous phase angiogram showing that the tortuous retinal vessels begin to fluoresce and show laminar flow (*arrow*). *C,* late venous phase angiogram showing a retinal vessel on the disc dipping into the optic nerve head (*arrow*); this vessel is not emptying into the central retinal vein. *D,* late phase angiogram shows that the collateral does not leak. Retinal venous-ciliary venous collaterals at the optic nerve head fill slowly and do not leak. Neovascularization at the nerve head virtually always shows leakage, and shunts in this area exhibit fast flow.

Suggested Readings

Archer, D.D., Deutman, A., Ernest, J.T., and Krill, A.E.: Arteriovenous communications of the retina. *Am J Ophthalmol, 75:* 224, 1973.

Henkind, P. and Wise, G.N.: Retinal neovascularization, collaterals and vascular shunts. *Brit J Ophthalmol, 58:* 413, 1974.

Schatz, H., Burton, T.C., Yannuzzi, L.A., and Rabb, M.F.: Interpretation of Fundus Fluorescein Angiography, C.V. Mosby, St. Louis, 1978.

Schatz, H., Justice, J., Yannuzzi, L.A., and Rosen, E.: Congenital arterio-venous shunts. *Trans Am Acad Ophthalmol Otolaryngol,* in press.

Wise, G.N., Dollery, C.T., and Henkind, P.: The Retinal Circulation. Harper & Row, New York, 1971

Wyburn-Mason, R.: Arteriovenous aneurysm of mid-brain and retina, facial nevi and mental changes. *Brain, 66:* 163, 1943

PART III

Pigment Epithelial-Bruch's Membrane-Choroidal Diseases

CHAPTER 13

Central Serous Chorioretinopathy

Lawrence A. Yannuzzi, M.D., Howard Schatz, M.D., and Kurt A. Gitter, M.D.

The exact pathogenesis of central serous chorioretinopathy, or idiopathic detachment of the sensory retina of the macula, is unknown. Although von Graefe described the clinical aspects of this disease in 1866 [1], it was nearly 100 years later that Maumenee, utilizing fluorescein angiography, first noted that serous detachment resulted from a leak at the level of the retinal pigment epithelium [2]. Since this observation, numerous reports have been published regarding its etiology, natural history, and treatment [3–6]. No one has yet been able to obtain a case that correlates the fluorescein angiographic and clinical observations with the underlying histopathology in such a way as to reveal the exact site and mechanism of the detachment. The definitive natural history of the disease also remains obscure, principally because of: (1) a poor clinical definition of the entity, as pointed out by George Wise in 1968 [6], and (2) the absence of any large-scale prospective study on untreated cases employing frequent examinations rather than relying on clinical history.

Some of the data reported in this chapter are based on observations made in a long-term study on the natural course of untreated cases of central serous chorioretinopathy employing an absolutely strict clinical definition of the disease carried out by one of the authors (L.A.Y.) and Dr. Robert Wallyn [17]. The majority of patients were examined every 4 weeks when visually symptomatic and at least every 4 months during asymptomatic periods. From an original total of 111 patients, exclusions were made for treatment with steroids (15), photocoagulation (6), age (4), fluorescein angiographic character of the leak (3), other macular pathology such as hemorrhage or exudate (2), and poor follow-up (16), leaving a total of 65 cases (Table 13.1). Patients had been selected for treatment (steroids or photocoagulation) because of decisions by their referring physicians rather than the clinical severity or their subjective response to their visual impairment. The period of follow-up was an average of 3.4 years, with a range of 2–8 years.

Definition

In the study, central serous chorioretinopathy was strictly defined to meet the following criteria:

1. Age between 30 and 55.
2. Sensory retinal detachment of the macula that was not associated with: subretinal hemorrhage, exudate, intraretinal cystoid edema, disc or retinal vascular pathology.
3. Fluorescein angiographic evidence of a pinpoint leak or leaks from the level of the retinal pigment epithelium, with pooling into the subsensory retinal space.

It is true that central serous chorioretinopathy seldom occurs in patients who are less than 30 or more than 55 years of age. In general, sensory retinal detachments in patients who fall outside of this age bracket are produced by other primary or secondary macular disorders. Hemorrhage, exudate, cystoid intraretinal edema, and optic nerve or retinal vascular leakage are manifestations incompatible with the strict definition of this entity. In addition, the fluorescein angiographic character of the leak is of extreme importance. Any leak that is not pinpoint in nature and lacks discrete pooling of fluorescein from the level of the pigment epithelium into the subsensory retinal space, may originate from some other subretinal disturbance such as subretinal neovascularization. Patients with pure serous pigment epithelial detachments that were not associated with a sensory retinal detachment were also excluded from this study, although these detachments are frequently a part of the overall central serous chorioretinopathy syndrome.

Table 13.1. Natural history central serous chorioretinopathy

Patient selection	No.
Referred Cases	111
Exclusions	
Treated Cases	
Steroids	15
Photocoagulation	6
Age	4
Character of Leak	3
Other Macular Pathology	2
Poor Follow Up	16
Total cases in study	65

Incidence

The typical patient is a male between the ages of 40 and 45. In our study, 42 was both the mean and the mode age. Approximately 85% of the patients were males. Our patient population was skewed in that it failed to indicate the known tendency for this disease to occur in Orientals. Only a few Orientals and no blacks were included in our study. There were, however, a significant number of Hispanic patients. It seems that this group, like Orientals, is predisposed to this disorder. Since its completion, however, a total of six black patients have been seen with a strictly defined form of central serous chorioretinopathy and with manifestations indistinguishable from their Caucasian counterparts.

History

The typical patient first notices reduction in central vision, acuity or field. The central defects may include micropsia and metamorphopsia as well as a positive scotoma. Four of our patients had definite histories of antecedent blunt ocular trauma, although the association between such an injury and the onset of central serous chorioretinopathy has not been substantiated clinically. The medical, family, and additional ocular history were usually negative. Most ophthalmologists are of the opinion that the classic central serous chorioretinopathy patient is "super charged" with high levels of energy, repressed hostility, anxiety, and is often involved in a highly pressured occupation. While this is largely true, numerous exceptions were encountered in our patients implying that additional factors play a role in predisposing particular individuals to the disease. The presence of associated medical ailments in the category of "psychosomatic disorders" has been suggested by some, but evidence in support of this was not present in our study.

Ocular Examination

The presenting visual acuity varied widely, ranging from 20/20 to 20/100 in the primary case. Improvement in the visual acuity can usually be achieved by refraction with the addition of plus spheres to accommodate for the anterior displacement of the sensory retina. Central field examination often revealed a small central scotoma, particularly on testing either with a small blue test object, or, preferably, by the use of the Amsler grid. This latter test is an extremely useful and sensitive tool to document, as well as to monitor, the course of the scotoma in the patient.

The rest of the ocular examination usually was completely normal, except for the presence of low hyperopia. This refractive state persists even in the period following resolution of the sensory detachment. The vast majority of patients ranged between plano and plus 1.50 with an occasional low myope or high hyperope, and no high myopes. This is, therefore, a disease predominantly of patients with low hyperopia. Otherwise there is no evidence of other ocular pathology in the anterior segment, the vitreous, the retinal vasculature, or the optic nerve.

The presence of a sensory retinal detachment is best recognized first by using the indirect ophthalmoscope with a Nikon plus 20 or plus 14 examining lens. The detachment itself varies widely from a small elevation that encircles only the foveal region to a large one that may appear bullous in nature with typical sloping margins (Fig. 13.1). The morphology of the sensory retinal detachment gives no absolute clue to the location of the leak, although it is

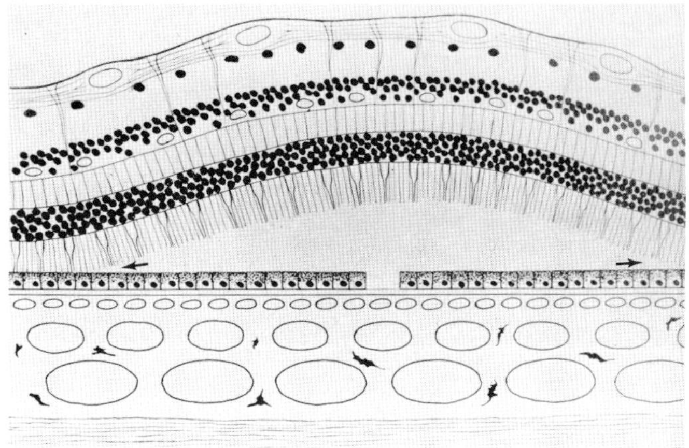

Figure 13.1. Schematic representation of a typical sensory retinal detachment in central serous chorioretinopathy in the macula. Note the shallow angle created by the detached sensory retina with the underlying pigment epithelium (*arrows*). These margins are typically sloping in nature and are probably produced by loose bonds between the outer layers of the retina and the pigment epithelium. The gap in the pigment epithelium centrally represents the presently unknown defect that is central serous chorioretinopathy. It is most likely produced by alterations in the terminal bars or junctional complexes between the pigment epithelial cells with serous detachment of the pigment epithelium itself, although focal inflammatory and ischemic factors, and choroidal tumors may also play a role. (From H. Schatz, T. C. Burton, L. A. Yannuzzi, and M. F. Rabb: Interpretation of Fundus Fluorescein Angiography, 1978, © C. V. Mosby Co., St. Louis; reprinted with permission.)

frequently in the upper portion of the detachment. In some instances, a localized detachment of the sensory retina in the inferior macula may be associated with a pigment epithelial leak that is superiorly located and which is apparently not in communication with the sensory retinal elevation below. Only careful examination of the macula with the slit-lamp biomicroscope and the Goldmann lens will reveal the full extent of the detachment and differentiate marked and shallow elevations from the flat, normal retina. Elevation of the retinal vessels and splitting of the slit beam accompanied by an anterior bowing of the slit beam are features of the slit-lamp biomicroscopic exam in these macula detachments.

Occasionally, underlying pigment epithelial atrophic changes or subsensory retinal precipitates serve as a guide to the full extent of a flat detachment, delineating the total possible area in which the leak may be found. When a zone of pigment epithelial atrophy in the macula is not associated with an overlying sensory retinal detachment but there is a sensory retinal elevation elsewhere in the posterior pole, there are usually two possible explanations—either the patient had a previous sensory retinal detachment which resulted in the atrophy or the existing subsensory retinal fluid shifts toward the macula area when the patient is in a supine position, for example during sleep.

Small or even large detachments that do not involve the fovea may be "silent" or visually asymptomatic. On the other hand, virtually all detachments involving the fovea are symptomatic. Sensory retinal detachments nasal to the disc are probably more common than is generally realized because they only produce symptoms when they are sufficiently extensive to involve the fovea.

Tiny, round, yellow specks, thought to be small proteinaceous precipitates, are often seen deposited on the posterior aspect of the sensory retina, particularly in detachments of long duration (Fig. 13.2). Pigment epithelial detachments beneath the sensory retinal detachment, or elsewhere in the macula, are frequently observed. Retinal pigment epithelial areas of hypopigmentation and pigmentary stippling are also seen in the chronic stages, particularly by means of slit-lamp biomicroscopy with a contact lens and indirect illumination. Directing the slit beam to one area of the macula and observing the pigment epithelial layer in another area reveals the more subtle alterations in the pigment epithelium.

Central serous chorioretinopathy has a distinct tendency toward bilaterality. In our study, 10% of the patients had a concomitant acute sensory retinal detachment in the fellow eye that seldom involved the foveal region. A detachment in the fellow eye on a separate occasion developed in an additional 12% of the patients. Recurrences were noted in 40% of the patients. This figure is slightly higher than comparable figures in other studies, but it is likely explained by the longer duration of follow-up in our study. On the other hand, retinal pigment epithelial atrophic and pigmentary changes in the fellow eye were seen in approximately 80% of our patients, and this finding emphasized the bilateral nature of this disease (Table 13.2).

Table 13.2. Natural history central serous chorioretinopathy*

Spontaneous resolution of detachment (average 4.4 months)	
	%
Bilaterality	
Simultaneous detachment fellow eye	10
Separate detachment fellow eye	12
RPE changes fellow eye	80
Recurrences	40
Vision	
Field: persistent scotoma	77
Acuity:	
20/20–20/40	74
20/50–20/100	20
20/200–worse	6

* Duration of follow-up: average: 3.4 year; range: 2–8 years.

Fluorescein Angiography

The fluorescein angiogram typically shows a very early pinpoint leak at the level of the pigment epithelium beneath the sensory retinal detachment. This leak is barely evident in the very early stages of the angiogram. During the mid-phases of the angiogram the leak gradually increases, as pooling of the dye occurs in the subsensory retinal space. In the later stages of the angiogram, the dye continues to pool in the subsensory retinal space but never completely fills it. Frequently, enough dye enters the subsensory retinal space to make the margin of the detachment discernible, but total filling is virtually never seen. In some cases the margins of the sensory retinal detachment are also evident as a gray shadow in the early stages of the angiogram, but this is less evident than in sensory retinal detachments of other types involving a more turbid fluid such as those associated with subretinal neovascularization.

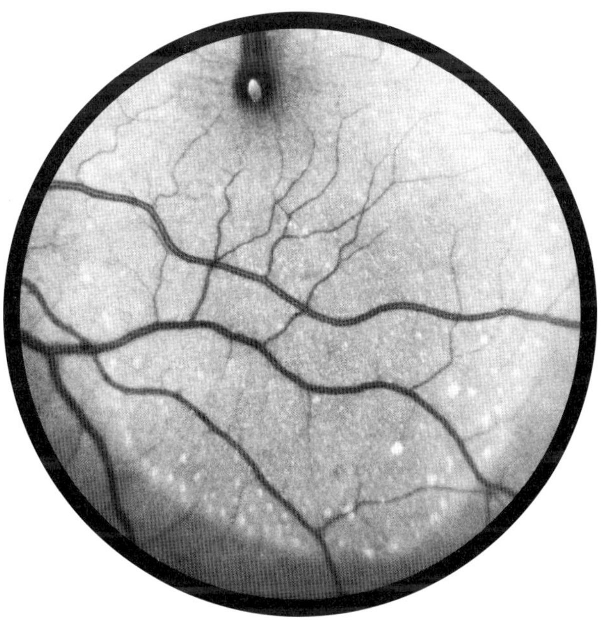

Figure 13.2. Ophthalmoscopic photograph of proteinaceous precipitates beneath sensory retinal elevation in central serous chorioretinopathy. Note the multiple yellowish-white deposits on the posterior aspect of the detached sensory retina commonly seen in long-standing detachments. A fixation target can be seen in the foveal region.

In general, this "classic" leak may manifest itself in three ways. The most frequent, often described as an "ink blot" variety, occurs in approximately 60% of the cases (Fig. 13.3). It starts as a pinpoint leak that gradually gets larger during the mid-phase of the angiogram and continues to expand with fuzzy margins in the late stages of the study.

The second variety of leak is referred to as a "smokestack," "umbrella," or "mushroom" type of leak. It occurs in approximately 20% of the cases (Fig. 13.4). It too, begins as a pinpoint leak from the pigment epithelium which becomes larger in the mid-phases of the angiogram and begins to ascend rapidly in the subsensory retinal space to the superior limits of the sensory retinal detachment. When it reaches a point close to the upper limit of the detachment, it continues to expand nasally and temporally, thereby forming its characteristic mushroom or umbrella appearance. Occasionally it will reach the superior limits of the subsensory retinal detachment and extend either nasally *or* temporally (but not in both directions) in such a way as to resemble a smokestack.

Finally, in the remaining 20% of the cases, there is a discrete, discernible retinal pigment epithelial detachment

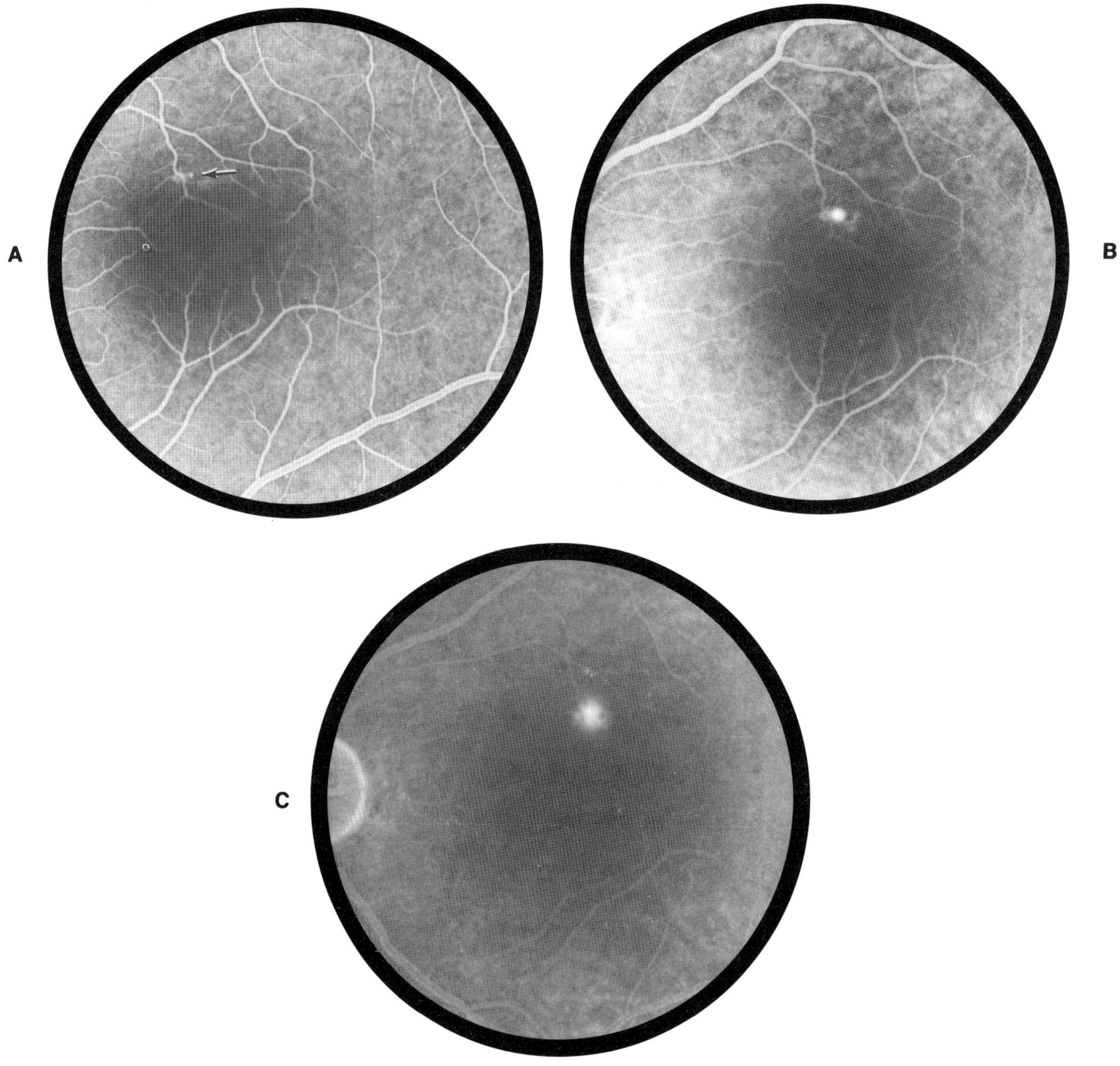

Figure 13.3. Central serous chorioretinopathy with an ink blot leak. *A*, arteriovenous phase fluorescein angiogram. Note the barely evident pinpoint leak in the superior nasal macula (*arrow*). *B*, late venous phase fluorescein angiogram. The leak has increased in size with indistinct margins. *C*, late phase fluorescein angiogram. The focal leak continued to increase in size with fuzzy margins, producing late hyperfluorescence by pooling into the subsensory retinal space.

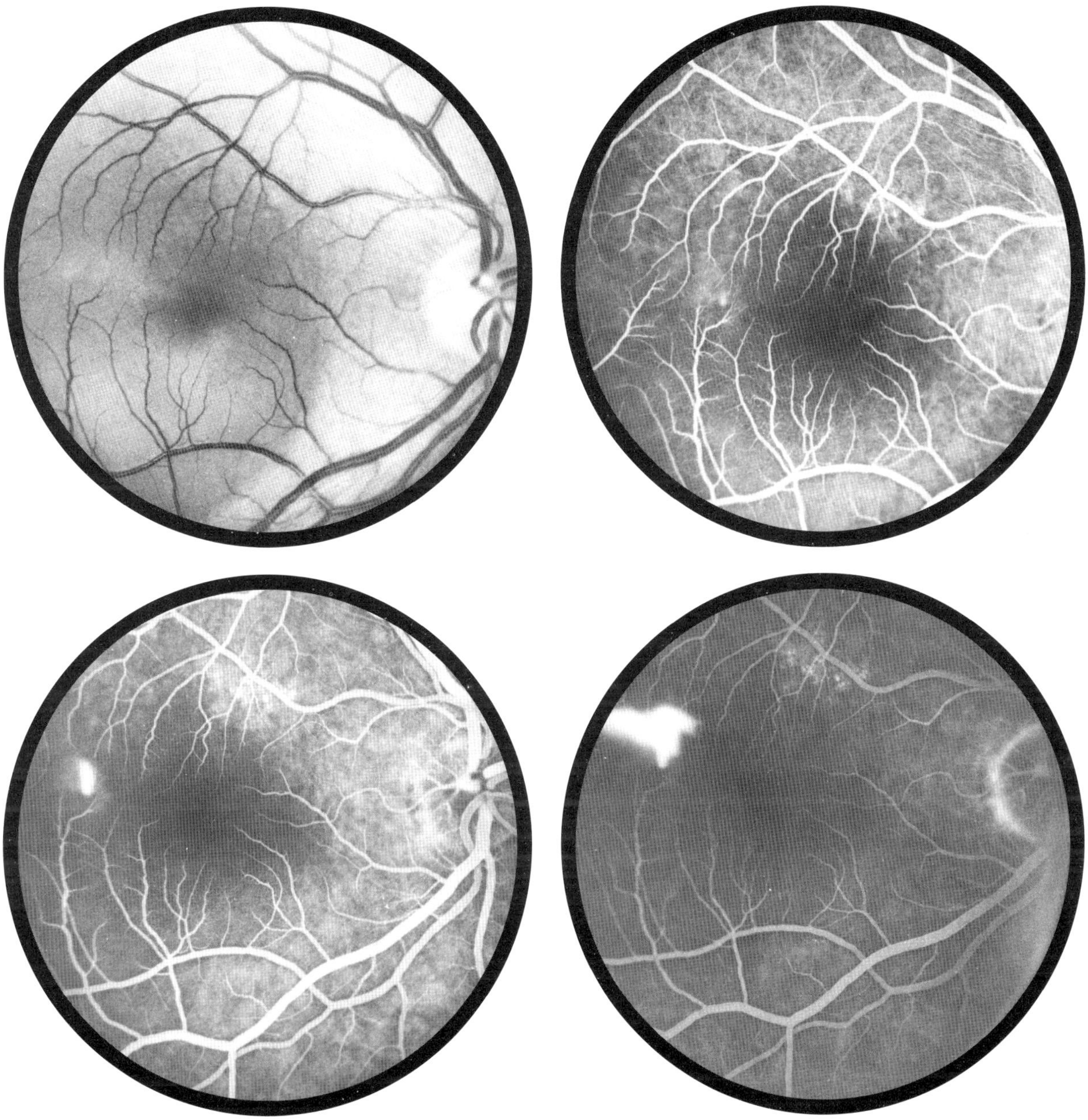

Figure 13.4. Central serous chorioretinopathy with smokestack or umbrella leak. *A*, ophthalmoscopic photograph. Note the sensory retinal detachment involving the macula and extending temporally and inferotemporally. *B*, early venous phase fluorescein angiogram. Note the focal hyperfluorescence temporal to the macula. *C*, late venous phase fluorescein angiogram. The hyperfluorescent focal leak has increased in size, extending superiorly from pooling under the neurosensory retina. *D*, late venous phase fluorescein angiogram. The leak has ascended to the superior limits of the detachment and extended both temporally and nasally to form a mushroom or umbrella configuration. The patchy hyperfluorescence in the superior macula, outside the region of the detachment, has faded indicating transmitted fluorescence from accentuation of the underlying choroidal circulation through defects in the pigment epithelium.

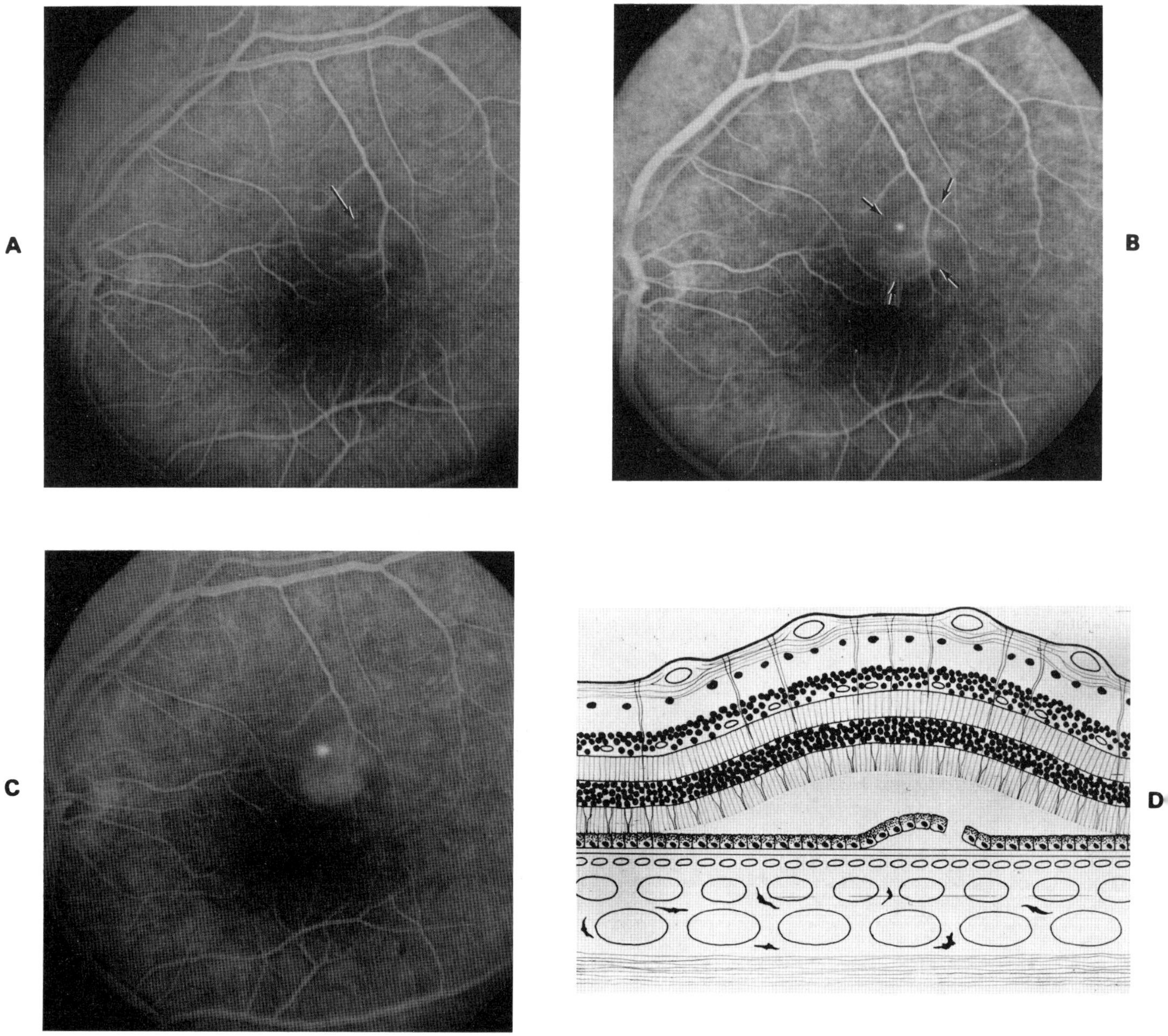

Figure 13.5. Central serous chorioretinopathy with leak from a discernible underlying pigment epithelial detachment. *A,* arteriovenous phase fluorescein angiogram. Note the focal leak *(arrow)* at the level of the retinal pigment epithelium. *B,* late venous phase fluorescein angiogram. There is diffuse homogeneous hyperfluorescence beneath a pigment epithelial detachment which has well demarcated borders (*arrows*). The focal leak has increased in size. *C,* late phase fluorescein angiogram. The focal leak continued to increase in size with fuzzy margins from pooling into the subsensory retinal space involving the entire macula. *D,* schematic representation of central serous chorioretinopathy associated with a discernible pigment epithelial detachment. (From H. Schatz, T. C. Burton, L. A. Yannuzzi, and M. F. Rabb: Interpretation of Fundus Fluorescein Angiography, 1978, © C. V. Mosby Co., St. Louis; reprinted with permission.)

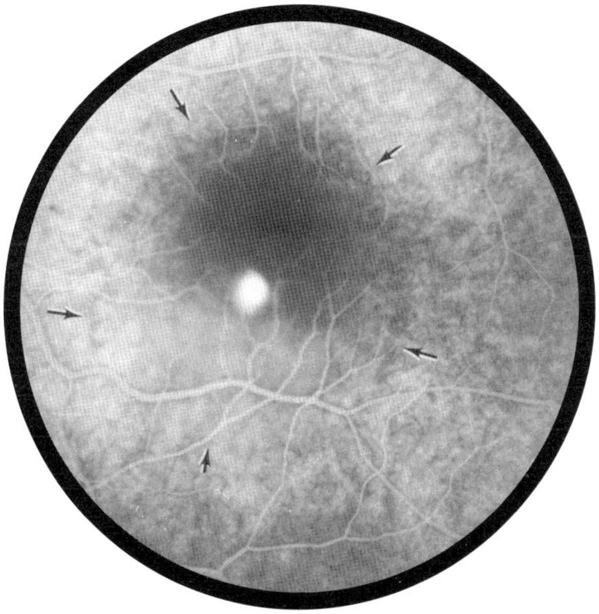
A

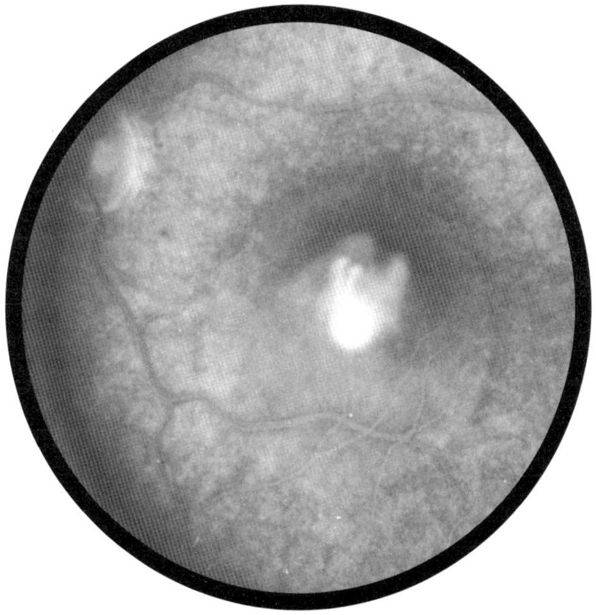
B

Figure 13.6. Central serous chorioretinopathy with discernible pigment epithelial detachment and multiple mushroom leaks. *A*, early venous phase fluorescein angiogram. Note the circumscribed area of hyperfluorescence in the inferior macula at the site of the serous detachment of the retinal pigment epithelium. The extent of the overlying sensory retinal detachment is barely evident as a faint ring of hypofluorescence (*arrows*). *B*, late venous phase fluorescein angiogram. Note the two linear areas of hyperfluorescence originating at the margin of the pigment epithelial detachment and ascending in the subsensory retinal space. *C*, late phase fluorescein angiogram. The dye has continued to pool into the subsensory retinal space, reaching the superior limit of the sensory retinal detachment and then coursing nasally and temporally to incompletely fill the sensory retinal detachment. However, sufficient fluorescein has pooled into the subsensory retinal space so that the full extent of the detachment is evident.

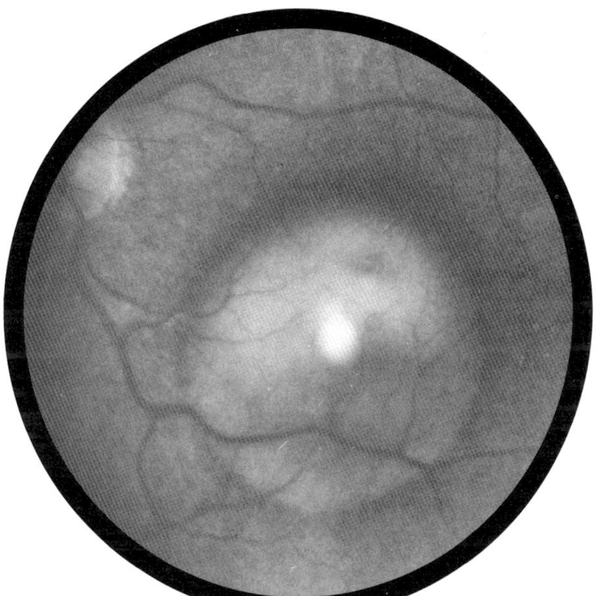
C

beneath the subsensory retinal detachment (Figs. 13.5 and 13.6). In these cases the pigment epithelial detachment is usually no larger than ¼ disc diameter in size. The pigment epithelial detachment fills first and, subsequently, there is leakage from it into the subsensory retinal space from one or more focal points, usually located at the margins of the retinal pigment epithelial detachment. This is the only form of central serous chorioretinopathy that has a clinically evident and fluorescein angiographic documentable pigment epithelial detachment. In the other forms the pigment epithelial detachment can only be presumed to be at the site of the leak, since it cannot be seen biomicroscopically.

The particular type of leak in central serous chorioretinopathy appears to have no definite value in terms of predicting the ultimate visual prognosis; however, it may indicate the duration of the detachment. Some ophthalmologists believe that a smokestack- or umbrella-type leak occurs in patients who have recently developed their sensory retinal detachments. Shimizu [11], however, has reported the conversion of a smokestack leak to an ink blot leak and vice versa. This suggests that at some stage in the disease the type of leak can shift regardless of the duration of the detachment. In our experience, however, an ink blot leak was never noted to convert to a smokestack leak but the opposite was true. This supports the impression that regardless of numerous exceptions, smokestack leaks tend to be acute and ink blot leaks chronic manifestations.

Some have explained the ascent of leak in the subsensory space as being produced by convectional currents induced by the warmer choroidal circulation. Others hold that the molecular weight differences between the low weight of the fluorescein molecule and the fluorescein albumin conjugate, on the one hand, and the heavier proteinaceous-laden subsensory retinal fluid, on the other, are largely responsible for this rise. In a simple experiment, a change in the position of the head can result in a correlative change in the direction of the fluorescein movement in the subsensory retinal space, always against gravity (Fig. 13.7). Although gravitational factors and weight differences do play a role, other unknown factors at the level of the pigment epithelium must also be of significance, because Shimizu has reported a case of a smokestack leak and an ink blot leak side by side, beneath the same sensory retinal detachment [11]. Unknown factors at the site of the pigment epithelium in such an eye must certainly contribute to the rapid ascent of the leak at one point and a more slowly moving leak at the other. Only one patient in our experience has ever been noted to have a descending leak (Fig. 13.8). In spite of the fact that all other criteria were met, he was not included in the natural course study because of the unique fluorescein angiographic findings.

The number of retinal pigment epithelial leaks beneath

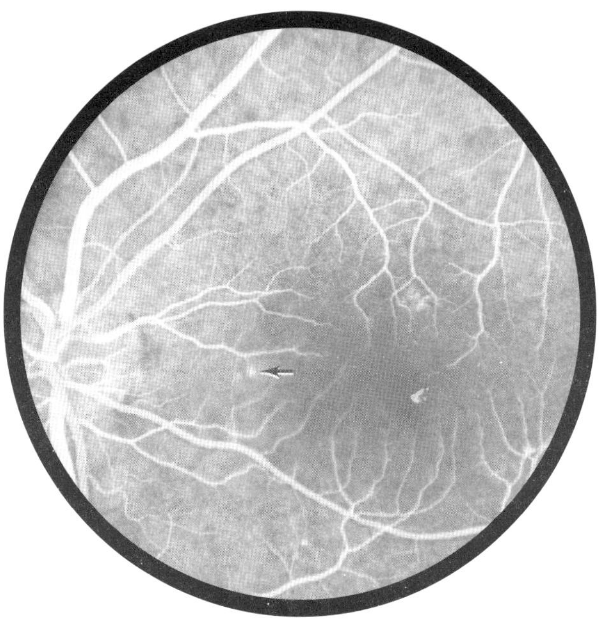

A

B

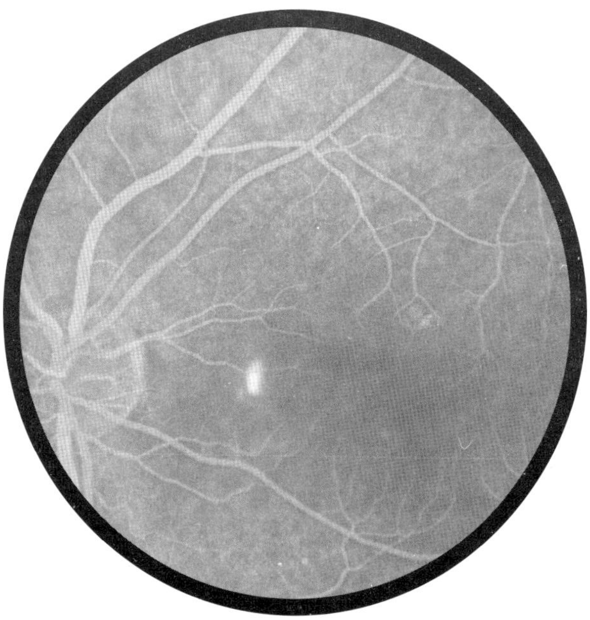

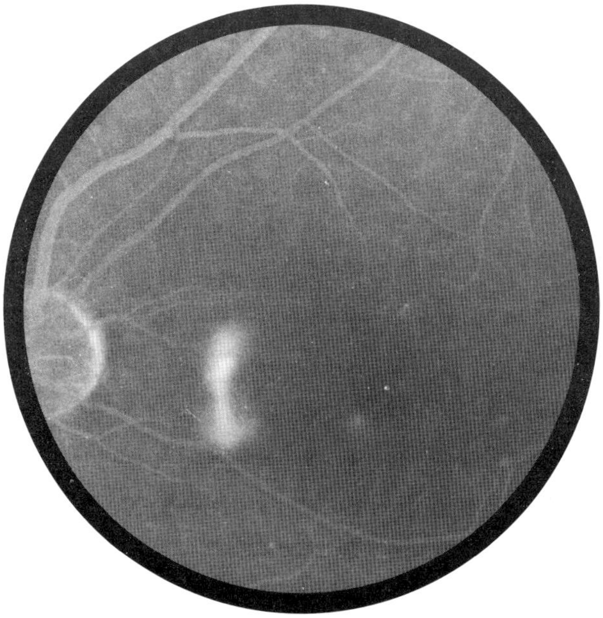

C

Figure 13.7. Central serous chorioretinopathy with reversal of a smokestack leak from change in head position. *A*, early venous phase angiogram. Note the focal leak in the nasal macula approximately at the horizontal raphe (*arrow*). Early hyperfluorescence is also present in the superior macula from transmitted fluorescence at the site of pigment epithelial atrophic changes. *B*, late venous phase fluorescein angiogram. The focal leak has begun to ascend in the subsensory retinal space. *C*, late phase fluorescein angiogram. Reversal of the smoke-stack leak. Note two apparent smokestack leaks, one seemingly ascending from the focal leak and one descending from it. The patient had placed his head between his legs after the venous phase of the angiograms, thereby reversing the direction of the dye pooling in the subsensory retinal space.

Figure 13.8. An unusual case of central serous chorioretinopathy with a descending leak. *A*, arteriovenous phase fluorescein angiogram. Note focal leak at the level of the pigment epithelium in the temporal macula. Early hyperfluorescence is also present in the nasal, inferior nasal, superotemporal macula, and the juxtafoveal region from atrophic changes in the pigment epithelium. *B* and *C*, early venous phase fluorescein angiograms. Note the increase in the size of the leak as it courses initially temporally and subsequently inferiorly in the subsensory retinal space. *D*, late venous phase fluorescein angiogram. The leak has continued to expand and descend inferiorly in the subsensory retinal space. *E*, late phase fluorescein angiogram. The dye has continued to expand in the subsensory retinal space to fill it completely with intense, homogeneous hyperfluorescence and with well demarcated margins resembling the fluorescein characteristics of a typical pigment epithelial detachment. This 40-year-old psychiatrist had had a previous attack of central serous chorioretinopathy with classic clinical and fluorescein angiographic features. The unusual features to his fluorescein angiogram (descent of the leak and complete filling of the sensory retinal space) are not typical of a central serous chorioretinopathy, suggesting that this patient may represent an unusual variant of the disease. (From H. Schatz, T. C. Burton, L. A. Yannuzzi, and M. F. Rabb: Interpretation of Fundus Fluorescein Angiography, 1978, © C. V. Mosby Co., St. Louis; reprinted with permission.)

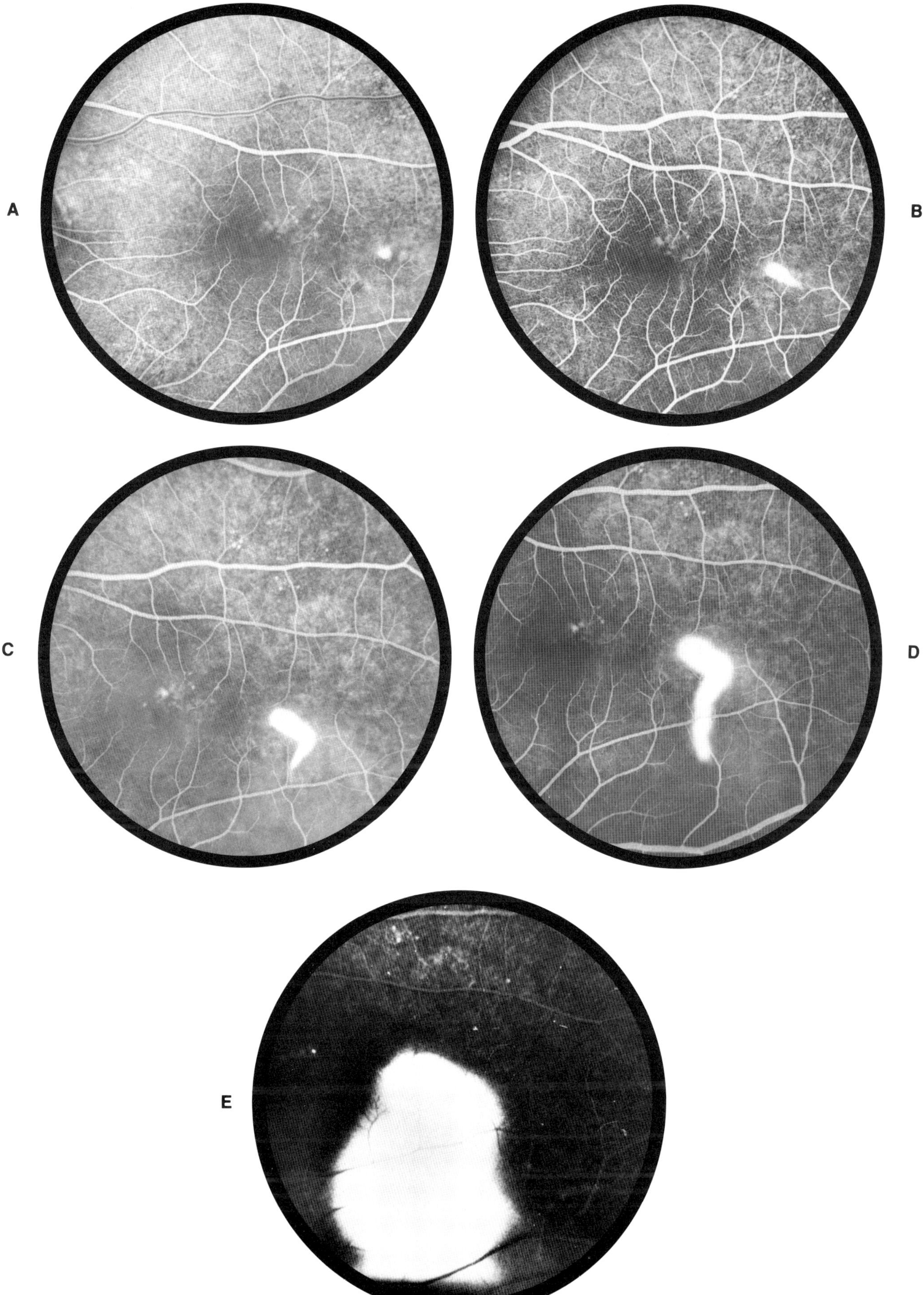

Figure 13.8

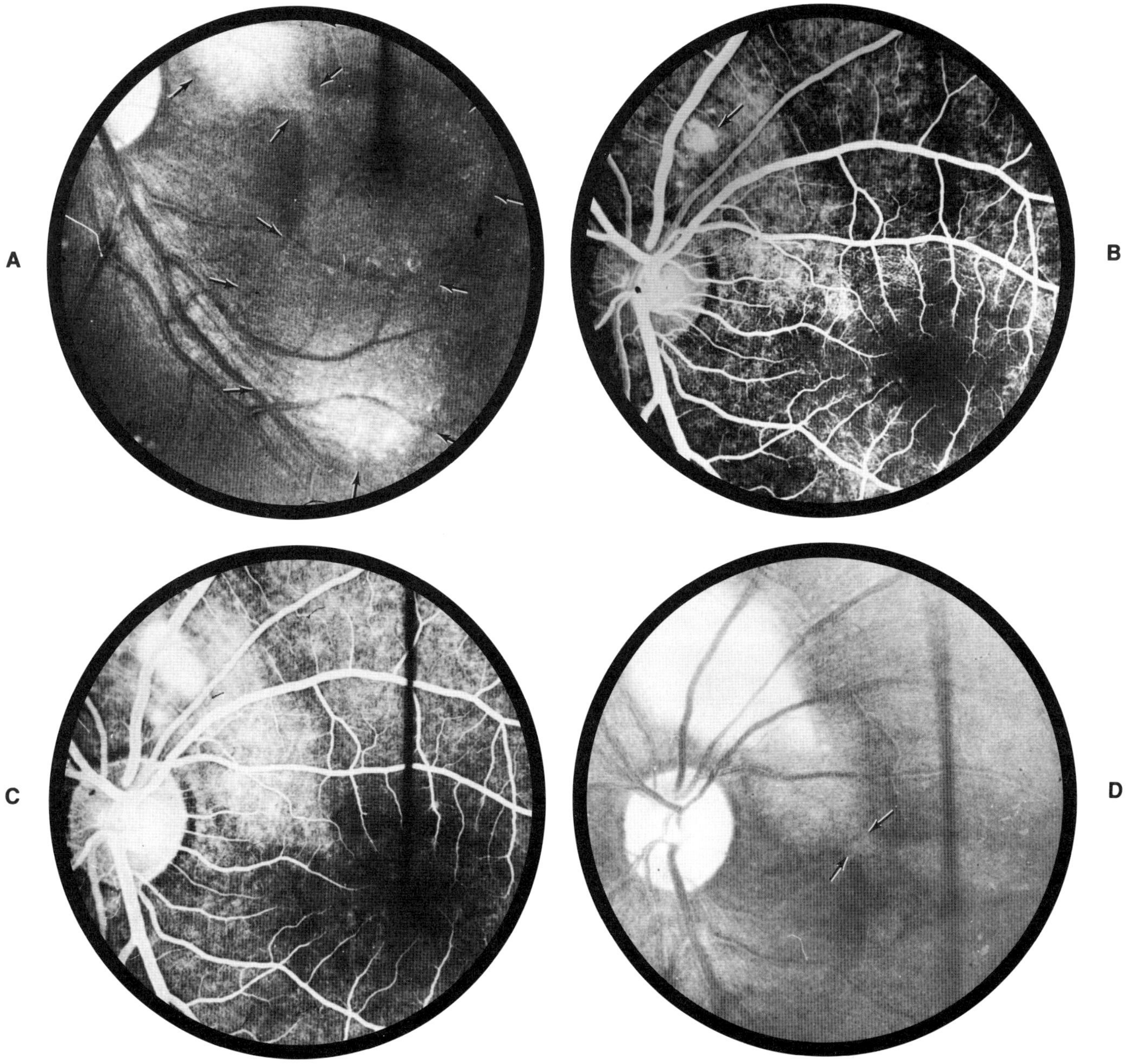

Figure 13.9. Central serous chorioretinopathy with eccentric leak superior to the disc. *A*, ophthalmoscopic photograph. There is a large sensory retinal detachment involving the macula and extending supranasally and inferiorly (*arrows*). Fixation target is at the fovea. *B*, early venous phase fluorescein angiogram. A focal pigment epithelial leak is evident just superior to the optic nerve (*arrow*). *C*, late venous phase fluorescein angiogram. The leak has begun to expand in the subsensory retinal space. *D*, late phase fluorescein angiogram. The late hyperfluorescence from pooling into the subsensory retinal space has continued to expand with some filling toward the macula. This case illustrates how an eccentric leak can involve the macula. The detachment pattern present in this patient has a segment resembling a strait (*arrows*), which connects two larger bodies of subsensory retinal detachment above and below. In order to ensure that all leaks are identified, photographic mapping of the posterior pole as well as fluorescein angioscopy should be carried out in all cases of central serous chorioretinopathy.

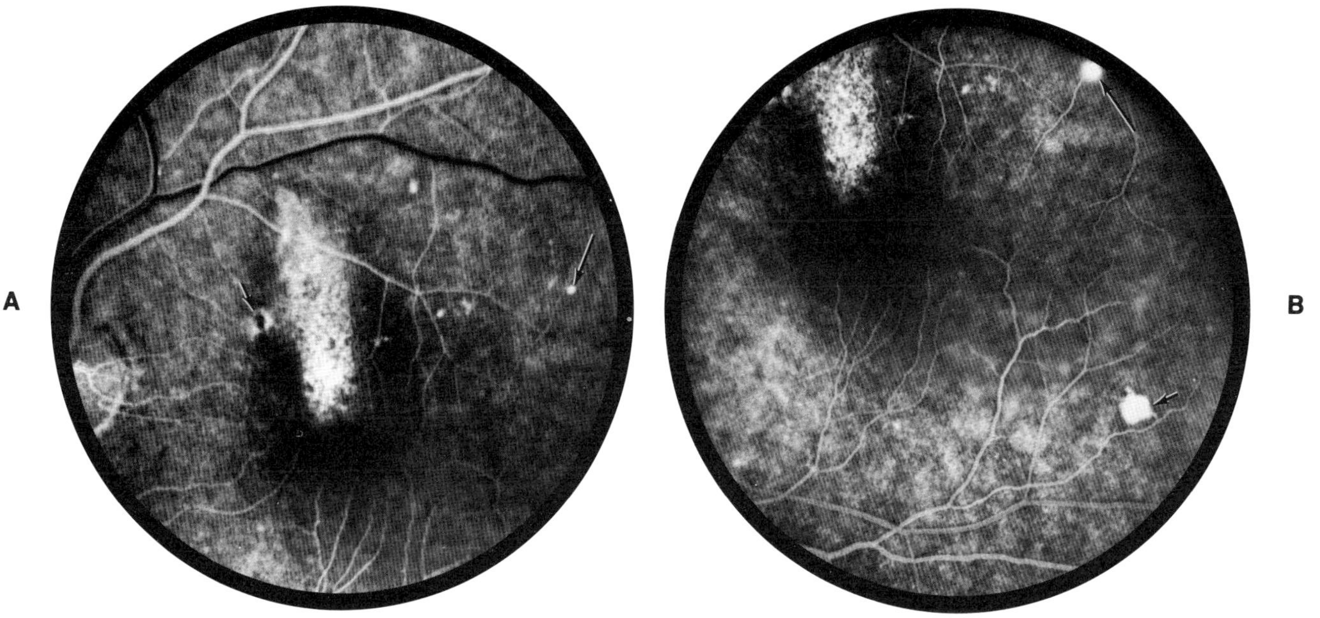

Figure 13.10. Central serous chorioretinopathy associated with multiple retinal pigment epithelial abnormalities. *A,* arteriovenous phase fluorescein angiogram shows a large patch of early hyperfluorescence associated with retinal pigment epithelial atrophy and representing choroidal transmission. At its nasal border is a small pigment figure overlying a chronic serous detachment of the retinal pigment epithelium (*small arrow*). The pigment epithelial leak responsible for the overlying sensory retinal detachment is evident in the temporal macula (*long arrow*). *B,* late venous phase fluorescein angiogram shows that the pigment epithelial leak has increased in size with fuzzy margins (*long arrow*). A serous detachment of the RPE in the inferotemporal macula is also noted and is unassociated with the sensory retinal detachment (*short arrow*). A photocoagulation burn along the inferotemporal vessels is present from prior treatment.

a detachment in our patients ranged from 1 to 5, with a mean of 1.4. Typographical analysis of these leaks indicated that approximately 60% of them occurred within a disc diameter of the fovea, and only 6% occurred within ¼ disc diameter of the foveola. Also, in the macular region, there was a random distribution of leaks with no particular predilection with respect to quadrants. Multiple isolated sensory retinal detachments were seen in a few patients. In some cases, definite macular detachments were produced by leaks located eccentrically outside of the arcades (Fig. 13.9). Nasal leaks also occur and can be associated with macular detachments. More commonly, they do not affect vision because their induced detachments do not involve the fovea. In order to ensure that all leaks are identified, photographic mapping of the posterior pole and fluorescein angioscopy should be carried out in all cases after preliminary photographs are taken. In any instance of macular detachment, careful examination by the fluorescein angioscopist and the motivated photographer, of the peripheral retina for primary pathology responsible for macular detachments is mandatory, to determine definitively that the actual diagnosis is that of central serous chorioretinopathy.

Examination of the chronic, recurrent acute eye with central serous chorioretinopathy reveals a myriad of fluorescein angiographic changes. These include hyperfluorescence from atrophy of the pigment epithelium following previous retinal detachment, focal leaks beneath an acute sensory retinal detachment, and leakage at the site of serous pigment epithelial detachments elsewhere in the fundus. Hypofluorescence is seen in areas of pigment epithelial proliferation and at the site of any photocoagulation treatment burns (Fig. 13.10). The fluorescein angiogram is also somewhat helpful in establishing a presumptive diagnosis of a previous sensory retinal detachment or episode of central serous chorioretinopathy even in a virtually asymptomatic eye (Fig. 13.11). Atrophic changes in the retinal pigment epithelium, forming an apron-like distribution inferior to the macula, are typical findings accentuated on the fluorescein angiogram. Unlike inflammatory and dystrophic disease of the choroid, the choriocapillaris is intact in the areas of retinal pigment epithelial atrophy resulting in a zone of early hyperfluorescence or transmitted fluorescence.

Although the exact defect in the pigment epithelium that is responsible for the disease has not been determined, alterations in the junctional complexes of the pigment epithelium, the so-called zonula occludens, have been implicated. Some have suggested that the primary event is that of an occlusive change in the choriocapillaris. This is supported by the presence of hypofluorescence presumably from nonperfusion, as the earliest manifestation on the fluorescein angiographic study at the site of the leak in some patients. Actually, it is true that the first change on an angiogram may occasionally be a small hypofluorescent spot prior to the appearance of a focal leak. However, it is as likely that a small pigment epithelial detachment and the fluid contained beneath it could serve to produce a minor form of localized blocked fluorescence until the dye has diffused through Bruch's membrane to fill the subpigment epithelial space.

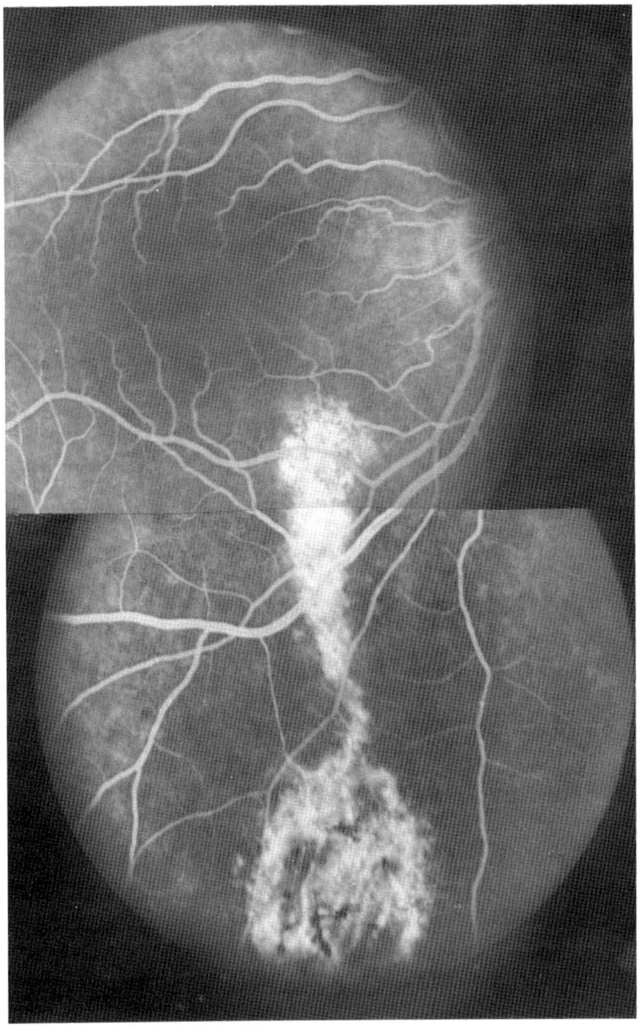

Figure 13.11. Fluorescein angiogram of presumed healed central serous chorioretinopathy. Note the early transmitted hyperfluorescence inferior to the macula. Most pigment epithelial leaks in central serous chorioretinopathy are in the upper third of the sensory retinal detachment. The subsensory retinal fluid gravitates inferiorly forming an apron-like pattern. In this eye the fovea was not involved, and vision was unaffected. These changes were found when the patient appeared with an acute macular detachment of his fellow eye.

Natural History

Virtually all leaks eventually heal spontaneously, although the duration of the detachment is extremely variable. In our experience, resolution of the detachment ranged from 3 weeks to nearly 1 year. Other cases have been known to last even longer. In our study, measurement of the recovery of central vision indicated that this is not a totally benign disease when left untreated. While 74% of the patients developed corrected vision of 20/40 or better, the acuity was often qualitatively less than the indicated level. More precisely, a 20/20 eye would have been accurately described as a "slow" 20/20 eye as minor central field disturbances persisted in spite of the 20/20 recorded acuity level. More discouraging was the fact that 20% of the patients had a vision of 20/50 to 20/100. In fact, 6% of the patients had vision of 20/200 or worse after refraction was carried out at least 2 months following resolution of the detachment (see Table 13.2).

A search for prognostic factors that would serve to predict which patients would undergo limited visual recovery revealed no definite indicators. Most ophthalmologists feel that the duration of the detachment, as well as the proximity of the leak to the fovea, are the principal factors in reducing the likelihood of a complete return of central vision, but statistical evidence in support of this impression is lacking. In our study, age, sex, race, onset acuity, systemic disease, additional ocular pathology, site, number and character of leaks, recurrence of leaks, and duration of detachment were all subjected to statistical analysis and none of these factors proved to be of significance in predicting a poor ultimate outcome. The one consistent finding in all patients who did poorly was the presence of retinal pigment epithelial atrophic changes in the juxtafoveal region following the resolution of their detachments (Fig. 13.12). Because of this, we have attempted to monitor the course of the juxtafoveal pigment epithelium during the acute stages of the detachments, in order to determine in advance, if possible, those patients who are beginning to develop these atrophic changes (Fig. 13.13). While monochromatic photography has proved to be superior to color photography or fluorescein angiography, in detecting early parafoveal retinal pigment epithelial degenerative changes, it has been somewhat disappointing because of the inability of various wavelengths employed to penetrate sensitively and consistently the subsensory retinal fluid in a number of patients. Still, this approach, which is designed to determine more accurately the state of the pigment epithelium beneath the detachment as a means of determining "when to treat," and which employs fluorescein angiography as a guide to photocoagulation to determine "where to treat," may prove useful in the future.

Recurrence was specifically not a definitive indicator of a poor prognosis. A number of patients had excellent vision following multiple recurrences, suggesting that this factor is not in itself an indication for treatment. All recurrences developed at new pigment epithelial sites. No recurrence developed exactly at a previous site, although frequently the recurrence site was very close to a formerly active leak.

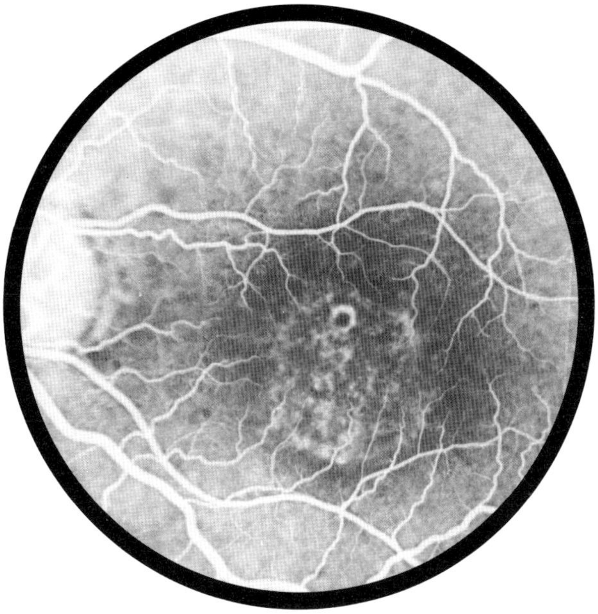

Figure 13.12. Retinal pigment epithelial atrophic change secondary to central serous chorioretinopathy. Note the circumscribed area of patchy hyperfluorescence secondary to atrophic changes in the retinal pigment epithelium in this patient with a previous attack of central serous chorioretinopathy. The visual acuity is 20/200. The presence of retinal pigment epithelial atrophic changes in the juxtafoveal region is the one consistent finding in patients who have a poor visual result in this disease.

A

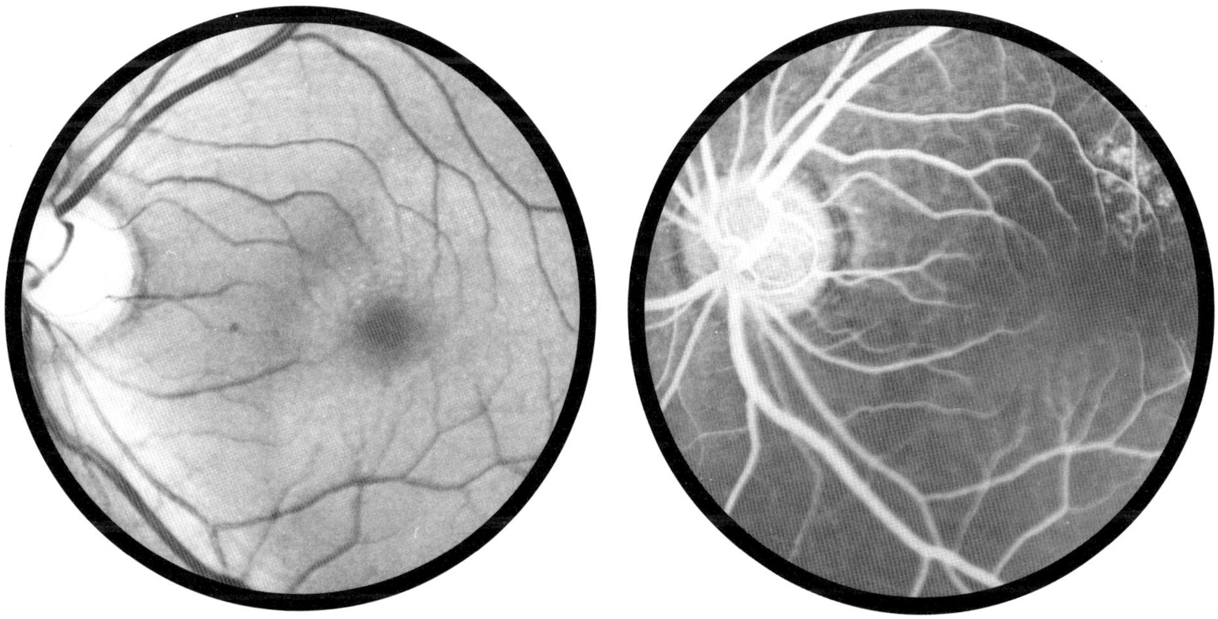

B

Figure 13.13. A comparison of monochromatic photography and fluorescein angiography in a patient with central serous chorioretinopathy and pigment epithelial atrophy. *A*, monochromatic photograph, 570 nm (yellow-green), showing extent of retinal pigment epithelial atrophy in the superior, supratemporal, inferior, and infratemporal macula. A large sensory retinal detachment of the macula and temporal macula is present. *B*, early venous phase fluorescein angiogram. Note the patchy hyperfluorescence which is evident only in the supratemporal portion of the macula and does not indicate the full extent of the pigment epithelial atrophy seen on the monochromatic photograph. The retinal vessels in the macula are somewhat out of focus because of the sensory retinal elevation.

Differential Diagnosis

The presence of a macular detachment, even in a patient between the ages of 30 and 55, does not mean absolutely that the involved disorder is that of central serous chorioretinopathy. As mentioned above, if there is hemorrhage, exudate, cystoid macular edema, or optic nerve or retinal vascular pathology, an alternative diagnosis is likely. One way of considering the overall differential is to determine from the fluorescein angiogram whether the macular detachment is associated with a subretinal leak similar to that seen in central serous chorioretinopathy. Some macular detachments resembling central serous chorioretinopathy are associated with such leaks; other such detachments are not.

MACULAR DETACHMENTS ASSOCIATED WITH SUBRETINAL LEAKS

Certain disorders such as multiple detachments of the retinal pigment epithelium associated with a bullous sensory retinal detachment, Vogt-Koyanagi-Harada's syndrome, malignant hypertension, toxemia of pregnancy, and subretinal neovascularization, are among the disease entities that produce leaks from the level of the pigment epithelium beneath a sensory retinal detachment. Some of these macular diseases can be differentiated from central serous chorioretinopathy because they exhibit optic nerve and/or retinal vascular involvement (Fig. 13.14). In the case of multiple pigment epithelial detachments with associated bullous sensory retinal detachment, bilateral shifting fluid with marked turbidity are both characteristics of this uncommon disorder which may be a variant of central serous chorioretinopathy [18] (Fig. 13.15). The identification of subretinal neovascularization in terms of its fluorescein angiographic manifestations, as well as of the disease entities predisposing to it, is useful in differentiating this entity from central serous chorioretinopathy (Fig. 13.16).

The association of macular detachments overlying choroidal tumors, particularly nevi, with a focal leak or leaks from the retinal pigment epithelium resembling central serous chorioretinopathy appears to be more than coincidence because of its relative frequency (Fig. 13.17). This suggests that any disturbance in the retinal pigment epithelium may predispose to leaks and overlying sensory retinal detachments. This is also true for pigment epithelial detachments and subretinal neovascularization as well.

MACULAR DETACHMENTS WITH NO SUBRETINAL LEAKS

This category includes rhegmatogenous detachments that are associated with peripheral tears, full thickness macular holes with posterior detachments, optic pits with sensory retinal detachments and peripheral choroidal tumors with detachments in the macular region. In peripheral choroidal tumors and rhegmatogenous peripheral tears, no leakage is seen beneath the sensory retinal detachment in the macula, although an acute tear may leak at its margin and a choroidal tear has associated hyperfluorescence of its own. Full thickness macular holes with posterior detachments in high myopia and, less commonly, following trauma, are not associated with leakage, although defects in the underlying pigment epithelium at the site of the hole may reveal hyperfluorescence from choroidal transmission. Optic pits are recognized by their characteristic appearance at the nerve head. The early phases of the fluorescein angiogram revealed hypofluorescence at the site of the pit and pooling of the dye within the pit, but the dye does not extend beneath the sensory retinal detachment.

A faint foveal leak, often seen with a small serous detachment around the fovea, is a variant of central serous chorioretinopathy. It is produced by a small leak, masked or hidden by the normally dark zone of the macula. In some instances only the very highly resolved, sensitive negative strip on the angiogram will reveal the presence of such a faint foveal leak. The so-called nonleaking variety of central serous chorioretinopathy, that has been subjected to the indirect form of photocoagulation at the margins of sensory retinal detachments because of no demonstrable leak, probably represents cases with very faint foveal leaks that have not been detected. Possibly a case of resolving central serous chorioretinopathy may produce a similar situation with no apparent leak, but in our experience all patients with strictly defined central serous chorioretinopathy have been found to have an active leak or leaks.

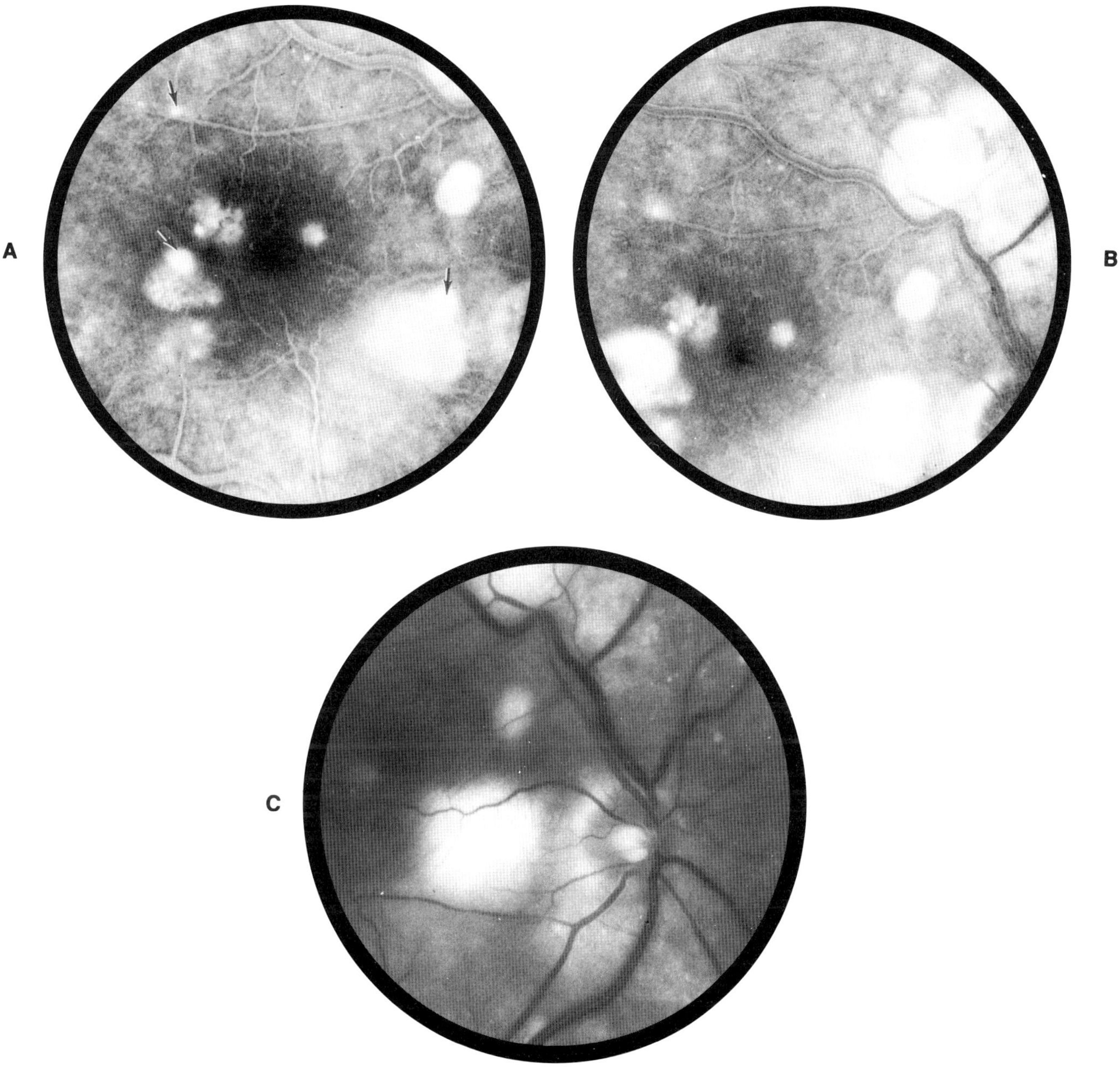

Figure 13.14. Multiple detachments and leaks of the retinal pigment epithelium associated with bullous sensory retinal detachment. *A*, early venous phase fluorescein angiogram shows homogeneous fluorescence in the subpigment epithelial space beneath multiple pigment epithelial detachments. Some of the pigment epithelial detachments are associated with focal leakage into the subsensory retinal space (*arrows*). *B*, late venous phase fluorescein angiogram shows more extensive pooling into the subsensory retinal space from multiple pigment epithelial detachments, late phase angiogram. Fuzzy hyperfluoresecence is evident from incomplete filling of the subsensory detachments by the multiple pigment epithelial leaks. *C*, the presence of bilateral bullous sensory retinal detachments associated with a markedly turbid shifting fluid and multiple pigment epithelial detachments are characteristic of this disorder which may represent a variant of central serous chorioretinopathy.

A 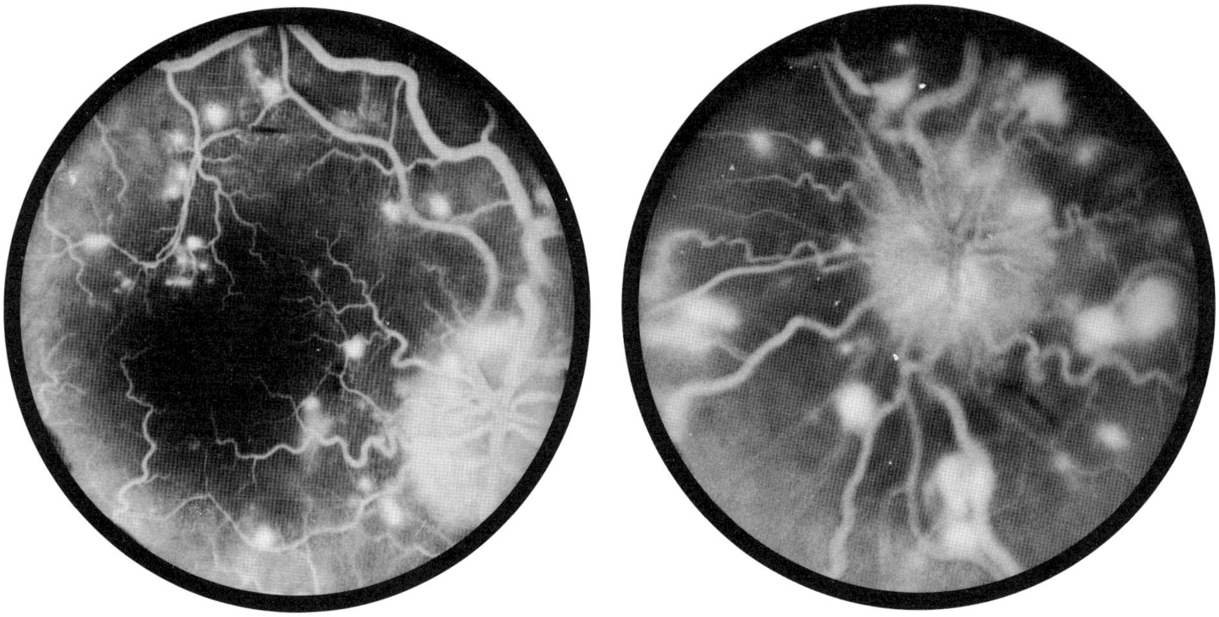 B

Figure 13.15. Sensory macular detachment and malignant hypertension. *A*, early venous phase fluorescein angiogram. Note multifocal hyperfluorescent subretinal leaks from the level of the pigment epithelium pooling into the subsensory retinal space and staining of optic nerve. *B*, late venous phase fluorescein angiogram. Note similar leaks scattered throughout the fundus and late staining of optic nerve. The retinal vascular and disc abnormalities aid in differentiating this detachment from central serous chorioretinopathy.

A 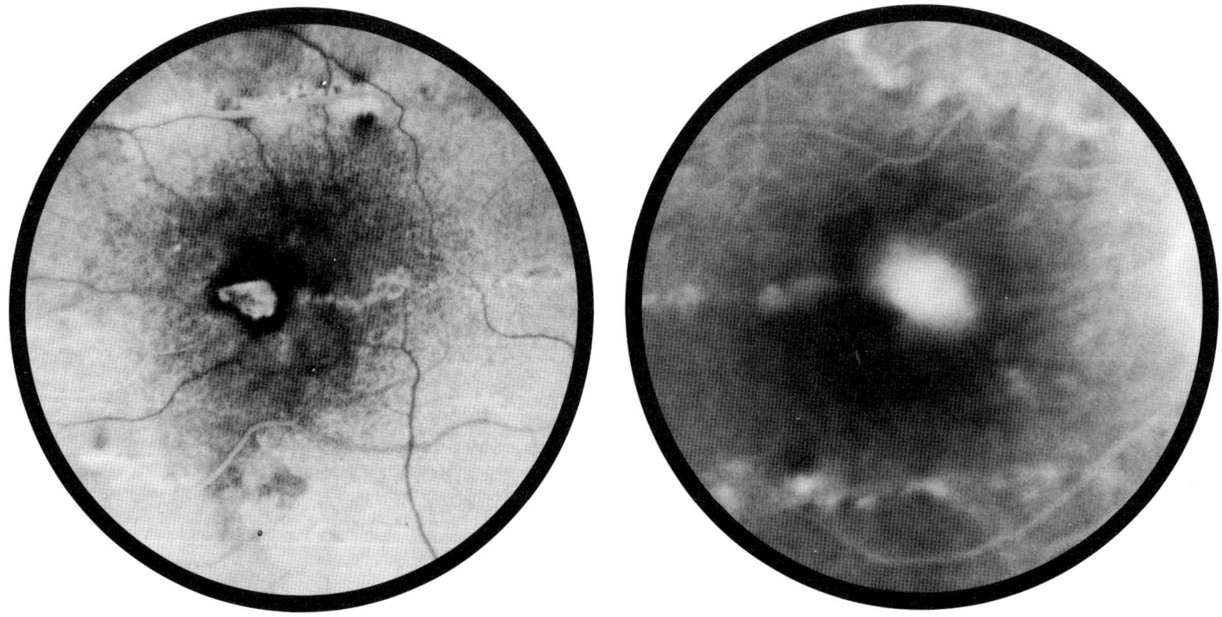 B

Figure 13.16. Macular detachment with subretinal leak due to subretinal neovascularization. *A*, arterial venous phase fluorescein angiogram. Note the lacy hyperfluorescence subretinally, surrounded by a dark zone indicative of subretinal neovascularization. *B*, late phase fluorescein angiogram. Note the late hyperfluorescence with fuzzy margins from leakage of vessels into subsensory retinal space. Irregular bands of hyperfluorescence are also seen at site of angioid streaks. The fluorescein angiographic characteristics of subretinal neovascularization can often differentiate it from macular detachments seen in central serous chorioretinopathy.

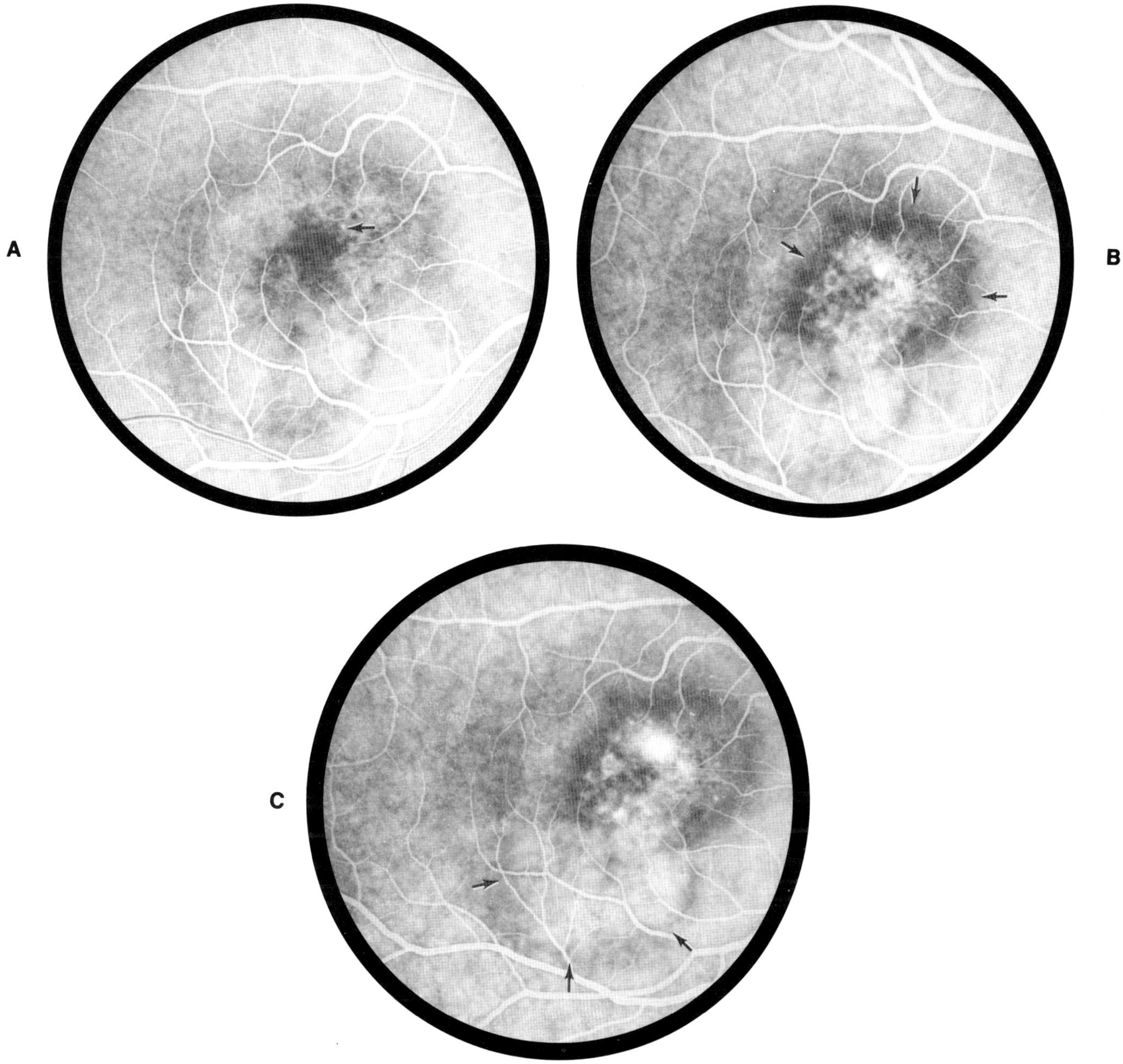

Figure 13.17. Serous detachment of the sensory retina overlying a pigmented tumor of the choroid presumed to be a nevus. *A*, arteriovenous phase fluorescein angiogram. Note focal leak (*arrow*) barely evident overlying a flat choroidal nevus. *B*, early venous phase fluorescein angiogram. Note the pigmented tumor of the choroid with hypofluorescence along its indistinct margins (*arrows*). Patchy hyperfluorescence is present overlying the central portion of the lesion secondary to atrophic changes in the pigment epithelium. The focal leak has increased in size. *C*, late venous phase fluorescein angiogram. Note the increase in size of the focal leak as it pools into the subsensory retinal space. The overlying sensory retinal detachment has gravitated inferiorly producing a zone of pigment epithelial atrophy beneath it from long-standing sensory retinal elevation (*arrows*).

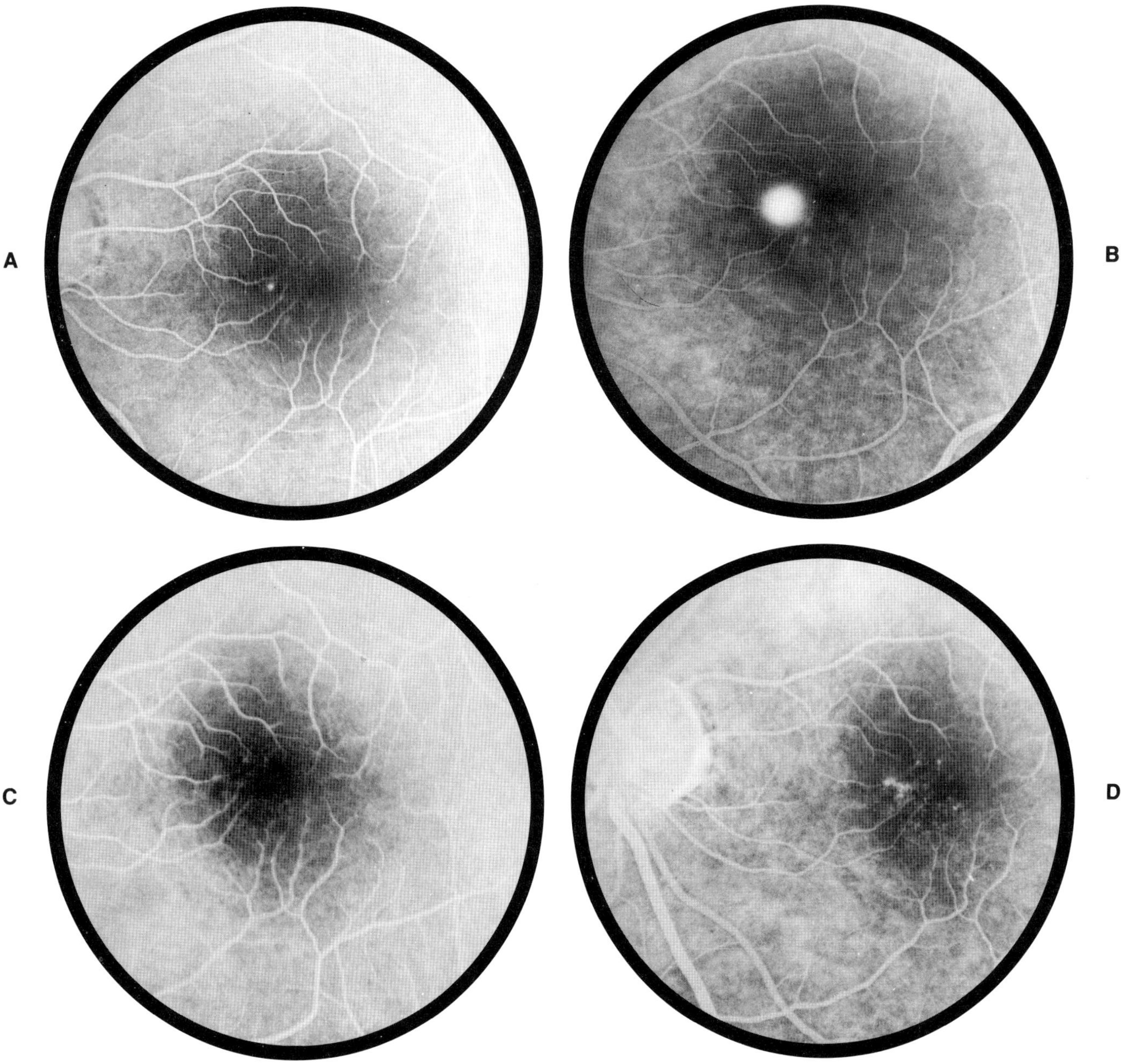

Figure 13.18. Photocoagulation treatment of central serous chorioretinopathy. *A*, and *B*, pretreatment fluorescein angiogram showing focal pigment epithelial leak with pooling into the subsensory retinal space. *C* and *D*, postphotocoagulation fluorescein angiograms showing obliteration of the leak and resolution of the macular detachment. Faint hyperfluorescence is due to scleral stain at the border of the photocoagulation burn.

Photocoagulation Treatment

Photocoagulation treatment, utilizing any of the available modalities, has been found to shorten the duration of the sensory retinal detachment [2, 4, 5, 7, 12, 19–21]. In our study, the average duration of detachment lasted 4.4 months before resolution. Following photocoagulation, resolution of subsensory retinal fluid usually occurs between 1 and 3 weeks following therapy (Fig. 13.18). Full visual recovery lags behind by approximately the same period of time. A mild reaction at the site of the pigment epithelium (gray) is usually sufficient to seal the leak and may then produce resolution of the detachment. However, there is no definite evidence yet, that shortening the duration of the detachment with photocoagulation, actually serves a useful purpose in the ultimate visual recovery. Until this controversy is resolved, photocoagulation is recommended for a leak or leaks that are remote from the foveal region and after the detachment has been present for a period of 3 months.

The risks of photocoagulation with such leaks are extremely minimal, and the treatment itself does shorten the duration of the detachment which, in turn, is likely to reduce the tendency toward atrophy of the pigment epithelium and limited visual recovery. However, the risks of photocoagulation treatment in the juxtafoveal region are considerable. We have never heard of an accidental foveal burn or preretinal membrane formation produced from argon laser photocoagulation in the treatment of central serous chorioretinopathy; we have never seen, although we have heard of two macular holes associated with such treatment; we have seen proteinaceous precipitation into the foveal region following photocoagulation with transient visual decline in three patients; however, we have also reported on a number of patients who have experienced hemorrhage and proliferation of subretinal neovascularization following photocoagulation for central serous chorioretinopathy (Fig. 13.19). These patients have been referred to as cases of subretinal neovascularization "masquerading" as central serous chorioretinopathy [21]. This is a distinct complication of photocoagulation in this disease and by no means rare. Since our original description of this phenomenon, a number of additional cases have been reported involving classic, pinpoint leaks which were treated with photocoagulation and which ultimately resulted in subretinal neovascularization. It is not clear whether or not the photocoagulation itself disrupts the rentinal pigment epithelium-Bruch's membrane-choriocapillaris complex to in some way provide an ischemic focus for neovascularization to begin, *or* whether there is pre-existing subretinal neovascularization in the form of a fine or delicate fibrovascular membrane which has produced a focal leak in the overlying pigment epithelium and which is, subsequently, "fertilized" by incomplete thermal obliteration particularly with a small, short burn. Because these cases appear almost exclusively in parafoveal leaks, a conservative form of management should be entertained in these cases unless there is evident visual decline associated with retinal pigment epithelial changes or a poor history in the fellow eye. A minimum of 6 months should be allowed to elapse before considering photocoagulation of such leaks.

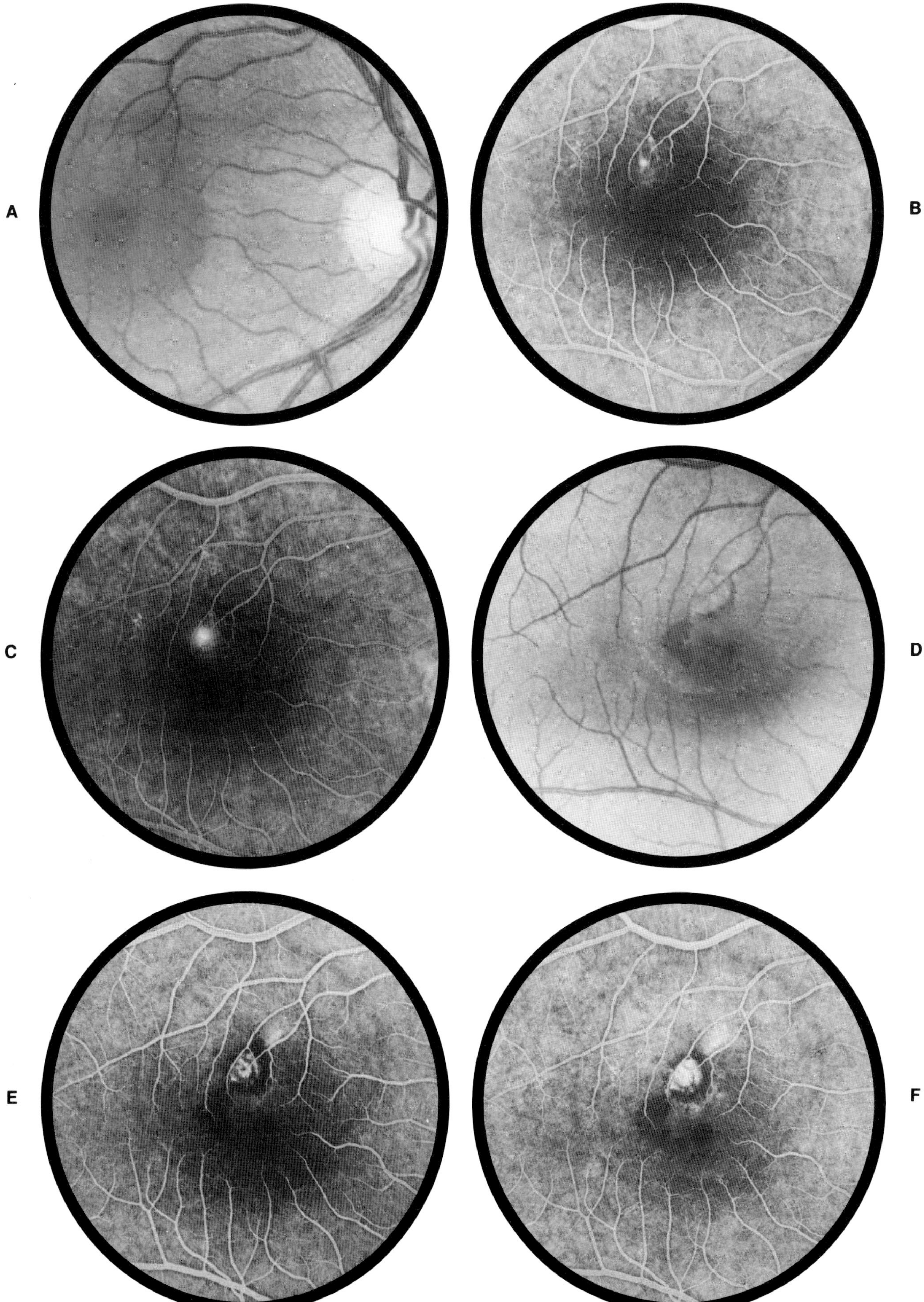

Figure 13.19

References

1. von Graefe, A.: Über centrale Recidivirende Retinitis. *Albrecht von Graefes Arch Ophthalmol, 12*: 211, 1866.
2. Maumenee, A.E.: Pathogenesis [of macular disease]. *Trans Am Acad Ophthalmol Otolaryngol, 69*: 691, 1965.
3. Straatsma, B., Allen, P.A., and Petit, T.H.: Central serous retinopathy. *Trans Pac Coast Otoophthalmol Soc, 47*: 107, 1966.
4. Gass, J.D.M.: Pathogenesis of disciform detachment of the neuroepithelium. II. Idiopathic central serous choroidopathy. *Am J Ophthalmol, 63*: 587, 1967.
5. Spalter, H.F.: Photocoagulation of central serous retinopathy. *Arch Ophthalmol, 79*: 247, 1968.
6. Wise, G.N., Campbell, C.J., Wendler, P.F., and Rittler, M.C.: Photocoagulation of vascular lesions of the macula. *Am J Ophthalmol, 66*: 452, 1968.
7. Peabody, R.R., Zweng, H.C., and Little, H.L.: Treatment of persistent central serous retinopathy. *Arch Ophthalmol, 79*: 166, 1968.
8. Nørholm, I.: Central serous retinitis: a follow-up study. *Acta Ophthalmol, 47*: 890, 1969.
9. Gass, J.D.M.: Stereoscopic Atlas of Macular Diseases: A Funduscopic and Angiographic Presentation, C.V. Mosby, St. Louis, 1970, p. 20.
10. Burton, T.C.: Central serous retinopathy. *Curr Concepts Ophthalmol, 3*: 1, 1972.
11. Shimizu, K.: Fluorescein Microangiography of the Ocular Fundus. Igaku Shoin Ltd., Tokyo, 1973, p. 113.
12. Watzke, R.C., Burton, T.C., and Leaverton, P.E.: Ruby laser photocoagulation therapy of central serous retinopathy. I. A controlled clinical study. II. Factors affecting prognosis. *Trans Am Acad Ophthalmol Otolaryngol, 78*: 205, 1974.
13. Annesley, W.H., Tasman, W.S., LeWin, D.P., *et al.*: A retrospective evaluation of photocoagulation for idiopathic central serous choroidopathy. *Mod Prob Ophthalmol, 12*: 234, 1974.
14. Klein, M.L., van Buskirk, E.M., Friedman, E., Gragoudas, E., and Chandra, S.: Nontreatment of central serous choroidopathy. *Arch Ophthalmol, 91*: 247, 1974.
15. Berrochal, J.A.: Current world-wide management of central serous retinopathy. *Mod Prob Ophthalmol, 12*: 239, 1974.
16. Schatz, H.: Central serous choroidopathy. *Int Ophthalmol Clin, 15* (1): 159, 1975.
17. Yannuzzi, L.A., and Wallyn, R.: Observations in untreated cases of central serous choroidopathy. Unpublished data.
18. Gass, J.D.M.: Bullous retinal detachment: an unusual manifestation of idiopathic central serous choroidopathy. *Am J Ophthalmol, 75*: 810, 1973.
19. Wessing, A.: Central serous retinopathy and related lesions. *Mod Prob Ophthalmol, 9*: 148, 1971.
20. Gass, J.D.M.: Photocoagulation of macular lesions. *Trans Am Acad Ophthalmol Otolaryngol, 75*: 580, 1971.
21. Schatz, H., Yannuzzi, L.A., and Gitter, K.: Subretinal neovascularization following argon laser photocoagulation treatment for central serous chorioretinopathy. *Trans Am Acad Ophthalmol Otolaryngol, 83*: 893, 1977.

Figure 13.19. Subretinal neovascularization masquerading as central serous chorioretinopathy. *A*, ophthalmoscopic photograph showing sensory retinal detachment. *B*, early venous phase angiogram revealing a focal leak at the level of the pigment epithelium. *C*, late phase angiogram revealing pooling into the subsensory retinal space with fuzzy margins. *D*, ophthalmoscopic photograph of same patient following photocoagulation with subretinal hemorrhage and exudate. *E*, arteriovenous phase angiogram reveals area of lacy hyperfluorescence, indicative of subretinal neovascularization at the site of the photocoagulation. *F*, late venous phase angiogram. Pooling has occurred into the subretinal space.

CHAPTER 14

Detachment of the Retinal Pigment Epithelium

Lawrence A. Yannuzzi, M.D., Kurt A. Gitter, M.D., and Howard Schatz, M.D.

Detachment of the retinal pigment epithelium is a histopathologic response in the macula which may occur as an isolated entity or as a manifestation of a variety of primary macular disorders [1–4]. When it occurs alone or in association with an overlying sensory retinal detachment in patients less than 55 years of age, it is thought by some to be either a variant or a basic part of the central serous chorioretinopathy syndrome. Serous detachments of the retinal pigment epithelium in older patients are most frequently encountered as exudative manifestations of involutional macular degeneration. Actually, it appears that any disturbance in the pigment epithelium, originating from a variety of retinal pigment epithelial-Bruch's membrane-choroidal disorders, may predispose to serous detachment of the pigment epithelium at any age. Typical predisposing factors include choroidal tumors, inflammation, and subpigment epithelial neovascularization.

History

The presenting symptomatology of serous detachments of the retinal pigment epithelium is extremely variable, depending on the size and location of the detachment, the age of the patient, the accompanying manifestations such as blood and exudate, the precipitating factors such as choroidal tumor or subretinal neovascularization, and the state of the overlying sensory retina. When the fovea is involved, when there is an overlying sensory retinal detachment, or when pigment epithelial atrophy and pigment migration have occurred in the juxtafoveal region, central vision may be reduced. The medical and family histories are usually negative unless the macular manifestation is related to an underlying systemic disease such as Harada's disease or pseudoxanthoma elasticum.

Examination

Often a serous pigment epithelial detachment in a young patient will be incidentally noted on a routine examination. When it is located eccentric to the fovea, the patient will be visually asymptomatic. In eyes exhibiting overlying sensory retinal detachment, the initial examination and visual testing is similar to that seen in central serous chorioretinopathy. Large pigment epithelial detachments in the juxtafoveal region, or small ones that are foveal in orientation, may themselves be sufficient to produce metamorphopsia, micropsia, a positive scotoma, or even reduced acuity. Changes in the pigment epithelium such as atrophy and pigment dispersion are also characteristic of visually symptomatic individuals.

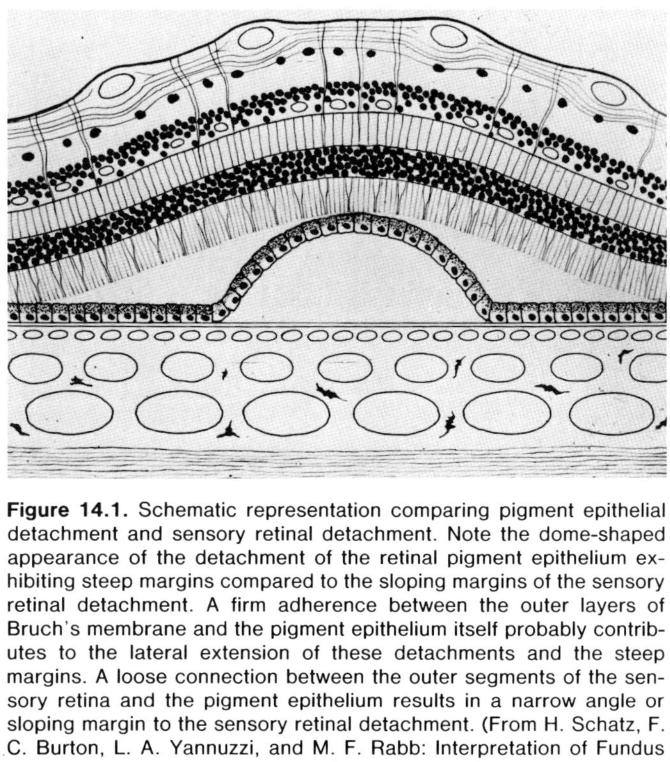

Figure 14.1. Schematic representation comparing pigment epithelial detachment and sensory retinal detachment. Note the dome-shaped appearance of the detachment of the retinal pigment epithelium exhibiting steep margins compared to the sloping margins of the sensory retinal detachment. A firm adherence between the outer layers of Bruch's membrane and the pigment epithelium itself probably contributes to the lateral extension of these detachments and the steep margins. A loose connection between the outer segments of the sensory retina and the pigment epithelium results in a narrow angle or sloping margin to the sensory retinal detachment. (From H. Schatz, F. C. Burton, L. A. Yannuzzi, and M. F. Rabb: Interpretation of Fundus Fluorescein Angiography, 1978, © C. V. Mosby and Co., St. Louis; reprinted with permission.)

On slit-lamp biomicroscopic examination with the Goldmann contact lens, retinal pigment epithelial detachments reveal anterior bowing of the entire slit beam. In the presence of an overlying secondary sensory retinal detachment, the beam splits. Typical pigment epithelial detachments are dome-shaped, in contrast to the more sloping margins of a sensory retinal detachment (Fig. 14.1). The steep margins, which are obvious and consistently evident in pigment

A

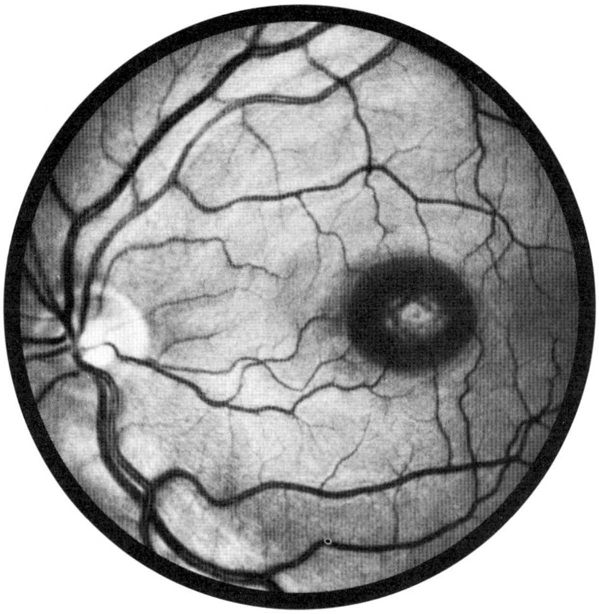

B

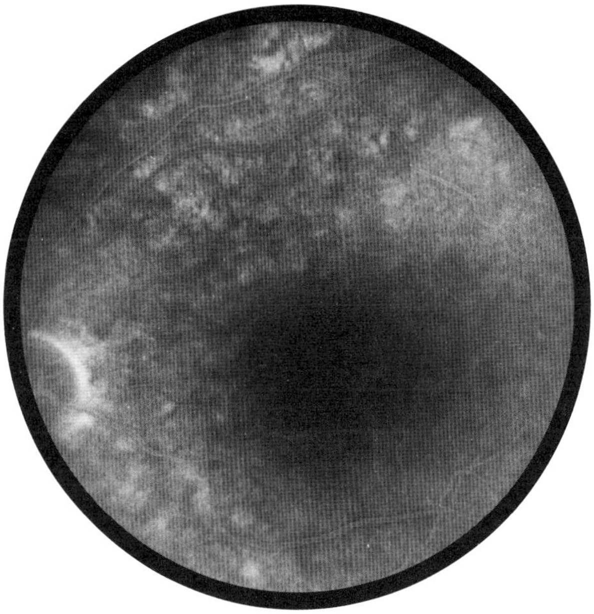

Figure 14.2. Vitelliform detachment of the macula. *A*, ophthalmoscopic photograph. Note the dome-shaped elevation in the macula, resembling a pigment epithelial detachment. *B*, late phase fluorescein angiogram. Note the absence of fluorescence in the macula, differentiating this lesion from a serous pigment epithelial detachment.

epithelial detachments, are probably produced by the rather firm adherence between the collagenous fibers of Bruch's membrane and the pigment epithelium itself, limiting lateral extension of the detachment. Sensory retinal detachments may also occasionally appear dome-shaped, (when they are: (1) small and parafoveal, (2) of acute onset in the macula, or (3) gravity-dependent) extending from a shallow base of the macula to an apron-like distribution toward and below the inferior arcade. The vitelliform lesion in the macula in Best's disease may on occasion clinically resemble a typical serous pigment epithelial detachment. These are easily differentiated from serous detachments of the pigment epithelium by fluorescein angiography in that they reveal no hyperfluorescence (Fig. 14.2). Frequently, an orange ring, completely encircling the margins of a retinal pigment epithelial detachment, is noted (Fig. 14.3). Although the exact character of this ring is unknown, its presence is virtually pathognomonic of the presence of the pigment epithelial detachment. Some observers have suggested that it represents a small area of sensory retinal detachment surrounding the base of the pigment epithelial detachment. This seems unlikely since some orange encircled retinal pigment epithelial detachments have much larger overlying sensory detachments that extend far beyond the orange ring. Others have theorized that the ring represents edema of the pigment epithelium or even an optically induced effect produced by a rotation of the pigment epithelial cells, themselves. We believe that the orange ring represents lipofuscin deposition, the same pigment seen overlying choroidal tumors. This correlates well with the frequently observed fluorescein angiographic pattern of "slight shrinkage" of the pigment epithelial detachment when compared to the ophthalmoscopic view [3], possibly accounted for by the propensity of lipofuscin to produce blocked fluorescence, thereby producing a hypofluorescent ring surrounding the detachment, i.e., "shrinkage" (Fig. 14.3).

Like the ring seen commonly around serous detachments of the pigment epithelium, lipofuscin is orange on the ophthalmoscopic view or the color photograph. The marked degree of hypofluorescence produced by lipofuscin is seen only with melanin pigment or blood on a fluorescein angiogram. On the monochromatic photograph or red-free view of the fundus, melanin and blood appear dark whereas lipofuscin is barely evident because of its orange color. Thus, a lesion that is extremely dark or hypofluorescent on a fluorescein angiogram and also dark on a monochromatic photograph, contains either melanin or blood. Similarly, a lesion that is extremely hypofluorescent on a fluorescein angiogram and barely evident on the monochromatic photograph, most likely contains lipofuscin. This simple comparison lends support to the impression that the ring around a serous pigment epithelial detachment is lipofuscin in origin (Fig. 14.4).

Pigment epithelial detachments in a given eye vary widely in their size, location, number, and natural course. Solitary detachments are frequently encountered; however, multiple detachments are more common. Some eyes contain multiple pigment epithelial detachments scattered widely throughout the posterior fundus (Fig. 14.5). In younger patients the pigment epithelial detachments tend to be smaller and associated with a clear subpigment epithelial fluid.

Older patients tend to have larger detachments (greater than 1 disc diameter) with markedly turbid subpigment epithelial fluid as well as other degenerative changes including: lipid exudate, pigment epithelial proliferation, pigment deposition (melanin and lipofuscin), pigment epithelial atrophy, hemorrhage, and even subretinal neovascular-

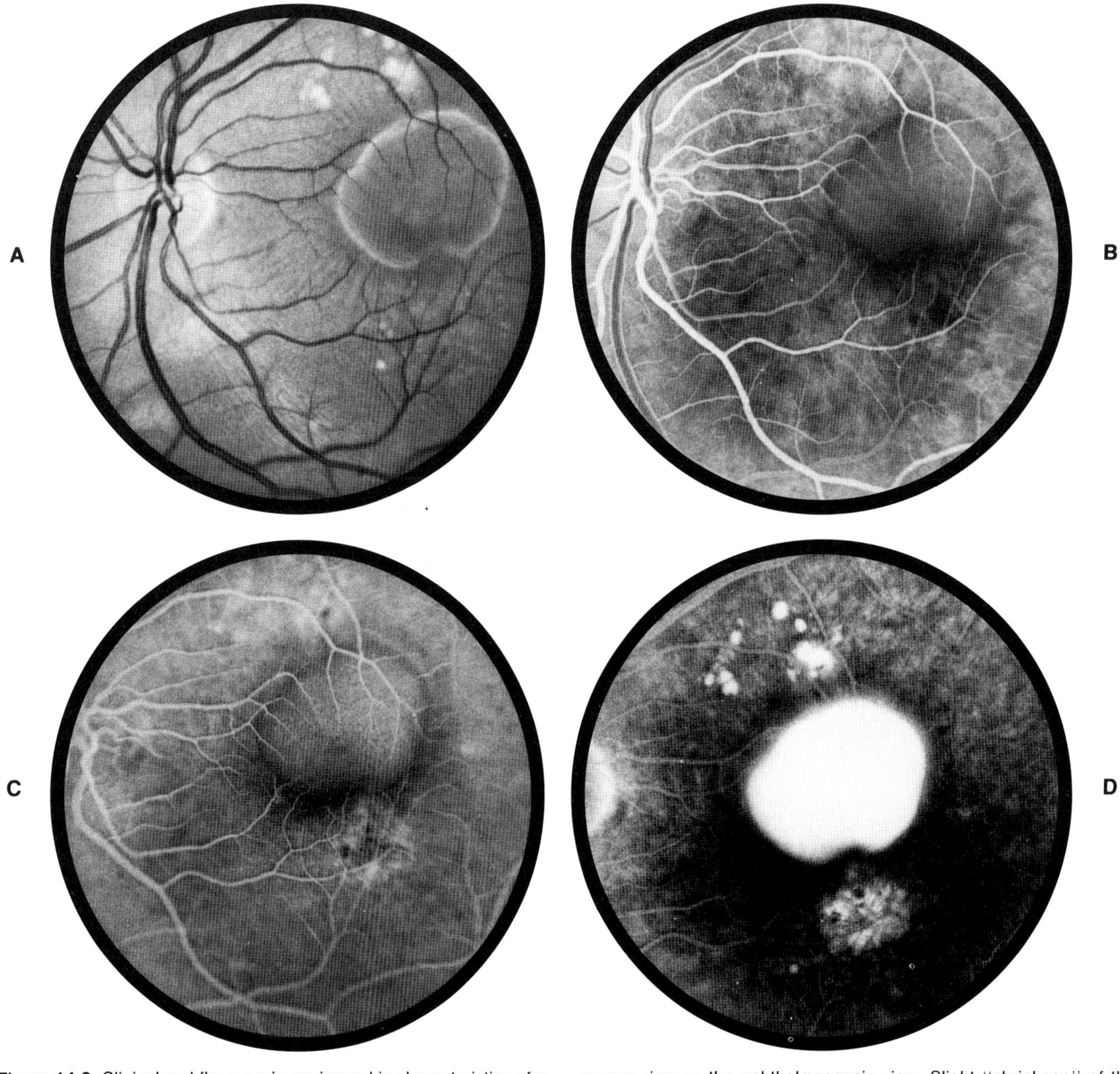

Figure 14.3. Clinical and fluorescein angiographic characteristics of a serous detachment of the retinal pigment epithelium. *A*, ophthalmoscopic photograph. Note dome-shaped elevation in the macula at the site of serous detachment of the retinal pigment epithelium. An orange ring encircles the detachment. Fine retinal folds are seen radiating from the pigment epithelial detachment, and a number of scattered drusen are visible. *B*, arterial phase fluorescein angiogram. Note the very faint, diffuse, homogeneous hyperfluorescence beneath the serous detachment of the pigment epithelium. A dark zone encircles the pigment epithelial detachment at its margins and corresponds to the orange ring on the ophthalmoscopic view. Slight "shrinkage" of the pigment epithelial detachment is suggested by the hypofluorescent ring surrounding it. *C*, arteriovenous phase fluorescein angiogram. The hyperfluorescence beneath the serous detachment of the pigment epithelium has increased in intensity but not in size. *D*, late phase fluorescein angiogram. Hyperfluorescence continues to increase in intensity as the dye concentration pools beneath the detached pigment epithelium. There is complete, homogeneous hyperfluorescence beneath the pigment epithelial detachment with well demarcated margins.

A B

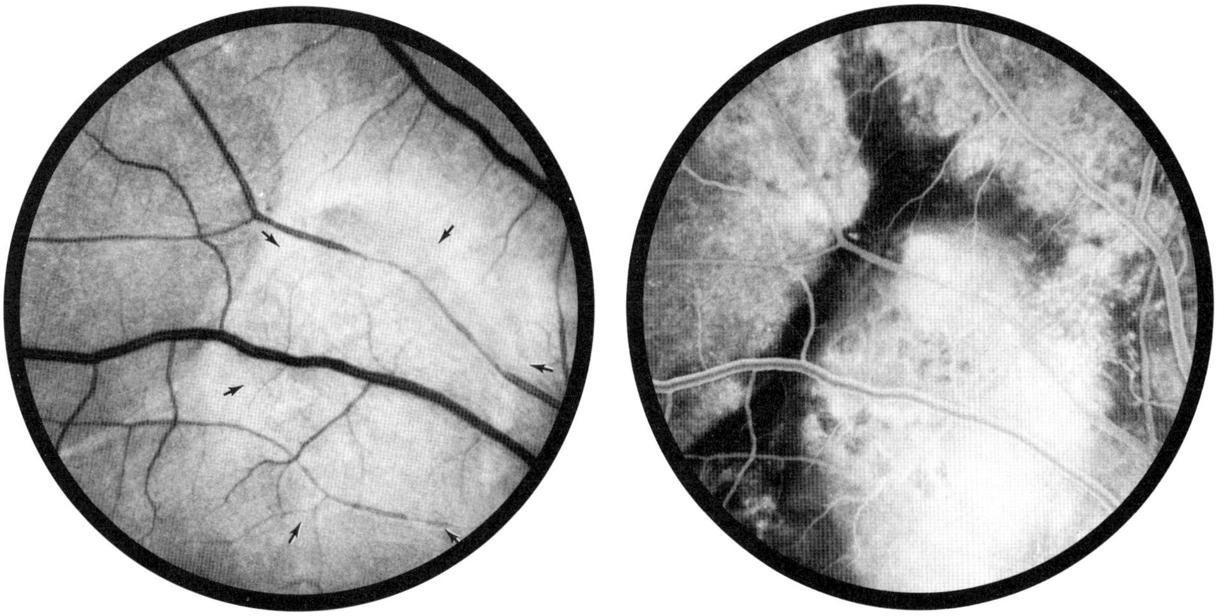

Figure 14.4. Orange pigment surrounding a pigment epithelial detachment. *A*, monochromatic or red-free photograph (560 nm yellow green). Note the pigment epithelium detachment (*arrows*) with an irregular surrounding band of pigmentation extending inferiorly. On the monochromatic photograph, the orange pigment is barely visible as a whitish margin. *B*, arteriovenous phase fluorescein angiogram, same eye. Note the diffuse hyperfluorescence beneath the detached pigment epithelium except for some circumscribed areas of hypofluorescence corresponding to previous photocoagulation burns. The orange pigment is markedly hypofluorescent surrounding the margins of the pigment epithelial detachment and tapers superiorly and inferotemporally. Blocked fluorescence of this degree is produced only by melanin, blood, or lipofuscin pigment. Melanin pigment and blood are easily identified on the monochromatic or red-free photograph as dark areas, while lipofuscin pigment is barely evident as in this case.

A B

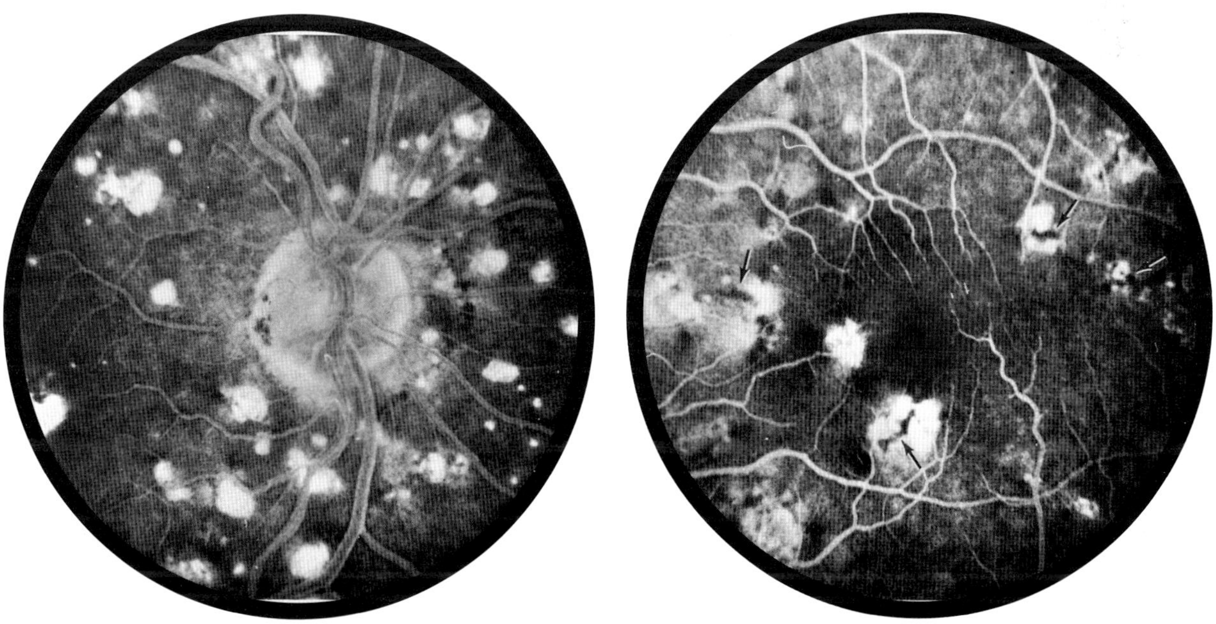

Figure 14.5. Bilateral multiple retinal pigment epithelial detachments. *A*, late phase fluorescein angiogram, right eye. *B*, late phase fluorescein angiogram, left eye. Note the multiple areas of late hyperfluorescence from pooling beneath serous detachments of the retinal pigment epithelium scattered in a widespread distribution throughout the posterior fundus. Many long-standing pigment epithelial detachments are associated with linear bands of hypofluorescence secondary to pigment fissures on the surface of the detachments (*arrows*).

A

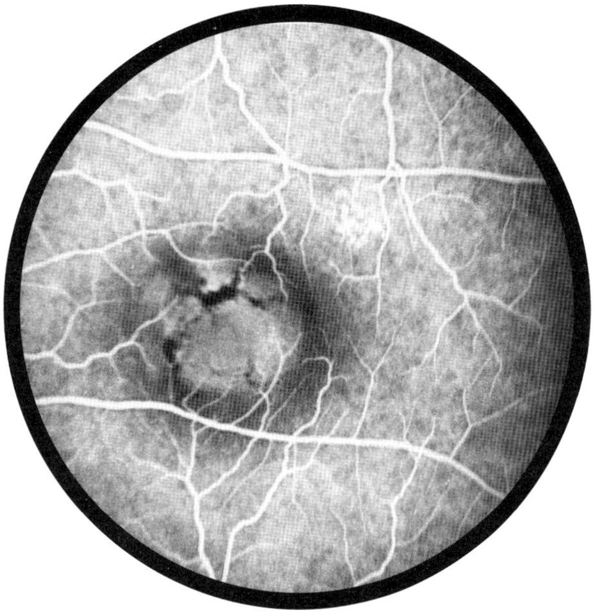

B

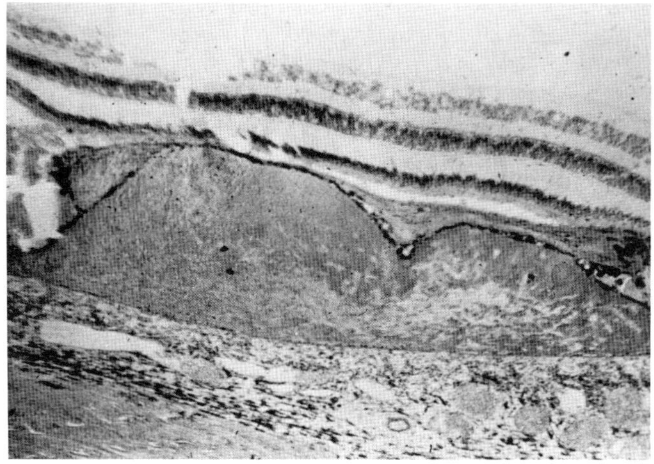

Figure 14.6. Chronic pigment epithelial detachment associated with overlying pigment figures. *A*, early venous phase fluorescein angiogram showing circumscribed area of hyperfluorescence from pooling beneath the serous detachment of the retinal pigment epithelium. Irregular bands of hypofluorescence are present on the surface of the detachment secondary to pigment proliferation and deposition. *B*, histopathologic specimen of a serous detachment of the retinal pigment epithelium with overlying pigment epithelial proliferation and pigment figures. (Courtesy of Lorenz Zimmerman, M.D., Armed Forces Institute of Pathology.)

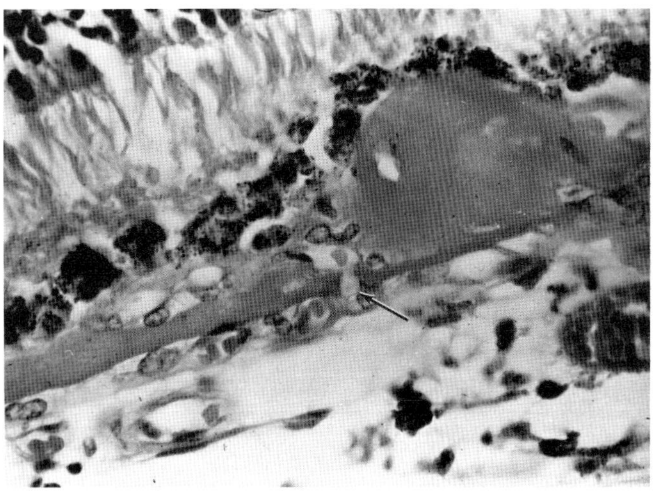

Figure 14.7. Histopathology of subretinal neovascularization beneath a drusen. Note the break in Bruch's membrane (*arrow*) with fibrovascular ingrowth into the subpigment epithelial space adjacent to a drusen. Drusen are often difficult to differentiate histopathologically from small serous detachments of the pigment epithelium. Occasionally, multiple adjacent drusen will become confluent to form discernible serous detachments of the pigment epithelium. Subretinal neovascularization from fibrovascular ingrowth through a break in Bruch's membrane may complicate either drusen or pigment epithelial detachments. (Courtesy of William R. Green, M.D.)

ization. Often there is a characteristic pigment band(s) along the dome of the pigment epithelial detachment, forming linear figures not infrequently resembling a "hot cross bun" (Fig. 14.6). The presence of such pigmentation is indicative of longevity [5]. Examination of this pigment with the slit-lamp biomicroscope often reveals an orange color suggesting lipofuscin pigment. Again, the pigment figures are markedly hypofluorescent on the angiogram and frequently less evident on the monochromatic photograph suggesting that they are predominantly lipofuscin in nature.

The view that a drusen in older patients is a micropigment epithelial detachment deserves consideration because of histopathologic similarities. Drusen have been described as being associated, in some instances, with subretinal neovascularization [6] (Fig. 14.7). If drusen may harbor a fine, delicate vascular complex beneath, and if is histopathologically indistinguishable from a micropigment epithelial detachment, then it is reasonable to assume that any pigment epithelial detachment may potentially be associated with an underlying fibrovascular membrane. In addition to subpigment epithelial neovascularization, other subretinal conditions such as choroidal tumors, inflammations, and virtually any disturbance in the pigment epithelium, may predispose to a detachment in the retinal pigment epithelium.

Fluorescein Angiography

The beginning phases of the fluorescein angiogram of a serous retinal pigment epithelial detachment show early hyperfluorescence diffusely beneath the entire detachment. During the mid-phase, the hyperfluorescence beneath the pigment epithelial detachment increases in intensity, but not in size. Finally, in the late stages of the angiogram the dye pools homogeneously into the subpigment epithelial space, completely filling the pigment epithelial detachment with well demarcated or sharp margins (see Fig. 14.3). This is considerably different from the fluorescein angiographic findings seen in a sensory retinal detachment such as in central serous chorioretinopathy where the sensory retinal detachment fills incompletely from a focal leak or leaks from the level of the pigment epithelium, and results ultimately in an area of late hyperfluorescence with fuzzy margins (Table 14.1)

There are certain histopathologic characteristics of pigment epithelial detachments that will alter the typical homogeneous well demarcated pattern (Table 14.2). Some of these factors tend to produce localized areas of hyperfluorescence; others produce areas of hypofluorescence.

Retinal pigment epithelial atrophy induced by stretching of the pigment epithelial cells may produce a heterogeneous area of hyperfluorescence in the detachment or at the margins. This comes about because of a reduction in the shielding or masking of the choroidal fluorescence normally produced by the pigment epithelium (transmitted fluorescence or so-called pigment epithelial window defect). When the atrophy is at the margins of a pigment epithelial detachment, irregular late hyperfluorescence or staining of visible sclera alters the normally sharp margins of the detachment in the late phase angiogram. The same is true for any drusen present at the margins of the pigment epithelial detachment.

Subretinal pigment epithelial neovascularization may also produce a localized area of hyperfluorescence beneath the pigment epithelial detachment. This is manifested by a zone of hyperfluorescence that is far more intense than the adjacent areas of hyperfluorescence beneath the detachment, and it is commonly referred to as a "hot spot" (Fig. 14.8).

Table 14.1. Fluorescein angiography characteristics

Stage	Central serious chorioretinopathy	Serous detachment of retinal pigment epithelium
Early	Barely evident focal leak(s) from level of retinal pigment epithelium	Diffuse homogeneous hyperfluorescence beneath entire retinal pigment epithelial detachment
Mid	Increase in size of hyperfluorescence	Increase in intensity of hyperfluorescence but not size
Late	Incomplete filling of subsensory retinal space with fuzzy margins	Complete filling of subpigment epithelial space with well demarcated margins

Table 14.2. Detachment of the retinal pigment epithelium

Factors affecting the typical fluorescein angiography characteristics	
Hypofluorescence	Hyperfluorescence
Hemorrhage	Atrophy of the retinal pigment epithelium
Hyperpigmentation	Hot spot
Normal macular pigments	Subretinal neovascularization
	Combined sensory retinal detachment

A

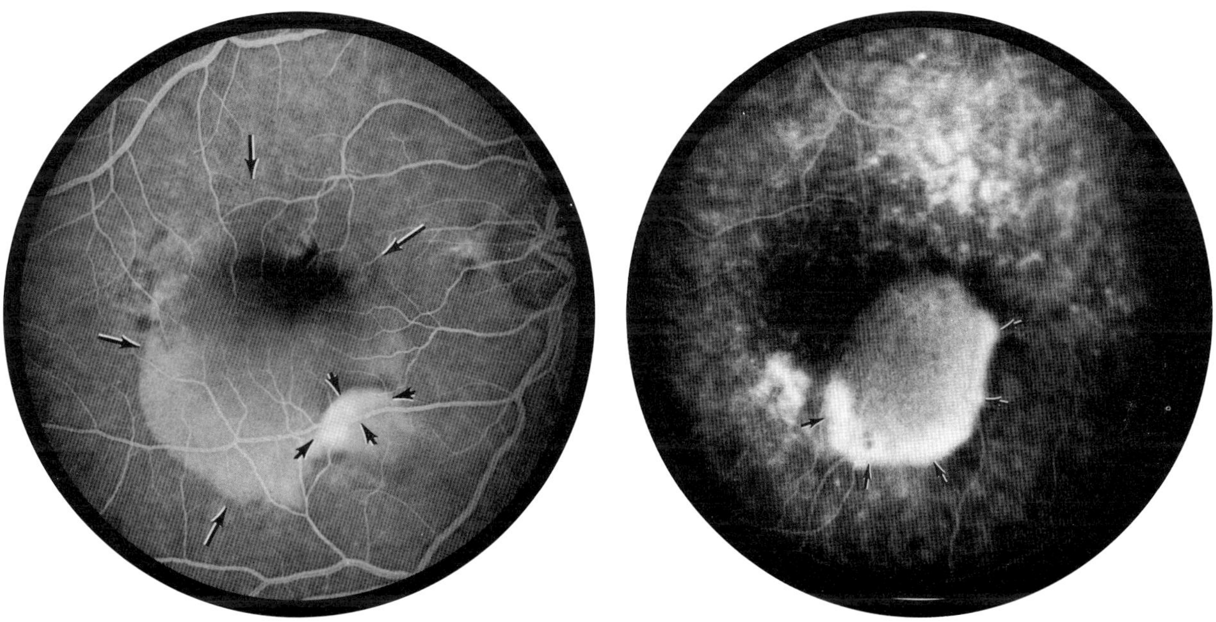

B

Figure 14.8. Detachment of the retinal pigment epithelium. *A*, note the heterogeneous hyperfluorescence produced by a serous detachment of the retinal pigment epithelium (*large arrows*). There is hypofluorescence in the foveal region and a localized area of intense hyperfluorescence or hot spot, corresponding to neovascularization (*small arrows*). When a serous detachment of the pigment epithelium involves the macular region, the normal macular pigments (melanin and lipofuscin in the pigment epithelium and xanthophyll in the outer layers of the sensory retina) serve to mask the underlying hyperfluorescence of the detached pigment epithelium, making the macular area relatively hypofluorescent. Subretinal neovascularization and normal macular pigments serve to alter the typical hyperfluorescence of a serous detachment of the retinal pigment epithelium. (Courtesy of Robert K. Abraham, M.D.) *B*, venous phase fluorescein angiogram on another eye with a pigment epithelial detachment and more extensive hot spot along its inferotemporal border (*arrows*). Subpigment epithelial neovascularization can produce focal areas of intense hyperfluorescence or hot spots. The early lacy-like hyperfluorescence is often absent at the site of a hot spot because of a masking effect created by the turbid subpigment epithelial fluid.

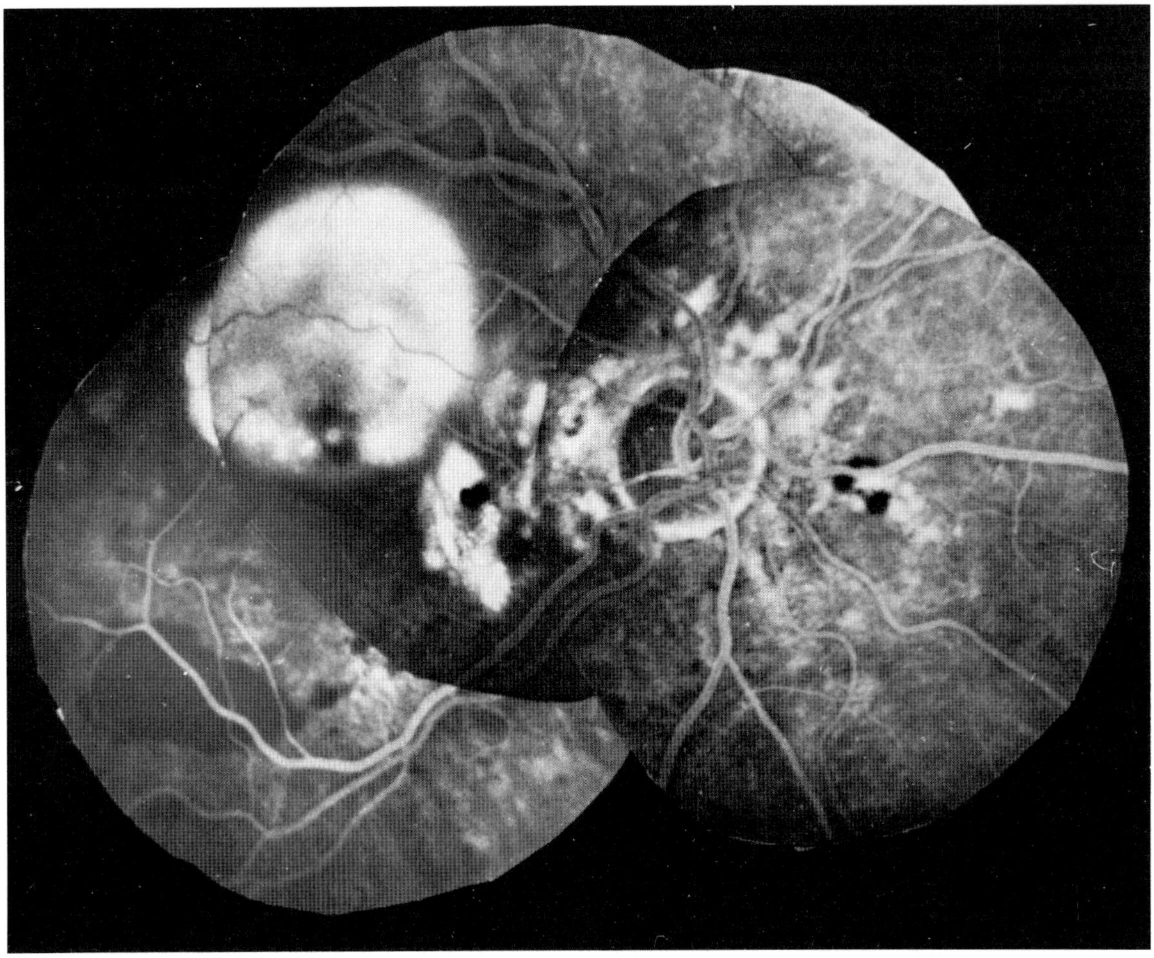

Figure 14.9. Venous phase fluorescein angiogram composite of a serous detachment of the retinal pigment epithelium in a patient with angioid streaks. Note the circumscribed globular area of hyperfluorescence from pooling beneath a serous detachment of the retinal pigment epithelium in the superior macula. There is a patch of hypofluorescence near the lower aspect of the pigment epithelial detachment and inferior macula corresponding to hemorrhage. Radiating bands of hyperfluorescence corresponding to the angioid streaks are seen originating from the optic nerve mainly in the nasal retina.

Finally, a localized area of intense hyperfluorescence may be seen in an area above a pigment epithelial detachment where there is a combined sensory retinal detachment as seen in central serous chorioretinopathy. When leakage occurs from a pigment epithelial detachment into the subsensory retinal space, from focal or multifocal points of origin, the site of leakage is usually present near the margins of the pigment epithelial detachment. This is true in central serous chorioretinopathy, involutional macular degeneration, and even in Harada's disease, where multiple pigment epithelial leaks may be seen to line up along the margin of pigment epithelial detachments with subsequent pooling into the subsensory retinal space. Of course, some leaks may be occurring from the dome of the pigment epithelial detachment but are not as evident because of the lack of contrast from the homogeneously fluorescing pigment epithelial detachment to its rear. In spite of this possibility, there seems to be a predilection for focal leakage at the margins of pigment epithelial detachments when they are complicated by overlying sensory retinal detachments.

It can be extremely difficult to differentiate the hyperfluorescence produced by subpigment epithelial neovascularization beneath pigment epithelial detachment (hot spot) from that of a focal leak in an eye with a combined pigment epithelial detachment and sensory retinal detachment. It is best achieved by stereoscopic analysis of the fluorescein angiogram since the subretinal neovascularization produces an area of hyperfluorescence beneath the pigment epithelium, whereas the leak due to a combined detachment results in hyperfluorescence above the pigment epithelial detachment. Also, the hot spot associated with subpigment epithelial neovascularization may sometimes fade late in the angiogram leaving a silhouette of larger vessels present in the vascular complex. In some cases, atrophy of or erosion through the retinal pigment epithelium makes the fibrovascular complex and its lacy-like pattern more visible in the early stages of the angiogram.

Localized areas of hypofluorescence associated with serous pigment epithelial detachments may be produced by pigment proliferation and migration (Fig. 14.6), by subpigment epithelial hemorrhage (Fig. 14.9), and by the normal macular pigment epithelium and the yellow retinal pigment, xanthophyll (Fig. 14.8). All these factors tend to block fluorescence by partially obscuring a portion of the hyperfluorescence beneath the pigment epithelial detachment (table 14.2).

A

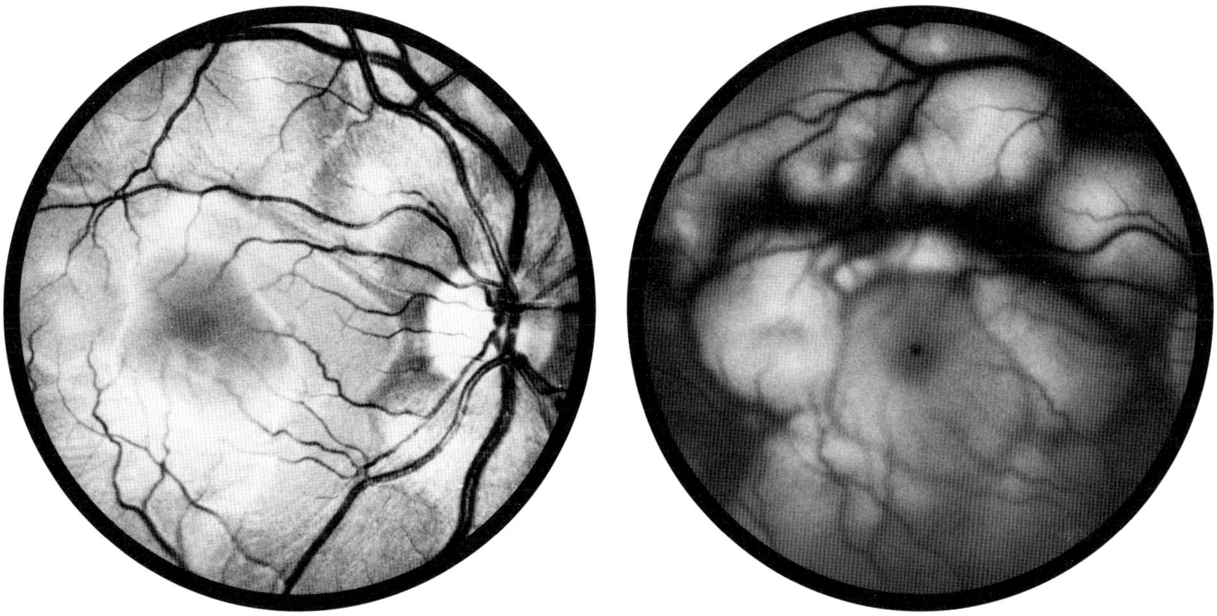

B

Figure 14.10. Multiple pigment epithelial detachments overlying a bullous sensory retinal detachment in Harada's disease. *A*, ophthalmoscopic photograph. Note multiple detachments of the retinal pigment epithelium, surrounded by a ring of orange pigment. *B*, late phase fluorescein angiogram. Note complete pooling beneath the multiple pigment epithelial detachments with well demarcated margins. A large bullous sensory retinal detachment was present and shifted from the macula inferiorly.

A

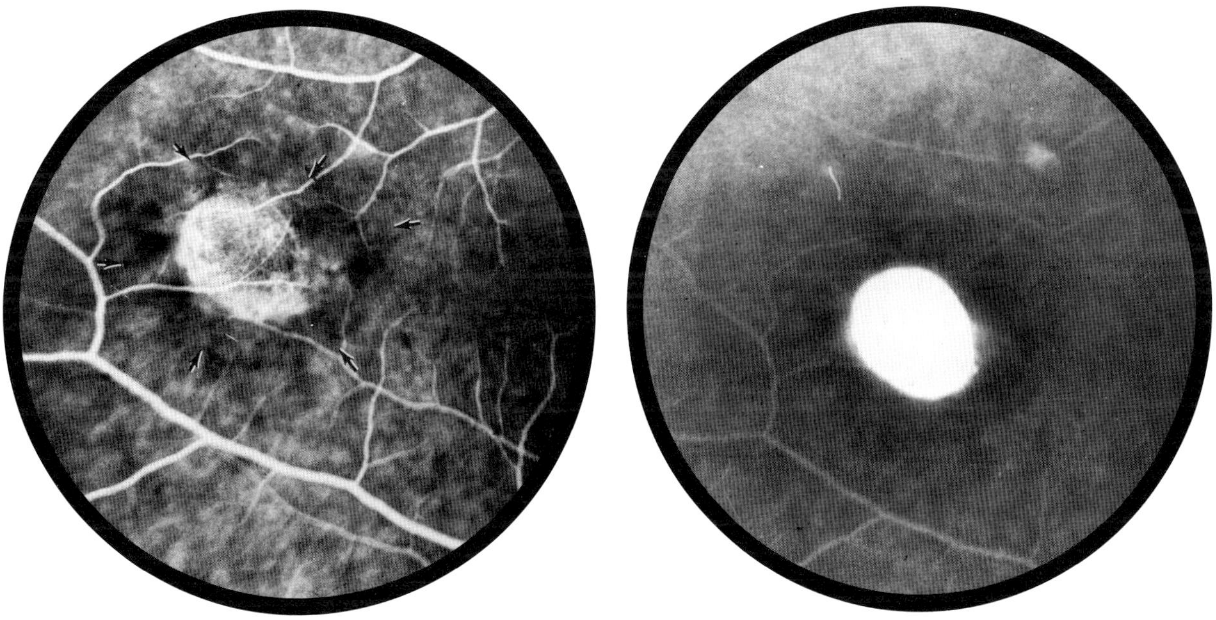

B

Figure 14.11. Serous detachment of the pigment epithelium overlying a tumor. *A*, venous phase fluorescein angiogram. Note the circumscribed hyperfluorescence due to a pigment epithelial detachment (*arrows*) overlying a flat pigmented choroidal tumor (presumably a choroidal nevus). *B*, late phase fluorescein angiogram. Note the well demarcated hyperfluorescence of the pigment epithelium detachment surrounded by a ring of hypofluorescence corresponding to the choroidal nevus. (Courtesy of Johnny Justice and The Wills Eye Hospital Retina Service.)

While choroidal inflammations such as Harada's disease (Fig. 14.10) and choroidal tumors (Fig. 14.11) can predispose to detachment of the retinal pigment epithelium, the most important overall consideration in a retinal pigment epithelial detachment is whether it is complicated by sub-pigment epithelial neovascularization. In short, the question is whether or not the retinal pigment epithelial detachment is vascular or avascular.

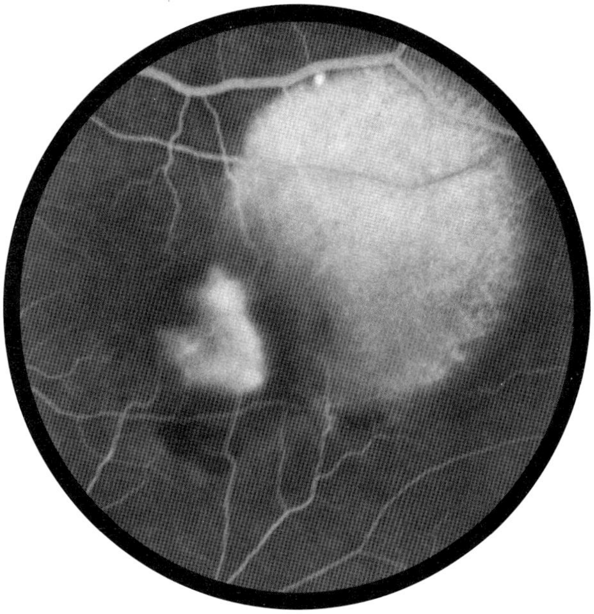

Figure 14.12. Venous phase angiogram of a serous detachment of the retinal pigment epithelium complicated by subretinal neovascularization. Between the fovea and the retinal pigment epithelial detachment, there is a triangular area of subretinal neovascularization with hemorrhage.

In some instances the presence of neovascularization is apparent on the fluorescein angiogram (Fig. 14.12). Less frequently it is evident on clinical examination. However, neovascularization cannot always be determined with reasonable clinical assurance on either ophthalmoscopic, slit-lamp biomicroscopic, or even fluorescein angiographic examination. There are some helpful considerations to keep in mind, however, when evaluating a retinal pigment epithelial detachment for the possibility of subpigment epithelial neovascularization. In general, there is a distinct tendency for all, a marked predisposition for some, and a virtually absolute certainty for others to harbor neovascularization even in the absence of fluorescein angiographic documentation. For example, alterations in the normally sharp margins of the fluorescence of a serous pigment epithelial detachment late in the angiogram suggest the possibility of subretinal neovascularization when these alterations are not due to marginal drusen or retinal pigment epithelial atrophic changes. When the margins are "scalloped," and particularly when they are "beaded," an underlying fibrovascular membrane with an advancing convex edge is probable. Such vascular networks typically produce "nodular" areas of hyperfluorescence at the margins of the detachment in a scalloped and/or beaded configuration. These nodular beads of hyperfluorescence correspond to the immature capillary buds on the advancing convex edge of the neovascularized complex (Fig. 14.13). In some instances atrophy of the pigment epithelium may produce greater visibility of these fibrovascular membranes in the subpigment epithelial space.

A

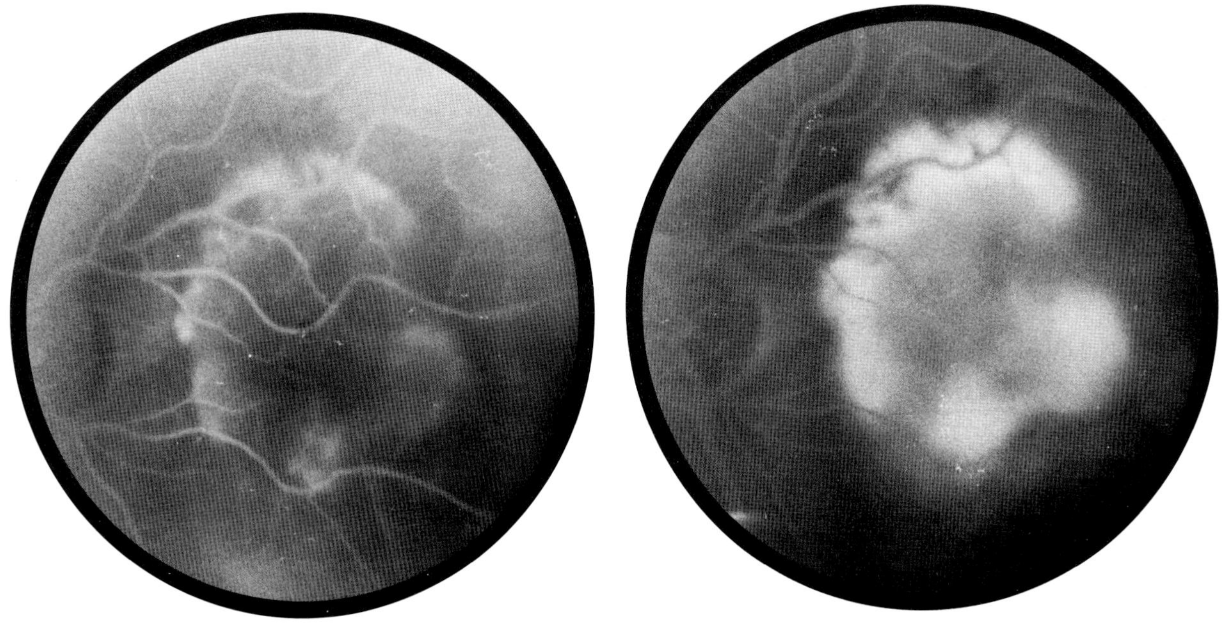

B

Figure 14.13. Serous detachment of pigment epithelium (vascular). *A*, early venous phase fluorescein angiogram. Note the scalloped margins of the serous detachment of the retinal pigment epithelium, which presumably are produced by proliferating vascular complexes. They are angiographically visible because of atrophy of the overlying pigment epithelium. The scalloped margins and small beads of fluorescence represent advancing convex fibrovascular membranes forming a cartwheel appearance characteristic of subretinal neovascularized membranes. *B*, late phase fluorescein angiogram. Note the accentuation of the scalloped margins as dye pools from the pigment epithelial detachment into an overlying sensory retinal detachment. There is an intense area of hyperfluorescence corresponding to each scalloped edge and underlying fibrovascular membrane, resembling hot spots.

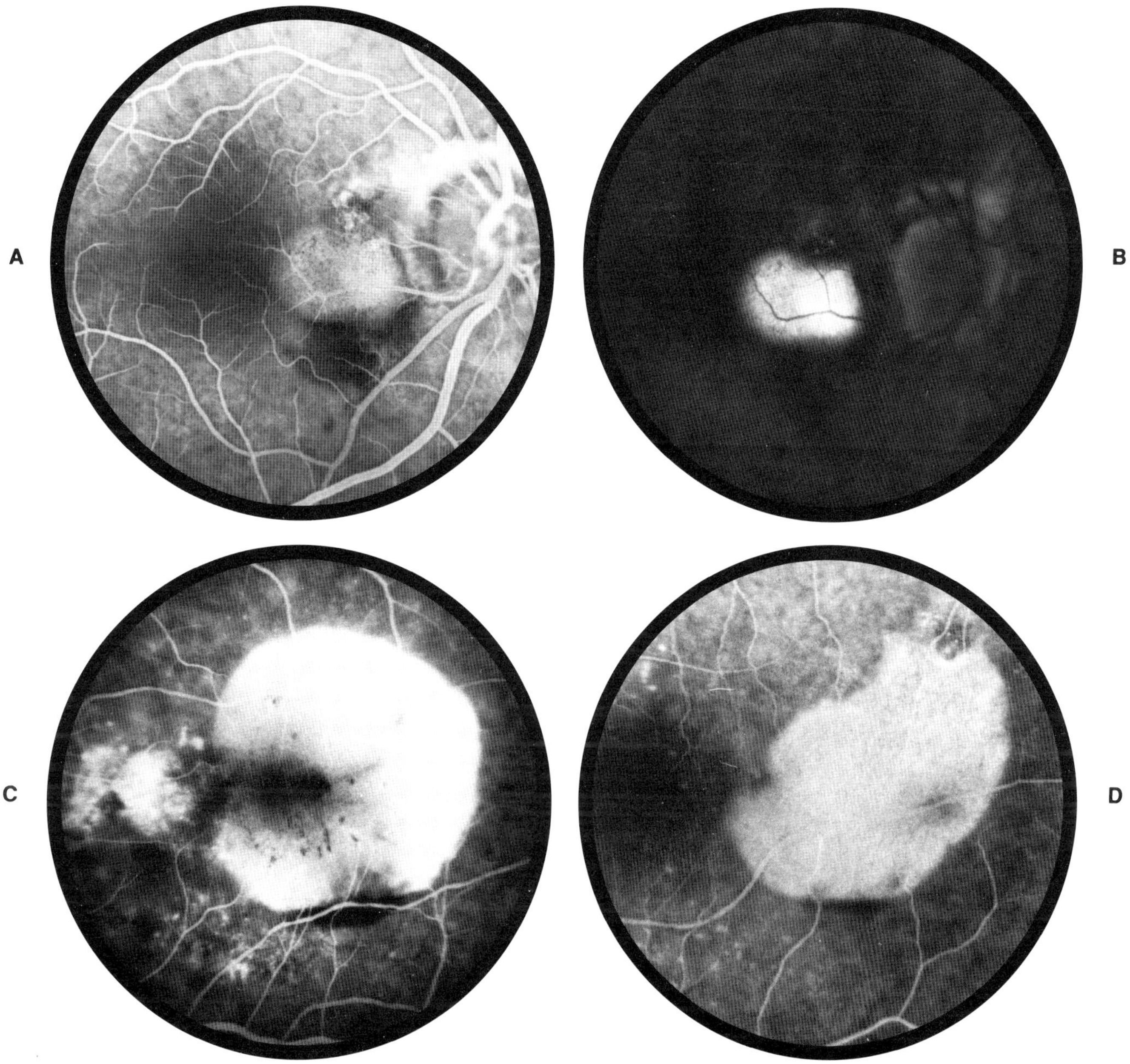

Figure 14.14. Detachment of pigment epithelium (vascular). *A*, early venous phase fluorescein angiogram. Note the homogeneous hyperfluorescence of the serous detachment of the pigment epithelium. Early hyperfluorescence secondary to atrophic changes in the pigment epithelium is seen at its superior margins. Inferior to the pigment epithelial detachment is a patchy area of hypofluorescence corresponding to a subretinal hemorrhage. *B*, late phase fluorescein angiogram. Note the homogeneous, well demarcated fluorescence of the pigment epithelial detachment. *C* and *D*, late phase fluorescein angiograms of two patients with large pigment epithelial detachments and with a hypofluorescent zone at their inferior margins, corresponding to a meniscus of subpigment epithelial blood. Although there was no early evidence of lacy hyperfluorescence or other late staining suggestive of subretinal neovascularization, the presence of the subretinal hemorrhage in association with a pigment epithelial detachment is sufficient clinical evidence to classify these pigment epithelial detachments as vascular.

In general, a pigment epithelial detachment is likely to contain underlying subretinal neovascularization under any of the following circumstances: (1) when the patient is elderly; (2) when the detachment is large; (3) when there is a markedly turbid subpigment epithelial fluid; (4) when the eye contains widespread retinal pigment epithelial atrophic and/or drusen changes or when there is subretinal neovascularization and/or a disciform scar in the fellow eye; and (5) when the detachment has scalloped or beaded margins with nodular fluorescence on the fluorescein angiogram. A pigment epithelial detachment with any of these characteristics should be suspected of harboring subretinal neovascularization even if the fluorescein angiogram fails to reveal a "hot spot" beneath the pigment epithelium for a lacy-like network of vessels originating from the choroidal circulation.

There are certain other clinical and fluorescein angiographic manifestations that are definitely evidence of subretinal neovascularization complicating a serous pigment epithelial detachment. These include: (1) lipid exudation; (2) subretinal hemorrhage (Fig. 14.14); (3) a subretinal "pigment ring"; (4) a "dirty gray" membrane; and (5) intraretinal cystoid edema. The presence of any one of these ophthalmoscopic findings or fluorescein angiographic evidence of a lacy-like vascular pattern or a hot spot is virtually pathognomonic of underlying subretinal neovascularization (Table 14.3).

Table 14.3. Detachment of the retinal pigment epithelium

Factors related to subretinal neovascularization	
Suspicious	Virtually pathognomonic
Older patients	Lipid
Large detachments	Hemorrhage
Markedly turbid fluid	Pigment ring
Widespread RPE atrophy, drusen, or disciform scar in fellow eye	Dirty gray membrane Cystoid edema
Fluorescein angiography	Fluorescein Angiography
Beaded or scalloped margins	Lacy-like vascular pattern
Nodular fluorescence at margins	Hot spot

Natural Course

The natural course of pigment epithelial detachments is extremely variable. In some people they may persist "silently" or asymptomatically for years, even when the fovea is involved, with no alteration in central vision. They may disappear in some instances after many years as mysteriously as they originally appeared. They may also become associated with overlying sensory retinal detachments and develop into a syndrome similar to that of central serous chorioretinopathy. Resolution of the pigment epithelial detachments, even when they become combined with sensory retinal detachments, has been known to occur spontaneously without residual effects on central vision (Fig. 14.15). Spontaneous resolution of a large detachment in elderly patients is, however, rare. The same risks that are inherent in any sensory retinal detachment of the macula exist when these pigment epithelial detachments begin to leak producing sensory retinal detachments.

Some pigment epithelial detachments have been observed to increase in size without affecting the central vision (Fig. 14.16). In other cases, particularly in elderly patients, subretinal hemorrhage from fibrovascular membranes evolving into disciform scars occurs with marked irreversible loss of macular function. In general, avascular lesions in patients under 50 years of age seem to have a fairly good prognosis with little tendency for progression to the more dreaded vascular complications, and with a maintenance of reasonably good central vision. In older patients, the tendency toward neovascularization with hemorrhage is greater although spontaneous resolution is unlikely.

Once a pigment epithelial detachment becomes vascular the prognosis for central vision appears to be extremely poor with 75% of the patients developing 20/200 or less in one preliminary study [7]. Unfortunately, the problem with natural course studies to date has been that they have not been purely prospective in nature, and that they have been faced with the task of differentiating vascular from avascular serous detachments of the pigment epithelium, a process that cannot always be determined definitively on a clinical or even fluorescein angiographic basis.

Figure 14.15. Multiple detachments of the retinal pigment epithelium with neurosensory detachment and spontaneous resolution. *A*, late venous phase fluorescein angiogram. Note four discrete detachments of the retinal pigment epithelium. *B*, early venous phase fluorescein angiogram. *C*, late venous phase fluorescein angiogram and *D*, late phase fluorescein angiogram of the same patient 3 years later. A sensory retinal detachment developed from leakage of one of the pigment epithelial detachments producing a classic mushroom leak. In the late phase angiogram, the entire sensory retinal detachment is evident as dye circulates through the subsensory retinal space. *E*, late venous phase fluorescein angiogram on the same patient 4 weeks later. Note the spontaneous resolution of the sensory retinal detachment as well as two of the four serous pigment epithelial detachments seen in (*A*).

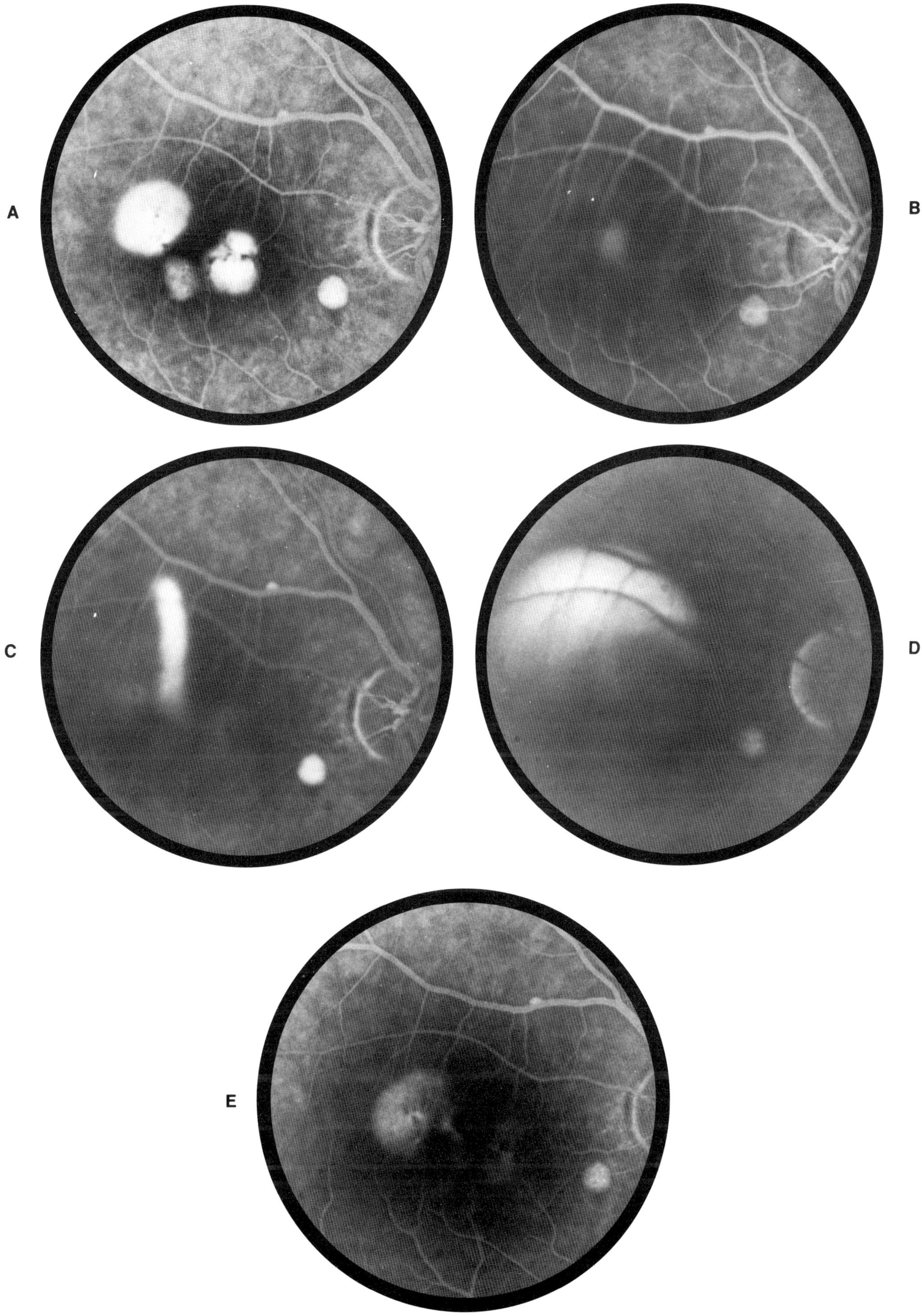

Figure 14.15

A 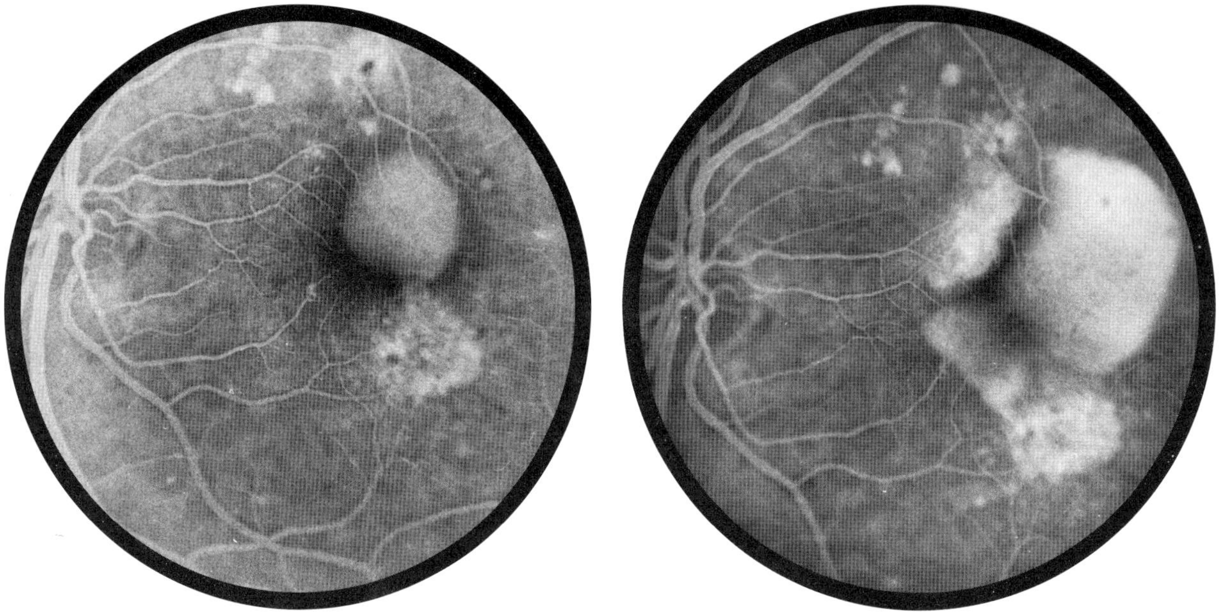 B

Figure 14.16. Serous detachment of the pigment epithelium with change in size over time. *A*, late venous phase fluorescein angiogram. Note the serous detachment of the retinal pigment epithelium in the central macula. *B*, late venous phase fluorescein angiogram, same patient 2½ years later. Note the increase in the size of the serous detachment of the pigment epithelium. Visual acuity remained unaltered at 20/20.

A 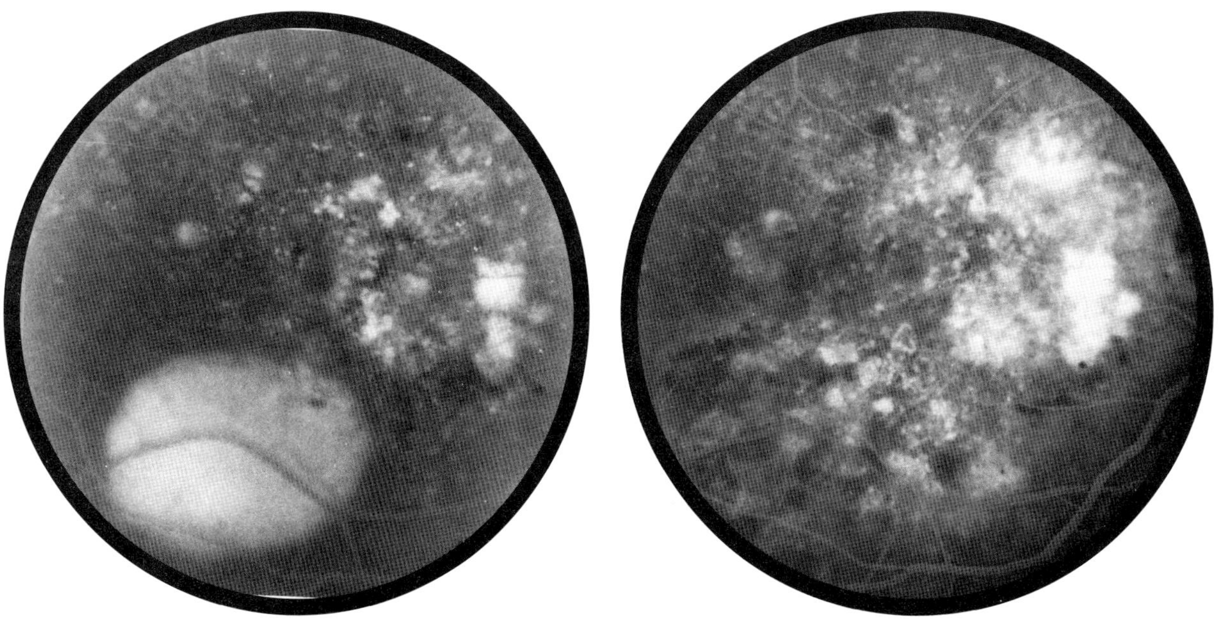 B

Figure 14.17. Photocoagulation treatment of a serous detachment of the retinal pigment epithelium with an overlying sensory retinal detachment in an eye with involutional macular degeneration. *A*, late phase fluorescein angiogram, pretreatment. Note the well demarcated diffuse hyperfluorescence beneath a large serous pigment epithelial detachment along the inferior temporal arcade. A retinal vessel overlying the pigment epithelial detachment is out of focus because of an associated widespread sensory retinal detachment. Patchy hyper- and hypofluorescence is present in the macular region from other nonexudative and exudative involutional degenerative changes. *B*, late phase fluorescein angiogram, postphotocoagulation therapy. Note the resolution of the serous detachment of the retinal pigment epithelium as well as the widespread sensory retinal detachment. There was improvement and stabilization of the visual acuity from 20/100 to 20/40 with no subsequent detachment of the sensory retina over the past 2½ years, in spite of the widespread degenerative disease.

Treatment

No clear-cut feasibility study has yet been carried out with strict patient definition, randomized selections of treatment and control, and independent prospective analysis of results. Even so, there is no question that photocoagulation can seal a leaking pigment epithelial detachment, producing resolution of the pigment epithelial detachment and combined sensory retinal detachment even in an eye with widespread disease (Fig. 14.17). Whether this form of treatment is beneficial to vision in the long run and whether the potential benefits outweigh the risks, are questions which have not yet been answered. Preliminary results in one well designed prospective study involving "treatment-nontreatment control eyes," have been encouraging (i.e., in favor of treatment) but not yet definitive [8].

For the present, when pigment epithelial detachments are not associated with combined sensory retinal detachments, or when they are visually asymptomatic in the macular region, particularly in the young, they should not be treated with photocoagulation. Only rarely does a young patient with these symptoms show progressive reduction in central vision. This fact, combined with the intrinsic risks of photocoagulation in the macular area, including accidental foveal burns, preretinal membrane formation, and stimulation of unsuspected neovascularization, collectively dictate a conservative approach to management until clearer guidelines evolve from scientific clinical studies.

Combined detachments in young patients should be handled along the guidelines suggested in central serous chorioretinopathy. In older patients, combined detachments without presumptive or definitive evidence of subretinal neovascularization (avascular) should be considered for photocoagulation utilizing 100 to 200-μ spot size burns of moderate intensity scattered nonconfluently throughout the retinal pigment epithelial detachment. Vascular retinal pigment epithelial detachments with overlying sensory detachments should be treated conservatively because of the extreme risk of fertilizing the existing vascular complex or unidentified neighboring vessels, until more definitive, carefully designed feasibility studies make available better treatment guidelines. If the neovascularization can be identified with reasonable clinical assurance and if it is eccentric to the fovea, argon laser photocoagulation should be considered, employing the same technique utilized in the management of subretinal neovascularization with intense, large, confluent burns of long duration to the entire vascular complex.

In summary, serous detachment of the retinal pigment epithelium may occur: (1) as an idiopathic response in young patients; (2) as a part of the central serous chorioretinopathy syndrome; (3) in association with choroidal inflammation, ischemia, necrosis, tumors, or neovascularization; and (4) as an avascular exudative manifestation of involutional macular degeneration. Differentiation between pure pigment epithelial detachments and those complicated by subpigment epithelial neovascularization (avascular vs. vascular) continues to be the principal problem in the diagnosis and treatment of these fundus disorders.

References

1. Gass, J.D.M., Norton, E.W.D., and Justice, J., Jr.: Serous detachment of the retinal pigment epithelium. *Trans Am Acad Ophthalmol Otolaryngol, 70:* 990, 1966.
2. Wessing, A.: Fluorescein Angiography of the Retina, C.V. Mosby, St. Louis, 1969.
3. Shimizu, K.: Fluorescein Microangiography of the Ocular Fundus. Igaku Shoin Ltd, Tokyo, 1973, pp. 113–135.
4. Schatz, H.: Central serous chorioretinopathy and serous detachment of the retinal pigment epithelium. *Int Ophthalmol Clin, 15:* (1): 159, 1975.
5. Robinson, P., and Gitter, K.: Multiple detachments of the retinal pigment epithelium: a stage of disciform macular degeneration. *In* Proceedings of the International Symposium on Fluorescein Angiography, ed. by K. Shimizu, Igaku Shoin Ltd, Tokyo, 1974, pp. 170–173.
6. Sarks, S.H.: New vessel formation beneath the retinal pigment epithelium in senile eyes. *Brit J Ophthalmol, 57:* 951, 1973.
7. Klein, M.L., Patz, A., et al.: The natural course of untreated serous detachments of the retinal pigment epithelium. In preparation.
8. Bird, A.: Moorfield's study on photocoagulation treatment of serous detachments of the pigment epithelium. Personal communication.

CHAPTER 15

Subretinal Neovascularization

Howard Schatz, M.D., Lawrence A. Yannuzzi, M.D., and Kurt A. Gitter, M.D.

Subretinal neovascularization is a histopathologic manifestation associated with a number of macular diseases. Approximately 5 years ago, only four or five disorders were thought to be associated with subretinal neovascularization. This list had steadily grown and, as of this date, includes at least 17 conditions. There are:

(1) Involutional macular degeneration (senile macular degeneration, exudative degeneration, maculopathy of aging)
(2) Histoplasmosis
(3) Angioid streaks
(4) Choroidal rupture
(5) Myopic maculopathy (Fuchs' spot)
(6) Heredodegenerative disease (Best's, Dominant Drusen, Peorsky's maculopathy)
(7) Optic nerve head drusen
(8) Over benign choroidal tumors
(9) Inflammation
(10) Post-photocoagulation
(11) Rubella retinopathy
(12) Retinal and pigment epithelial hamartoma
(13) Geographic helicoid peripapillary choroidopathy (GHPC)
(14) Osseous choroidoma
(15) Acute multifocal posterior placoid pigment epitheliopathy (AMPPPE)
(16) Harada's disease
(17) Idiopathic causes

The clinical recognition of subretinal neovascularization is important in terms of diagnosis, prognosis, and management of these entities. This chapter focuses on the recognition of subretinal neovascularization through clinical examination and fluorescein angiography.

For many years ophthalmic pathologists have been aware of the presence of fibrovascular membranes in various macular disorders. Their histopathologic findings were not appreciated by clinicians, even though the clinical manifestations of subretinal neovascularization could be observed quite simply with the ophthalmoscope. A major advance in clinical ophthalmology occurred when fluorescein angiography allowed the clinician to realize that certain ophthalmoscopic findings were indicative of the presence of subretinal neovascularization. The correlation of these clinical findings with known histopathologic changes has greatly facilitated the diagnosis and management of the various diseases of the macula, especially macular degeneration. The entire pathogenic cycle of subretinal neovascularization from the early vascular state to disciform scar can now be appreciated clinically. It is important to realize that subretinal neovascularization has many clinical appearances and an extremely variable pathogenic nature. Despite this variability, there are consistent and important ophthalmoscopic indicators of its presence and important fluorescein angiographic findings confirming these indicators.

Histopathology

Before a discussion of the clinical findings and fluorescein angiographic characteristics of subretinal neovascularization is presented, it is important that the histopathology of this condition is understood. Subretinal neovascularization starts as a break in Bruch's membrane, followed by a growth of capillaries from the choriocapillaris through the break toward the pigment epithelium (Fig. 15.1 and 15.2). The new vascular growth proliferates and grows under the pigment epithelium (Fig. 15.3). These new vessels often destroy the involved pigment epithelium or damage it to a degree that it cannot be discerned histopathologically (Fig. 15.4 and 15.5). The vessels may bleed and cause hemorrhagic detachment of the pigment epithelium and/or sensory retina; leakage from the vessels may result in serous detachment of the pigment epithelium and/or sensory retina. In fact, fluid pressure may develop under the sensory retina to such an extent that some fluid will penetrate the sensory retina, resulting in cystoid edema of the overlying retina. Some of the components of this fluid may become absorbed, leaving a precipitate of intraretinal and subretinal exudate.

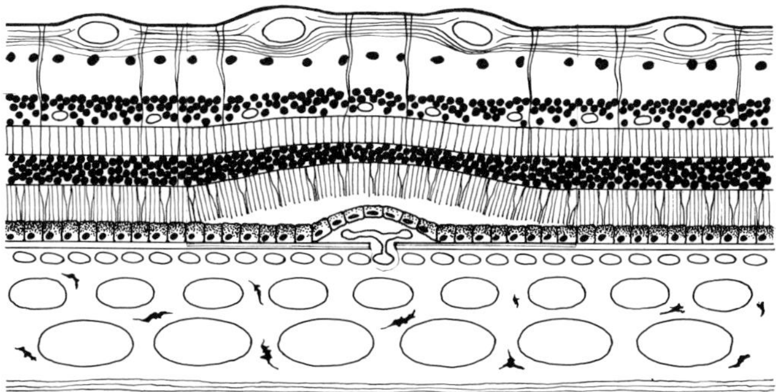

Figure 15.1. Subretinal neovascularization. This schematic illustrates a capillary tuft from the choriocapillaris proliferating under the pigment epithelium through a break in Bruch's membrane. (From H. Schatz, T. C. Burton, L. A. Yannuzzi, and M. F. Rabb: Interpretation of Fundus Fluorescein Angiography, 1978, © C. V. Mosby Co., St. Louis; reprinted with permission).

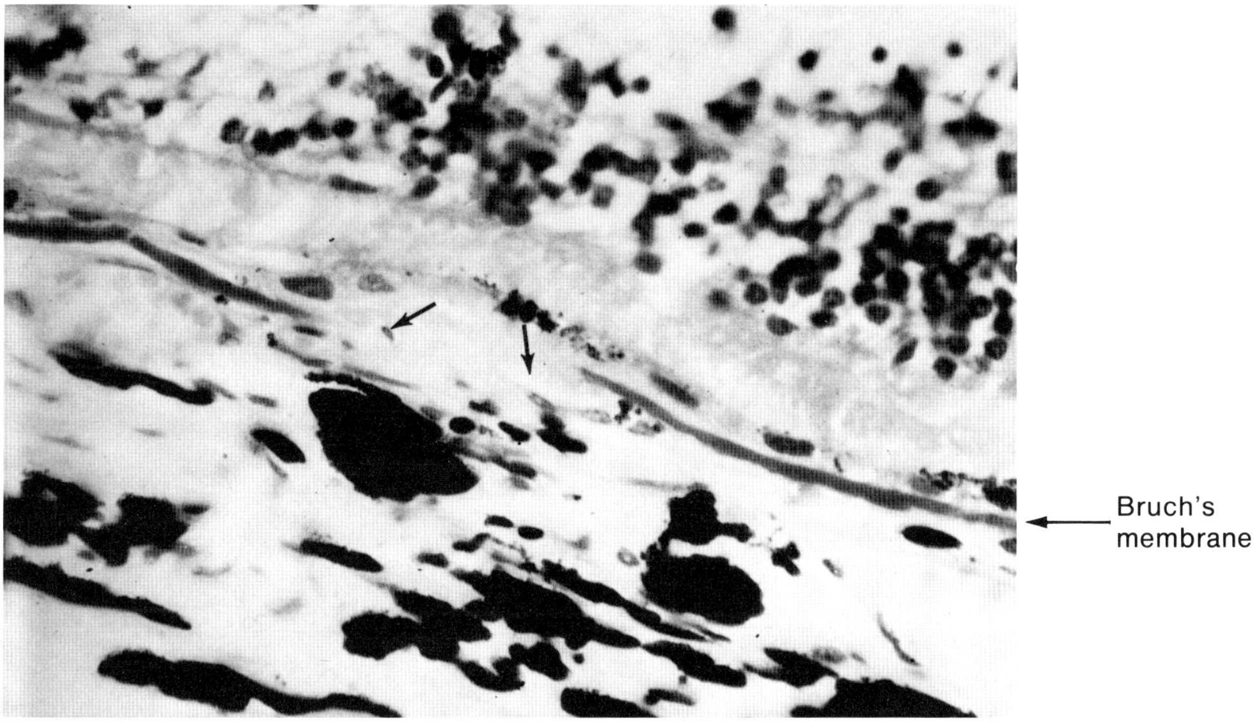

Figure 15.2. Subretinal neovascularization. Note a tuft of capillaries (*arrows*) extending through a gap in Bruch's membrane to proliferate under the pigment epithelium.

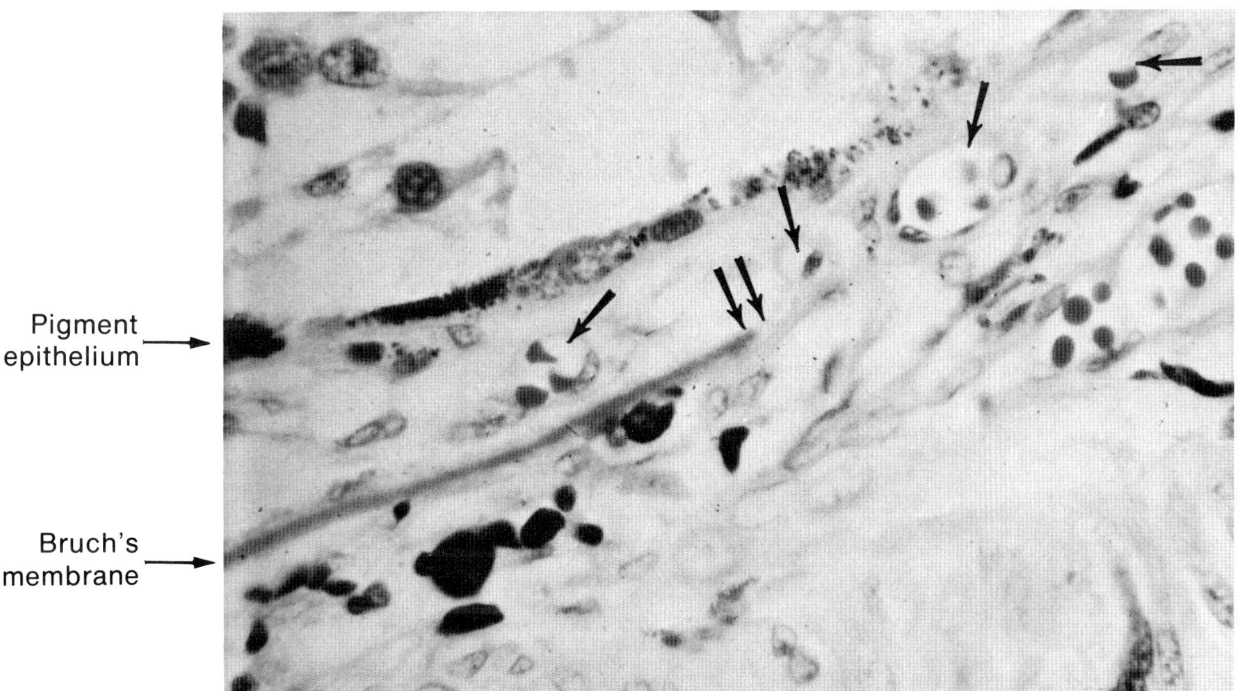

Figure 15.3. Subretinal neovascularization. Note the capillaries (*single arrows*) emanating from the choriocapillaris and growing through a break in Bruch's membrane (*double arrows*) to proliferate under the pigment epithelium.

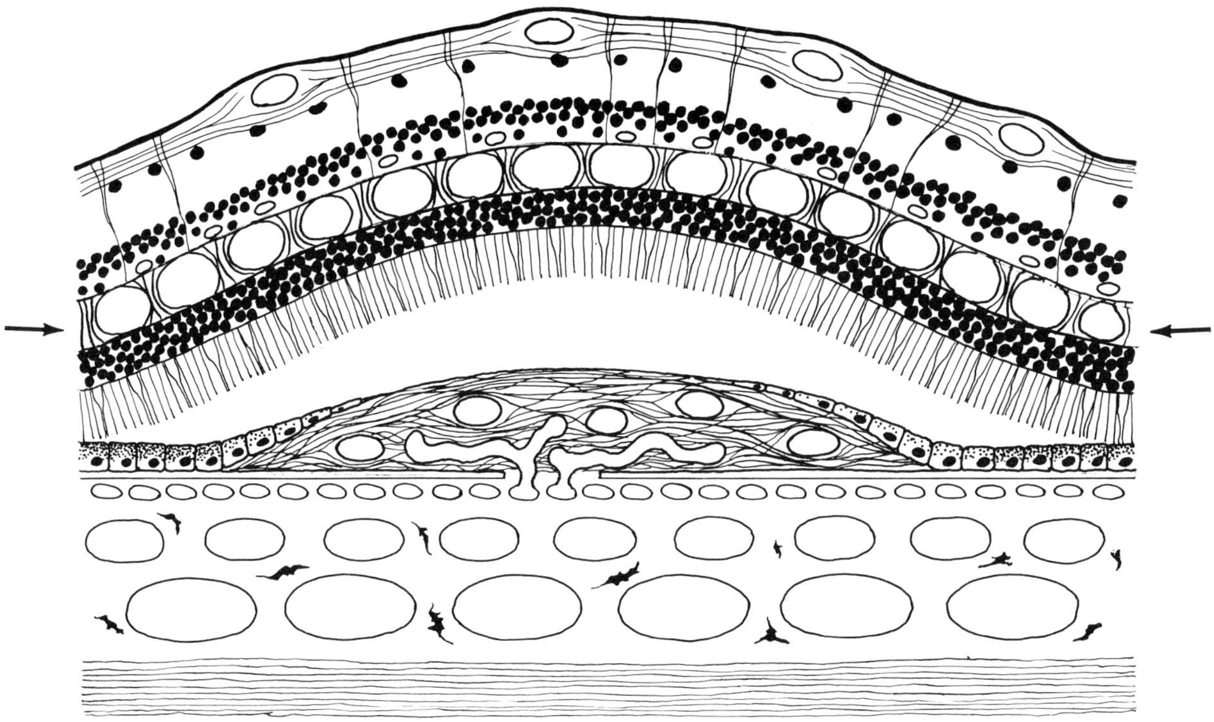

Figure 15.4. Subretinal neovascularization. In this schematic note the proliferative capillaries that have grown from the choriocapillaris through a break in Bruch's membrane. Accompanied by fibrous tissue, the fibrovascular membrane has destroyed the pigment epithelium. Detachment of the sensory retina and cystoid edema, represented as circular spaces in the outer plexiform layer of the retina (*arrows*), frequently accompany subretinal neovascularization and are also represented.

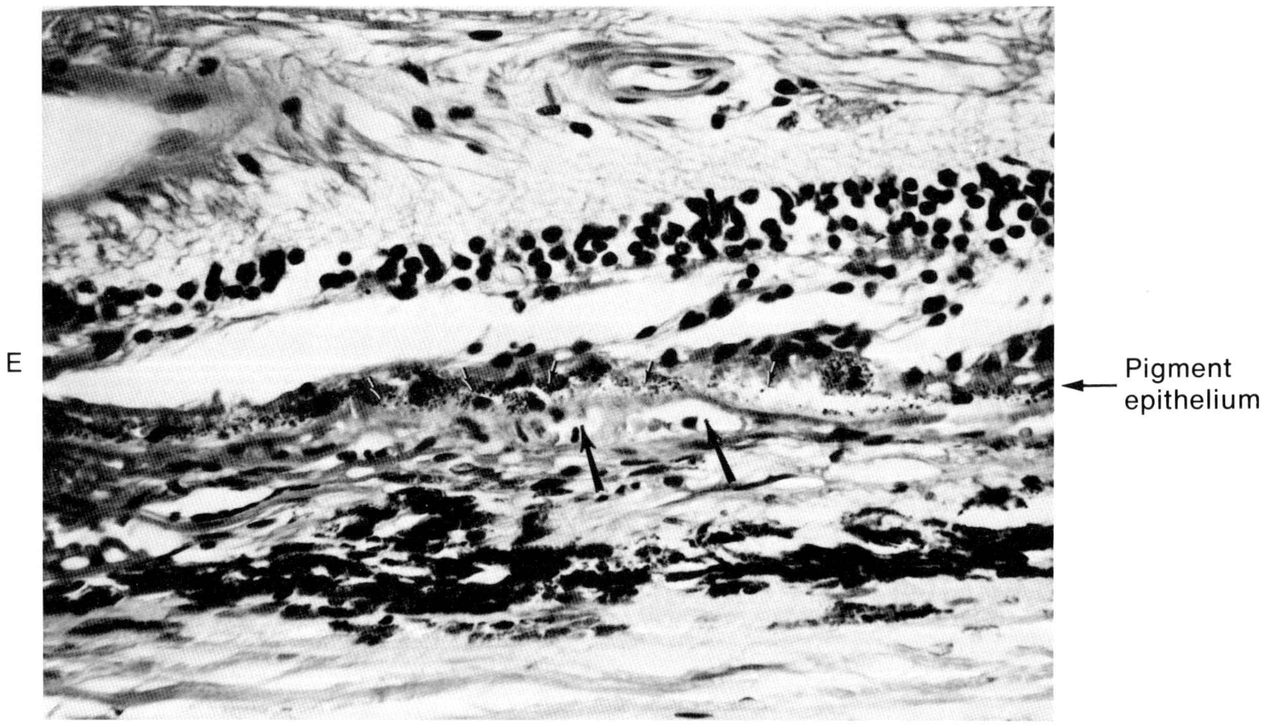

Figure 15.5. Subretinal neovascularization. Note that a tuft of capillaries (*long arrows*) proliferating from the choriocapillaris has grown through a break in Bruch's membrane, damaging the pigment epithelium (*short arrows*).

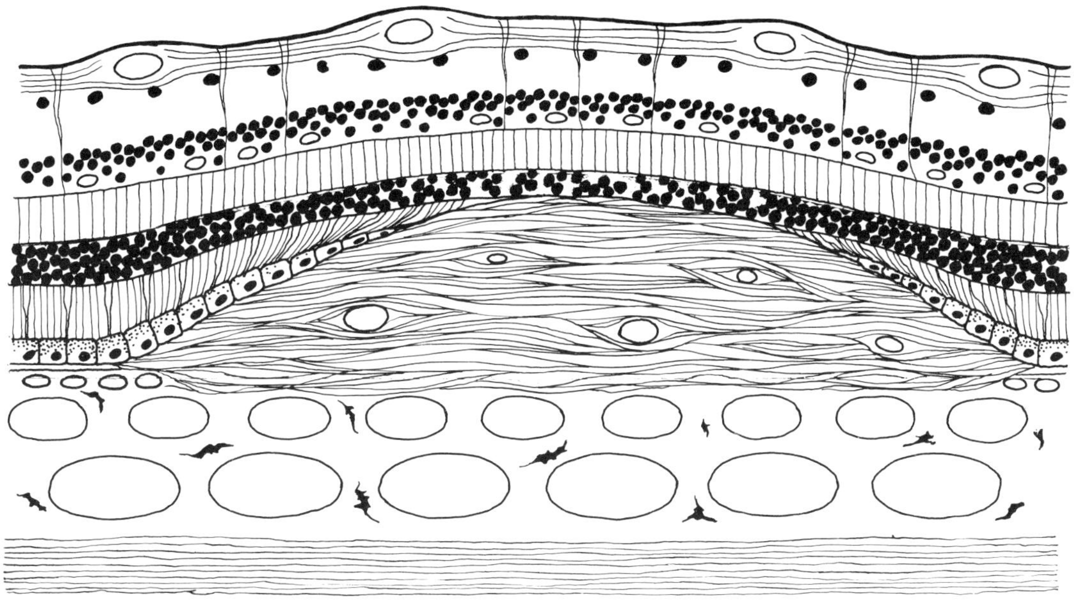

Figure 15.6. Subretinal neovascularization, disciform scar. Note on this schematic that the outer retina is destroyed by a fibrous disciform scar.

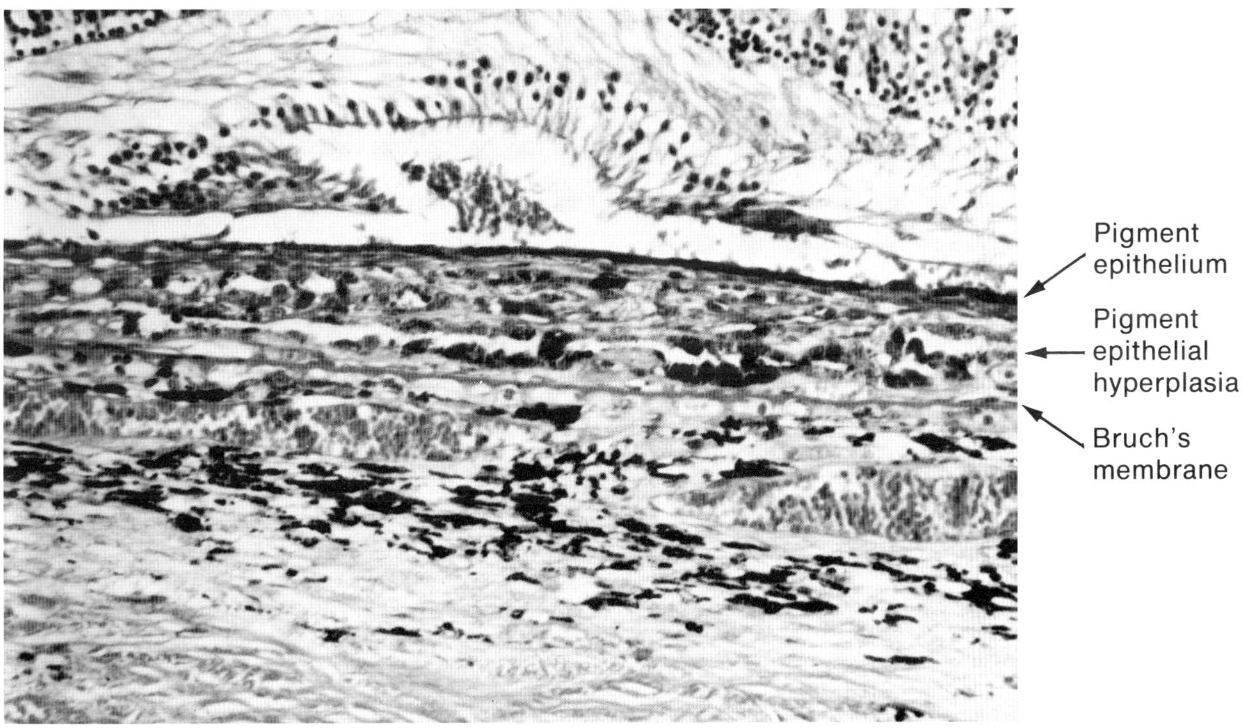

Figure 15.7. Pigment epithelium hyperplasia. Note how the pigment epithelium has undergone hyperplasia secondary to an underlying subretinal neovascular growth.

Whenever new vessels proliferate under the retina, fibrous tissue eventually accompanies them. The fibrous tissue ultimately becomes the dominant pathologic change and results in disciform scar formation which is associated with destruction of the outer layers of the retina and the pigment epithelium (Fig. 15.6). In some cases the pigment epithelium undergoes hyperplasia (Fig. 15.7).

Knowledge of the histopathogenesis of subretinal neovascularization will now enable us to develop a more thorough understanding of the clinical characteristics of this disease.

Clinical Examination

Various ophthalmoscopic methods are available for examination of the macula:

(1) Direct ophthalmoscope: yields an excellent view of the macula with good magnification, although the view is monocular, rather than stereoscopic.

(2) Indirect ophthalmoscope: yields a stereoscopic view, but the low magnification prevents detailed examination of the macula.

(3) Hruby lens with slit-lamp biomicroscope: yields a stereoscopic view, but it is minified and is not as well resolved in comparison with the alternate slit lamp-contact lens system.

(4) Diagnostic fundus contact lens with slit-lamp biomicroscope: yields a stereoscopic well illuminated view with reasonably good magnification. Also, placement of the lens on the eye is easily accomplished, facilitating a troublefree examination.

Therefore, the most accurate and exact examination of the macula yielding the most detailed results is achieved with the diagnostic fundus contact lens and the slit-lamp biomicroscope.

Clinical Findings

Various specific clinical findings from contact lens ophthalmoscopy are indicators of the presence of subretinal neovascularization. These ophthalmoscopic findings include:

(1) Dirty-gray or yellow-green discoloration
(2) Pigmented ring
(3) Hemorrhage
(4) Exudate
(5) Sensory retinal detachment with turbid fluid
(6) Pigment epithelial detachment
(7) Cystoid edema

DIRTY-GRAY OR YELLOW-GREEN DISCOLORATION

The presence of a subretinal dirty-gray or yellow-green discoloration indicates subretinal neovascularization (Fig. 15.8). The dirty-gray appearance is caused by a small amount of fibrous tissue associated with the new vessels and their blood flow. As the subretinal neovascular membrane becomes older, more fibrosis develops and the amount of vessels reduces proportionately, the dirty-gray color turns yellow-green and eventually the entire membrane becomes a hard yellow disciform scar (Fig. 15.9). The membrane at first generally has convex margins as the vascular network proliferates. When the scar ages, it tends to contract at its edges forming irregular concave margins.

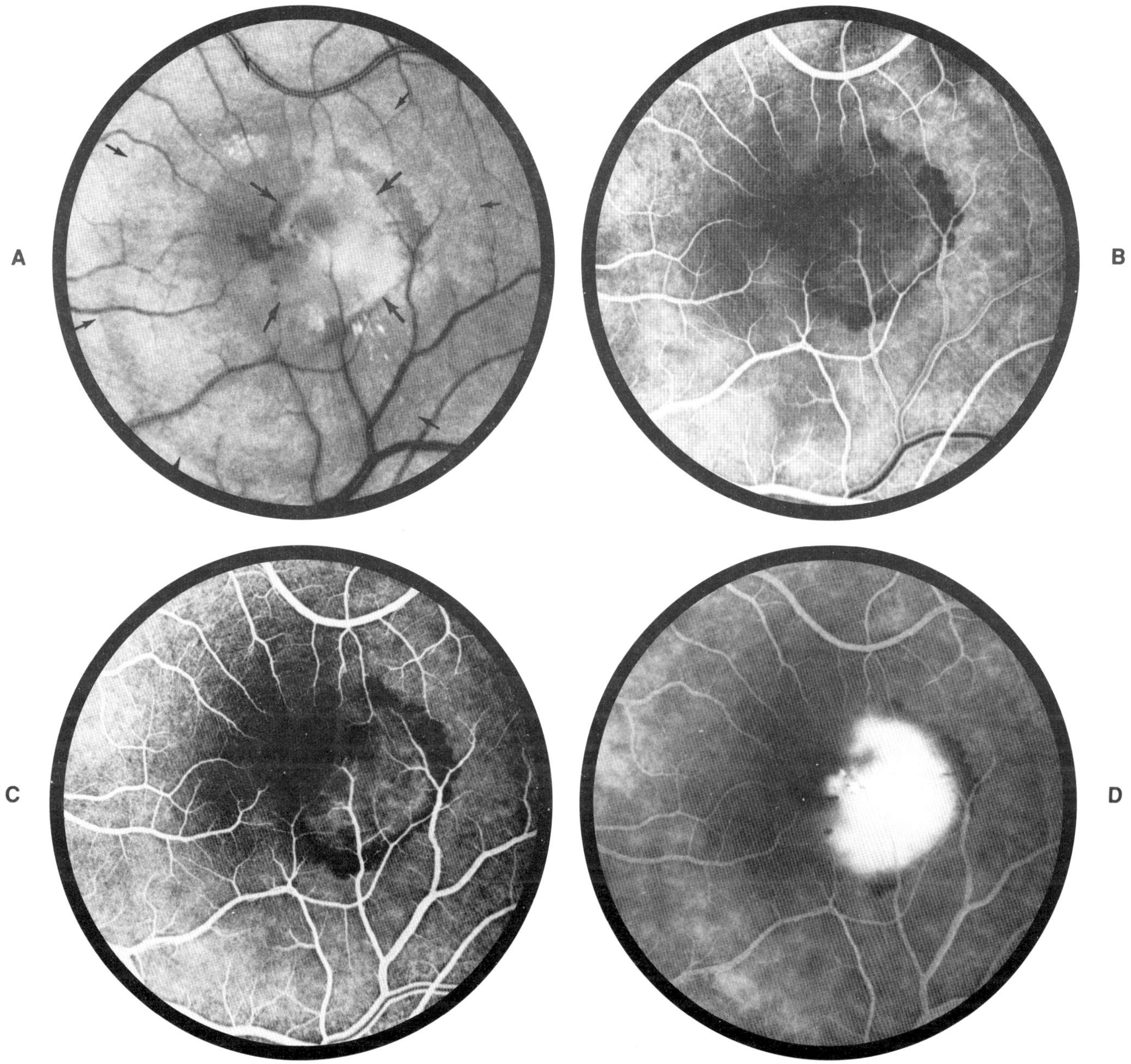

Figure 15.8. Dirty-gray discoloration indicating subretinal neovascularization. *A*, ophthalmolscopic photograph of the left macula demonstrating a dirty-gray membrane (*large arrows*) involving the central portion of the macula. Subretinal hemorrhage and exudate and a sensory retinal detachment (*small arrows*) are also apparent. *B*, arteriovenous phase angiogram showing irregular hyperfluorescence surrounded by a zone of hypofluorescence in the area corresponding to the membrane seen ophthalmoscopically. *C*, increased fluorescence in the macula is apparent a few seconds later. *D*, late phase angiogram showing marked hyperfluorescence under the detached sensory retina, as the fluorescein dye pools into the subsensory retinal space from the neovascularization.

PIGMENTED RING

Frequently, when subretinal neovascularization is present in the macula, a ring of pigment encircles the border of the dirty-gray membrane. This ring of pigment is caused either by hyperplasia of the pigment epithelium or pigment migration secondary to damage of the pigment epithelium overlying the center of the subretinal neovascular membrane. Occasionally the pigmented ring may represent subretinal hemorrhage associated with hyperplasia of the pigment epithelium (Fig. 15.10).

HEMORRHAGE

In the absence of retinal vascular disease, a trauma, or a choroidal tumor, the presence of hemorrhage in the macula (especially subretinal or subpigment epithelial hemorrhage) should be considered caused by subretinal neovascularization, unless proven otherwise. Diseases such as central serous chorioretinopathy and uncomplicated serous detachments of the pigment epithelium do not cause hemorrhage; Therefore, subretinal neovascularization must be suspected when subretinal hemorrhage is seen. From the subsensory retinal space or subpigment epithelial space, the hemorrhage may work its way up into the retina and in rare cases may break through, causing a vitreous hemorrhage. In macular pigment epithelial disease, hemorrhage (especially subretinal or subpigment epithelial) is a strong indicator of the presence of subretinal neovascularization (Fig. 15.11).

A

B

C

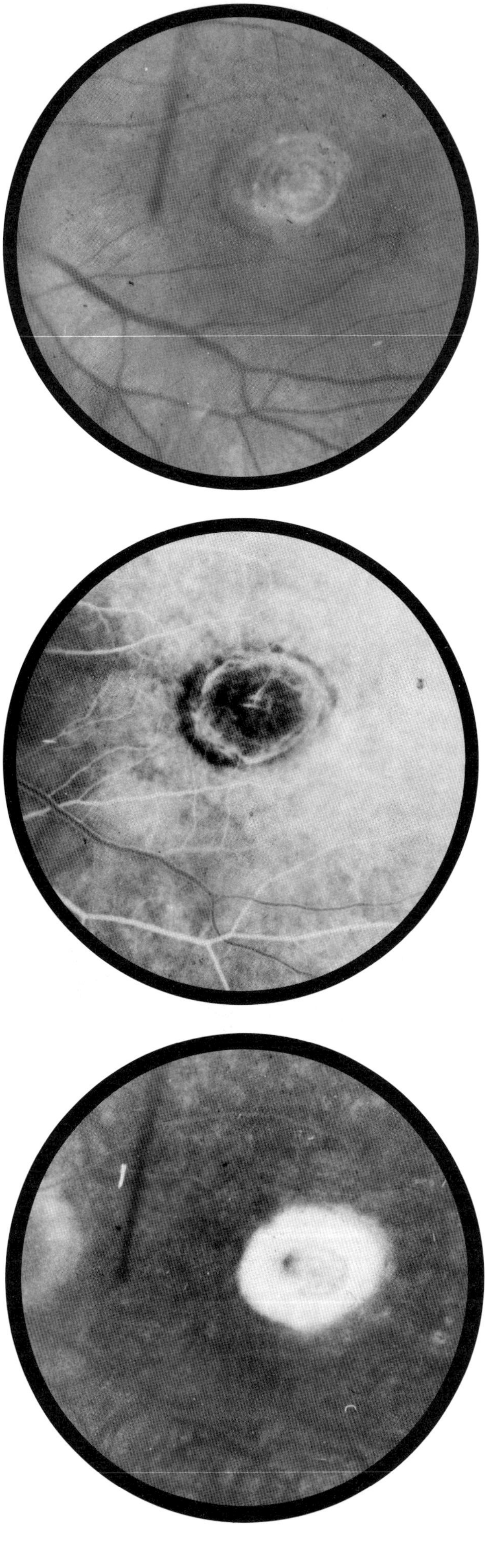

Figure 15.9. Yellowish disciform scar of macula. *A*, ophthalmoscopic photograph of left macula, showing a 1 disc-diameter sized yellowish disciform scar. *B*, arteriovenous phase angiogram showing vessels within the scar. *C*, late phase angiogram showing staining of the scar. (From Schatz, H: *Perspect Ophthalmol 1:* 59, 1977; reprinted with permission.)

Figure 15.10. A dark ring encircling subretinal neovascularization. *A*, ophthalmoscopic photograph of the macula showing a ring (*arrows*) around a dirty-gray membrane. There is also an associated detachment of the sensory retina of the macula. *B*, arteriovenous phase angiogram showing hyperfluorescence of the membrane indicating subretinal vessels. A hypofluorescent ring encircles the lesion. *C*, late phase angiogram showing staining of the lesion. In this lesion, a dark ring composed of a mixture of hemorrhage, exudate, and hyperplasia of the pigment epithelium encircles a patch of subretinal neovascularization. This is a frequent clue to the identification of subretinal neovascularization on a fluorescein angiogram.

Figure 15.11. Subretinal neovascularization with subretinal hemorrhage. *A*, ophthalmoscopic photograph of the right macula demonstrates a dirty-gray membrane (*arrows*) encircled by subretinal hemorrhage. *B*, early arteriovenous phase of the angiogram shows lacy hyperfluorescence indicating subretinal neovasculariaztion. The margins of the membrane are convex and scalloped in nature, typical of a fresh lesion. Nodular beads of hyperfluorescence are most evident at the margins of the membrane, the site of the most immature capillary buds. The subretinal hemorrhage block choroidal fluorescence, producing hypofluorescence. At one site, it even blocks part of the membrane itself (*arrow*). *C*, late angiogram shows hyperfluorescence of the lesion. The hemorrhage continues to block fluorescence.

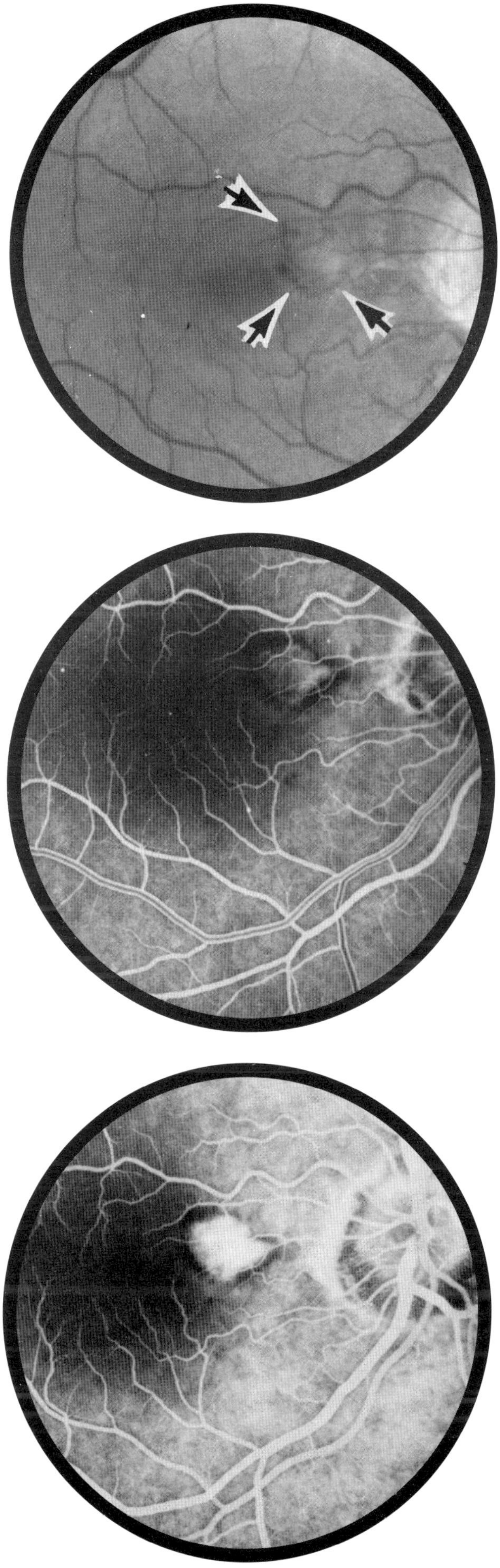

A

B

C

Figure 15.10

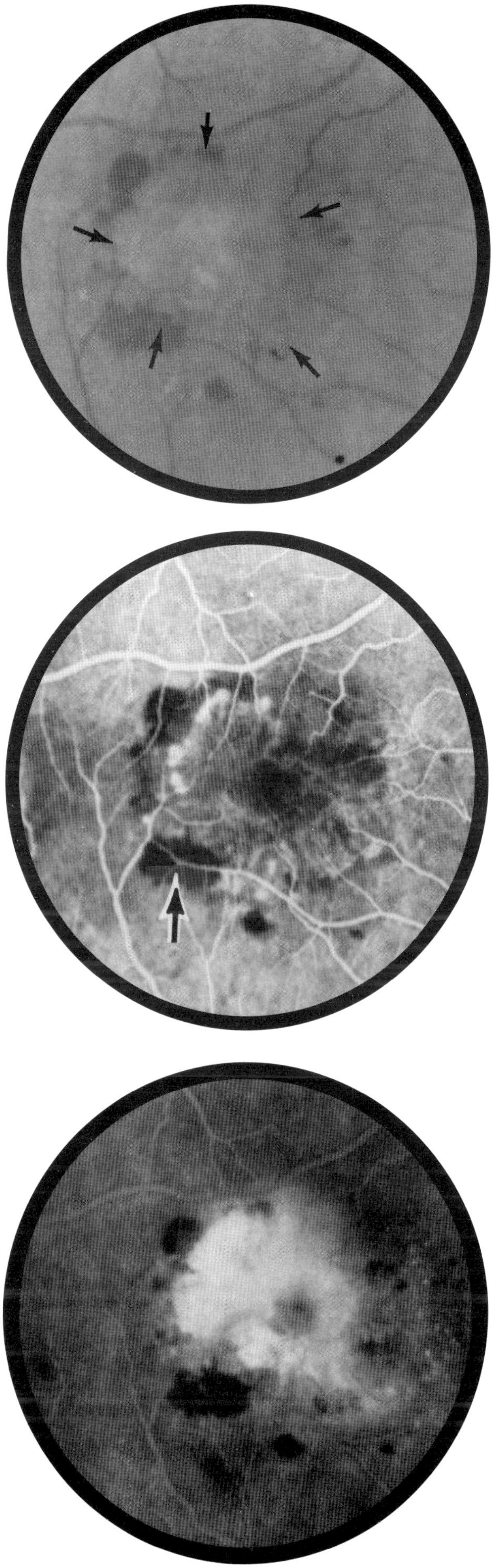

A

B

C

Figure 15.11

EXUDATE

The presence of subretinal or intraretinal exudate in any macular choroidal pigment epithelial disease is another indicator of subretinal neovascularization. Lipid deposition in the presence of normal retinal vessels indicates that subretinal neovascularization is present, unless proven otherwise (Fig. 15.12). The exudate may be scattered in an irregular pattern or may surround the area of macular detachment. The exudate may become extremely thick and form a confluent circle around the subretinal macular lesion, resulting in a circinate ring of lipid called "Coats' response" (Fig. 15.13). The importance of exudate in signaling the presence of subretinal neovascularization is especially apparent in very subtle macular exudative disease. Occasionally, all that may be seen in such cases is a miniscule amount of exudate. However, upon careful slit-lamp and contact lens examination, other findings associated with subretinal neovascularization may be seen. Even the smallest amount of intraretinal or subretinal exudate should alert the clinician to the presence of subretinal neovascularization.

A

B

C

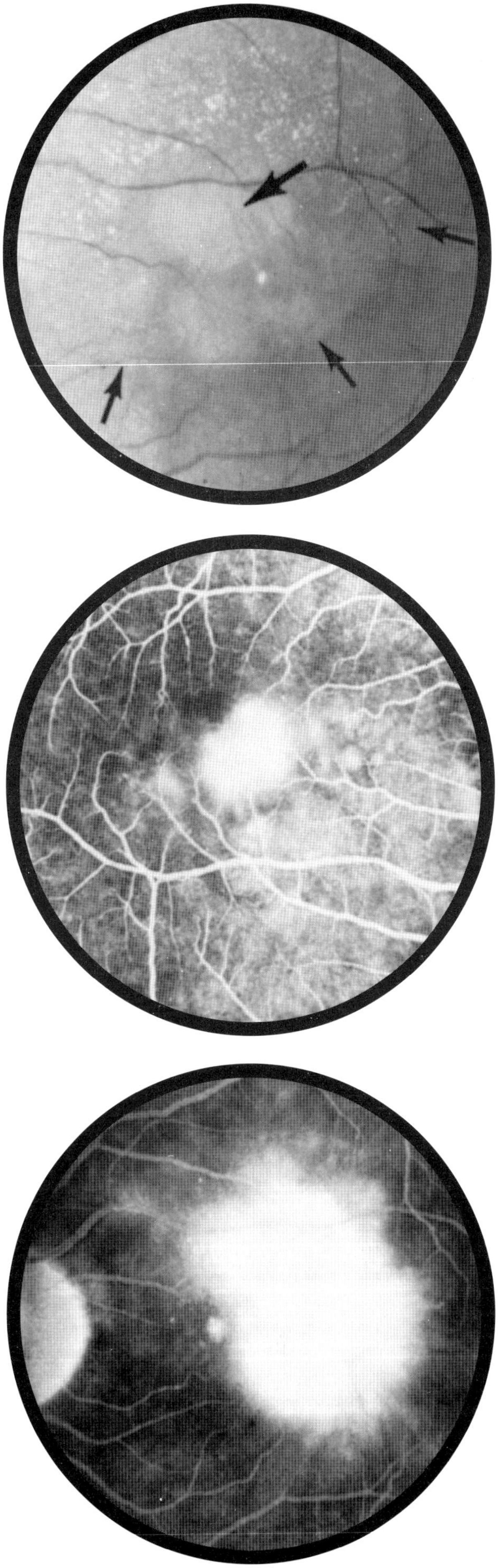

Figure 15.12. Subretinal neovascularization with lipid deposition. *A*, ophthalmoscopic photograph of macula shows a detachment of the superior portion of the macula (*small arrows*). There is a dirty-gray membrane just above and nasal to the fovea (*large arrow*) with lipid deposition scattered throughout the area. *B*, arteriovenous phase angiogram showing marked hyperfluorescence of the membrane. *C*, late phase angiogram showing marked hyperfluorescence, as the dye extends under the sensory retinal detachment.

A

B

C

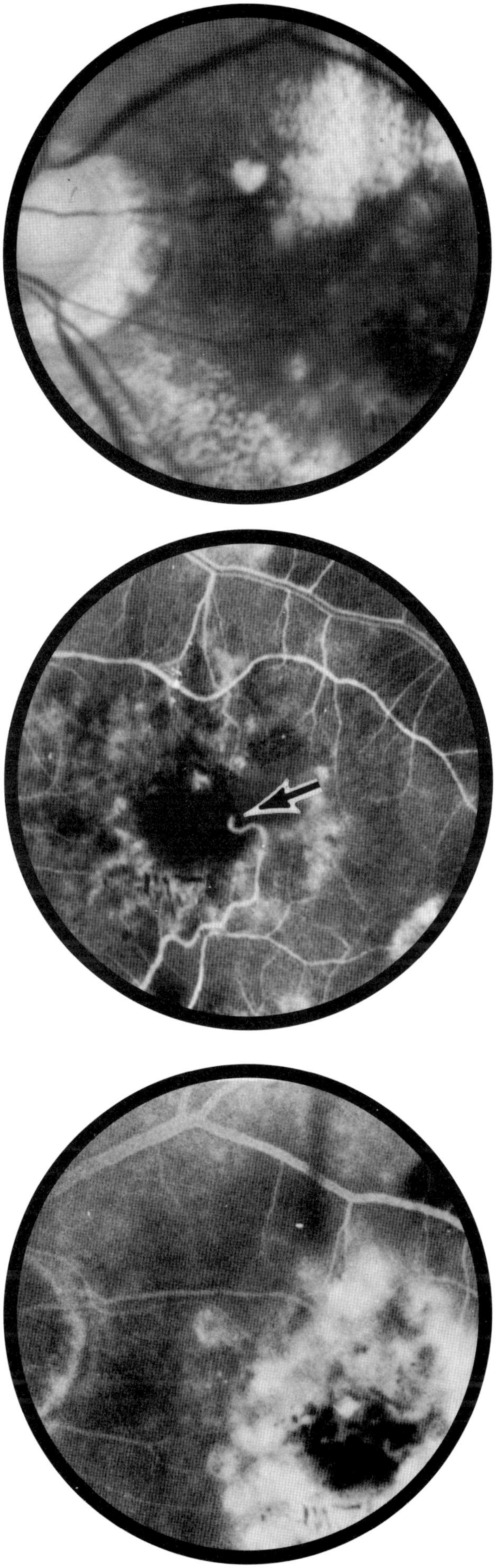

Figure 15.13. Coats' response with subretinal neovascularization. *A*, ophthalmoscopic photograph of macula demonstrates a thick ring of exudate encircling the macula. *B*, arteriovenous phase angiogram showing irregular hyperfluorescence of the central macular lesion. A chorioretinal anastomotic channel is seen emptying blood from the subretinal lesion (*arrow*). *C*, late phase angiogram showing marked hyperfluorescence of the lesion and fluorescence of the fluid under the detached sensory retina. The exudate itself appears to block fluorescence throughout the angiogram. This patient had a massive disciform response which resulted in a large sensory detachment and a considerable amount of hard exudate deposited in the area.

SENSORY RETINAL DETACHMENT WITH TURBID FLUID

Although there are many causes of sensory retinal detachment in the macula, including various pigment epithelial diseases, choroidal tumors, and even retinal vascular diseases, the presence of subretinal neovascularization should be considered in the differential diagnosis. When the fluid under the sensory retina is turbid, one must strongly suspect the presence of new subretinal vessels (Fig. 15.14). The subretinal fluid appears turbid due to a large concentration of protein, fibrin, exudate, and, in some cases, small amounts of blood; all are products of abnormal leaking subretinal vessels. In central serous chorioretinopathy, in which there is usually a single pigment epithelial leak with no subretinal vessels, the fluid is usually clear. An exception to this rule is the rare condition, bullous sensory retinal detachment associated with multiple pigment epithelial detachment. This is probably a variant of central serous chorioretinopathy with turbid subretinal fluid and is not associated with subretinal neovascularization.

PIGMENT EPITHELIAL DETACHMENT

Although there are several causes of pigment epithelial detachment, a common one, especially in patients over 50 years of age, is subretinal neovascularization. Pigment epithelial detachment can occur primarily in or associated with central serous chorioretinopathy, in choroidal inflammatory or ischemic disease, or over choroidal tumors. It may also be associated with a confluence of drusen. However, when a pigment epithelial detachment is present, especially in a patient who has clinical signs of other diseases that cause subretinal neovascularization such as exudative maculopathy, histoplasmosis, and angioid streaks, subretinal neovascularization should be suspected. When the fluid under the pigment epithelial detachment is turbid, the degree of suspicion that subretinal neovascularization is present should be even greater (Fig. 15.14). If the detached pigment epithelium is atrophic from stretching and chronic elevation, underlying subretinal neovascularization can more readily be identified on fluorescein angiography (Fig. 15.15).

A

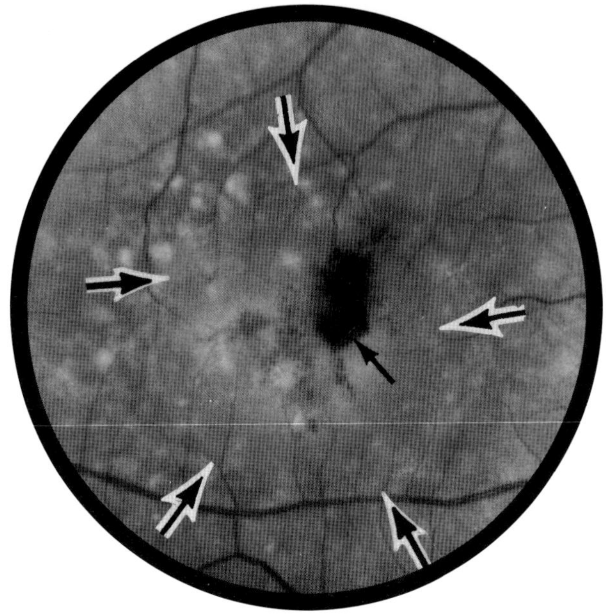

B

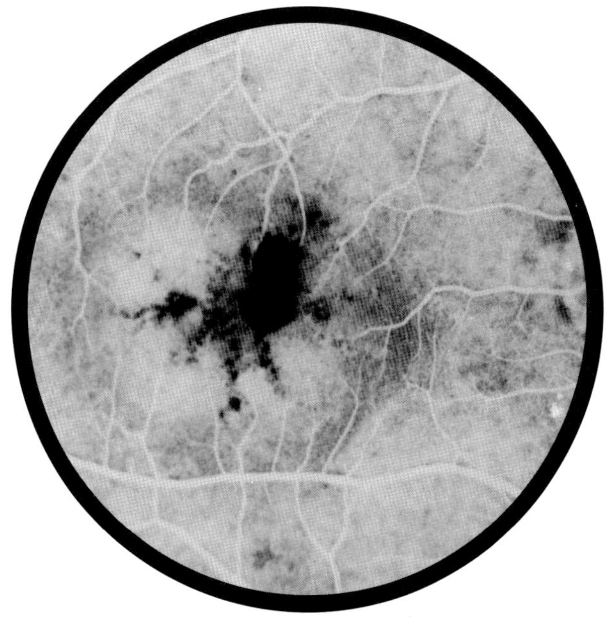

C

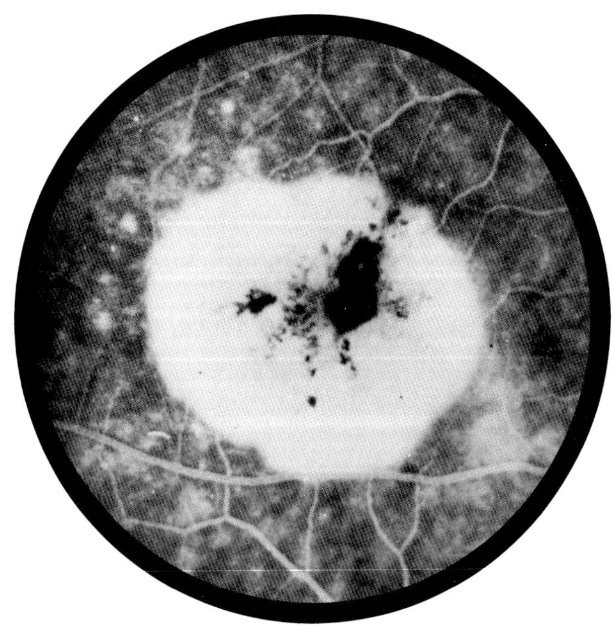

Figure 15.14. Turbid pigment epithelial detachment indicating subretinal neovascularization. *A*, ophthalmoscopic photograph of the macula showing a detachment of the pigment epithelium with turbid fluid (*black and white arrows*). In addition to pigment, there is a spot of hemorrhage on the surface of the detachment (*small black arrow*). *B*, early arteriovenous phase angiogram showing diffuse hyperfluorescence of the pigment epithelial detachment. The pigment and hemorrhage block fluorescence. *C*, late phase angiogram showing marked hyperfluorescence of the entire fluid space under the detachment. This patient had a turbid pigment epithelial detachment and hemorrhage, indicating that subretinal neovascularization is present, even though the fluorescein angiogram could not definitively identify the vascular complexes.

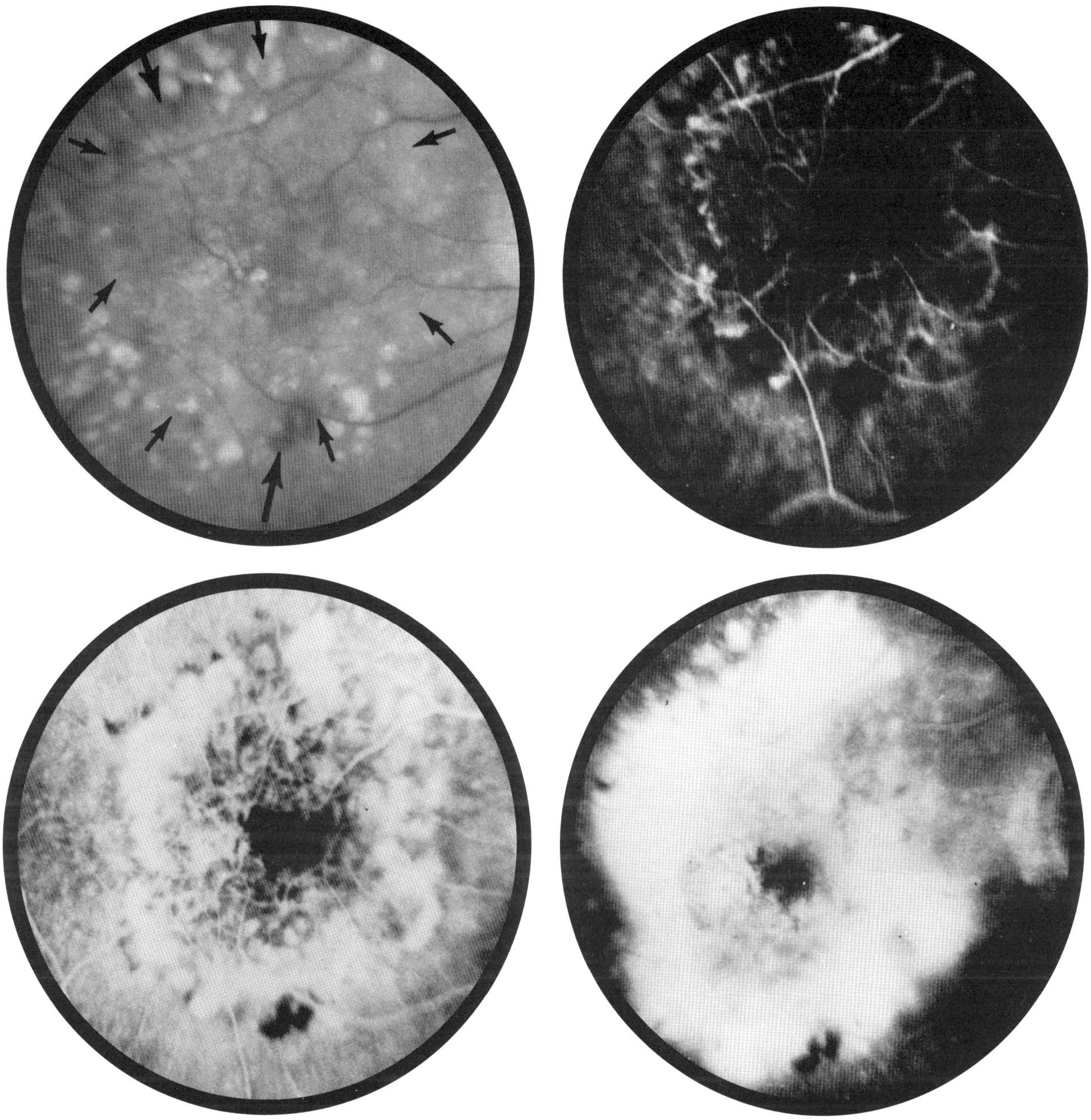

Figure 15.15. Atrophic pigment epithelial detachment with underlying subretinal neovascularization. *A*, ophthalmoscopic photograph of the macula. Note the large irregular pigment epithelial detachment (*small arrows*) associated with a turbid subpigment epithelial fluid and a few areas of hemorrhage (*large arrows*). There is also a larger overlying sensory retinal detachment and multiple drusen scattered elsewhere in the posterior pole. *B*, early venous phase angiogram showing a widespread lacy hyperfluorescence beneath the pigment epithelial detachment. The full extent of the vascular network is visible because the pigment epithelium is atrophied from stretching and chronic detachment. *C*, late venous phase angiogram. The immature capillaries show nodular leakage and the margins of the detachment are beaded or scalloped in nature. These findings are characteristic of neovascularization. *D*, late phase angiogram in which dye leakage from the neovascularization pools beneath the detached pigment epithelium and sensory retina.

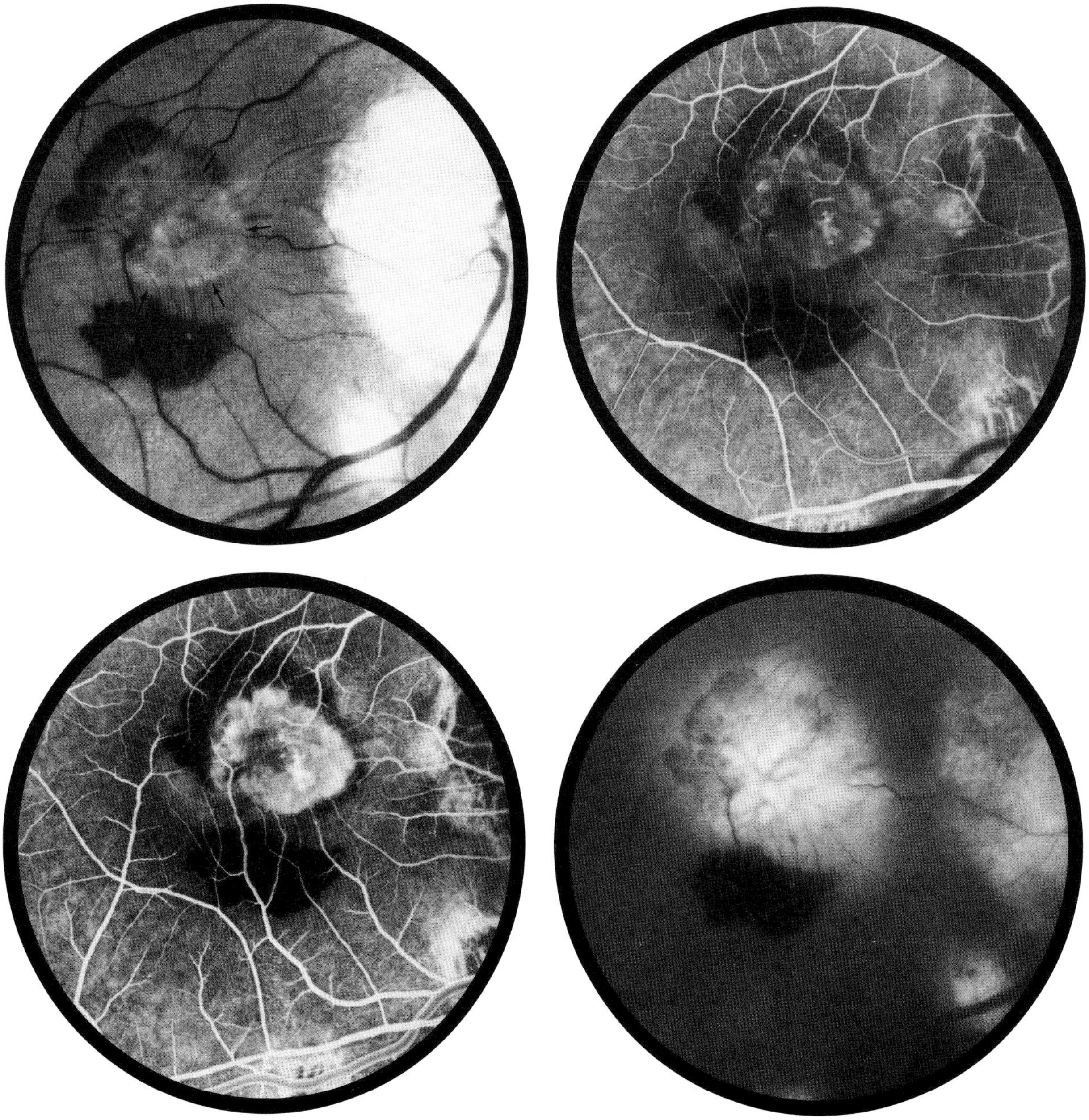

Figure 15.16. Cystoid edema secondary to subretinal neovascularization. *A*, ophthalmoscopic photograph of macula showing a dirty-gray membrane in the macula (*arrows*), with subretinal hemorrhage. Slit-lamp biomicroscopy revealed cystoid edema within a detached sensory retina. *B*, arterial phase angiogram showing lacy hyperfluorescence of the membrane. *C*, arteriovenous phase angiogram showing increased fluorescence of the membrane. Hemorrhage is blocking fluorescence. *D*, late phase angiogram showing marked cystoid edema in the overlying detached sensory retina. This patient not only had cystoid edema and subretinal hemorrhage, but also a turbid sensory retinal detachment, all secondary to subretinal neovascularization in the macula.

CYSTOID EDEMA

Many retinal vascular diseases as well as choroidal and vitreous diseases may result in cystoid edema. Another major cause of cystoid edema is intraocular inflammation. When cystoid edema is present in the macula and there is no retinal vascular disease and/or intraocular inflammation, subretinal neovascularization should be suspected. Cystoid edema almost always accompanies sensory retinal detachment overlying the subretinal neovascularization (Fig. 15.16). This is most evident by careful examination with the Goldmann lens and slit-lamp biomicroscopy. It is difficult to see on the angiogram because of the absence of contrast produced by the subretinal and intraretinal hyperfluorescence.

These seven clinical findings:

(1) dirty-grey or yellow-green subretinal discoloration,
(2) pigmented ring,
(3) hemorrhage,
(4) exudate,
(5) sensory retinal detachment with turbid fluid,
(6) pigment epithelial detachment, and
(7) cystoid edema,

are changes occurring as a result of subretinal neovascularization. The optimum examination method for finding these changes is carried out with slit-lamp and diagnostic fundus contact lens. When one or more of these changes is found, the presence of a subretinal new vessel membrane ought to be strongly suspected. The differential diagnosis should, therefore, include the many macular diseases that are associated with subretinal neovascularization.

Fluorescein Angiographic Characteristics

For many years histopathologists have known that disciform macular scars contained vessels. However, the fluorescein angiogram and sophisticated developments in its interpretation have provided the clinician with a diagnostic tool which more vividly and accurately delineates the full extent and character of the vascular complexes. In the following section the fluorescein angiographic findings of subretinal neovascularization will be discussed.

Fluorescein angiography has been very effective in teaching ophthalmologists the histopathologic meaning of various clinical changes. Therefore, since the fluorescein angiogram has become more readily predictable, the ophthalmoscopic examination is often sufficient for a proper diagnosis. In many cases it is possible to make a diagnosis of subretinal neovascularization with ophthalmoscopic examination alone. However, the fluorescein angiogram provides the clinician with a more exact location of subretinal neovascularization. This is essential to determine if argon laser photocoagulation can be of potential benefit in the obliteration of the neovascularization. The fluorescein angiogram, therefore, is necessary as a guide for laser treatment.

The angiogram can be divided into the early (vascular) phase and the later (extravascular) phase. A few angiographic abnormalities help indicate the presence of subretinal neovascularization. The angiographic findings are as follows:

(1) Vascular phase: early, lacy, nodular, irregular hyperfluorescence
(2) Extravascular phase: late hyperfluorescence (leak)
  (a) Dense staining (of fibrovascular membrane)
  (b) Fuzzy fluorescence (of fluid under detached sensory retina)
  (c) Cystoid edema (of overlying sensory retina)
(3) Hot spot in pigment epithelial detachment
(4) Meniscus of hemorrhage in pigment epithelial detachment
(5) Hypofluorescence (blockage due to hemorrhage or pigment ring surrounding vessel complex)

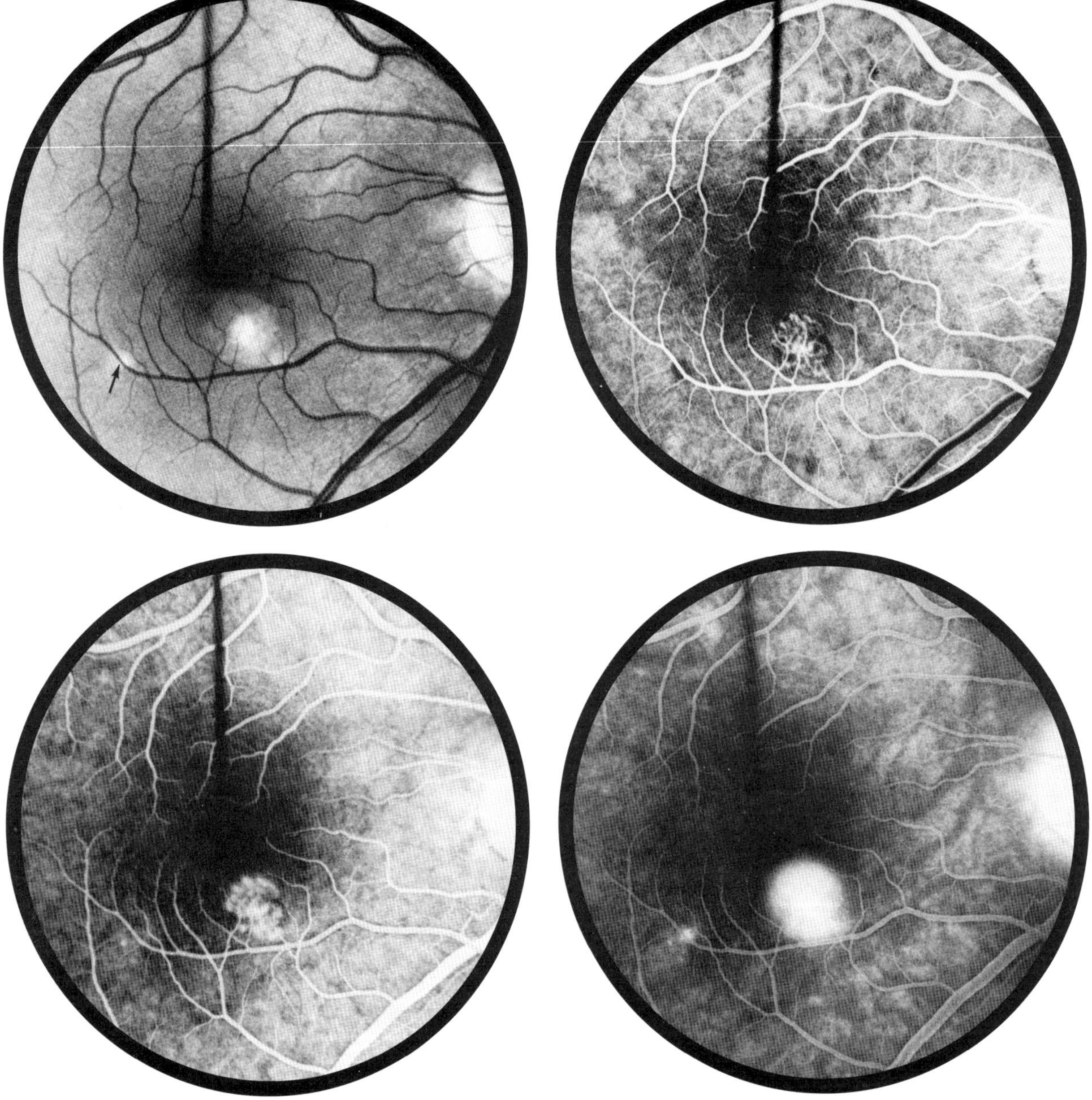

Figure 15.17. Lacy, early hyperfluorescence indicating subretinal neovascularization. *A*, ophthalmoscopic photograph of the macula showing a pale membrane under the retina, just inferior to the fovea. A small atrophic scar is also present in the inferior-temporal macula (*arrow*). *B*, arteriovenous phase angiogram showing lacy hyperfluorescence of the membrane, indicating subretinal neovascularization. *C*, venous phase angiogram showing leakage from the vessels. *D*, late phase angiogram showing hyperfluorescence under the detached sensory retina overlying the subretinal neovascularization. There is also late hyperfluorescence or staining of the small scar in the inferior-temporal macula. The early lacy hyperfluorescence indicated the presence of subretinal neovascularization in this patient with presumed ocular histoplasmosis.

VASCULAR PHASE: EARLY, LACY, NODULAR, IRREGULAR HYPERFLUORESCENCE

When subretinal neovascularization is present, the early (vascular) phase of the angiogram will show lacy subretinal hyperfluorescence. The lacy effect is caused by fluorescence of the capillaries of the neovascular membrane (Fig. 15.17). In some cases, small capillaries cannot be seen as vascular channels, especially when they are under an intact and well pigmented pigment epithelium. In these cases the presence of vessels is indicated by scalloped and/or irregular edges of the vascular membrane (Fig. 15.18). The vessels begin to hyperfluoresce in an intense and irregular fashion. The newer less mature vessels tend to leak more than the older growth and, therefore, fluoresce to a greater extent.

A single spot of hyperfluorescence, although often seen in central serous chorioretinopathy may be indicative of a small capillary tuft breaking through Bruch's membrane. However, without other findings it may be difficult or impossible to determine if the small spot of hyperfluorescence is a bud of subretinal neovascularization or a pigment epithelial leak characteristic of central serous chorioretinopathy. In other words, a small spot of hyperfluorescence should be highly suspect when the diagnosis of central serous chorioretinopathy is not obvious (Fig. 15.19) or in any macular disease associated with subretinal neovascularization.

A

B

C

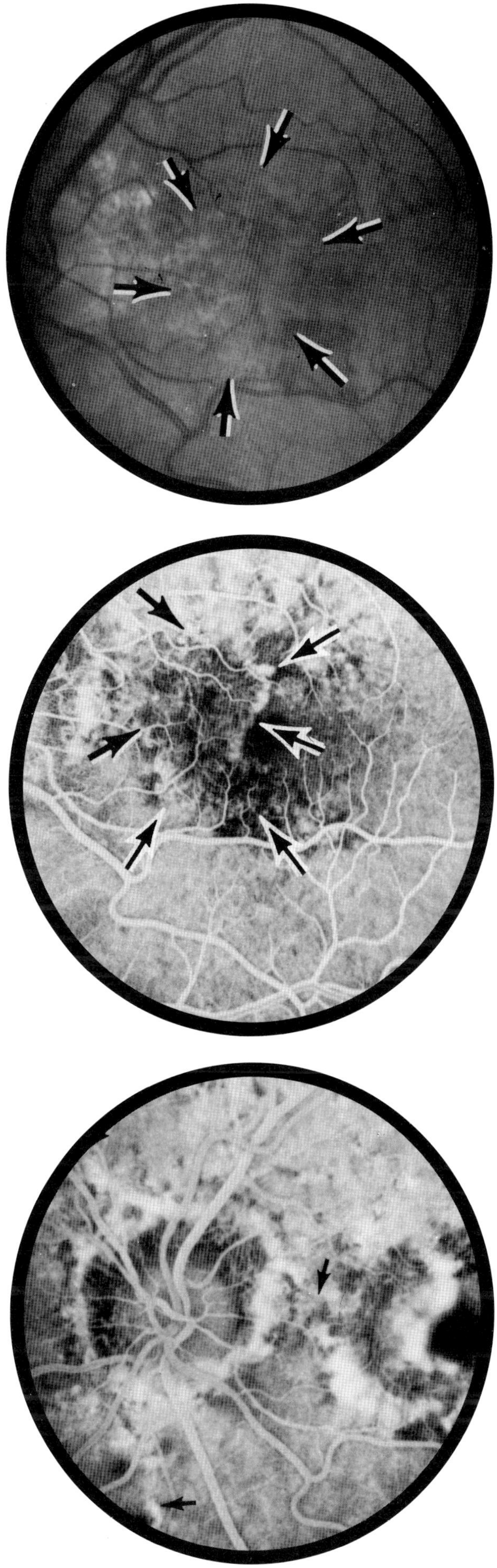

Figure 15.18. Nodular early hyperfluorescence indicating subretinal neovascularization. *A*, ophthalmoscopic photograph of the left macula showing some subretinal hemorrhage below the fovea and a dirty-gray membrane (*arrows*) in the papillomacular bundle. *B*, arteriovenous phase angiogram showing nodular hyperfluorescence immediately nasal to the fovea (*arrows*). *C*, late phase angiogram showing leakage from the subretinal neovascularization in the papillomacular bundle. Angioid streaks can be seen emanating from the optic nerve head (*arrows*). Scalloped or irregular early hyperfluorescence clearly indicated that this patient had subretinal neovascularization which was associated with angioid streaks.

A

B

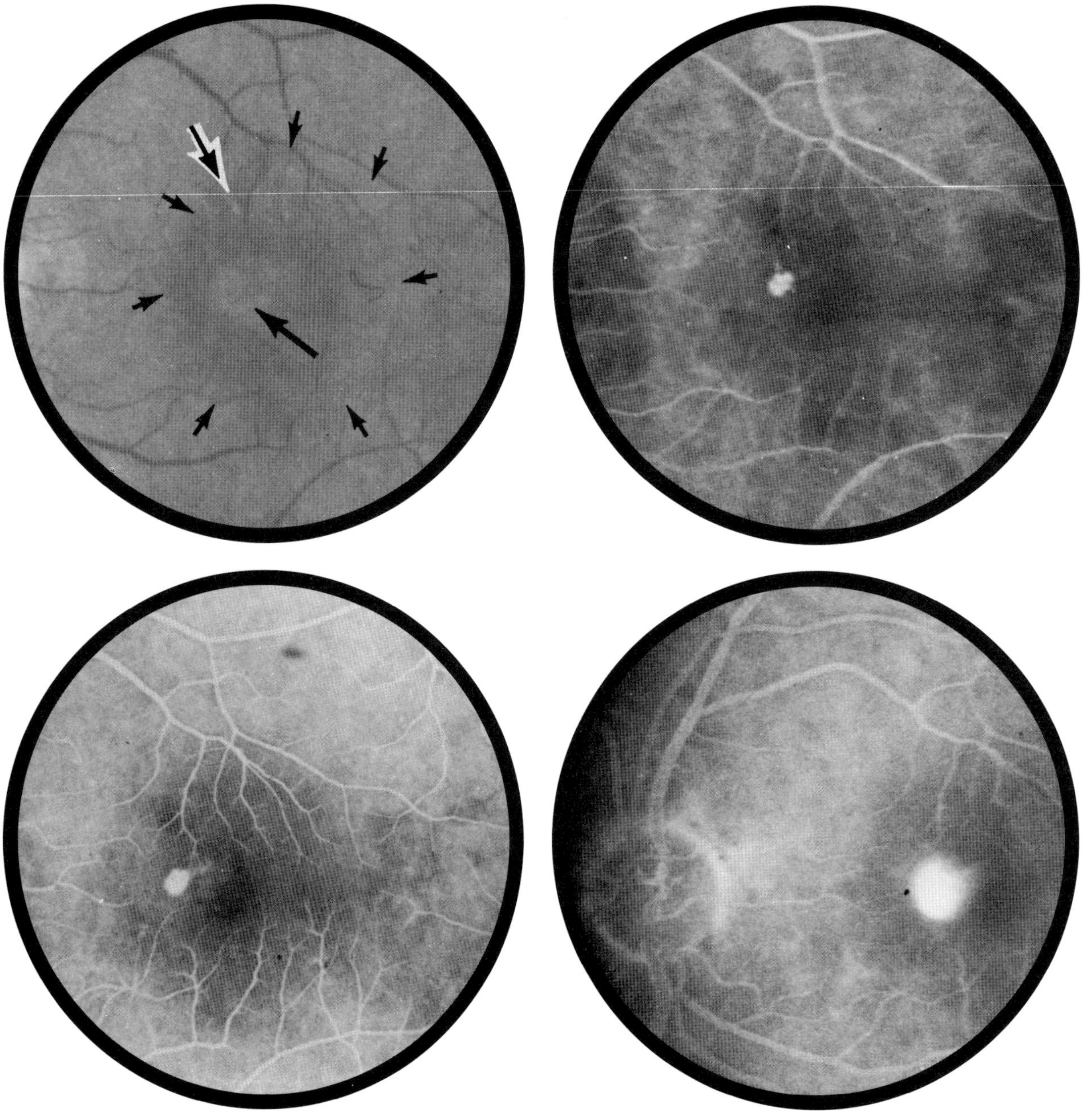

C

D

Figure 15.19. A small spot of hyperfluorescence due to a small tuft of subretinal neovascularization. *A*, ophthalmoscopic photograph of the macula showing a turbid sensory detachment in the center of the macula (*small black arrows*), overlying a grayish subretinal disturbance (*large black arrow*). There is a small amount of exudate just above the fovea (*black and white arrow*). *B*, arteriovenous phase angiogram showing a small, slightly nodular spot of hyperfluorescence. *C*, venous phase angiogram showing that the spot has increased in fluorescence. *D*, in the late phase angiogram, fluorescein has leaked under the detached sensory retina. Although this case could possibly be interpreted as central serous chorioretinopathy, there are several findings which are also indicative of subretinal neovascularization: the turbid detachment, a slightly gray color to the lesion, and the presence of exudate noted in ophthalmoscopic examination. Nodular irregular fluorescence on the angiogram also indicates subretinal vessels.

EXTRAVASCULAR PHASE: LATE HYPERFLUORESCENCE (LEAK)

The late phase of the angiogram represents the extravascular phase. When fluorescence is present in the late angiogram, leakage of fluorescein has occurred. There are three causes of late hyperfluorescence: (a) staining of the fibrous tissue of the subretinal neovascular membrane; (b) pooling in the fluid under the detached pigment epithelium and/or sensory retina; (c) fluorescence of the cystoid spaces in the overlying sensory retina.

Since subretinal noevascularization has fibrous tissue associated with it, and because the vessels within the subretinal neovascular membrane leak, dense fluorescein staining of the fibrous tissue occurs. Even when very little fluid is present, dense hyperfluorescent staining of the subretinal neovascular membrane occurs because of absorption of fluorescein by the fibrous tissue component and/or fibrous scar (Fig. 15.10).

Fuzzy late hyperfluorescence, on the other hand, indicates leakage from the vessels into a fluid space which most often suggests that there is a sensory retinal detachment (Figs. 15.12 and 15.17). Often the leakage is great enough to completely fill the subsensory retinal space with fluorescein. The fluorescent edges of the subsensory retinal fluid are feathered or fuzzy and somewhat irregular and not as clearly demarcated as those of a pigment epithelial detachment (Fig. 15.20).

Finally, the leakage from the new vessels is usually great enough to cause fluorescence of the cystoid edema in the overlying sensory retina, as well as fluorescence under the retina. Occasionally, the retinal vessels of the overlying sensory retinal detachment are abnormal and leak, adding to the cystoid edema fluid. However, the fluid comprising the cystoid macular edema generally originates from the subretinal tissue (Fig. 15.16). Because of an absence of an intervening zone of hypofluorescence, there is very little contrast between the hyperfluorescence in the subretinal space and the hyperfluorescence produced by the cystoid edema. As a result, the cystoid edema is often very difficult to demonstrate on the fluorescein angiogram in patients with sensory detachments and subretinal neovascularization.

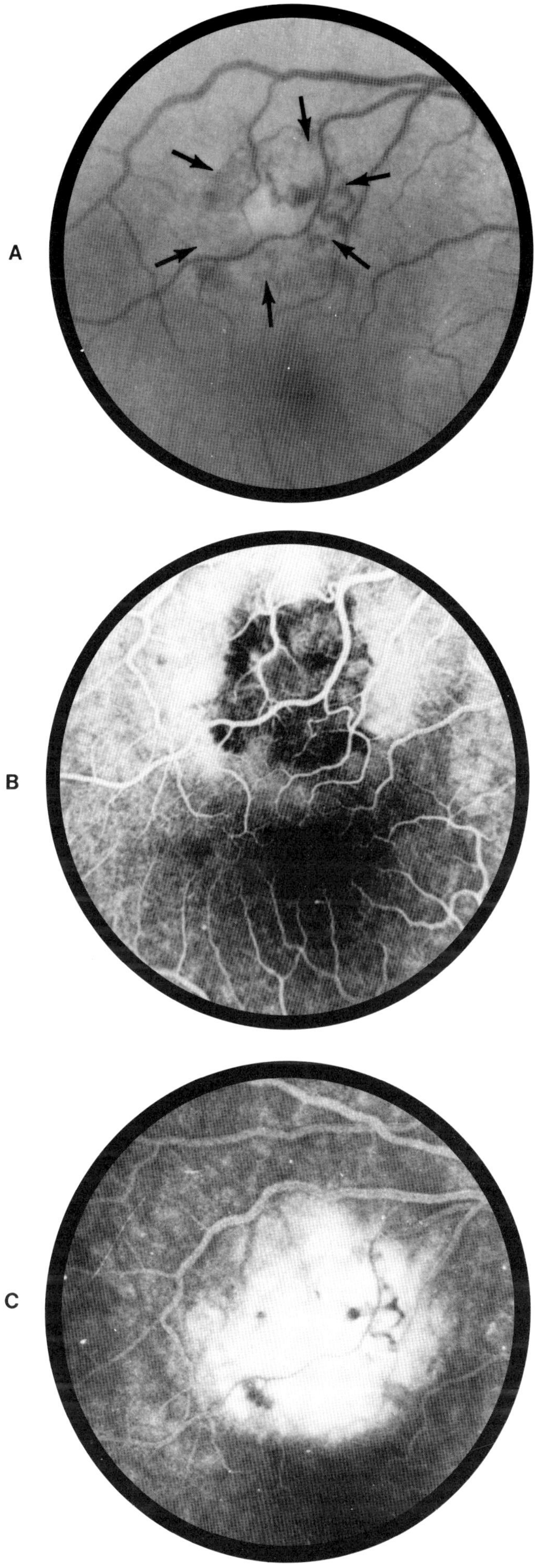

Figure 15.20. Late hyperfluorescence with irregular fuzzy edges, indicating sensory retinal detachment associated with subretinal neovascularization. *A*, ophthalmoscopic photograph of the right macula showing a sensory retinal detachment with a discolored membrane above the fovea (*arrows*) and associated subretinal hemorrhage. *B*, arteriovenous phase angiogram showing irregular hyperfluorescence of the lesion, surrounded by a dark, hypofluorescent zone. *C*, late phase angiogram showing fuzzy or irregular margins of hyperfluorescence under the detached sensory retina.

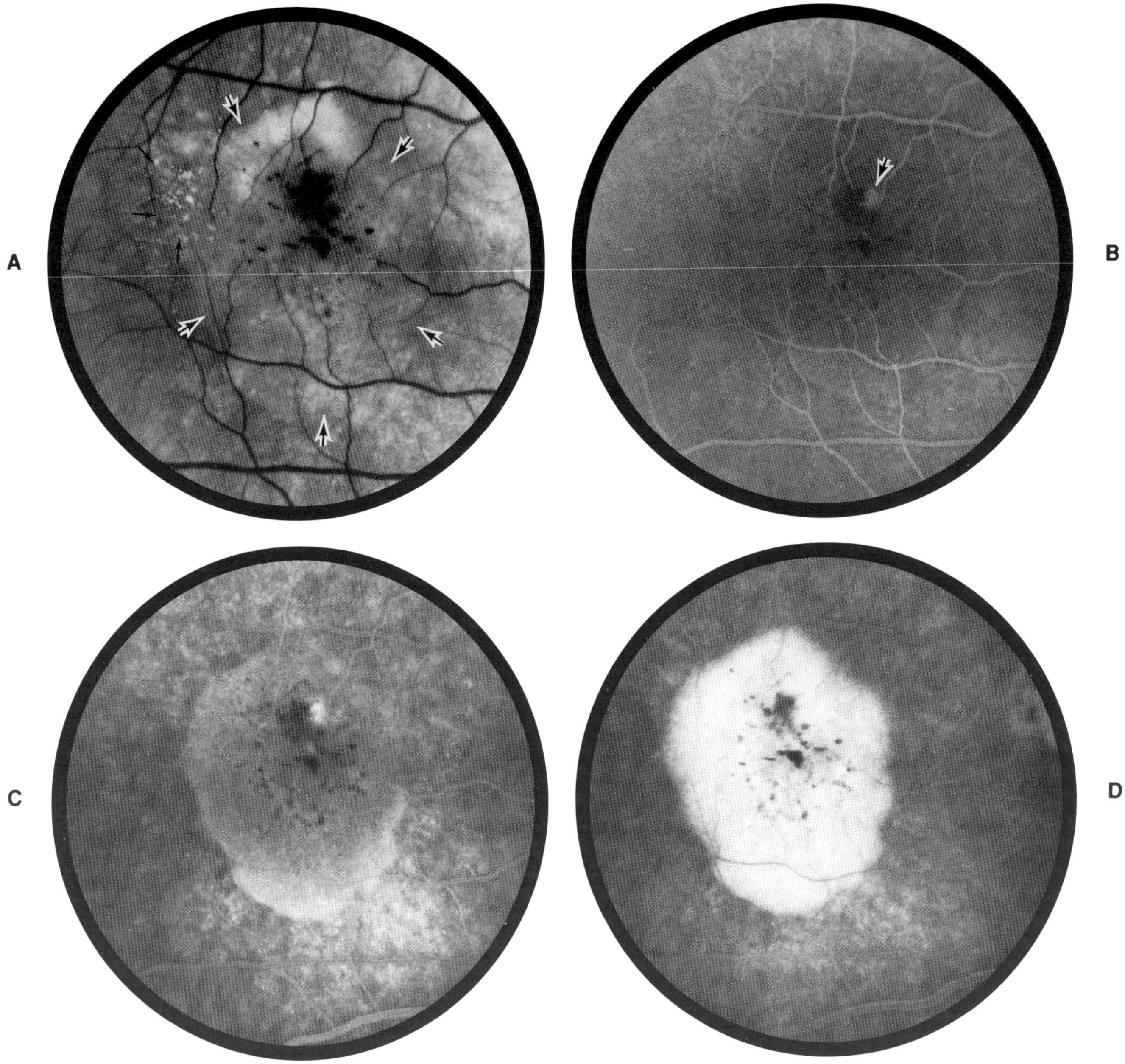

Figure 15.21. Pigment epithelial detachment with a hot spot of hyperfluorescence, indicating subretinal neovascularization. *A*, ophthalmoscopic photograph of the right macula showing a large turbid pigment epithelial detachment (*encircled by wide arrows*), with hemorrhage scattered over its surface, and exudate at its temporal aspect (*small arrows*). *B*, early venous phase angiogram showing that the pigment epithelial detachment has not yet fluoresced. A hyperfluorescent spot (*arrow*) is located above the fovea. C, late venous phase angiogram shows beginning fluorescence of the pigment epithelial detachment. The hyperfluorescent spot also shows increased fluorescence. *D*, late phase angiogram showing that the pigment epithelial detachment has become completely hyperfluorescent with scalloped margins. This patient had a turbid pigment epithelial detachment with hemorrhage and exudate, all of which were indicative of subretinal neovascularization. The hot spot seen in the early phases of the angiogram indicates the presence of the vessels beneath the detached pigment epithelium. Less indicative but still suggestive of subretinal neovascularization is the scalloped appearance to the margins of the detachment.

HOT SPOT IN PIGMENT EPITHELIAL DETACHMENT

The fluid beneath a detached pigment epithelium begins to hyperfluoresce evenly in the early phase of the angiogram. It is usually impossible to discern whether or not there are vessels beneath such a detachment. When vessels are present, occasionally a hot spot of greater hyperfluorescence within the usually hyperfluorescing fluid beneath the detached pigment epithelium can be seen (Fig. 15.21). This hot spot is a strong indicator of the presence of subretinal new vessels within the pigment epithelial detachment. As mentioned above if the pigment epithelium is atrophic from chronic stretching and elevation, neovascularization beneath it is more readily visible on the fluorescein angiogram.

A B C D

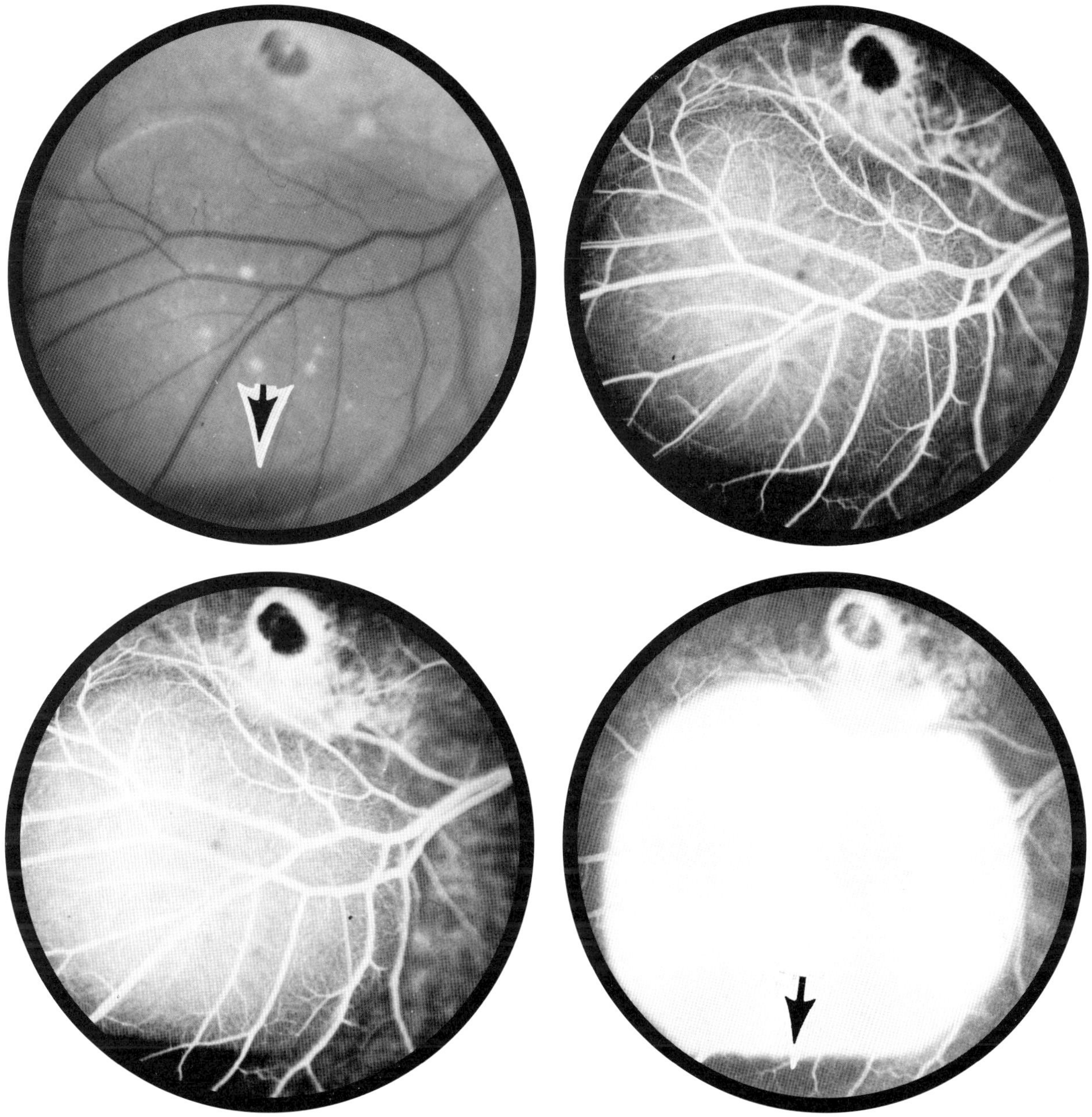

Figure 15.22. Meniscus of hemorrhage in the pigment epithelial detachment, indicating subretinal neovascularization. *A*, ophthalmoscopic photograph of an area just inferior to the right macula, showing a large pigment epithelial detachment bordered by an orange ring, typical of this lesion. There is a meniscus of hemorrhage at its inferior margin (*arrow*). A pigmentary scar is also present above the detachment. *B*, arteriovenous phase angiogram showing hyperfluorescence of the pigment epithelial detachment and hypofluorescence at the site of the pigmentary scar. *C*, late venous phase angiogram showing marked hyperfluorescence of the pigment epithelial detachment. *D*, late phase angiogram showing marked hyperfluorescence of the pigment epithelial detachment. The meniscus of hemorrhage can be seen inferiorly as an area of hypofluorescence (*arrow*) due to blockage of the choroidal circulation. This patient had a large pigment epithelial detachment with a meniscus of hemorrhage at its inferior margin. The hemorrhage indicates the presence of subretinal neovascularization even though the fluorescein angiogram failed to demonstrate the vessels. (From Schatz, H: *Perspect Opthalmol, 1*:8, 1977.)

MENISCUS OF HEMORRHAGE IN PIGMENT EPITHELIAL DETACHMENT

Finally, a pigment epithelial detachment may be seen with a meniscus or fluid level of hemorrhage at the bottom (Fig. 15.22). As stated in the section on the ophthalmoscopic appearance, hemorrhage and pigment epithelial disease are strong indicators of subretinal neovascularization. Even when the vessels cannot be discerned by fluorescein angiography, the presence of a meniscus of hemorrhage seen on the angiogram (or possibly seen clinically) indicates the presence of vessels.

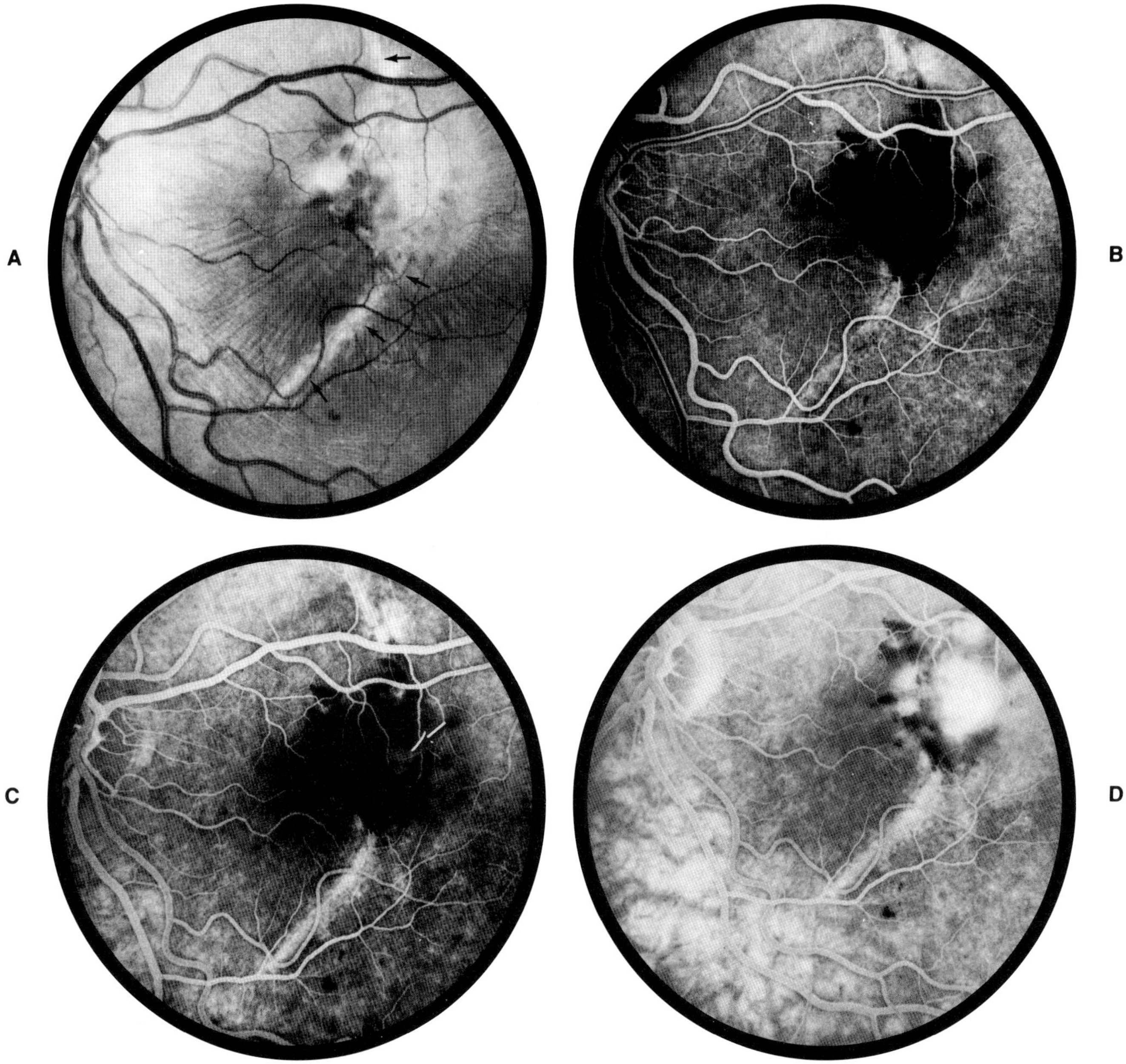

Figure 15.23. Subretinal neovascularization partially blocked by subretinal hemorrhage in an eye with a choroidal rupture. *A*, ophthalmoscopic photograph shows, in the temporal macula, a semilunar choroidal rupture (*arrows*) concentric with the disc. It is associated with a sensory retinal detachment, retinal folds, subretinal hemorrhage, and a subretinal pigmentary disturbance. *B*, arteriovenous phase angiogram showing early hyperfluorescence of the rupture, except for a large area of hypofluorescence corresponding to the hemorrhage. *C*, early venous phase angiogram showing a small patch of hyperfluorescence in the center of the hemorrhage. *D*, in the late phase angiogram, the hyperfluorescence in the center of the hemorrhage increases as dye pools into the subsensory retinal space. Subretinal neovascularization has complicated this choroidal rupture, producing a detachment and hemorrhage. The lacy vascular hyperfluorescence, typical of neovascularization, is not evident on the fluorescein angiograms because it is obscured, and in some areas, completely concealed by the blood.

HYPOFLUORESCENCE (BLOCKAGE DUE TO HEMORRHAGE OR PIGMENT RING)

Often accompanying subretinal neovascularization is a pigment ring or hemorrhage. Both tend to obscure choroidal fluorescence, creating an area of hypofluorescence on the angiogram that corresponds ophthalmoscopically in shape, size, and location to the pigment ring or hemorrhage. This blockage of choroidal fluorescence surrounding the neovascularization, caused by hemorrhage exudate or pigment is simply a confirmation of the pathologic changes associated with subretinal neovascularization (see Figs. 15.10 and 16). It is important to keep in mind that blood and pigment may serve to shield the neovascularized membrane to a variable degree (Fig. 15.23).

In summary the recognition of subretinal neovascularization is important in the diagnosis and management of many macular diseases. The presence of a subretinal neovascular membrane may be strongly suspected clinically by the findings on contact lens- and slit-lamp biomicroscopic examinations and is confirmed by fluorescein angiography. The ophthalmologist's knowledge of the presence of subretinal neovascularization in a patient is important for the purposes of diagnosis, prognosis, and specific management of the patient's macular disease. However, it is of paramount importance to keep in mind, based on histopathologic studies, that subretinal neovascularization may be present even when the clinical and fluorescein angiographic examination is negative. Early subpigment epithelial neovascularization in an eye with nonexudative changes can be concealed by an intact pigment epithelium, and there may be no evidence of late hyperfluorescence (leak) since there is relatively no staining of scar or pooling into an anatomic space.

Suggested Readings

Gass, J.D.M.: Choroidal neovascular membranes: their visualization and treatment. *Trans Am Acad Ophthalmol Otolaryngol, 77:* 310, 1973.

Sarkes, S.H.: New vessel formation beneath the retinal pigment epithelium in senile eyes. *Brit J Ophthalmol, 57:* 951, 1973.

Schatz, H.: The senile maculopathies and the retinal pigment epithelium. *Int Ophthalmol Clin, 15* (1): 169, 1975.

Schatz, H.: Other retinal pigment epithelial diseases. *Int Ophthalmol Clin, 15* (1): 181, 1975.

Schatz, H.: Subretinal neovascularization: clinical findings and fluorescein angiographic characteristics. *Perspect Ophthalmol, 1:* 59, 1977.

Teeters, W., and Bird, A.C.: A Clinical study of the vascularity of senile disciform macular degeneration. *Am J Ophthalmol, 75:* 53, 1973.

Teeters, W., and Bird, A.C.: The development of neovascularization and senile macular degeneration. *Am J Ophthalmol, 76:* 1, 1973.

Yannuzzi, L., and Gitter, K.: The fluorescein angiographic characteristics of subretinal neovascularization. *In* Proceedings of the First International Symposium on Photocoagulation, (1974), ed. by P. Amalric, In press.

CHAPTER 16

Involutional Macular Degeneration

Emanuel S. Rosen, M.D.

Involutional macular degeneration (maculopathy of aging, macular degeneration, and senile macular degeneration) is the most common maculopathy and one of the most severe in terms of visual function. When referring to this problem, the author prefers to use the term involutional, which is a pathologic term indicating degeneration caused by aging, rather than the word senile which has an undesirable connotation. It would be helpful to define other terms that have been applied to the maculopathies and in particular to the aging form of macular degeneration.

Abiotrophy is a term coined by Gowers in 1902 [1]; he called it a "premature disintegration of highly differentiated tissues as a result of defective vitality." This term was applied to hereditary retinal anomalies by Collins in 1919 [2] and 1 year later, Behr [3] utilized the term *heredodegeneration* to indicate the close relationship between all degenerative and familiar anomalies in the nervous system. In 1934 Sorsby [4] suggested that the term *abiotrophy* be reserved as a general concept in pathology. He preferred the term *dystrophy* to indicate a localized manifestation of an abiotrophy, in this case, of the retina.

Several authors, including Waardenburg [5], Blodi [6], Duke-Elder [7], and Deutman [8] used the term dystrophy to indicate premature cell changes and death caused by hereditary factors. Deutman [8] suggested that dystrophies of the posterior pole of the eye became manifest at a certain age as a result of genetically determined disorders of enzymatic and metabolic functions.

The term *disciform degeneration* of the macula was first used by Oeller in 1900 [9]. Similar cases were described in the literature by Pagenstecher in 1875 [10], by Michel in 1877 [11], and by Doyne in 1904 [12]. Junius and Kuhnt [13], in 1926, described the juvenile form of this degnerative process.

Involutional degeneration of the macula is synonymous with the terms: senile macular degeneration, senile disciform macular degeneration, exudative senile maculopathy, senile macular choroidal degeneration, maculopathy of aging, and disciform disease of the macula in the over-50 age group. Involutional degeneration of the macula, therefore, can be considered either: (1) a dystrophy, or (2) an aging phenomenon to which all people may succumb according to their exposure to undetermined environmental influences.

The disciform response in macular disease is characterized by hemorrhagic, exudative, and tissue organization phenomena resulting from invasion of the subpigment epithelial and subretinal space by a proliferation of vessels from the choriocapillaris through a break in Bruch's membrane. Subretinal neovascularization is a feature frequently occurring with involutional macular degeneration; it is found also in the maculopathies of pseudoxanthoma elasticum and other cases of angioid streaks, myopia, trauma, histoplasmosis, toxocariasis, Harada's disease, tumors, photocoagulation lesions, and other conditions.

Various changes are understood as precursors of the involutional disciform macular degenerative process: retinal pigment epithelium—atrophy, hyperplasia and drusen formation; Bruch's membrane—hyalinization, calcification, thickening and breaks; choroid—atrophy, thinning and hyalinization of intercapillary tissue. These changes are often seen in one eye in which the fellow eye is affected with involutional disciform macular degeneration. These changes have been investigated histopathologically particularly by Sarks [14].

Bruch's membrane thickens with age, and in some aging eyes, may increase to 15 times normal thickness. Accumulation of phagosomal and basement membrane material, replication of the basement membrane, and hyalinization account for thickening. Electron microscopic studies of aging Bruch's membranes have shown that phagosomes contain cone material. Physiologically, the number of cones in the retina declines with age, and the presence of cone material in Bruch's membrane indicates the fate of degenerated cones. The decrease in the number of cones that accompanies aging correlates with the slight decline in visual acuity of aging eyes which are otherwise normal. Accumulation of phagosomal material in Bruch's membrane seems to follow the physiologic decline of the number of cones in the retina. It has been suggested by Sarks [14], among others, that this accumulated material could be a stimulus to neovascularization. However, postmortem studies of aging eyes have shown that multifocal penetration of Bruch's membrane by new vessels from the choroid without any disciform macular degenerative process is a frequent finding (Fig. 16.1). Patchy calcification of Bruch's membrane occurs which leads to fractures of these more rigid areas. The fractures of Bruch's membrane are the sites of proliferating new vessels from the choriocapillaris into the subpigment epithelial space. The penetration of Bruch's membrane by blood vessels does not necessarily lead to the disciform response. The disciform response occurs when the vascular network proliferates and hemmorhages. Fluorograms of normal aging eyes may show multifocal punctate

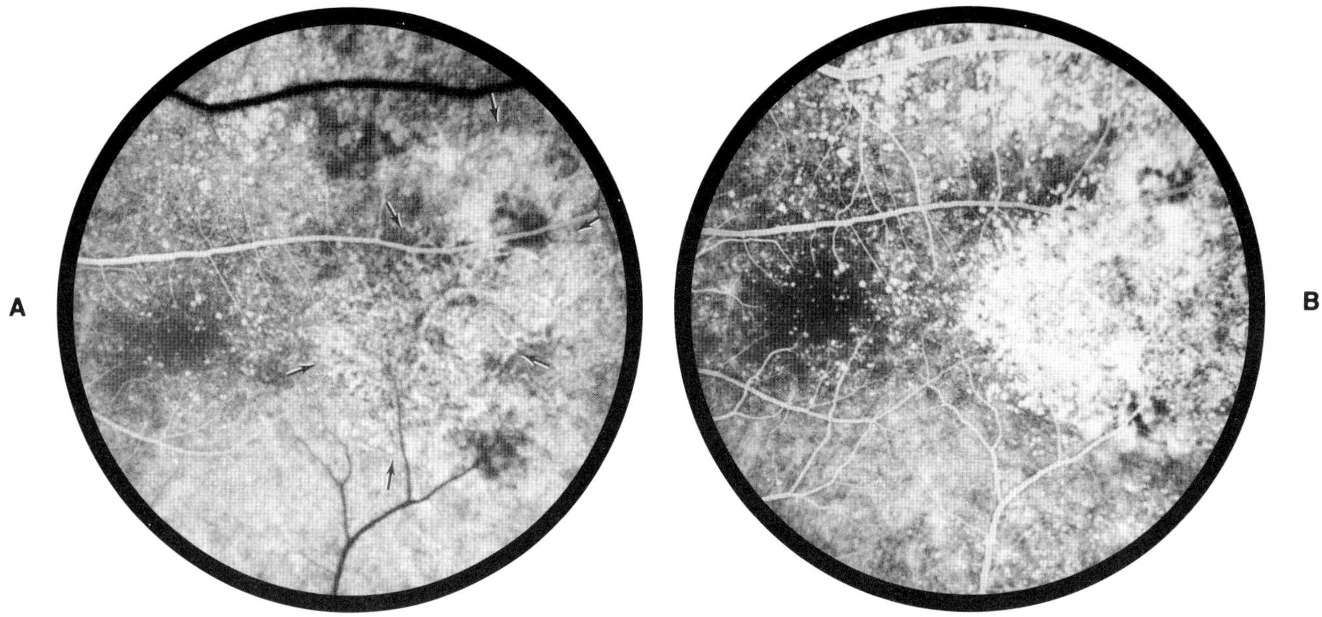

Figure 16.1. *A*, arteriole phase angiogram of a 65-year-old patient. Note the transmitted hyperfluorescence at sites of drusen. Subretinal lacy hyperfluorescence suggests subretinal neovascularization (*arrows*). *B*, early venous phase angiogram. Note the hyperfluorescence at drusen and leakage from the subretinal neovascularization temporal to the macula.

areas of fluorescence. Correlated with pathologic reports, these findings suggest end-on views of vessels perforating Bruch's membrane.

Ischemic changes in the choroid and retina may be a more important pathologic factor in the genesis of vascular proliferation in involutional disciform macular degeneration. Hayreh [15] has shown that the macula is the watershed of the choroidal circulation. Sclerosis of the choroidal vessels associated with aging may reduce perfusion of the choriocapillaris in the macula and provide a stimulus for neovascular growth. This phenomenon occurs in the retinal circulation, e.g., in diabetic retinopathy, as new vessels proliferate from the optic nerve head or elsewhere and seem to grow adjacent ischemic areas. Is it possible that ischemia of the choriocapillaris at the macula may, in a similar manner, stimulate the growth of new blood vessels from beneath the retina? This hypothesis has not been proved, but the concept remains an important one in the consideration of the pathogenesis of the development of subretinal neovascularization.

Drusen in the macula are an important finding in elderly patients, but significant loss of central vision in patients with macular drusen rarely occurs before the sixth or seventh decade of life. Under fluorographic examination, drusen will hyperfluoresce early because of the associated atrophy of the retinal pigment epithelium and transmission of the choriocapillaris. Some larger drusen may show late hyperfluorescence from staining of the subpigment epithelial space similar to detachments of the retinal pigment epithelium.

Degenerative phenomena can conveniently be divided into a dry or nonexudative form, and a wet or exudative form. In the nonexudative form, atrophy takes place in the outer layers of the neurosensory retina, the retinal pigment epithelium, and the choriocapillaris. The condition is usually slowly progressive. Islands of tissue within the area of atrophy or tissue surrounding the area may survive for a long period of time. The macula shows irregular or clustered pigmentation and is pale in appearance. Hemorrhage, exudate, and fluid are absent and localized detachment of the neurosensory retina or the retinal pigment epithelium does not occur. The visual prognosis in this type of involutional process is rarely predictable and, in some cases, may be good. When the choriocapillaris and pigment epithelium are atrophic, fluorography demonstrates late hyperfluorescence due to scleral staining.

The exudative or wet manifestations of involutional macular degeneration usually result from the presence of subretinal neovascularization. Serous and/or hemorrhagic detachment of the pigment epithelium can occur with secondary detachment and cystoid edema of the overlying sensory retina. Table 16.1 illustrates diagrammatically the histopathologic factors which play a role in the pathogenesis of involutional macular degeneration and in its evolution to a disciform stage.

Among the clinical signs that indicate the presence of subretinal neovascular tissue in the macula are: subretinal hemorrhage, subretinal or intraretinal lipid accumulation, a grayish discoloration under the retina, and cystoid edema of the overlying detached sensory retina. The fluorographic signs include early lacy hyperfluorescence of the subretinal neovascular tissue. In common with new vessels elsewhere, subretinal neovascularization is incontinent to fluorescein (leaks); therefore, late phase fluorograms are characterized by confluent hyperfluorescence of the neovascular membrane, subretinal space, and adjacent tissues (Fig. 16.2). Study of the natural history of such a membrane over a period of weeks in an individual eye shows its extension in an ameboid fashion with convex advancing fronts. The membrane tends to extend and may grow to several disc diameters in size, and may involve the entire macula (Fig. 16.3).

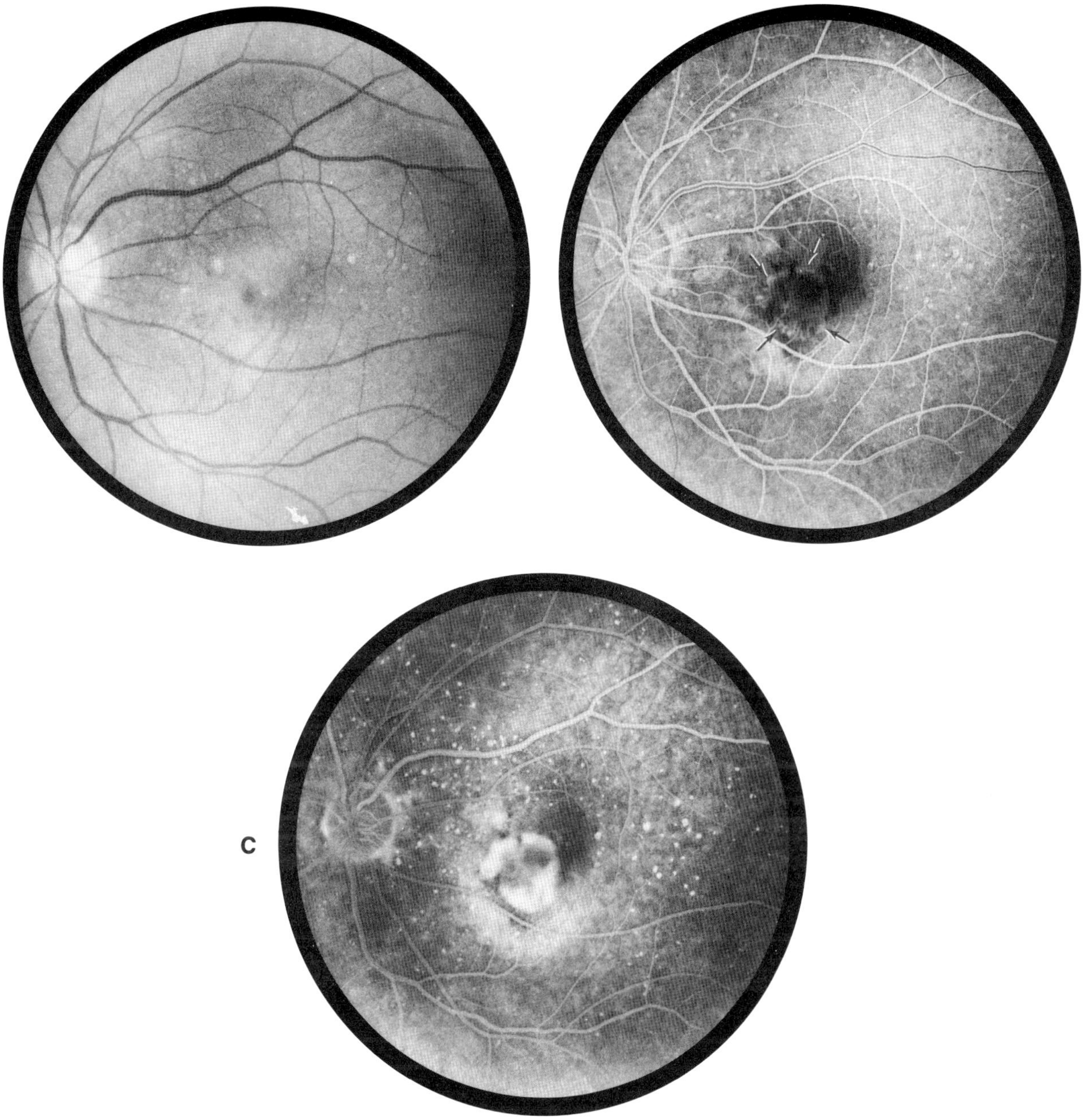

Figure 16.2. *A*, ophthalmoscopic photograph of a 62-year-old patient. Note the macular detachment and the scattered drusen. *B*, arteriovenous phase angiogram. Note the lacy hyperfluorescence in the central macula corresponding to a subretinal neovascularized membrane (*arrows*). Scattered dots of hyperfluoresence are also seen at drusen. *C*, late phase angiogram. Note the late hyperfluorescence from staining of the membrane and pooling into the subsensory retinal space. Some of the larger drusen also stain similar to retinal pigment epithelial detachments.

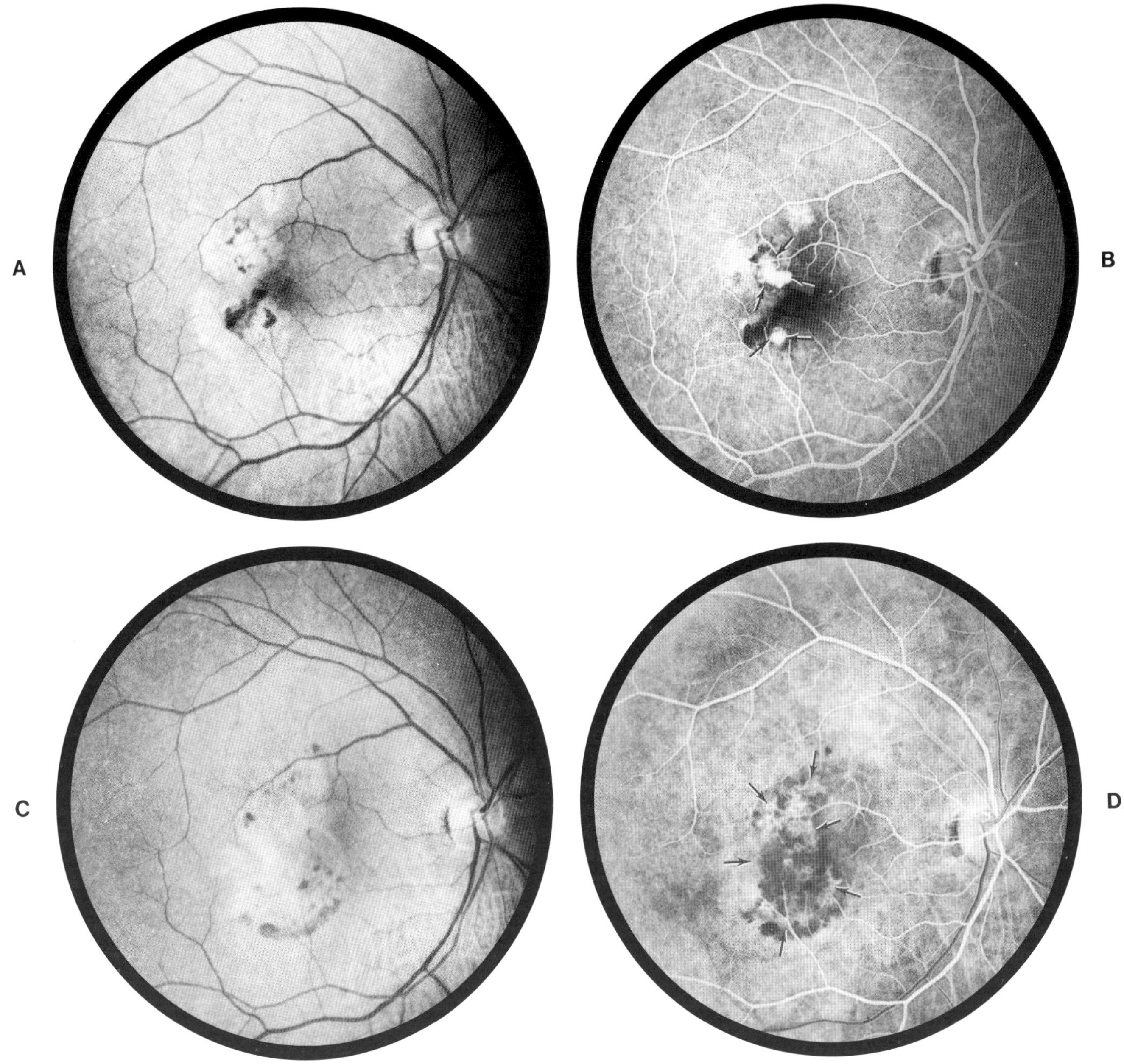

Figure 16.3

E

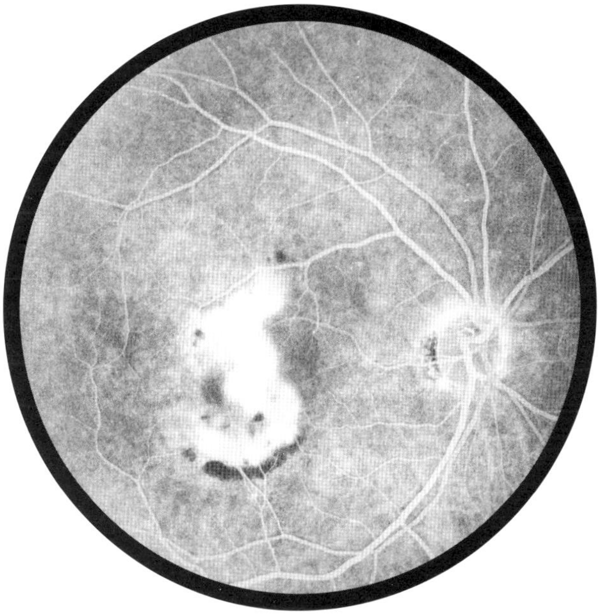

F

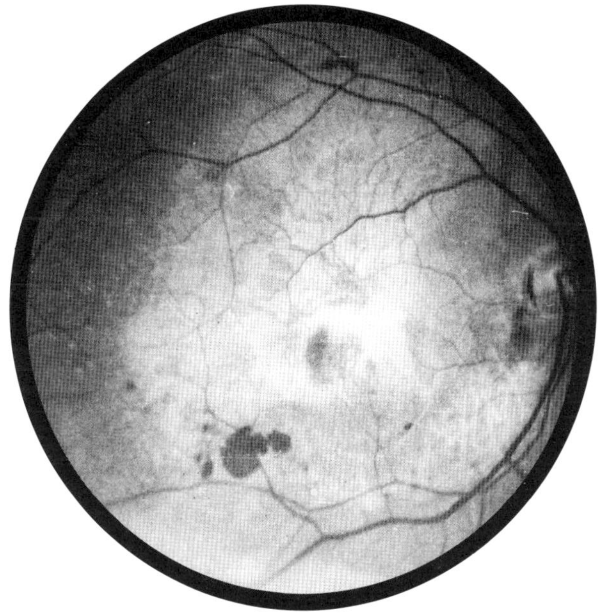

G

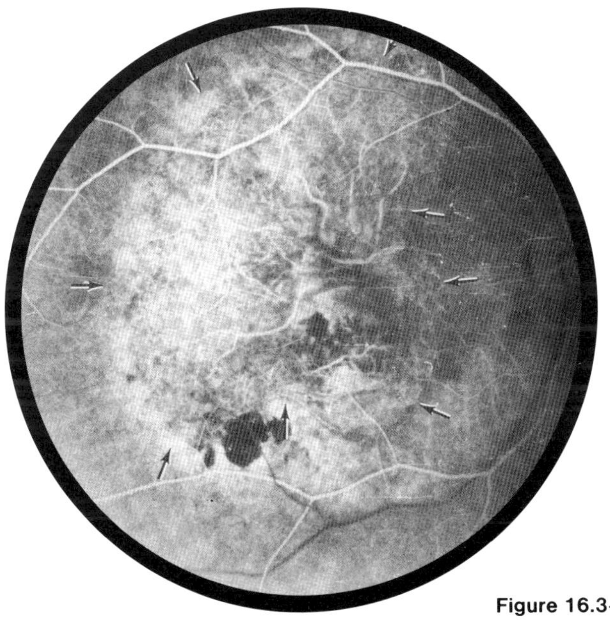

H

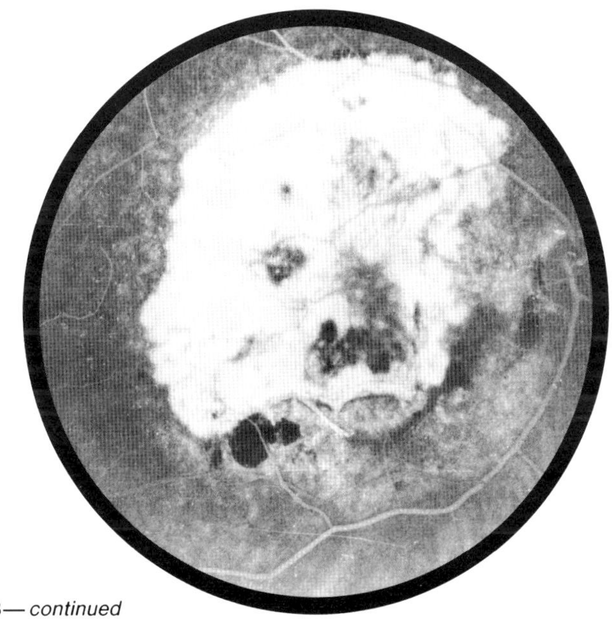

Figure 16.3—*continued*

Figure 16.3. Evolution of involutional macular degeneration. *A*, ophthalmoscopic photograph of a 72-year-old patient. Note the multifocal subretinal hemorrhage. *B*, arteriovenous phase angiogram. Note the hyperfluorescence of the subretinal neovascularization (*arrows*). Patchy hyperfluorescence elsewhere in the macula is seen at the site of retinal pigment epithelial atrophy. *C*, ophthalmoscopic photograph of the same eye, 1 month later. Note the more widespread hemorrhage, the subretinal membrane and the exudative detachment in the macula. *D*, arteriovenous phase angiogram shows a large area of lacy hyperfluorescence corresponding to the subretinal neovascularized membrane (*arrows*). A more widespread hyperfluorescence is evident surrounding the vascular network. This corresponds to retinal pigment epithelial atrophy and probably to extensive subpigment epithelial neovascularization as well. *E*, late venous phase angiogram. Note the diffuse hyperfluorescence from stains of the subretinal neovascular membrane and pooling into the overlying subretinal space. The hypofluorescence is due to the subretinal hemorrhage. *F*, ophthalmoscopic photograph of the same eye, 4 months later. Note the massive increase in size of the subretinal neovascular membrane occupying most of the posterior pole. *G*, arteriolar phase angiogram. Note the early lacy hyperfluorescence of the subretinal neovascular membrane, with advancing convex margins (*arrows*). *H*, late phase angiogram. Note the staining of the subretinal scar. The extent of the scar suggests that widespread neovascularization may have been present earlier beneath the retinal pigment epithelium but not absolutely evident on the fluorescein angiogram in (*D*).

The prognosis for vision is related to various factors including size and especially location. When the membrane is located in the fovea, the long-term prognosis for central vision is poor. Neovascularization beneath the fovea is, however, compatible with good central vision (up to 6/12 or 20/40) for periods of months in some patients. Hemorrhagic detachment of the retinal pigment epithelium in the fovea represents a poor prognostic sign. Hemorrhage may break through to all levels in the retina and may even rarely result in vitreous hemorrhage. Exudate forming circinate patterns around the neovascular tissue may be so extensive that the term Coats' response is warranted. Ultimately, these tissues become organized to form a disciform scar involving the retina (see Table 16.1).

Involutional macular degeneration is a bilateral disorder; there is approximately a 12% chance per year that the fellow eye will be similarly affected. Thus, within 5 years of onset of signs in the first eye, 60% of the fellow eyes will also be affected [16].

The hereditary and environmental roles in relationship to the involutional process have not yet been defined. Gass [17] concluded that there was no clinical fluorographic or electrophysiologic evidence to differentiate patients with macular drusen from those who have an autosomal dominant heredodegenerative disorder.

The condition is a major cause of blindness in Caucasians and thus, is deserving of consideration for therapy. It is the leading cause of new blindness after the age of 60. The present concept of therapy is to try to control the subretinal neovascular process. If the lesion is juxtafoveal with a clearance of 200 μ from the center of the fovea, there is then the potential for therapeutic obliteration of the membrane by argon laser photocoagulation. If this can be achieved, hemorrhage, exudation, and subsequent reorganization of the tissues that result in the destruction of the macula may be prevented or delayed. Obliteration of the subretinal neovascular lesion does not necessarily cure the condition, but it may preserve vision for an indeterminate period of time. Clinical experience suggests that involutional macular degeneration is a diffuse progressive process that deserves careful periodic examination and fluorographic monitoring to control the pathology as it evolves.

Table 16.1

INVOLUTIONAL DEGENERATION OF THE MACULA
PATHOGENESIS

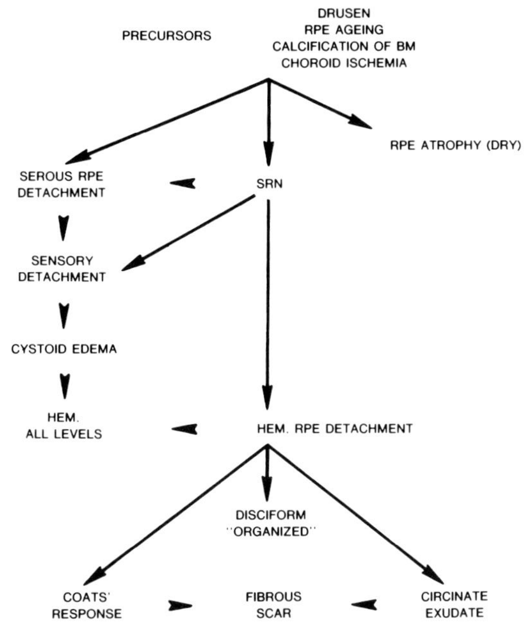

References

1. Gowers, W.R.: A lecture on abiotrophy. *Lancet, 1:* 1003, 1902.
2. Collins, E.T.: Diseases of the retina. I. Abiotrophy of the retinal neuroepithelium or "retinitis pigmentosa." *Trans Ophthalmol Soc U K, 39:* 165, 1919.
3. Behr, C.: Die Heredodegeneration der Makula. *Klin Monatsbl Augenheilkd, 65:* 465, 1920.
4. Sorsby, A.: Diseases of the retina. I. Retinal abiotrophy. *Trans Ophthalmol Soc U K, 54:* 160, 1934.
5. Waardenburg, P.J., Franceschetti, A., and Klein, D.: Genetics and Ophthalmology, Blackwell Scientific Publications, Oxford, part I, 1961 and part II, 1963.
6. Blodi, F.C.: The pathology of central tapeto-retinal dystrophy (hereditary macular degenerations). *Trans Am Acad Ophthalmol Otolaryngol, 70:* 1047, 1966.
7. Duke-Elder, S.: System of Ophthalmology, vol. 10: Diseases of the Retina, C.V. Mosby, St. Louis, 1967, p. 576.
8. Deutman, A.F.: The Hereditary Dystrophies of the Posterior Pole of the Eye, Royal van Gorum, Assen, The Netherlands, 1971.
9. Oeller, J.N.: Atlas Seltener Ophthalmoskopischer Befunde. J.F. Bergmann, Wiesbaden, 1900.
10. Pagenstecher, H.E. and Genth, A.: Atlas der Pathologischen Anatomie des Augapfels. C.W. Kreidel, Wiesbaden, 1875.
11. Michel, J.: Über Geschwülste des Uvealtractus. *Albrecht von Graefes Arch Ophthalmol, 24:* 131, 1878.
12. Doyne, R.W.: Diseases of the retina and choroid. I. Varicose veins in the retina. *Trans Ophthalmol Soc U K, 24:* 91, 1904.
13. Junius, P., and Kuhnt, H.: Die Scheibenförmige Entartung der Netzhautmitte (degeneratio maculae luteae disciformis), S. Karger, Berlin, 1926.
14. Sarks, S.H.: New vessel formation beneath the retinal pigment epithelium in senile eyes. *Brit J Ophthalmol, 57:* 951, 1973.
15. Hayreh, S.S.: Segmental nature of the choroidal vasculature. *Brit J Ophthalmol, 59:* 631, 1975.
16. Teeters, V.W., and Bird, A.C.: The development of neovascularization of senile disciform macular degeneration. *Am J Ophthalmol, 76:* 1, 1973.
17. Gass, J.D.M.: Pathogenesis of disciform detachment of the neuroepithelium. IV. Fluorescein angiographic study of senile disciform macular degeneration. *Am J Ophthalmol, 63:* 645, 1967.

CHAPTER 17

Presumed Ocular Histoplasmosis

Arnall Patz, M.D., and Stuart L. Fine, M.D.

The presumed ocular histoplasmosis syndrome is a major cause of visual impairment in selected areas of the United States. In recent years, the diagnosis and understanding of this ocular disorder has improved with the use of fluorescein angiography. A rationale exists for the use of photocoagulation in the treatment of the exudative manifestations that develop in the macula. This chapter reviews the epidemiology, pathogenesis, clinical and fluorescein angiographic findings, and our current method of management.

Epidemiology

Histoplasmosis capsulatum is a dimorphic fungus which grows in the soil in the mycelial or spore phase. It is resistant to extremes of humidity and temperature, and in animals, exists in the yeast phase [1, 2]. In mammals histoplasma infection occurs by the inhalation of spores [1, 2]. Other portals of entry such as vulvovagina, conjunctiva, or accidental injection are extremely rare [3].

Damp soil, located in darkness, is prominently associated with the fungus as are old chicken houses, barns, parks, forests, caves, and the excreta of bats and birds. At room temperatures of 25°C and below, the organisms exist in the spore form, but at body temperatures of 37°C (*in vivo* and *in vitro*) they transform into the yeast phase [4]. The spore forms consist of macroconidia (chlamydospores) 8–15 μ in diameter, and microconidia 2–4 μ in diameter. When both are inhaled, intact macroconidia are too large to enter the alveoli; however, fragments of macroconidia and microconidia may pass into alveoli and serve as a source of infection [4]. In mammals the intracellular oval budding yeast phase is ingested by macrophages and, thus, makes its way into the reticuloendothelial system.

Clinically, systemic histoplasmosis presents in a myriad of guises, ranging from an asymptomatic illness to a flu-like illness to disseminated disease in the very young, the aged, and the immune-incompetent [2].

Systemic histoplasmosis is found worldwide in river valleys, primarily in the temperate and tropical zones. It exists in the major river valleys of North, Central, and South America; India; Pakistan; Burma; Southwest Asia; and western tropical Africa. Europe is unscathed, save for a small localized area in Italy. In the United States, histoplasmosis is endemic in the eastern and central states and in 31 of the 48 continental states. The largest area of endemic histoplasmosis occurs in the Ohio and Mississippi River valleys. In endemic areas of the eastern half of the United States, approximately 75–80% of the population show a positive skin test to the histoplasmin antigen, which is interpreted to represent prior exposure to the histoplasma organism [5].

Recently, an article on patients in Britain with a clinical picture of presumed ocular histoplasmosis syndrome in a country with essentially no positive histoplasmin skin tests suggests strongly that this clinical syndrome may not always be related to histoplasmic infection [6].

It is significant that other investigators have described lesions identical with those found in the ocular histoplasmosis syndrome in patients having no prior exposure to histoplasma infection. Wessing [7] and de Laey [8] have observed a number of patients under 50 years of age who reported to them with choroidal neovascularization in the macula and who had the classic peripapillary and peripheral atrophic punched-out lesions. These patients were not from endemic areas and, above all, they had no systemic or clinico-serologic evidence of the disease.

Clinical Appearance and Course

The triad of findings for the clinical diagnosis of presumed ocular histoplasmosis syndrome is atrophic choroidal scars in the retinal periphery, peripapillary choroidal scars, and macular disciform lesions in eyes with no anterior segment or vitreous inflammation (Fig. 17.1).

The peripheral "punched-out" white atrophic choroidal scars located posterior to the equator range from 0.1 to 0.7 disc diameters in size (Fig. 17.2). Their borders are irregular and the lesions are often circumferential or linear in pattern. Occasionally there is pigment clumping in the center or at the edges of the choroidal scars [9].

The circumpapillary choroidal lesions occur in four morphologic patterns as reported by Schlaegel and Kennedy [10] in 1966. In 80 eyes of 54 patients, the patterns were as follows: diffuse scarring, 50% nodular scarring, 30%; mixed scarring (diffuse and nodular), 10%; and hemorrhagic peripapillary lesions, 10% [10].

The elevated hemorrhagic disciform macular lesions secondary to subretinal neovascularization usually occur between the second and fifth decades with a peak incidence in the fourth decade [11, 12] (Fig. 17.3). Clinically, patients are usually aware of metamorphopsia first, with a gradual progression to a relative paracentral, followed by a central scotoma. The subretinal fluid or active gray-white choroiditis is present, usually adjacent to or under an old macular scar or "histo spot" (Fig. 17.4). This progresses in a majority of cases (60%) to the hemorrhagic phase, and 50–60% of these have permanent central visual loss. Formation of a central glial scar often is the final stage of the macular lesion [13]. Lesions with serous subretinal fluid have a better prognosis than those with hemorrhage [14]. Subsensory retinal hemorrhage is more favorable than subpigment epithelial hemorrhage, which has a uniformly poor prognosis when the fovea is involved. The number of macular

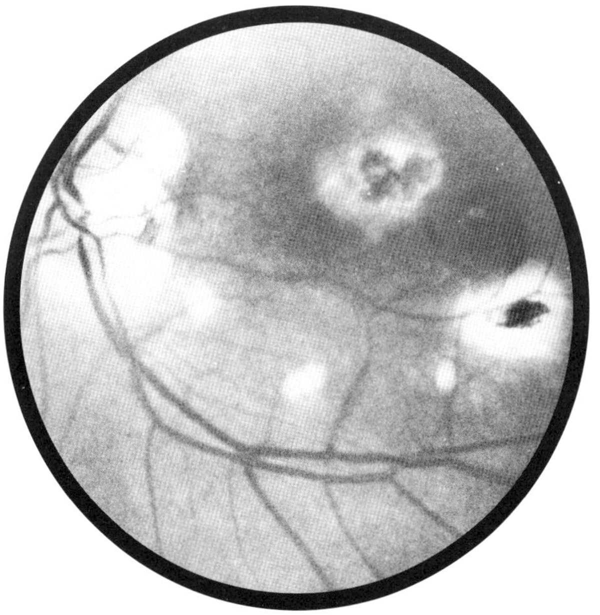

Figure 17.1. Ophthalmoscopic photograph of an eye with inactive paramacular choroidal atrophic spots and peripapillary choroidal atrophic scarring, in a patient with presumed ocular histoplasmosis.

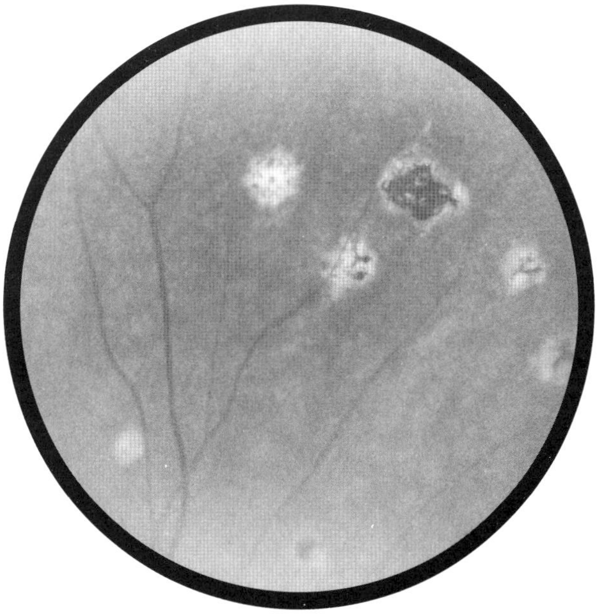

Figure 17.2. Ophthalmoscopic photograph of peripheral ("punched out") atrophic choroidal spots in presumed ocular histoplasmosis.

A

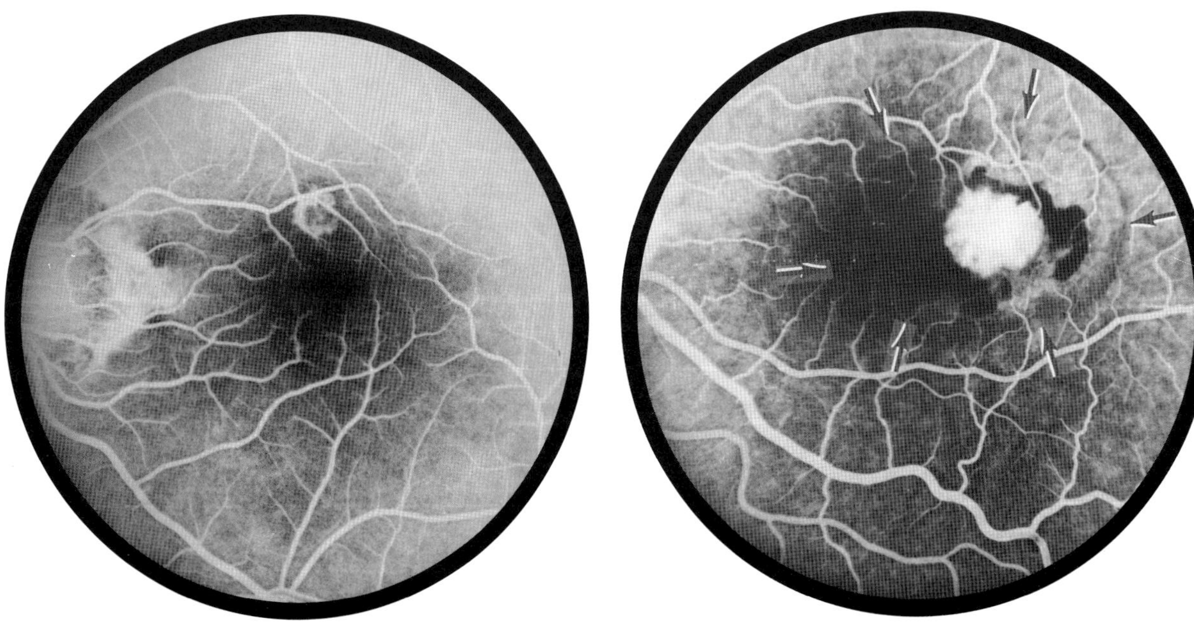

B

Figure 17.3. Fluorescein angiograms of subretinal neovascularization in presumed ocular histoplasmosis. *A*, note the lacy hyperfluorescence subretinally in the superior macula corresponding to subretinal neovascularization. *B*, note the hyperfluorescence of the subretinal neovascularized complex with blocked hypofluorescence due to hemorrhage at its margins. An overlying sensory retinal detachment involves the macula (*arrows*).

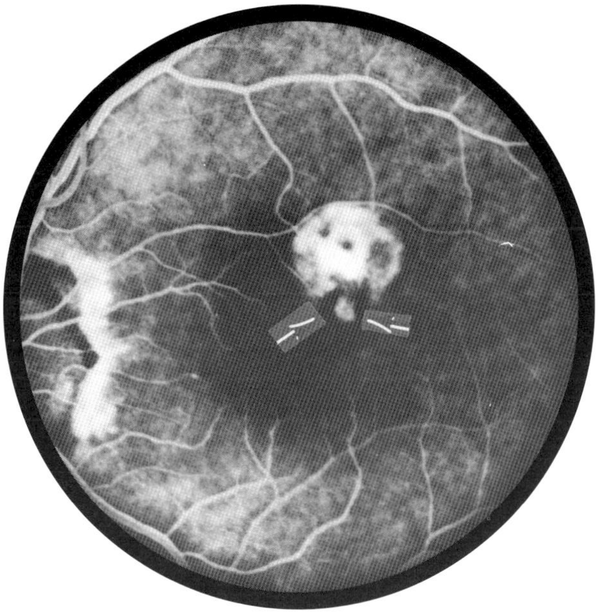

Figure 17.4. Active subretinal neovascular membrane arising from prior atrophic choroidal lesion with associated hemorrhage and macular detachment (*arrows*). Peripapillary scarring is also evident in this patient with presumed ocular histoplasmosis.

histo spots does not, however, seem to be related to the chances of reactivation [12, 14].

The general prognosis for vision is poor when active disciform lesions are present. The final visual acuity in various series reported in the literature run as follows: visual acuity of 20/200 or worse, 50–60%; vision of 20/100 to 20/40, 15–20%; vision of 20/30 or better, 20–30% [15]. Bilateral macular scars with loss of macular function occur in 20–30% of patients with this syndrome [16, 17].

For some unknown reason, the macula of the patient's second eye fares much better than the eye that was first involved. Final visual acuity of 20/200 or worse occurs in approximately 80% of first affected eyes, while only approximately 30% of second eyes have such poor vision [18]. The risk of an active macular lesion in the second eye containing a histo spot of patients with macular disciform lesions in the first eye is approximately 20% over a 2- to 2 ½-year period [12, 17, 18]. The risk of an active macular lesion arising in a second eye with a peripapillary scar (without a paramacular atrophic spot) and a macular disciform lesion in the first eye is approximately 5% over a 2- to 2 ½-year period [12, 17, 18].

White patients with presumed ocular histoplasmosis syndrome are affected at least 20 times more frequently than black patients [19].

Fortunately, only a small number of patients with atrophic histo spots near the macula develop neovascularization. Our experience has been that if a patient has a choroidal neovascular membrane develop in one eye and has inactive histo spots in the other, in the course of a 3- to 4-year follow-up, approximately ⅓ of the patients will develop active neovascularization in the second eye from histo spots in that eye. We have never observed neovascularization developing *de novo* in the second eye, although a case has been reported.

Pathophysiology

Clinical and experimental evidence suggests that the peripheral punched-out atrophic choroidal lesions result from a focal choroiditis following *Histoplasmosis capsulatum* fungemia [20, 21].

Debate exists, however, over the etiology of the exudative macular lesions in the presumed ocular histoplasmosis syndrome. There are presently four major theories proposed, each with its own vocal and adamant followers.

The hypersensitivity theory first suggested by Woods and Wahlen [22] hypothesized the presence of a highly sensitized uveal tissue in the areas of the focal choroiditis. Later on, following resensitization by histoplasmosis antigens, an amnestic immunologic reaction occurs with secondary serous and hemorrhagic inflammatory response. Ganly [23] believes that the immunity system of these patients has a genetically determined overactivity to any antigen introduced into the patients' immune systems.

Gass and Wilkinson [17] have proposed that old atrophic histoplasmosis scars become areas of "chronic choroidal vascular decompensation" with leakage into choroidal and retinal anatomic spaces and eventual development of a disciform lesion secondary to subretinal neovascularization.

Still others believe both these theories (the overactive immune response and the vascular ischemia) are, in part, correct and that the ocular lesions result from "a combination of a hypersensitivity reaction superimposed on an area of structurally and physiologically altered choroid" [24].

While the precise pathogenesis of the ocular histoplasmosis syndrome is still not clearly understood, the general consensus is that an infection with the histoplasma organism produces focal areas of granulomatous choroiditis [25]. These undergo spontaneous healing, leaving the patients with the histo spots. For reasons that are still not understood, in later years the histo spots near the macular area will be involved by choroidal neovascularization, breaking through Bruch's membrane to lie under the pigment epithelium. The natural history of the choroidal neovascularization in the macular histoplasmosis lesion is typical of other forms of subpigment epithelial neovascularization. Hemorrhage beneath the pigment epithelium occurs and the overlying pigment epithelium loses its competence as a choroidal-retinal barrier. Fluid leaks beneath the sensory retina to produce a detachment of the overlying sensory retina. The pigment epithelium may be grossly damaged and hemorrhage breaks through the detached pigment epithelium with blood lying beneath the sensory retina, or it may break into the sensory retina proper (Fig. 17.5). We have never observed a patient to have a major vitreal hemorrhage from a break-through of the subretinal hemorrhage through the sensory retina, as occasionally occurs in patients with senile subretinal neovascularization.

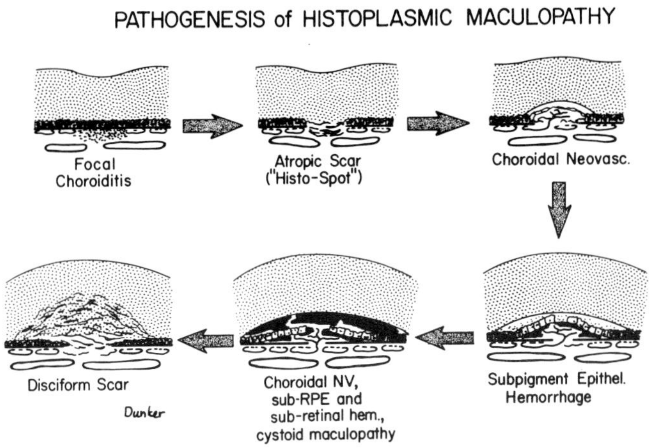

Figure 17.5. Schematic diagram showing course of the histoplasmosis lesion. During the initial infection with the histoplasma organism, a focal choroiditis occurs. This heals and leaves an atrophic scar (histo spot). Several years later the lesion becomes active with choroidal neovascularization growing through Bruch's membrane to proliferate beneath the pigment epithelium. The pigment epithelial barrier is damaged and fluid leaks beneath the sensory retina. Hemorrhage occurs beneath the pigment epithelium and may spread beneath the sensory retina; organization of the hemorrhage leaves a disciform scar in the final stage.

Therapy for the Active Histoplasmic Choroidal Neovascular Lesion

Some investigators have advocated the use of steroids, and the results are equivocal. A randomized prospective controlled study to test steroid therapy will be necessary to document the role of this or any other form of medical therapy. Photocoagulation has been commonly used in the late 1960's and early 1970's. Watzke and Leaverton [26] have reported on a randomized controlled study using xenon arc photocoagulation and found no significant difference in the treated and untreated eyes. Although the study was properly designed from a statistical standpoint, photographic documentation of cases indicates that many of the patients who were selected for treatment were those whose membrane extended too close to the center of the fovea to be considered as candidates for photocoagulation, according to the present criteria. Others have employed xenon photocoagulation with apparently more beneficial results. To date, however, there are no data available.

Photocoagulation Therapy

CRITERIA FOR SELECTION OR EXCLUSION OF PATIENTS

We have considered the distance of ¼ disc diameter of the choroidal neovascular membrane from the center of the fovea as the minimal safe distance to apply photocoagulation therapy [27–29]. Utilizing the average diameter of the avascular zone in the center of the macula as 500 μ, we find it convenient to use the diameter of the blood column in a retinal vein as it crosses the disc margin (125 μ) as a reference point. One vein width past the border of the perifoveal capillary ring is considered as the safe distance for treatment (Fig. 17.6). Because an intense white photocoagulation end-point is desired, it is necessary to have a sufficient distance from the edge of the choroidal neovascular membrane to the center of the fovea to prevent significant damage to the central foveal cones as the result of photocoagulation. This is especially important as the photocoagulation treatment should extend a distance of 125 μ past the edge of choroidal neovascular membrane in all directions. We have found that the placement of small spots of coagulation 125 μ past the foveal edge of the neovascular membrane provides a good visual landmark to prevent inadvertent extension of the photocoagulation closer to the center of the fovea than desired (Fig. 17.7). In the photocoagulation treatment, we apply these photocoagulation burns with 50- or 100-μ spot sizes at mild-to-moderate intensity to provide the visual landmark. The foveal edge of the neovascular membrane is then treated, utilizing 100-μ spot sizes and the timing of 0.2 second with an intense white retinal burn produced. The remainder of the peripheral border of the neovascular membrane is then treated, utilizing 200-μ spot sizes, 0.5-second exposure, and an intense white photocoagulation end-point. After completely surrounding the neovascular membrane and extending the photocoagulation burns 125-μ past the edge of the new vessels, the central portion of the lesion is treated with either 200- or 500-μ spot size settings, using 0.5-second exposure. We feel that it is extremely important to avoid small spot sizes and short exposures in direct treatment of the neovascularization as there is a tendency to break Bruch's membrane and also there is poor penetration for a deeper thermal effect beneath the retinal pigment epithelium.

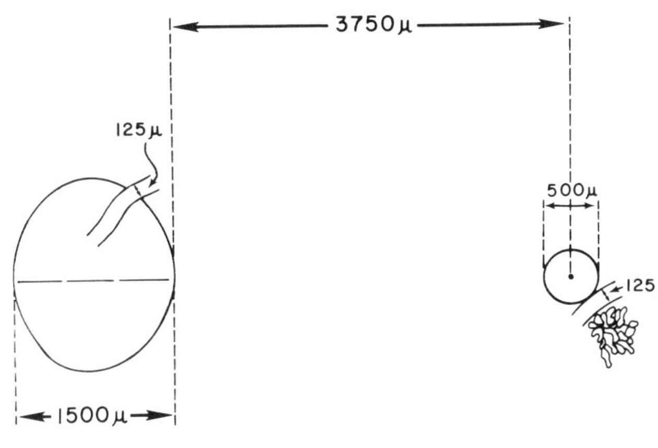

Sub-Pigment-Epithelial-Neovascularization

Figure 17.6. Schematic diagram showing the relationship of the optic disc measurement, blood column in retinal vein at disc margin, and the central avascular zone. Note that the neovascular membrane is one vein width (125 μ) past the edge of the capillary border ring of the avascular zone. Thus, the radius of the perifoveal capillary free zone, which is 250 μ, plus the width of the vein (125 μ) is equivalent to 375 μ, or ¼ the horizontal disc diameter. Neovascularization at this distance or further from the fovea is considered for photocoagulation.

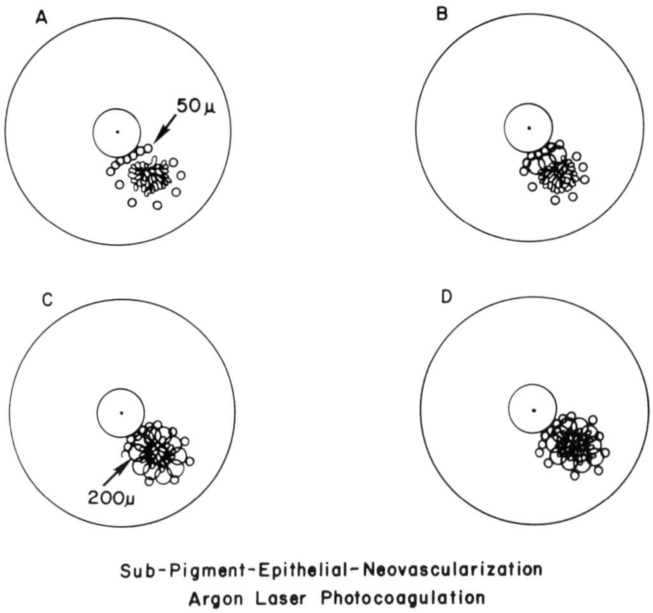

Figure 17.7. Technique of argon laser photocoagulation. *A*, 50-μ row of mild photocoagulation burns serve as a visual landmark to prevent inadvertent photocoagulation extending to the center of the fovea. These mild photocoagulation burns are 125 μ past the edge of the neovascularization. *B*, the foveal edge of the neovascularization is first treated, utilizing 100-μ spot sizes at a 0.2-second exposure time. An intense white burn is desired. *C*, the remainder of the border of the neovascular membrane is treated, utilizing 200-μ spot sizes at 0.5-second time exposure. An intense white burn is produced. *D*, the center is treated last, utilizing either 200- or 500-μ spot size settings with 0.5-second exposure. An intense white burn is produced. A retrobulbar anesthetic is recommended.

POSTPHOTOCOAGULATION FOLLOW-UP TREATMENT

We like to examine the patient within 1 week of the treatment and repeat the fluorescein angiogram. This is done primarily to see if the treatment has extended past the edges of the new vessel membrane. Generally, there is sufficient edema of the pigment epithelium to obscure any residual neovascularization in the center of the photocoagulation lesion. For this reason, we wait until approximately 2–3 weeks after the initial treatment to repeat the post-treatment angiogram, at which time the pigment epithelial edema will have subsided and any residual new vessel membrane beneath the pigment epithelium can be resolved. Even when no residual new vessels are noted, it is possible that residual new vessels are present but simply not filling with fluorescein at this stage. The patient is followed on a regular basis after the treatment.

Once the lesion is healed and the sensory retina flattened, we provide the patient with an Amsler grid to test at home every few days on a regular basis with the goal in mind that early sensory detachment can be detected sooner using the Amsler grid. Changes may be detected even before the patient has new subjective impairment or distortion of vision. In a patient with an active choroidal neovascular membrane in one eye, who shows old histo spots in the opposite eye near the macula, we also instruct him to use the Amsler grid periodically for the second eye. In view of the significant risk of approximately 30% of patients developing choroidal neovascular membranes where histo spots are present in the second eye, we feel that early detection of choroidal neovascularization with an overlying sensory elevation will permit better management.

When the choroidal neovascular membrane is in a peripapillary location, we advocate treatment if the edge of the membrane is sufficiently removed from the fovea to be at least ¼ disc diameter from the center of the fovea. Although there is concern for damage to the papillomacular bundle with the intense photocoagulation energy that is required, the patient has partial protection to the nerve fiber layer in the papillomacular bundle by virtue of the retina being thicker in this portion, and, secondly, the fluid beneath the sensory retina further removes the nerve fiber layer from the pigment epithelium where the energy is maximally absorbed. The same intense photocoagulation energy, as described above, is utilized in the peripapillary neovascularization and the photocoagulation is extended past the edge of the new vessel membrane in all directions. We treat up to the edge of the disc border to obliterate the neovascular membrane at that edge but do not extend the coagulation on to the disc itself, although there is some slight spread of energy onto the disc. Small peripapillary neovascular membranes, particularly in the papillomacular bundle, are watched and unless there is a significant sensory detachment which involves the center of the macula and causes visual impairment, we do not routinely advocate treatment.

Typical treated cases of active histoplasmosis choroidal neovascularization are presented in Figures 17.8 and 17.9.

Dr. Michael Klein, while at the Retinal Vascular Center, analyzed the fluorescein angiograms of all ocular histoplasmosis patients seen at the Wilmer Institute during a 7-year period. In approximately 450 angiograms studied, 30 eyes with choroidal neovascular membranes, at least ¼ disc diameter from the center of the fovea, and with good quality photographs and adequate follow-ups were found. These have been followed for a minimum period of 6 months up to 79 months, with a mean follow-up period of 30 months. Since these patients, with a choroidal neovascular membrane removed ¼ disc diameter or more from the center of the fovea, would be considered candidates for photocoagulation by present criteria, we compared the natural history with a group of 30 consecutive patients treated by photocoagulation. Of those eyes that did not receive photocoagulation therapy, 64% maintained visual acuity of 20/40 during the follow-up period. Of those eyes that were photocoagulated, 76% maintained 20/40 vision or better. The average follow-up in the treated cases was 2 years. The difference between these two groups is not statistically significant because of the small number of patients. The data justify a randomized prospective controlled clinical trial to document the role of photocoagulation in the management of the histoplasmosis choroidal neovascular membrane.

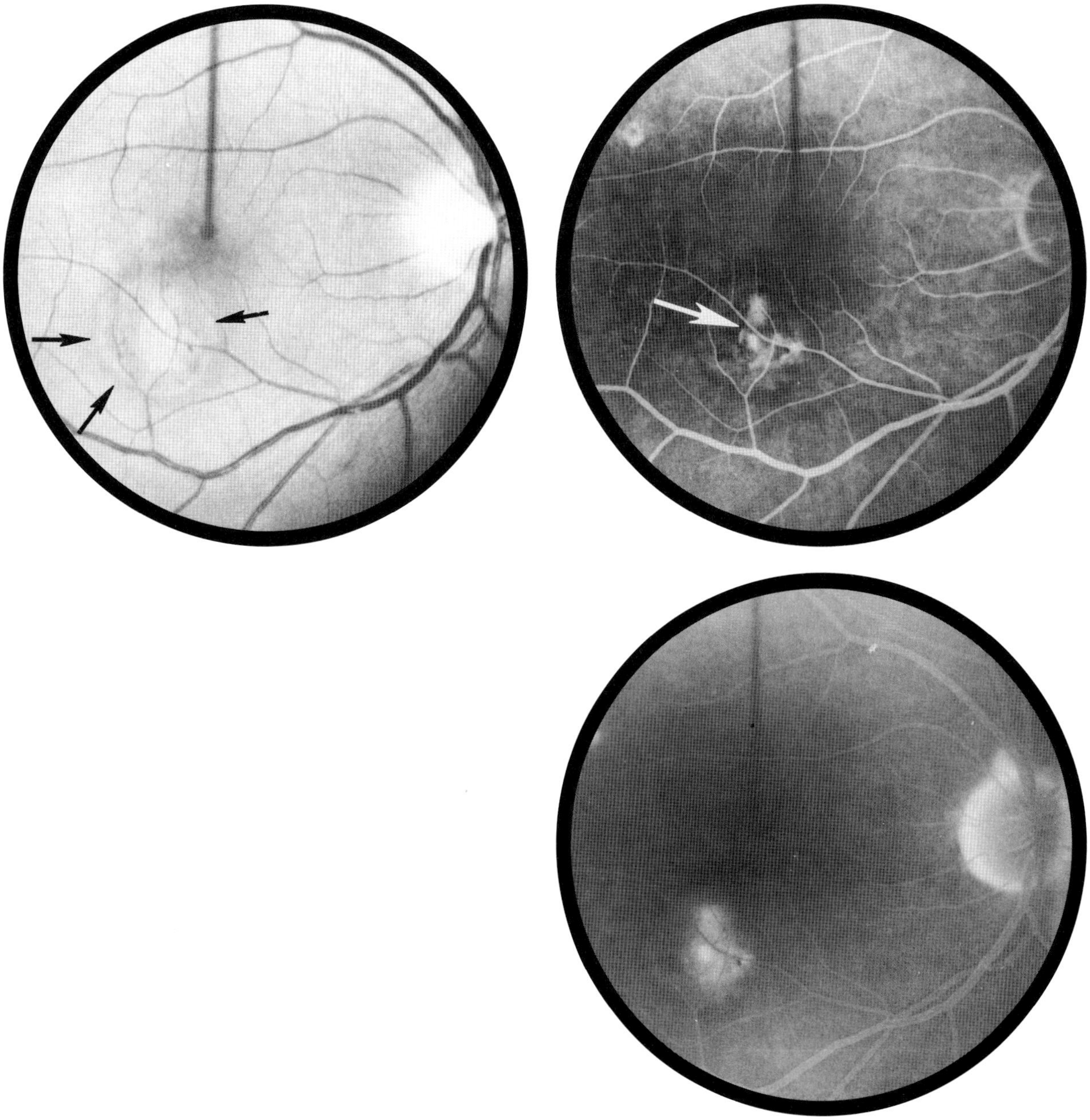

A

B

C

Figure 17.8

D

E

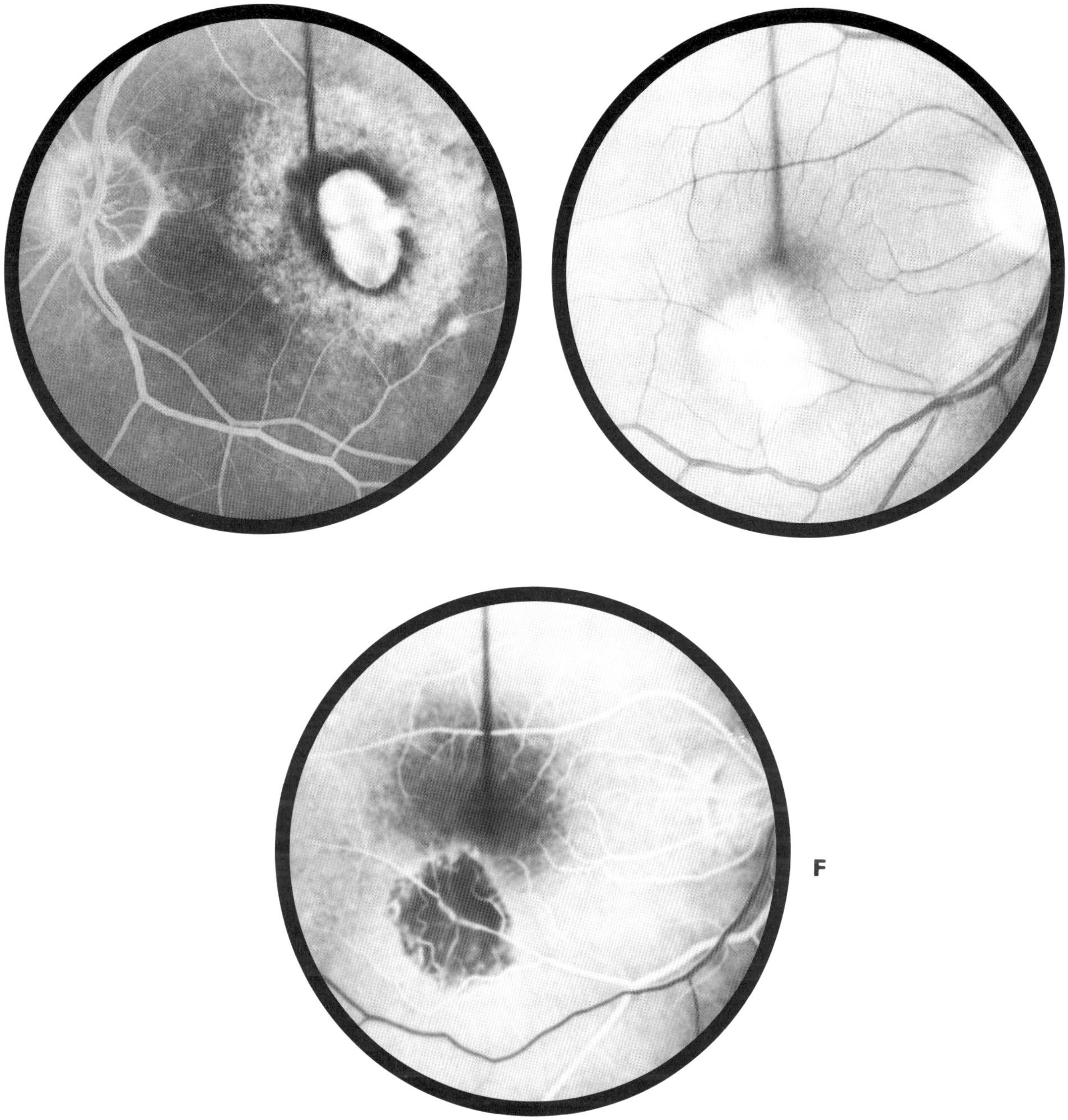

F

Figure 17.8—*continued*

Figure 17.8. *A*, ophthalmoscopic photograph of right eye of a 37-year-old physician with active histoplasmic macular lesion. *Arrows*, outline the area of sensory retinal detachment overlying the choroidal neovascularization. *B*, venous phase fluorescein angiogram shows choroidal neovascular membrane (*arrow*). *C*, late phase angiogram shows further leakage beneath the sensory retinal detachment. *D*, left eye of same patient showing hyperfluorescence of old disciform scar involving the left macula. Visual acuity: right eye, 20/20-2; left eye, 10/200. *E*, ophthalmoscopic photograph of the treated right eye 4 days after photocoagulation treatment. Intense white reaction is noted over the area of neovascularization. *F*, arterial stage of angiogram shows that photocoagulation has extended past the edge of the neovascular membrane in all directions.

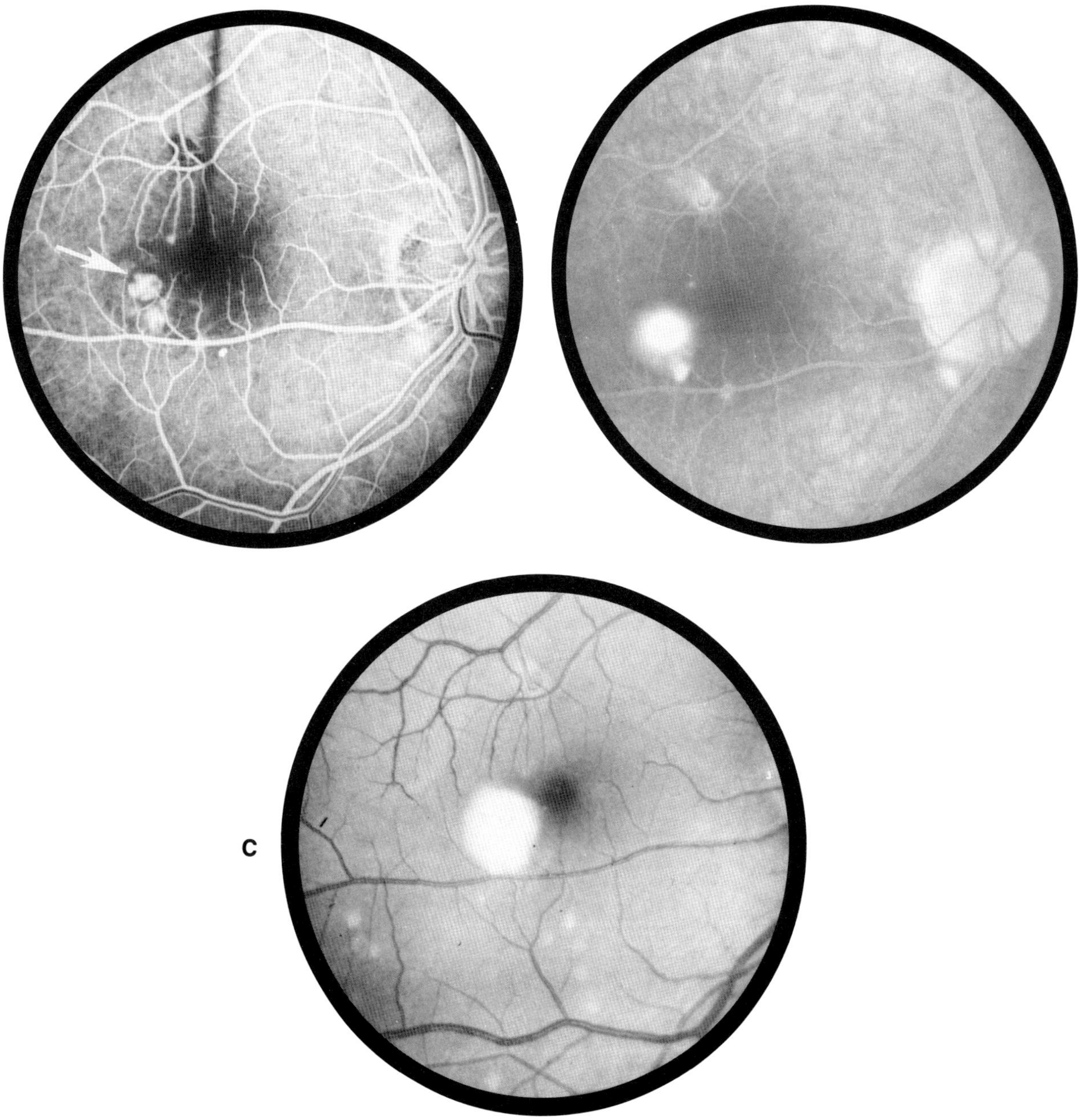

Figure 17.9. *A*, arteriovenous phase angiogram of active choroidal neovascular membrane (*arrow*) above an old histo spot. *B*, late phase angiogram showing marked dye leakage from neovascular membrane beneath the overlying detached sensory retina. There is no change of size in the "inactive spot" inferior to the choroidal neovascular membrane. *C*, ophthalmoscopic photograph taken immediately post-treatment shows intense white retinal burn used in treatment of choroidal neovascularization. The intense reaction extends at least 125 μ past the edge of the neovascular membrane in all directions.

References

1. Schlaegel, T.F., Jr.: Histoplasmic choroiditis. *Ann Ophthalmol, 6:* 237, 1974.
2. Mann, J.J.: Systemic histoplasmosis. *In* Selected Topics on the Eye in Systemic Disease, Grune & Stratton, New York, 1974, pp. 123–134.
3. Schwarz, J.: Granulomatous histoplasmosis of the eye: a rare disease. *Int Ophthalmol Clin, 15* (3): 65, 1975.
4. Wong, V.G., Kwon-Chung, K.J., and Hill, W.B.: Koch's postulates and experimental ocular histoplasmosis: panel discussion. *Int Ophthalmol Clin, 15* (3): 139, 1975.
5. Smith, R.E., and Ganley, J.P.: Presumed ocular histoplasmosis. I. Histoplasmin skin test sensitivity in cases identified during a community survey. *Arch Ophthalmol, 87:* 245, 1972.
6. Braunstein, R.A., Rosen, D.A., and Bird, A.C.: Ocular histoplasmosis syndrome in the United Kingdom. *Brit J Ophthalmol, 58:* 893, 1974.
7. Wessing, A.: Personal communication.
8. de Laey, J.J.: Personal communication.
9. Gass, J.D.M.: Stereoscopic Atlas of Macular Diseases, C.V. Mosby, St. Louis, 1970, pp. 48–61.
10. Schlaegel, T.F., Jr. and Kenney, D.: Changes around the optic nervehead in presumed ocular histoplasmosis. *Am J Ophthalmol, 62:* 454, 1966.
11. Schlaegel, T.F., Jr.: Introduction. *Int Ophthalmol Clin, 15* (3): 1, 1975.
12. Schlaegel, T.F., Jr.: The natural history of histo spots in the discmacular area. *Int Ophthalmol Clin, 15* (3): 19, 1975.
13. Schlaegel, T.F., Jr.: Essentials of Uveitis. Little, Brown & Co., Boston, 1969, pp. 135–163.
14. Krill, A.E., Chishti, M.I., Klien, B.A., Newell, F.W., and Potts, A.M.: Multifocal inner choroiditis. *Trans Am Acad Ophthalmol Otolaryngol, 73:* 222, 1969.
15. Elliott, J.H., and Jackson, D.J.: Presumed histoplasmic maculopathy: clinical course and prognosis in nonphotocoagulated eyes. *Int Ophthalmol Clin, 15* (3): 29, 1975.
16. Smith, R.E., and Ganley, J.P.: An epidemiologic study of presumed ocular histoplasmosis. *Trans Am Acad Ophthalmol Otolaryngol, 75:* 994, 1971.
17. Gass, J.D.M., and Wilkinson, C.P.: Follow-up study of presumed ocular histoplasmosis. *Trans Am Acad Ophthalmol Otolaryngol, 76:* 672, 1972.
18. Smith, R.E., Knox, D.L., and Jensen, A.D.: Ocular histoplasmosis: significance of asymptomatic macular scars. *Arch Ophthalmol, 89:* 296, 1973.
19. Schlaegel, T.F., Jr.: Panel discussion. *Int Ophthalmol Clin, 15* (3): 147, 1975.
20. Craig, E.L. and Suie, T.: *Histoplasma capsulatum* in human ocular tissue. *Arch Ophthalmol, 91:* 285, 1974.
21. Roth, A.M.: *Histoplasma capsulatum* in the presumed ocular histoplasmosis syndrome. *Am J Ophthalmol, 84:* 293, 1977.
22. Woods, A.C. and Wahlen, H.E.: The probable role of benign histoplasmosis in the etiology of granulomatous uveitis. *Trans Am Ophthalmol Soc, 57:* 318, 1959.
23. Ganley, J.P.: The role of the cellular immune system in patients with macular disciform histoplasmosis. *Int Ophthalmol Clin, 15* (3): 83, 1975.
24. Smith, R.E.: Ocular histoplasmosis. *In* Selected Topics on the Eye in Systemic Disease, Grune & Stratton, New York, 1974, pp. 135–165.
25. Wong, V.G., Kwon-Chung, K.J., Greeb, W.R., Anderson, R.R., Collins, E.M., and Hill, W.B.: Focal choroidopathy in experimental ocular histoplasmosis. *Trans Am Acad Ophthalmol Otolaryngol, 77:* 769, 1973.
26. Watzke, R.C., and Leaverton, P.E.: Light coagulation in presumed ocular histoplasmic choroiditis: a controlled clinical study. *Arch Ophthalmol, 86:* 127, 1971.
27. Patz, A., Ticho, U., and Kelley, J.S.: Some observations on argon laser photocoagulation for the presumed ocular histoplasmosis syndrome. *Mod Prob Ophthalmol, 12:* 288, 1974.
28. Fine, S.L., and Patz, A.: Comparison of xenon arc and argon laser photocoagulation in ocular histoplasmosis. *Int Ophthalmol Clin, 15* (3): 259, 1975.
29. Patz, A., Fine, S.L., and Orth, D.H.: Sights and Sounds in Ophthalmology, vol. 1, C.V. Mosby, St. Louis, 1975.

CHAPTER 18

Angioid Streaks

Jay L. Federman, M.D., Jerry A. Shields, M.D., Terrance L. Tomer, and William H. Annesley, M.D.

Angioid streaks are produced by pathologic alterations of the pigment epithelium, Bruch's membrane, and the choriocapillaris. The primary change appears to be linear, crack-like dehiscences in the collagenous and elastic portions of Bruch's membrane radiating from the peripapillary area with irregular or serrated margins throughout the fundus. Fibrovascular ingrowth from the choriocapillaris through Bruch's membrane into the subpigment epithelial space with secondary pigment proliferation, hemorrhage, exudation, and scar formation may become associated with some of the streaks, particularly those in the macular region. In their typical form, they have a characteristic ophthalmoscopic appearance presenting no diagnostic difficulties for the experienced ophthalmologist. In some instances, however, they may be subtle or may simulate other fundus conditions and the diagnosis may be more difficult. They also may exhibit variations in size, distribution, and color, and be associated with several fundus abnormalities. Angioid streaks are known to be associated with aging and a number of underlying systemic conditions, usually characterized by widespread degeneration of mesodermal tissue and generalized vascular disease. In recent years, fluorescein angiography has become useful in the evaluation of the clinical and histopathologic features of these streaks, and in their early recognition. The clinical and, in particular, the fluorescein angiographic characteristics of angioid streaks are reviewed in this chapter.

Clinical Features

The clinical significance and ophthalmoscopic features of angioid streaks have received considerable attention in the ophthalmologic literature [1–6]. Recently, the ophthalmoscopic variations were reviewed and discussed in a report based on the findings in patients with angioid streaks of the ocular fundus, who were evaluated and photographed by the Retina Service of the Wills Eye Hospital [7]. A total of 56 patients with angioid streaks were studied. All cases were bilateral, and the age ranged from 16–76 years, with a mean of 49 years. There were 50 white patients and 6 black patients; 32 women and 24 men. The visual acuities ranged from 20/20 to hand movements. No patient was completely blind, despite extensive macular involvement in some. One had chronic open angle glaucoma; otherwise, no other significant ocular abnormalities, such as refractive errors, defects in the ocular adnexae, anterior segment or vitreous, were present.

The fundus findings of the angioid streaks were variable (Table 18.1). The streaks demonstrated differences in distribution and color. In addition, several associated fundus findings were frequently present. In each case there was some degree of peripapillary chorioretinal degeneration. The angioid streaks radiated from the peripapillary region as irregular, serrated lines of variable size and shape, lying deep to the retinal vessels. They were confined to within 2 disc diameters of the optic nerve head (peripapillary region) in 15 of the 56 cases (27%). In 41 cases (73%), they were more widespread, radiating in an irregular manner from the optic disc for variable distances in the fundus. In all cases, they tapered to an end before reaching the equator. There was a distinct tendency for the streaks to involve the macula area.

The angioid streaks were gray in 18 cases (32%), and red in 13 (23%). Usually, however, they were an in-between color such as red-brown, or red-gray (Fig. 18.1*A*). In 8 instances (14%), there was pigment proliferation over the angioid streaks, producing a black appearance (Fig. 18.1*B*). The color of the angioid streak appeared to be unrelated to systemic disease, associated fundus changes, or prognosis. Rather it was most likely a function of the pigmentation of the individual eye. It was not uncommon, for example, for angioid streaks to be associated with extensive proliferation and migration of the retinal pigment epithelium in black patients. These marked pigmentary changes on occasion lead to diagnostic confusion, simulating toxoplasmosis.

Macular degeneration, usually bilateral, was present in 40 of the 56 patients (71%) (Fig. 18.1*C*). Nonexudative macular changes, characterized by pigmentary mottling, but no hemorrhages or exudation, were present in 32 cases. Exudative changes consisting of hemorrhage, exudate, serous detachment of the sensory retina and/or pigment epithelium, intraretinal cystoid edema, subretinal neovascularization or scar formation, were present in 8 patients. In 32 patients (57%), there were light areas along the margins of the streaks. These areas extended equidistant from either

Table 18.1. Fundus findings in angioid streaks

Fundus Findings	No.	%
Distribution of streaks		
Peripapillary region only	15	27
Widespread in posterior pole	41	73
Color of streaks		
Gray	18	32
Red	13	23
Combination	25	45
Pigment proliferation into streaks	8	14
Macular degeneration	40	71
Exudative	8	14
Nonexudative	32	57
Mottled fundus (peau d'orange)	34	61
Light margins along streaks	32	57
Peripheral focal lesions	24	43
Fresh hemorrhage	19	34
Paired red spots along streaks	10	18
Drusen of optic disc	5	9

edge of the streak to not more than 3 times the width of the streak.

In 10 cases (18%), poorly delineated, focal, reddish-brown spots, less than ½ disc diameter in size were present just outside the light-colored area along the margins of the angioid streaks. These always occurred in pairs, one on each side of the angioid streaks (Fig. 18.1*D*). Each affected eye had from one to ten pairs of such lesions. These lesions were often subtle and may be easily overlooked unless the fundus is carefully examined. Their exact significance is yet unknown.

Drusen of the optic disc were present in five cases (9%), and were bilateral in each instance (see Fig. 18.1*D*). This association was found in patients with pseudoxanthoma elasticum in every instance.

Focal chorioretinal lesions resembling those seen in presumed ocular histoplasmosis were observed in 24 cases (37%) (Fig. 18.1*E*). These lesions have been referred to as "salmon spots" by some observers. The number of such lesions in a single eye range from 5–30. They were often, but not always, located in close association with a streak. They varied from small, slightly elevated glistening yellow nodules without pigment to well delineated, partially pigmented spots.

Another characteristic finding, usually nasal to the optic disc, consisted of numerous short vertical lines concentric to the disc margin. These resembled a cracked egg shell and appeared to be more common in blacks and young patients.

A mottled appearance in the fundus (peau d'orange) was present in 34 patients (61%) (Fig. 18.1*F*). This consisted of a granular reddish-brown speckled area which usually extended from the macula toward the temporal equator. In two cases, it was more widespread, extending nasally to surround the optic disc. It appeared to be more common in patients with pseudoxanthoma elasticum. This finding was noted to precede the development of angioid streaks in some patients.

Fresh hemorrhages were present in 19 patients (34%). They were most often located in the macular region, but could occur anywhere in the fundus along the course of angioid streaks. There appears to be a relationship between ocular trauma and macular hemorrhage in patients with angioid streaks, although the presence of subretinal neovascularization often complicating this macular disorder in itself is sufficient to predispose to hemorrhage and is the most likely precursor to hemorrhage.

A number of systemic disorders are associated with angioid streaks (Table 18.2). The most frequently encountered systemic disorders are pseudoxanthoma elasticum, Paget's disease, sickle cell anemia, senile elastosis, Marfan's syndrome, Ehlers-Danlos syndrome, and cardiovascular elastorrhexis. They have also been described as associated with diffuse lipomatosis, dwarfism, acromegaly, pituitary tumor, epilepsy, lead poisoning, hypercalcinosis, thrombocytopenia, facial hemangioma, diabetes, systemic lupus erythematosus, exsanguination, and internal carotid aneurysm. These latter associations, however, have not always been clearly established and may indeed be coincidental. In the Wills Eye Hospital study, the diagnosis of pseudoxanthoma elasticum was made on the basis of clinical examination or by skin biopsy in 30 cases (54%). Two patients had sickle cell disease. A 16-year-old white male with angioid streaks and a confirmed diagnosis of pseudoxanthoma elasticum had physical features compatible with Marfan's syndrome. A few patients had mild cardiovascular disease. No patient was known to have Paget's disease. The remainder either had no evidence of medical disease or the medical data were insufficient. Aging is another factor related to the development of angioid streaks and probably represents a principal etiologic factor.

The hereditary aspects to the angioid streaks depend largely on the underlying disease present. In the case of pseudoxanthoma elasticum, angioid streaks are thus usually transmitted as an autosomal recessive characteristic, although there are a few pedigrees which seem to show an irregular dominance. In others, a sex-linked hereditary transmission has been implied. Paget's disease is transmitted as an incomplete autosomal dominant with variable penetrants; Ehlers-Danlos syndrome is usually dominant; sickle cell anemia shows either a dominant or recessive transmission.

The varied fundus findings in angioid streaks will occasionally pose certain problems in differential diagnosis. Angioid streaks are most often misdiagnosed as involutional macular degeneration when examining clinicians fail to recognize that the streaks were the underlying cause. The differentiation should not be difficult in most instances because the macular changes usually occur at a younger age in patients with angioid streaks. In addition, the degenerative process is usually more diffuse, often involving the papillomacular bundle.

On occasion, the fundus picture may be identical with so-called choroidal sclerosis. One of the Wills patients was initially thought to have this entity, but examination of the family revealed a sibling with typical angioid streaks. It is possible that the degeneration of the retinal pigment epithelium and the choriocapillaris may become wider and finally coalesce, so that the streaks become difficult or impossible to recognize even with the aid of fluorescein angiography.

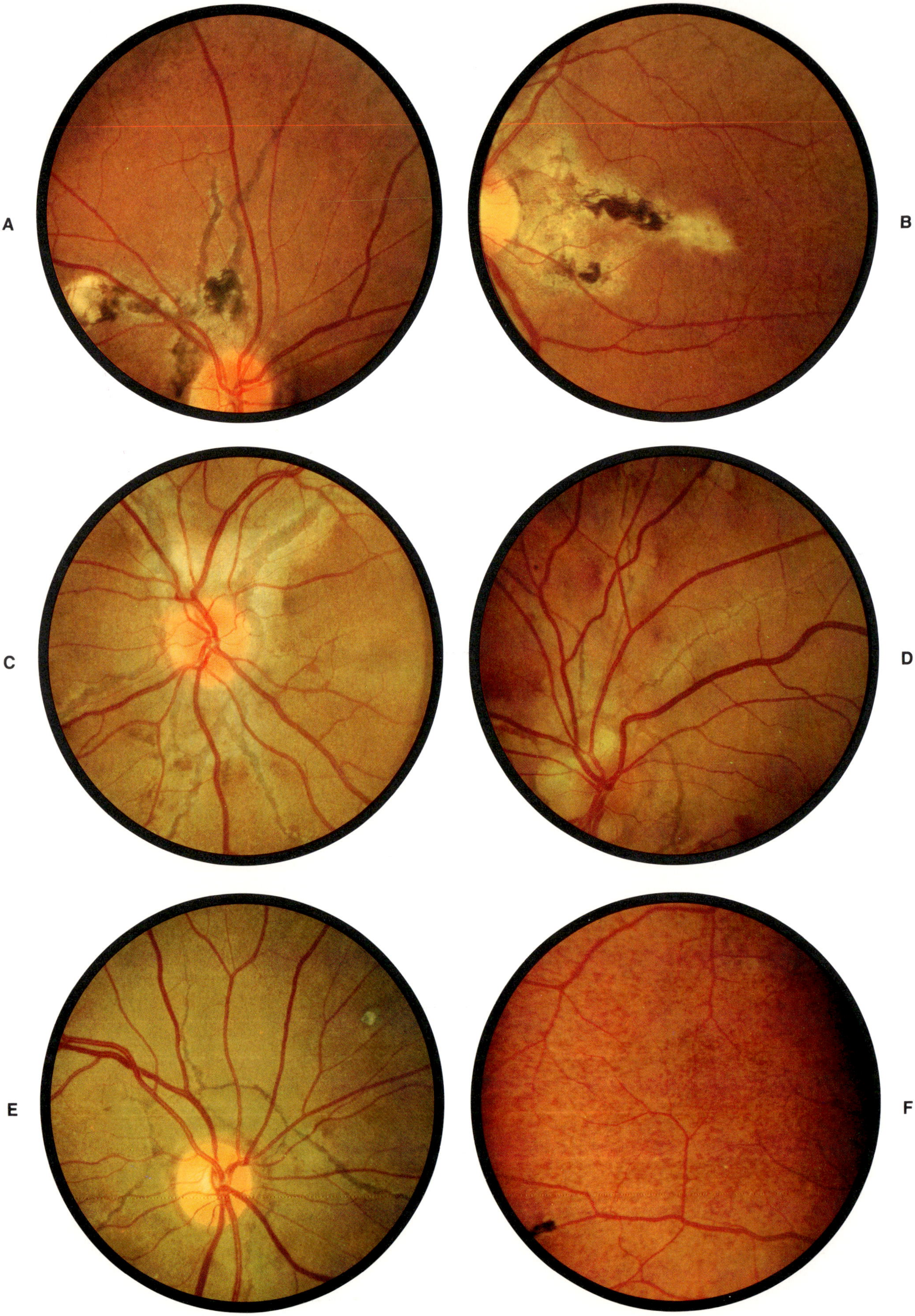
A
B
C
D
E
F

Table 18.2. Systemic conditions associated with angioid streaks

(1) Pseudoxanthoma elasticum
(2) Paget's disease
(3) Sickle cell anemia
(4) Aging
(5) Marfan's syndrome
(6) Ehlers-Danlos syndrome
(7) Cardiovascular elastorrhexis
(8) Diffuse lipomatosis
(9) Dwarfism
(10) Acromegaly
(11) Pituitary tumor
(12) Epilepsy
(13) Lead poisoning
(14) Thrombocytopenia
(15) Hypercalcinosis
(16) Facial hemangioma
(17) Systemic lupus erythematosus
(18) Diabetes
(19) Exsanguination
(20) Internal carotid aneurysm

The peripapillary and macular changes seen with angioid streaks may also simulate hereditary peripapillary choroidopathy or myopic chorioretinal degeneration. The large disc and temporal crescent of myopia, as well as the refractive error, should serve to differentiate the myopic fundus from angioid streaks. In addition, the macular lesion (Fuchs' spot) in myopia usually produces a small and discrete area of subretinal neovascularization in a young patient as opposed to a larger more diffuse fibrovascular membrane seen in angioid streaks. "Lacquer cracks" present in the posterior pole of a myopic eye may resemble angioid streaks, but they are usually isolated to the macular region, do not radiate from the peripapillary location, and are almost exclusively seen in eyes with posterior staphyloma.

Angioid streaks may occasionally simulate certain inflammatory conditions of the fundus. Peripapillary, macular, and peripheral changes may resemble those of ocular histoplasmosis. Most reports in the literature fail to note the close similarity between these two conditions, although in this series there was some degree of peripapillary change in 100% of the patients, macular degeneration in 71%, and focal chorioretinal lesions in 37%. In rare instances, angioid streaks may be confused with ocular toxoplasmosis. This is especially true in black patients in whom considerable pigment proliferation may occur along the margins of the streaks.

The treatment of angioid streaks centers around the possible use of photocoagulation in the management of induced exudative macular degeneration. The tendency for widespread macular involvement and foveal proximity of the subretinal neovascularized complex have led to discouraging experiences in selected cases that have been treated with argon laser. A few patients, however, have had seemingly beneficial results. Patient selection and treatment techniques employed follow the same guidelines presently available for involutional exudative macular degeneration.

Fluorescein Angiography

Fluorescein angiography has provided a new dimension in the study and understanding of angioid streaks [7–13]. In some cases, the streaks may be so subtle that they are not recognized clinically and only made evident on fluorescein angiography.

We have studied 31 patients with angioid streaks in an attempt to clinically evaluate the pathologic features of (1) the red and gray angioid streaks, (2) the light-colored adjacent areas, (3) the paired red-brown spots, (4) the peau d'orange, and (5) the focal lesions. Our findings are summarized below.

In the clinical evaluation of any fundus lesion with fluorescein, the sequential analysis may proceed in three separate phases:

(1) The early filling phase can be divided into two parts, intravascular and extravascular. The intravascular part is the filling of the choriocapillaris with fluorescein. This occurs within the first 8–12 seconds of the study and represents the first component of the background choroidal fluorescence. The fluorescein immediately leaks from the intravascular space into the extravascular stromal layers of the choroid [14, 15]. This extravascular component of the early filling phase is usually completed within the first 60 seconds of the dye study.

(2) As the recirculation phase begins, a greater concentration of fluorescein is found in the extravascular compartment of the choroid than within the choroidal vessels themselves. This usually occurs within 3 minutes, and at this stage of the study, all stromal layers of the choroid should have been saturated equally with fluorescein. By this stage, the fluorescein should be equally distributed throughout the entire body blood volume [14, 15].

(3) The elimination phase of the dye sequence begins early and reaches a peak by 45 minutes. During this stage, the intravascular fluorescein concentration is greatly reduced. The extravascular choroidal fluorescence is reduced similarly and persists in the outer stromal layers and inner scleral fibers. This corresponds to the so-called late phase angiogram.

Following this sequential format for angiographic analysis, there are no differentiating fluorescein characteristics

Figure 18.1. *A*, gray angioid streaks. Note the adjacent white areas. (Corresponds to black and white Fig. 18.2.) *B*, angioid streaks with a dense pigment proliferation and macular degeneration. (Corresponds to black and white Fig. 18.3.) *C*, angioid streaks with adjacent white areas. Note the faintly gray-colored streak that goes through the macula which is dry. (Corresponds to black and white Fig. 18.4.) This eye developed exudative disciform macular degeneration 4 years later. (See black and white Fig. 18.5.) *D*, angioid streaks with paired reddish-brown spots on either side. Note also the presence of drusen at the optic nerve. (Corresponds to black and white Fig. 18.6.) *E*, angioid streaks with a focal chorioretinal lesion ("salmon spot") resembling fundus findings in patients with presumed ocular histoplasmosis. Note the presence of paired reddish-brown spots. *F*, peau d'orange appearance of fundus in an eye with angioid streaks. Note also the presence of a tiny chorioretinal lesion. (Corresponds to black and white Fig. 18.8.)

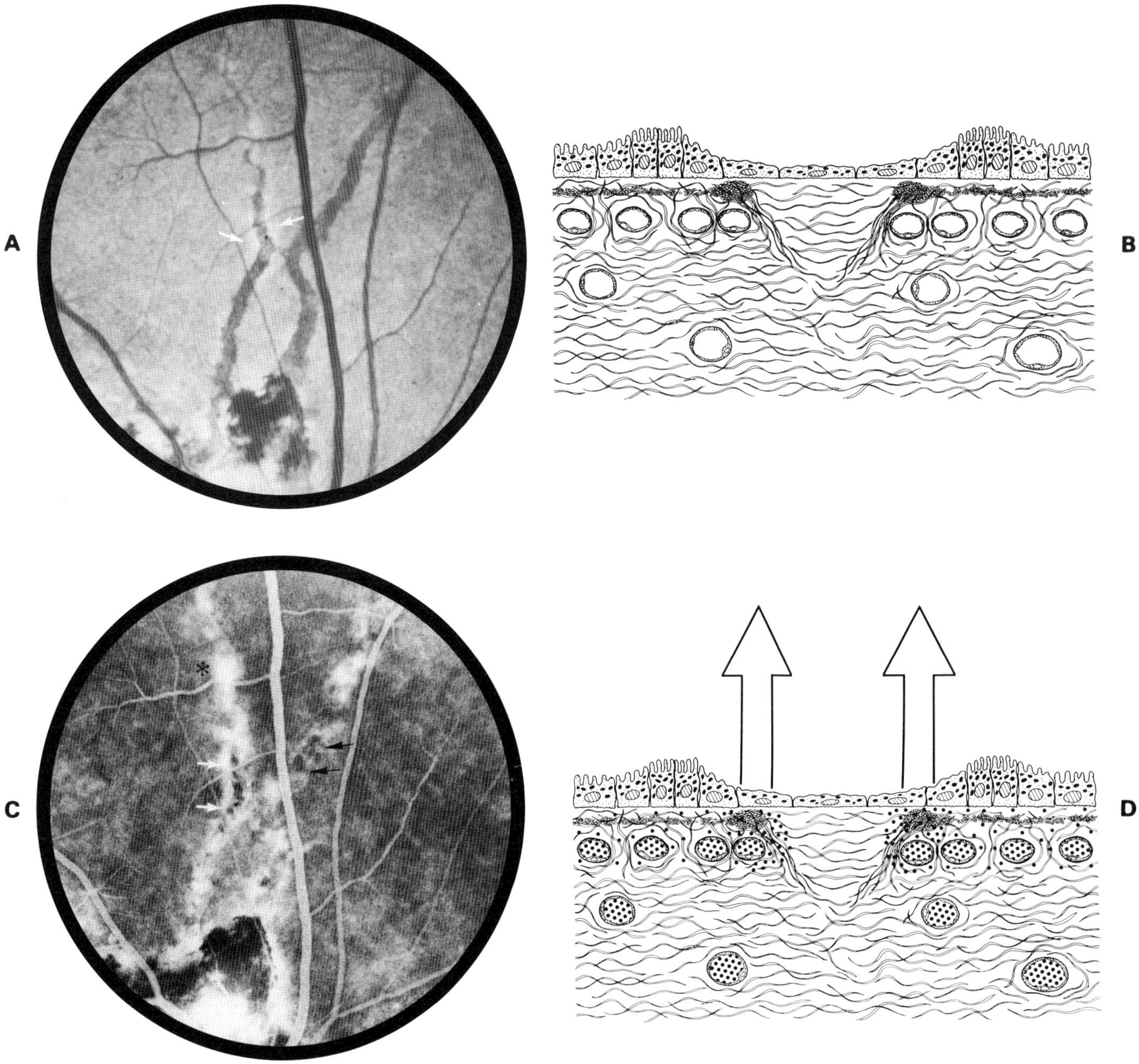

Figure 18.2. Fluorescein patterns of angioid streaks. *A*, ophthalmoscopic photo of typical angioid streaks. Note light-colored adjacent areas (*arrows*). *B*, suggested schematic cross-section of angioid streak in (*A*, *arrows*). Choriocapillaris is separated, corresponding to break in Bruch's membrane, which is not as wide as area of overlying retinal pigment epithelium. (RPE). Bruch's membrane is thickened at edges of break. *C*, early venous phase angiogram (intravascular filling phase). Note hypofluorescent areas (*white and black arrows*) running along central portion of streaks. Hyperfluorescent borders correspond to light-colored adjacent areas seen in (*A*). In some areas, central portion of streak is hyperfluorescent (*asterisk*). *D*, suggested schematic cross-section of streak in (*C*) depicting areas with central zone of hypofluorescence. Fluorescein (*black dots*) has filled intravascular space of choroid and is beginning to leak from choriocapillaris into surrounding extravascular inner choroidal stroma and Bruch's membrane. Absence of fluorescein (*black dots*) in area of streak itself explains hypofluorescent zone seen during this phase of dye study. At edges of streak, thickened Bruch's membrane and bunched-together choriocapillaris show denser accumulation of dye (*black dots*) through overlying thinned RPE and represents hyperfluorescent adjacent borders. *E*, late venous phase angiogram. (Extravascular filling phase and early recirculation phase of fluorescein study.) Area previously seen with central zone of hypofluorescence has now become hyperfluorescent (*white arrows*), due to extravascular leakage of dye. Other areas continue to

during any phase related to the color of the angioid streaks. Patients with red and gray streaks exhibit similar fluorescein patterns. It is interesting to note that, during the early filling phase, angioid streaks usually show an area of hypofluorescence (Figs. 18.2*C*, 18.3*C*, 18.4*B*, and 18.5*B*) corresponding with the central zone of the streak (Figs. 18.2*A*, 18.3*A*, 18.4*A*, and 18.5*A*). This comparative hypofluorescent zone remains throughout both the recirculation and elimination phases of the study (Fig. 18.2*E* and 18.2*G*, *black arrows*). These hypofluorescent zones may also be interrupted by

E

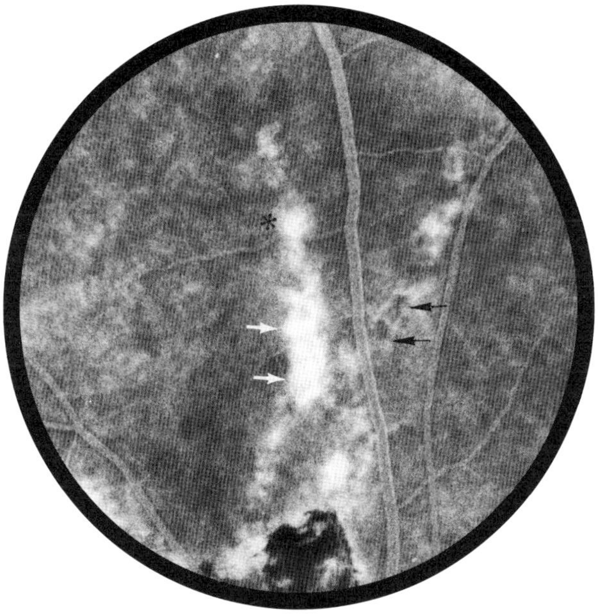

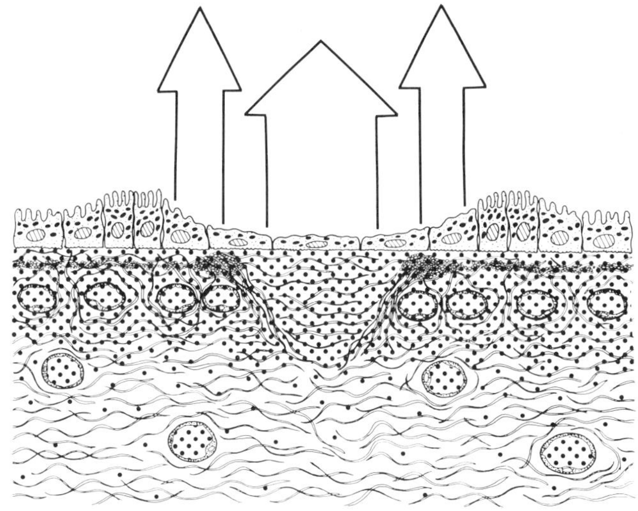

F

G

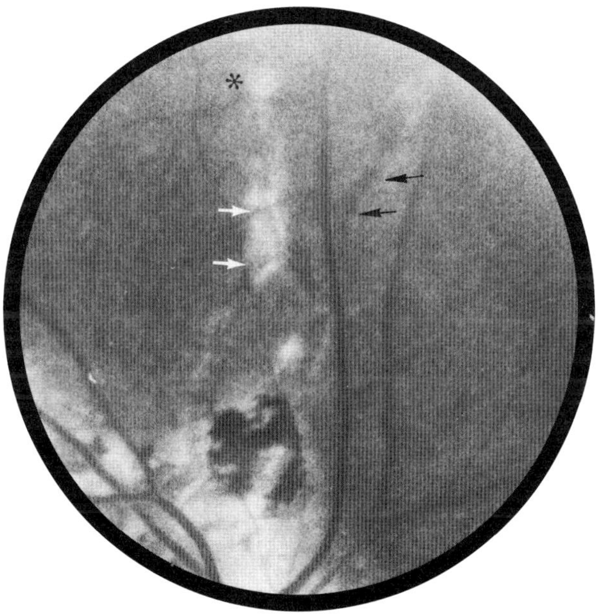

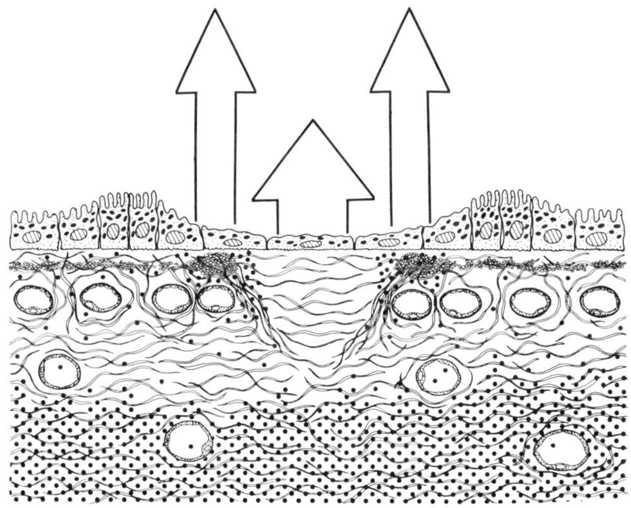

H

show hypofluorescence (*black arrows*) in central zone due to continued relative lack of fluorescein. Earlier fluorescent central zone continues to show hyperfluorescence (*asterisk*) during this phase, due to presence of dye. *F*, suggested schematic cross-section explaining mechanism of hyperfluorescent central zone in (*E*, *white arrows*). Note fluorescein (*black dots*) has now leaked from choriocapillaris into Bruch's membrane and entire inner choroidal extravascular stroma, filling space within break in Bruch's membrane. Fluorescence is transmitted through entire layer of thin RPE (*open large arrows*) while adjacent denser pigment layer within normal RPE continues to block underlying choroidal fluorescence. *G*, late phase angiogram showing relative hypofluorescence (*white arows*) in central zone of streak that was previously hyperfluorescent in (*E*) and hypofluorescent in (*C*). Note adjacent light-colored areas continue to show relative hyperfluorescence. Central zone of hypofluorescence (*black arrows*) of streak on right has continued throughout entire study because of persistent relative absence of dye. Apical portion of streak that showed hyperfluorescence earlier exhibits less intense fluorescence (*asterisk*). *H*, suggested schematic cross-section of streak in (*G*, *white arrows*). During elimination phase of study, fluorescein (*black dots*) persists in outer extravascular choroidal layers in thickened Bruch's membrane at edges of streak. Fluorescence is due to transmission (*open large arrows*) through thin RPE of underlying dye. Adjacent normal RPE continues to block out surrounding choroidal fluorescence.

focal areas of hyperfluorescence seen as one of three different sequential patterns:

(1) In some cases, a focal area of hyperfluorescence can be seen within the central zone of the streak during the early intravascular filling phase. This increases in intensity by the recirculation phase, and gradually diminishes during the late elimination phase (Figs. 18.2*C*, 18.2*E*, and 18.2*G*, *asterisks*).

(2) In other instances, intermittent areas of hyperfluorescence crossing some streaks, seen during the early intravas-

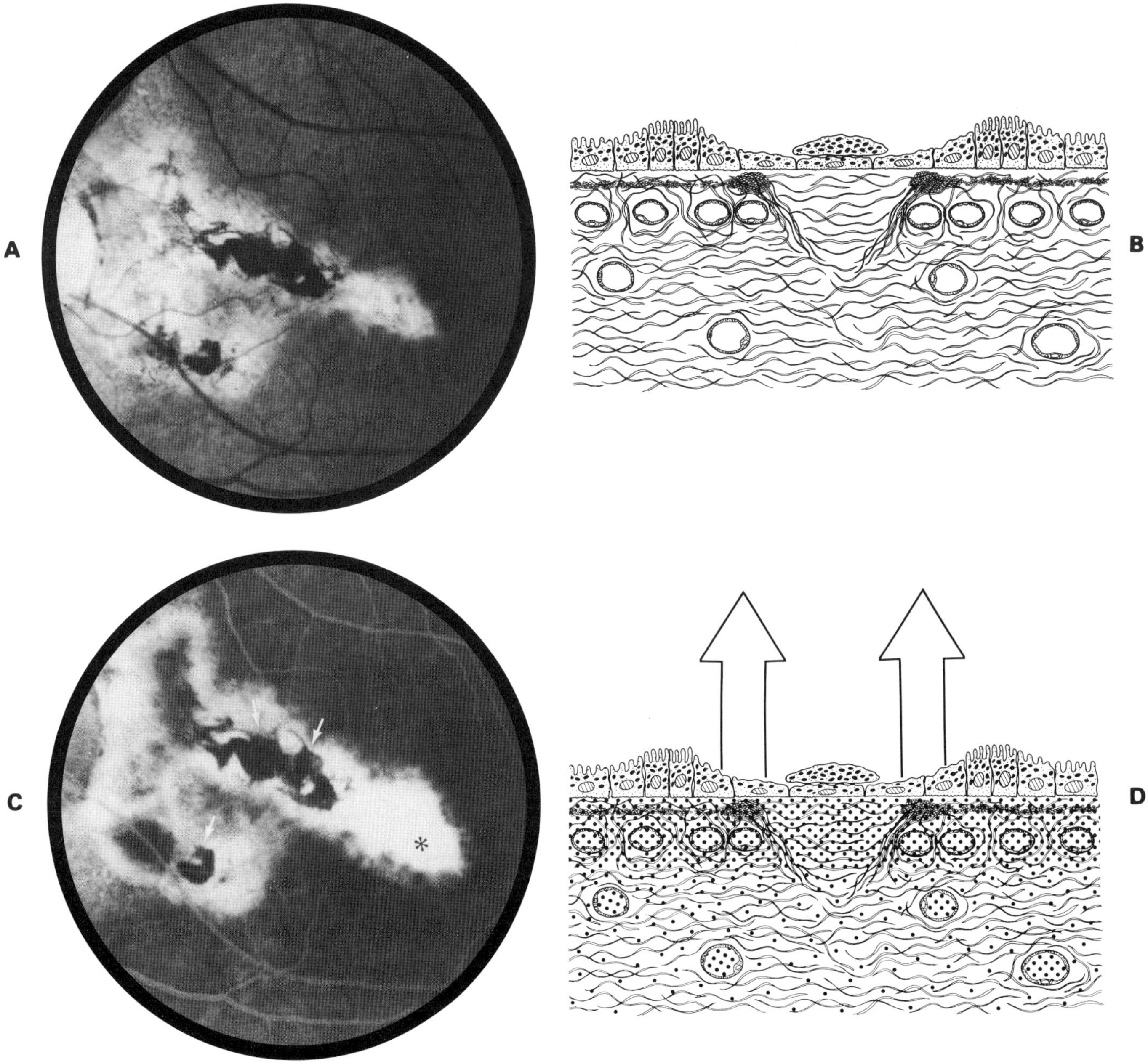

Figure 18.3. Hypofluorescence of angioid streak due to blockage. *A*, clinical appearance of streak with hyperpigmented central zone. *B*, suggested schematic cross-section of hyperpigmented streak in (*A*). In central zone overlying the streak, there is dense layer of pigment due to presence of pigmented macrophages or duplication of RPE. *C*, late venous phase angiogram (early extravascular filling phase) showing hypofluorescence (*white arrows*) in central zone of streak, corresponding to area of hyperpigmentation. Note hyperfluorescence (*asterisk*) at apex of streak in macular area presumably due to presence of patent vessels. *D*, suggested schematic cross-section of fluorescein (*black dots*) present in inner choroidal layers is blocked by dense pigmentation in central region of streak. Transmission (*large open arrows*) occurs through thin overlying RPE along both edges corresponding to hyperfluorescent borders. Surrounding normal RPE continues to block out normal background choroidal fluorescence.

cular filling phase, rapidly diminish by the recirculation phase (Fig. 18.4*B*, *upper streak*).

(3) While still in other instances, the areas of hyperfluorescence in some streaks do not appear until the extravascular filling of the inner choroidal stromal layers develops, replacing a previous zone of hypofluorescence. These hyperfluorescent areas gradually diminish again in the late elimination phase of the study (Fig. 18.2*C*, 18.2*E*, and 18.2*G*, *white arrows*).

One or a combination of several factors may be responsible for a hypofluorescent zone during an angiographic series: (1) the absence of dye in an area where it is normally found, (2) a weaker concentration of fluorescein than normal for that area, or (3) blockage of fluorescence by overlying tissue changes [15].

One can best explain the very early hypofluorescent patterns corresponding to the central portion of the streaks (Figs. 18.2*C*, 18.3*C*, 18.4*C*, and 18.5*B*) by a relative absence

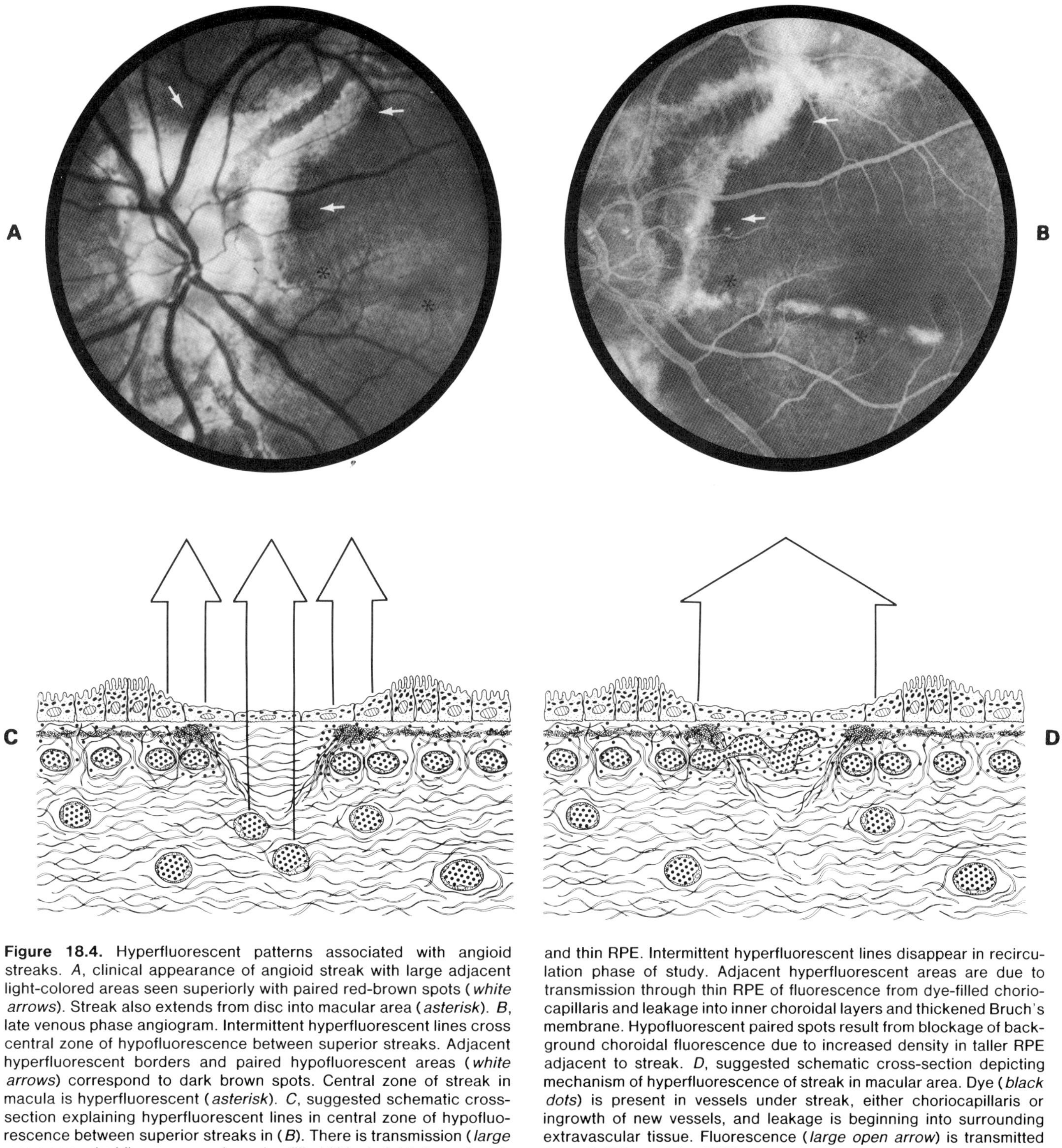

Figure 18.4. Hyperfluorescent patterns associated with angioid streaks. *A*, clinical appearance of angioid streak with large adjacent light-colored areas seen superiorly with paired red-brown spots (*white arrows*). Streak also extends from disc into macular area (*asterisk*). *B*, late venous phase angiogram. Intermittent hyperfluorescent lines cross central zone of hypofluorescence between superior streaks. Adjacent hyperfluorescent borders and paired hypofluorescent areas (*white arrows*) correspond to dark brown spots. Central zone of streak in macula is hyperfluorescent (*asterisk*). *C*, suggested schematic cross-section explaining hyperfluorescent lines in central zone of hypofluorescence between superior streaks in (*B*). There is transmission (*large open arrows*) of fluorescence from dye-filled (*black dots*) deep choroidal vessels through area void of Bruch's membrane, choriocapillaris, and thin RPE. Intermittent hyperfluorescent lines disappear in recirculation phase of study. Adjacent hyperfluorescent areas are due to transmission through thin RPE of fluorescence from dye-filled choriocapillaris and leakage into inner choroidal layers and thickened Bruch's membrane. Hypofluorescent paired spots result from blockage of background choroidal fluorescence due to increased density in taller RPE adjacent to streak. *D*, suggested schematic cross-section depicting mechanism of hyperfluorescence of streak in macular area. Dye (*black dots*) is present in vessels under streak, either choriocapillaris or ingrowth of new vessels, and leakage is beginning into surrounding extravascular tissue. Fluorescence (*large open arrow*) is transmitted through thin overlying RPE.

of dye from a filling defect in the choriocapillaris. During the early intravascular filling phase this takes place from nonperfusion of the choriocapillaris as a result of absent or atrophic capillaries (Figs. 18.2*B*, 18.2*D*, and 18.4*C*). It is generally agreed that angioid streaks represent actual breaks in Bruch's membrane with thinning or atrophy of the overlying retinal pigment epithelium (RPE). These changes in the RPE might lead one to expect hyperfluorescence due to transmission of the underlying choroidal fluorescence. However, close study of the published photographs in the earlier reports show several hypofluorescent zones that appear to correspond to the streaks. The absence of dye best explains the resulting hypofluorescence of the angioid streak in the presence of an overlying atrophic RPE. The

A 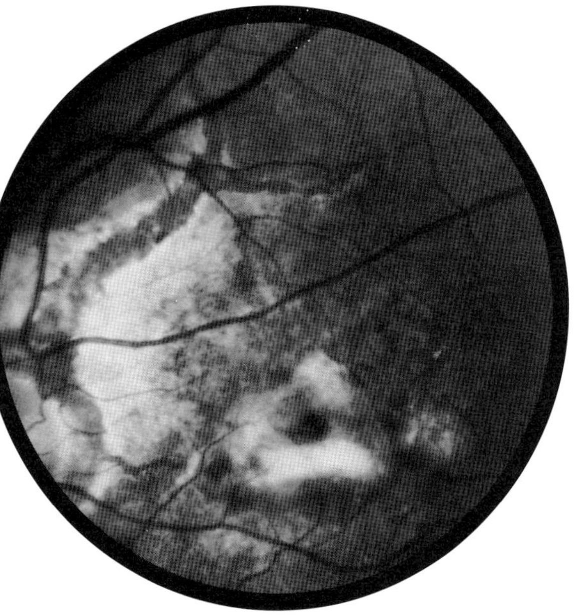 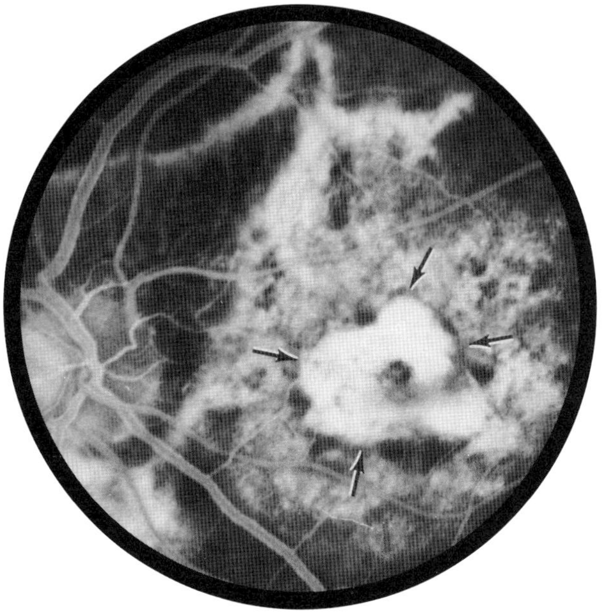 B

Figure 18.5. Development of disciform maculopathy over previous hyperfluorescent streak and disappearance of paired red-brown spots. *A*, clinical appearance of same area seen in Figure 18.4*A*, 3 years later. Disciform macular lesion is present where hyperfluorescent streak in Figure 18.4*B*, was seen. Paired red-brown spots visible in Figure 18.4*A* are no longer present. *B*, late venous phase angiogram of same eye 4 years after Figure 18.4*B*. Disciform macular lesion is hyperfluorescent and paired hypofluorescent areas depicted by *white arrows* in Figure 18.4*B* are absent. Note the diffuse hyperfluorescence of the subretinal neovascularized membrane (*arrows*) except for a central hypofluorescent spot which corresponds to the retinal pigment xanthophyll.

choriocapillaris has been reported to be absent, atrophic, or replaced by fibrous tissue below the break in Bruch's membrane [12, 20].

A break occurring in Bruch's membrane with a corresponding separation involving the choriocapillaris is what one would expect to occur knowing the fine structural relationship of the components comprising the inner choroidal layers. There is a complex arrangement between the elastic and collagen fibers in Bruch's membrane and the adjacent RPE, choriocapillaris, and choroidal layers. The inner and outer collagenous layers of Bruch's membrane are connected through spaces in the elastic layer (Fig. 18.6*A*). The collagen fibers run in many different directions, some parallel to the plane of the Bruch's membrane and others oriented 90 degrees away from this plane [23–25]. The fibers oriented in a plane running from the RPE to the sclera seem to wrap around the capillaries of the choriocapillaris and intermesh with the deeper collagen bundles of the choroidal stroma (Fig. 18.6*A*). The organization of this collagen meshwork holding the choroidal structures firmly in place is in agreement with earlier histologic studies showing a definite organization of the choroidal connective tissue around the vascular components. This histologic basis of an angioid streak represented by a break in Bruch's membrane most likely occurs due to defect of the elastic tissue components [17–22]. As the elastic component separates, since the more vertically oriented collagen fibers are intimately associated and intermeshed with the deeper stromal collagen (Fig. 18.6*A*), it is conceivable that these also separate and pull the choriocapillaris apart toward either edge of the break (Fig. 18.6, *B* through *D*). It would seem virtually impossible for the choriocapillaris to spread apart in the exact configuration of the angioid streak because the choriocapillaris itself is a complex monolayer of interconnected capillaries. Thus, there would be interrupted areas along the streak where patent capillaries of the choriocapillaris persist within the streak. This would help to explain some of the areas of hyperfluorescence seen in the central portion of the streak during the early intravascular filling phase (Figs. 18.2*C*, 18.2*C*, and 18.4*B, asterisks*).

LIGHT-COLORED ADJACENT AREAS

The light-colored adjacent areas straddling either side of the angioid streaks (Fig. 18.2*A*, 18.3*A*, 18.4*A*, and 18.5*A*) exhibit marked hyperfluorescence during the early filling phases of angiography (Figs. 18.2*C*, 18.3*C*, 18.4*B*, and 18.5*B*). This hyperfluorescence is seen to persist during recirculation, often becoming more intense (Fig. 18.2*E, arrows*). As the adjacent areas of hyperfluorescence intensify, they appear to encroach upon the hyperfluorescent streak itself (Fig. 18.2*C* and 18.2*E white arrows*). The area of the streak, however, most often remains relatively hypofluorescent (Fig. 18.2*C*, 18.2*E*, and 18.2*G, black arrows*). These adjacent areas of hyperfluorescence gradually diminish during the late elimination phases of the study (Fig. 18.2*G*).

The inner collagen network appears to end abruptly at the basal lamina of the RPE, and these collagen fibers are not seen to intermesh with the RPE cells [24]. As Bruch's membrane separates in the area of the streak, it may slide under and put gentle tension on the RPE. If there is tension pulling the RPE aside, the tight junctions (zonular occludens) at the apex of these cells may help to hold them together. The RPE over the streak becomes thin and atrophic (Fig. 18.6, *B* through *D*) perhaps due to tension on the cells exerted by the break in Bruch's membrane or, more important, by a lack of blood supply due to an absent choriocapillaris in the area of the streak. In some areas, the RPE may be completely absent. The area of thinned or atrophic RPE is often wider than the actual break in Bruch's membrane (Fig. 18.6, *B* through *D*).

As Bruch's membrane breaks, if the choriocapillaris separates and is pulled to either side of the streak, these capillaries may be more bunched together at the edges of the streak under a thickened Bruch's membrane (Fig. 18.6, *B* through *D*). Hyperfluorescence will occur as these vessels fill and leak during the early filling phase of the dye study (Figs. 18.2*D*, 18.2*F*, 18.2*H*, 18.3*D*, and 18.4*C*). This is exaggerated because the fluorescence is transmitted through a thinned and atrophic RPE. The thickened abnormal Bruch's membrane may retain a greater concentration of the dye longer than normal, explaining why these areas continue to show fluorescence in the very late phases of the study (Fig. 18.2*G*, and *H*). Another explanation might be the presence of fibrous tissue in these areas, which stain and fluoresce late.

RED-BROWN SPOTS

During the early filling phases of the angiographic sequence, the paired red-brown spots (Figs. 18.4*A* and 18.7*A*) are seen as focal areas of hypofluorescence with abrupt edges bordering the hyperfluorescent zone corresponding to the previously described light-colored areas (Figs. 18.4*B* and 18.7*C*). The opposite border of the hypofluorescent red-brown spot gradually blends with the general background choroidal fluorescence (Figs. 18.4*B* and 18.7*C*). A relative hypofluorescence corresponding to the red-brown spots remains through both the recirculation and elimination phases of the study. This hypofluorescence is due to blockage of the background choroidal fluorescence by an increased pigment density at the level of the RPE (Figs. 18.4*C* and 18.7*D*). When Bruch's membrane recoils to either side of the break, it stretches, thins, and sometimes even ruptures the overlying RPE. To accommodate these changes the adjacent RPE might bunch together, causing the cells to be taller adjacent to the streak and, thus, increasing the pigment density (Figs. 18.6, *B* through *D*, and 18.7*B*). This would explain the well demarcated hypofluorescent border facing the streak in these areas (Figs. 18.4*B* and 18.7*C*). According to this concept, as one moves away from the central zone of the streak, the tall RPE cells flatten and appear similar to the surrounding RPE (Fig. 18.7*B*). The hypofluorescence for the same reason becomes less intense

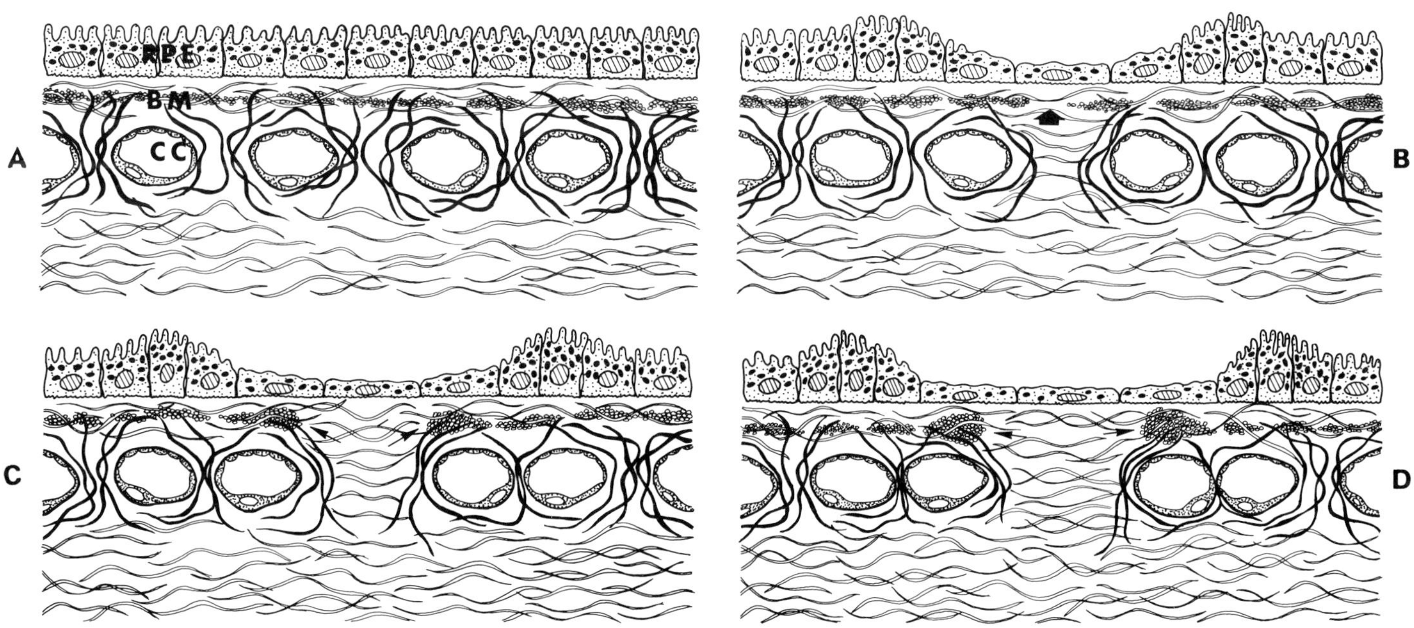

Figure 18.6. Schematic cross-section of RPE and inner choroidal layers depicting postulated development of angioid streaks. *A*, normal anatomic relationship of RPE and inner choroidal layers. Horizontal collagen bundles (*white fibers*) run parallel with plane of Bruch's membrane (*BM*). Vertical collagen bundles (*black fibers*) running through elastic portion (*small open circles*) of Bruch's membrane wind around capillaries of choriocapillaris (*CC*) and intertwine with horizontal collagen bundles above and below choriocapillaris. *B*, break occurs in Bruch's membrane (*arrow*) due to defective elastic tissue component. As elastic portion separates, vertical collagen fibers are pulled to either side of break. Because these fibers are tightly wound around capillaries, corresponding separation of choriocapillaris develops. Tension may also be exerted on overlying RPE, causing these cells to become wider and flatter, while adjacent cells become bunched together and, thus, taller. *C*, as break in Bruch's membrane (*arrows*) and resulting separation of choriocapillaris become wider, overlying pigment is seen to be less dense due to greater thinning and atrophy of RPE. Thinned RPE overlaps thickened abnormal Bruch's membrane (*arrows*) along edge of angioid streak. *D*, break in Bruch's membrane (*arrows*) with resulting separation of choriocapillaris and thinning of overlying RPE represents angioid streak. At edges of streak, capillaries of choriocapillaris are crowded together and abnormal components of Bruch's membrane are greatly thickened. Width of thin RPE overlaps edges of break and thickened Bruch's membrane (*arrows*) is white border along streak. Adjacent bunched-up taller RPE causes greater pigment density and may represent red-brown spots.

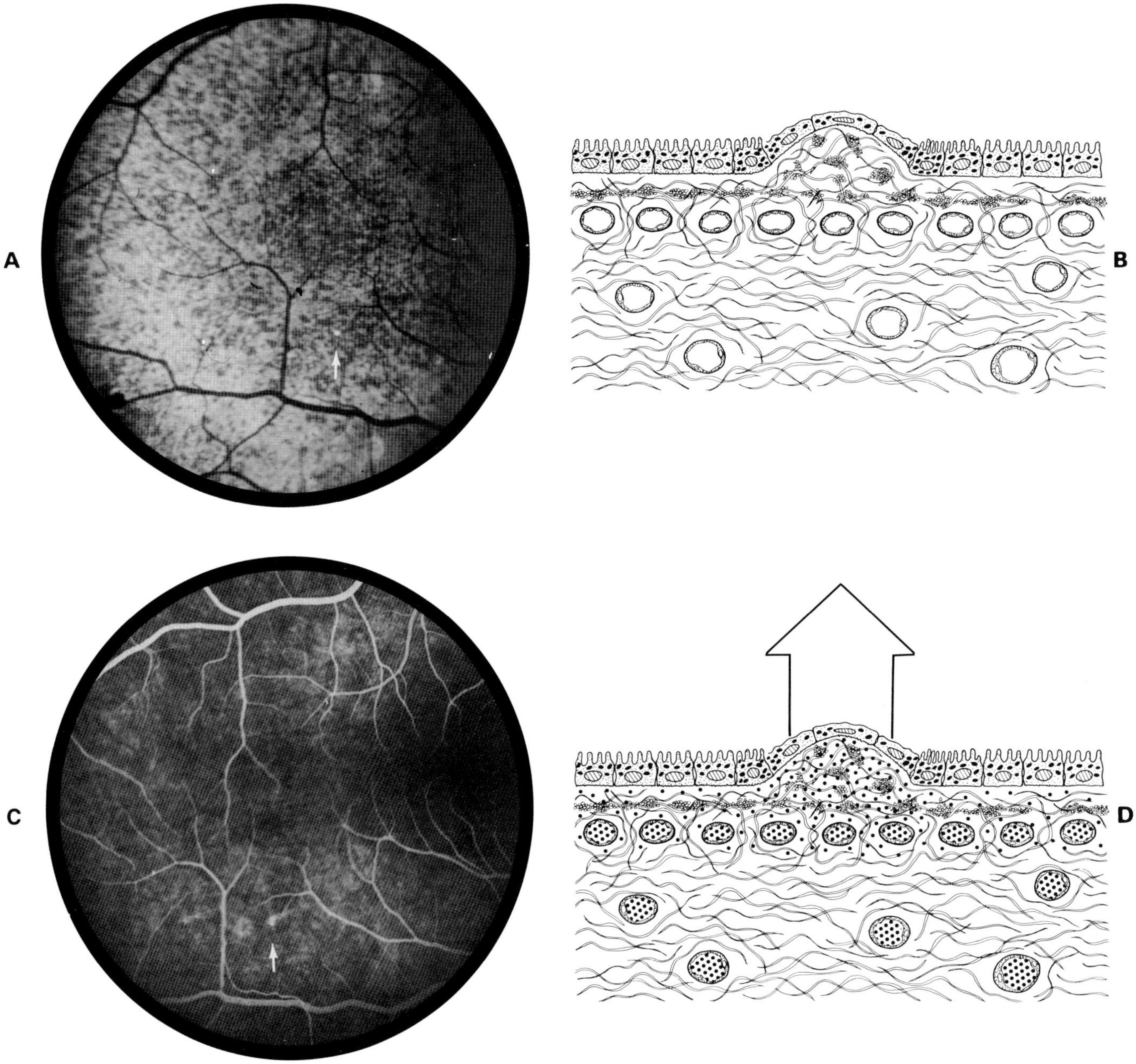

Figure 18.7. Hypofluorescence of paired red-brown spots. *A*, clinical appearance of red-brown spots (*white arrows*) usually occurring in pairs opposite each other along margins of light-colored adjacent areas of streaks. *B*, suggested schematic cross-section through streak with adjacent paired red-brown spots. As RPE stretches and thins over break in Bruch's membrane, adjacent areas of RPE bunch up and become crowded together. These taller than normal RPE cells (*black arrows*) have thicker pigment density and may represent paired red-brown spots. *C*, late venous phase angiogram (extravascular filling phase and early recirculation phase). Note hypofluorescent red-brown spots (*white arrows*) seen in (*A*). *D*, suggested schematic cross-section showing hypofluorescence of paired red-brown spots due to blockage of underlying choroidal fluorescence secondary to increased pigment density (*black arrows*). Angioid streak with overlying thin pigment epithelium fluoresces due to transmission (*open large arrow*) of extravascular choroidal dye (*black dots*).

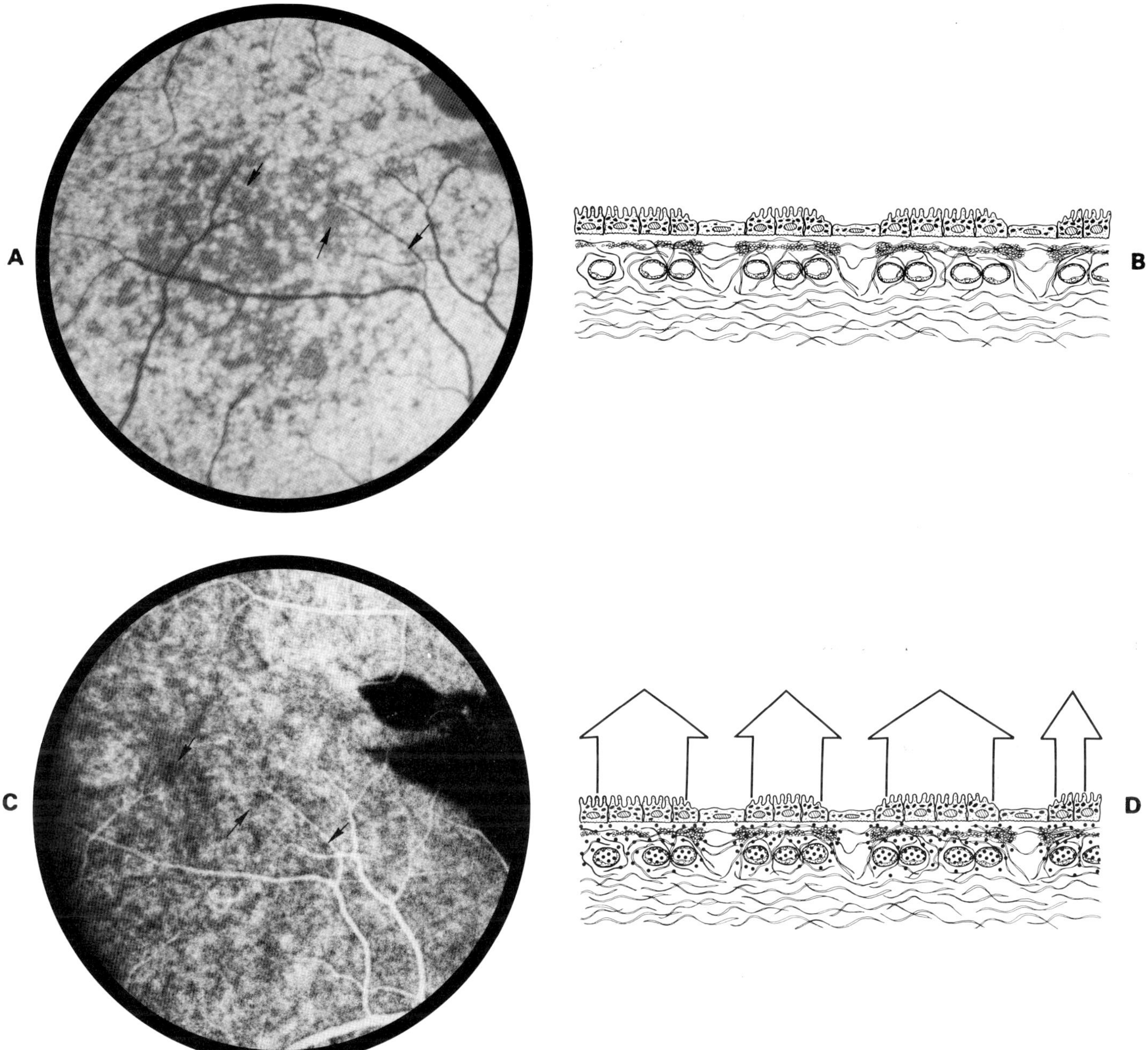

Figure 18.8. Fluorescein pattern of peau d'orange. *A*, clinical appearance of area of peau d'orange. Focal irregular dark spots (*arrows*) are of similar texture and color as streaks and correspond to hypofluorescent spots seen in (*C*). *B*, suggested schematic cross-section postulated to represent area of peau d'orange. Intermittent focal areas of thin RPE with underlying absence of Bruch's membrane and choriocapillaris correspond to dark spots seen clinically in (*A*). *C*, late venous phase angiogram area of peau d'orange. Note the multiple irregular hypofluorescent spots (*arrows*) that correspond to dark spots seen spots. *C*, late venous phase angiogram (extravascular filling phase and early recirculation phase). Note hypofluorescent red-brown spots (*white arrows*) seen in (*A*). *D*, suggested schematic cross-section showing hypofluorescence of paired red-brown spots due to blockage of underlying choroidal fluorescence secondary to increased pigment density (*black arrows*). Angioid streak with overlying thin pigment epithelium fluoresces due to transmission (*open large arrow*) of extravascular choroidal dye (*black dots*).

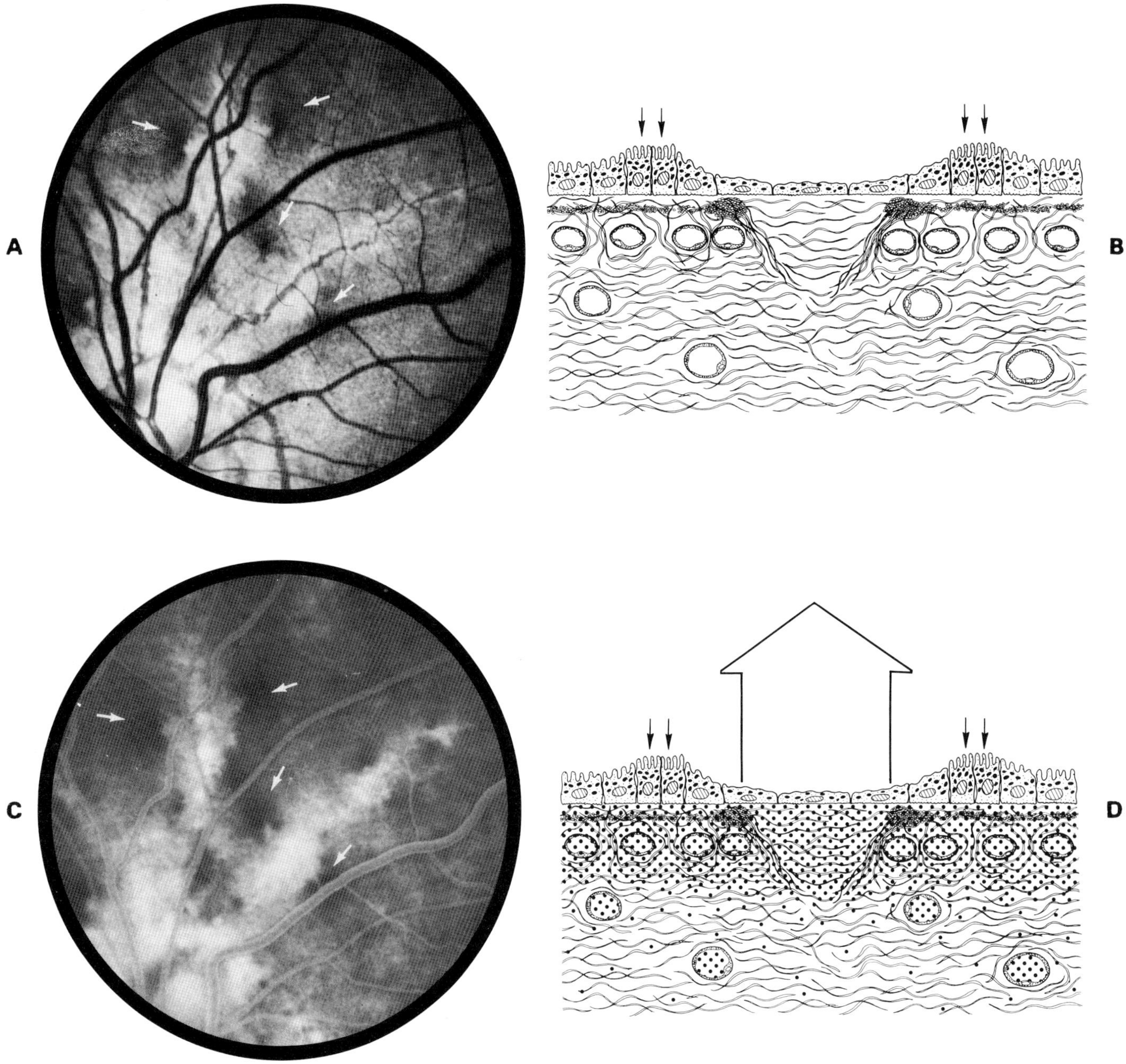

Figure 18.9. Hyperfluorescence of focal lesions. *A*, clinical appearance of small light-colored focal lesion (*arrow*). *B*, suggested schematic cross-section of focal lesion depicting this as thickened focal area of disrupted elastic and collagen fibers involving Bruch's membrane. Overlying RPE is stretched and thinned. *C*, late venous phase angiogram showing hyperfluorescence (*arrow*) of focal lesion. *D*, suggested schematic cross-section explaining mechanism of hyperfluorescence of focal lesion in (*C*). Dye (*black dots*) is present in extravascular tissue surrounding choriocapillaris due to leakage. Fluorescein (*black dots*) accumulating in focal lesion is transmitted (*large open arrow*) through overlying thin RPE.

and blends with the surrounding fluorescence (Fig. 18.7, *C* and *D*). These areas possibly may occur early in the development of angioid streaks (Fig. 18,4, *A* and *C*) and with time gradually disappear as the RPE adjusts itself (Fig. 18.5, *A* and *B*). These paired red-brown spots thus may be a sign that the break in Bruch's membrane has occurred recently.

PEAU D'ORANGE

Areas of peau d'orange (Fig. 18.8*A*) exhibit a similar pattern as seen with the angioid streaks, i.e. areas of hypofluorescence corresponding to the focal red or gray spots (Fig. 18.8, *B* and *C*). These areas of hypofluorescence are surrounded by zones of hyperfluorescence or normal fluorescence, often making it extremely difficult to correlate these findings with the clinical picture. This pattern essentially remains unchanged during the recirculation and elimination phases of the study. Since these areas are of the same color as the streaks and exhibit a similar fluorescein pattern, they may also represent focal breaks in Bruch's membrane and the choriocapillaris. These areas are usually seen temporal to the macula in the mid-periphery. It may be that the intraocular pressure exerted on Bruch's membrane differs geographically within the globe. Thus, a weakened Bruch's membrane may break with linear cracks posteriorly and small focal dehiscences in the mid-periphery (Fig. 18.8*B*). These hypofluorescent spots may be explained by focal areas of nonperfusion due to dehiscences in Bruch's membrane and the choriocapillaris (Fig. 18.8*D*).

FOCAL LESIONS

The isolated focal lesions seen in the fundus of patients with angioid streaks (Fig. 18.9*A*) show hyperfluorescence during early intravascular filling phase (Fig. 18.9*C*). This hyperfluorescence persists during the recirculation phase and gradually diminishes in the late elimination phase of the study. Thus, one would expect patent vessels in these areas, perhaps either the choriocapillaris or new vessels. Neovascularization might be present if these focal lesions represented tiny mounds of fibrous tissue. Another possibility is that these focal lesions are primary, occurring as a result of the same abnormality of Bruch's membrane that causes angioid streaks. It is conceivable that, with disorganization, thickening, and calcification of the components of Bruch's membrane, other changes in addition to angioid streaks might occur. A small focal disorganized mass of thickened elastic tissue and collagen fibers, with or without calcium deposition, could form and result in a thinning of the overlying RPE (Fig. 18.9*B*). If the choriocapillaris remained patent under such an area, clinically it would exhibit hyperfluorescence early during the intravascular filling phase (Fig. 18.9*C*). The hyperfluorescence would increase during the extravascular filling as the tissue mound itself filled with dye (Fig. 18.9*D*). Such a lesion would continue to fluoresce in the late elimination phases of the study, the same sequence as seen clinically in these isolated focal lesions.

In summary, an attempt has been made to correlate the fluorescein angiographic findings of angioid streaks and associated fundus abnormalities with the underlying histopathology. Hypofluorescence is explained on the basis of a relative absence of fluorescein due to loss of the choriocapillaris and, to a lesser degree, to tissue blockage. Early hyperfluorescence is explained on the basis of patent vessels visible through atrophic pigment epithelium. Late hyperfluorescence is due to leak from subretinal neovascularization and staining of visible sclera and scar tissue. Hopefully, careful evaluation of the fluorescein angiographic sequences in patients with angioid streaks will provide a better understanding of the pathogenesis of this condition. This, in turn, may lead to future therapeutic alternatives designed to prevent irreversible loss of central vision so commonly seen in these patients.

References

1. Doyne, R.W.: Choroidal and retinal changes: the results of blows on the eyes. *Trans Ophthalmol Soc U K, 9:* 128, 1889.
2. Scholz, R.O.: Angioid streaks. *Arch Ophthalmol, 26:* 677, 1941.
3. Geeraets, W.J., and Guerry, D.P., III: Angioid streaks and sickle-cell disease. *Am J Ophthalmol, 49:* 450, 1960.
4. Shimizu, K.: Mottled fundus in association with pseudoxanthoma elasticum. *Jpn J Ophthalmol, 5:* 1, 1961.
5. Percival, S.P.B.: Angioid streaks and elastorrhexis. *Brit J Ophthalmol, 52:* 297, 1968.
6. Shields, J.A., Federman, J.L., Tomer, T.L., and Annesley, W.H.: Angioid streaks. I. Ophthalmoscopic variations and diagnostic problems. *Brit J Ophthalmol, 59:* 257, 1975.
7. Federman, J.L., Shields, J.A., and Tomer, T.L.: Angioid streaks. *Arch Ophthalmol, 93:* 951, 1975.
8. Smith, J.L., Gass, J.D.M., and Justice, J., Jr.: Fluorescein fundus photography of angioid streaks. *Brit J Ophthalmol, 48:* 517, 1964.
9. Rosen, E.: Fundus in pseudoxanthoma elasticum. *Am J Ophthalmol, 66:* 236, 1968.
10. Kalina, R.E.: Facial angiomatosis with angioid streaks. Association of angioid streaks with a component of the Sturge-Weber syndrome. *Arch Ophthalmol, 84:* 528, 1970.
11. Patnaik, B., and Malik, S.R.K.: Fluorescein fundus photography of angioid streaks. *Brit J Ophthalmol, 55:* 833, 1971.
12. Gass, J.D.M. and Clarkson, J.G.: Angioid streaks and disciform macular detachment in Paget's disease (osteitis deformans). *Am J Ophthalmol, 75:* 576, 1973.
13. von Winning, C.H.O.M. and Oosterhuis, J.A.: A fluorographic study of reticular patterns in the fundus. *Am J Ophthalmol, 77:* 491, 1974.
14. Hyvarinen, L. and Maumenee, A.E.: Interpretation of choroidal fluorescence. *In* Proceedings of the International Symposium on Fluorescein Angiography, J. Karger, Basel, 1971, pp. 183–190.
16. Hagedoorn, A.: Angioid streaks. *Arch Ophthalmol, 21:* 746–774 and 935–965, 1939.
17. Verhoeff, F.H.: Histological findings in a case of angioid streaks. *Brit J Ophthalmol, 32:* 531, 1948.
18. Klien, B.A.: Clinical and histopathologic aspects of angioid streaks. *Am J Ophthalmol, 32:* 1134, 1949.
19. Geeraets, W.J., and Guerry, D.P., III: Elastic tissue degeneration in sickle-cell disease. *Am J Ophthalmol, 50:* 213, 1960.
20. Hogan, M.J., and Zimmerman, L.E.: Ophthalmic Pathology: An Atlas and Textbook, W.B. Saunders, Philadelphia, 1964.
21. Paton, D.: The Relation of Angioid Streaks to Systemic Disease, Charles C. Thomas, Springfield, Ill., 1972, pp. 11–32.
22. Hogan, M.J.: Pathogenesis: electron microscopy of Bruch's membrane. *Trans Am Acad Ophthalmol, 69:* 683, 1965.
23. Hogan, M.J.: Bruch's membrane and disease of the macula: role of elastic tissue and collagen. *Trans Ophthalmol Soc U K, 87:* 113, 1967.
24. Hogan, M.J., Alvardo, J.A., and Weddell, J.E.: Histology of the Human Eye: an Atlas and Textbook, W.B. Saunders, Philadelphia, 1971, pp. 320–395.
25. Wolter, J.R.: Histologic character of connection between Bruch's membrane and choriocapillaris of human eye: a study with silver carbonate technique. *Arch Ophthalmol, 53:* 208, 1955.

CHAPTER 19

Myopia

Brian J. Curtin, M.D.

Few ocular diseases have a variety of ophthalmoscopic changes the equal of pathologic myopia. The same may also be said of the range of severity of these changes. Two thoroughly distinct stages of pathologic myopia can be noted on ophthalmoscopic examination—an early development stage and a later degenerative stage. In the former, the ophthalmoscopic changes are a direct consequence of the increased axial diameter of the eye especially the presence of a posterior staphyloma. In the degenerative stage, the fundus lesions are principally vascular disturbances of either an occlusive (focal atrophy) or proliferative (subretinal neovascularization) nature. In degenerative changes both axial elongation and aging are primary pathogenetic factors.

The fundus examination in high myopia is best conducted with binocular indirect ophthalmoscopy and slit-lamp biomicroscopy. These methods, which utilize the indispensable feature of stereopsis, best reveal the great panorama of myopic changes. Direct ophthalmoscopy is of least value not only because it lacks stereopsis, but also because it introduces a high degree of magnification often with distortion. Nonetheless, it is useful in some instances in the assessment of fine details. Bothersome magnification can be eliminated by the use of special adapters, such as those available with the Keeler ophthalmoscope, or by the simpler technique of allowing the patient to wear his corrective lenses during the examination.

The importance of fluorescein angiography in the evaluation of high myopia should also be noted for it reveals many features of ocular hemodynamics beyond the capabilities of the unaided ophthalmoscope.

Developmental Fundus Changes

Although not as dramatic as the later changes, the early fundus alterations in pathologic myopia are both striking and unique. They can be attributed to the unusual development of the myopic eye with its great distention of the posterior segment. This 40% increase in posterior segment area [1] is not due to a normal process of growth. This is attested to by the characteristic changes this process produces in the appearance of the optic nerve, retinal pigment epithelium-Bruch's membrane-choriocapillaris complex, choroid, and sclera.

The fluorescein angiogram in the myopic eye with developmental changes shows a widespread accentuation of the choroidal fluorescence in the early phases of the angiogram because of reduction in pigment in the pigment epithelium. Late hyperfluorescence from staining of the visible sclera silhouetted by larger choroidal vessels is characteristic of the late stage angiogram (Fig. 19.1). The peripheral aspects of the photographs show poorer resolution of detail because of inherent focusing difficulties in the highly myopic eye, notably those with posterior staphyloma. This occurs in spite of a myopia neutralizing lens present in the optical system of most fundus cameras. In general, with a noncorneal contact lens fundus camera, the larger the field the more apparent the marginal distortion on the photographs in high myopia.

OPTIC NERVE AND RETINA

Crescent Formation

Crescent formation invariably present in pathologic myopia is also seen in physiologic myopia [2] in a wide variety of forms. In pathologic myopia, crescents tend to be larger, however, and often encompass the entire disc. Crescents of either type may appear white (scleral) or pigmented (choroidal). This appearance is determined by the degree of choroidal pigmentation. Therefore, "choroidal" crescents are usually seen in non-Caucasian races, although with age this pigmentation may lessen. The fluorescein angiogram at the site of a crescent reveals no early transmitted fluorescence, even though the retinal pigment epithelium is absent. This is because the choriocapillaris has been displaced with the retinal pigment epithelium and Bruch's membrane; these three tissues act as a complex. The choriocapillaris, therefore, is not present in the scleral crescent, and early hyperfluorescence produced by transmitted fluorescence depends on an intact choriocapillaris as well as defects in the retinal pigment epithelium. Larger choroidal vessels, present within the crescent, are visible throughout the filling phases of the angiogram and silhouette late as physiologic staining of the sclera within the crescent takes palce. The staining of the sclera usually is most evident at the margins of the crescent adjacent to the intact choriocapillaris (Fig. 19.2).

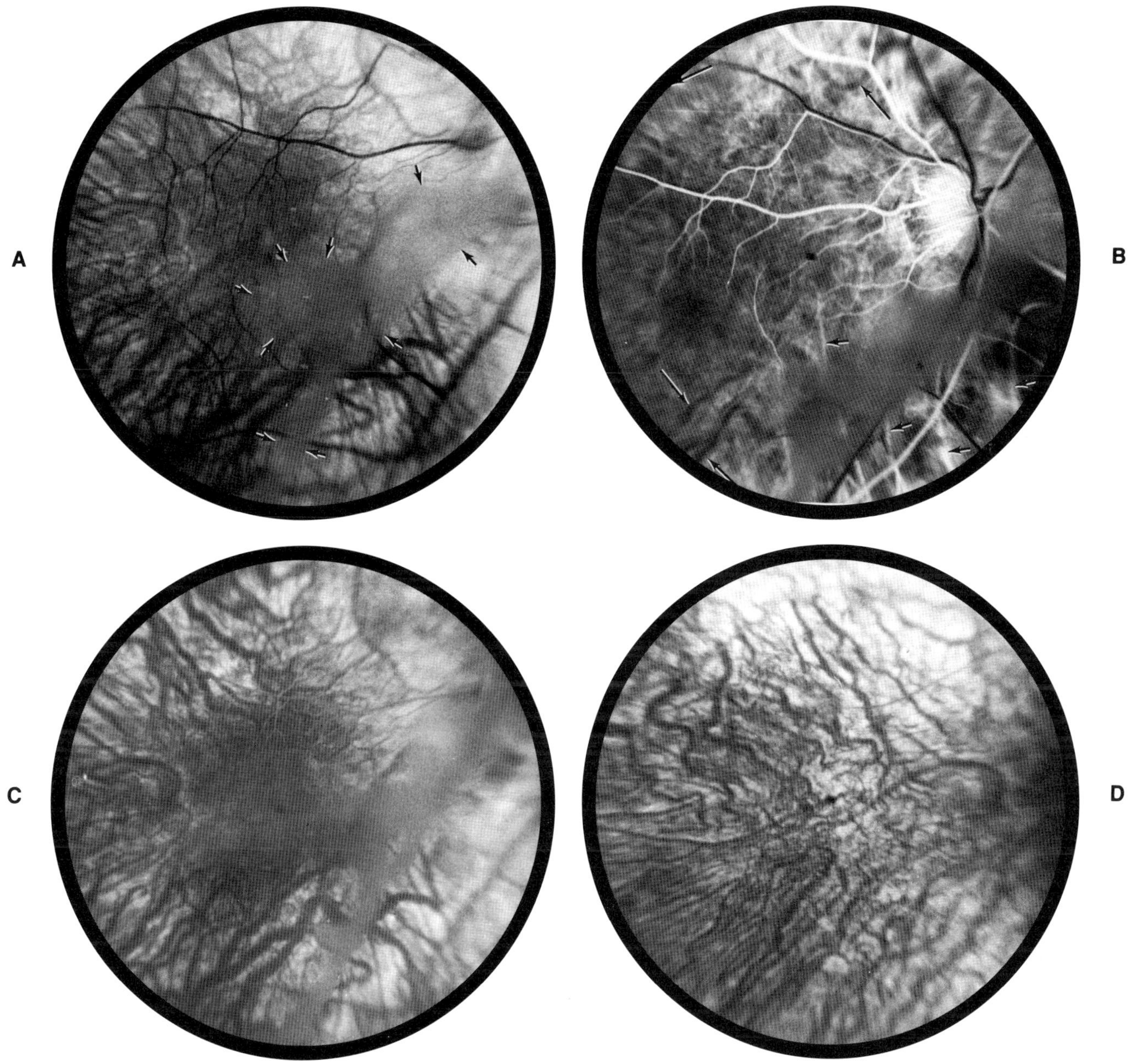

Figure 19.1. Fluorescein angiogram in developmental myopia. *A*, ophthalmoscopic photograph of -15 diopter myope with Wagner's disease. Note the visible choroidal vessels through the attenuated retinal pigment epithelium. A vitreous opacification (*arrows*) is also present. *B*, arterial phase angiogram. Note the filling of the choroidal arteries (*small arrows*). The choroidal veins (*large arrows*) are still hypofluorescent. The margins of the photograph are in poor focus, typical of any eye with a high refractive error. *C*, late phase angiogram of macula. *D*, late phase angiogram of peripheral retina. Note the choroidal vessels as they silhouette against the staining sclera. (Courtesy of Thomas C. Burton, M.D.)

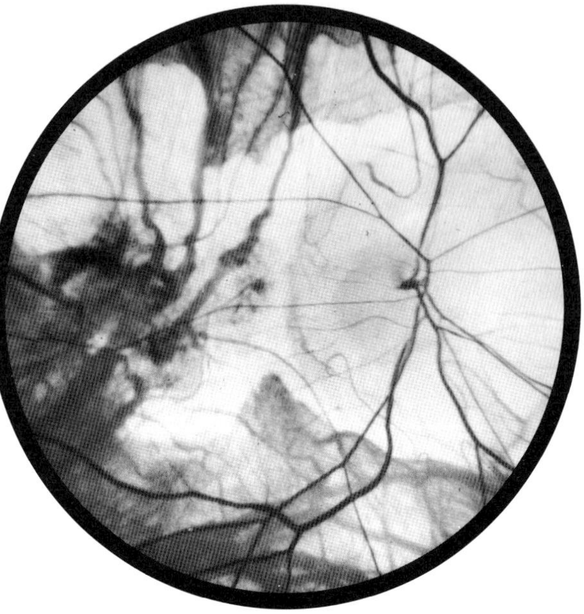

Figure 19.3. Ophthalmoscopic photograph of eversion of the inner aspect of the optic nerve with the "T" sign in myopia. Note the distal segment of the central retinal artery and vein as their bifurcation rests on the disc surface forming the letter T. The visualization of this 0.5 mm of the distal segment of these vessels is a consequence of eversion of the inner aspect of the optic nerve. Note the absence of normal tortuosity in the retinal vasculature as the arterioles and venules take a relatively straight course from the disc toward the macula.

A

B

C

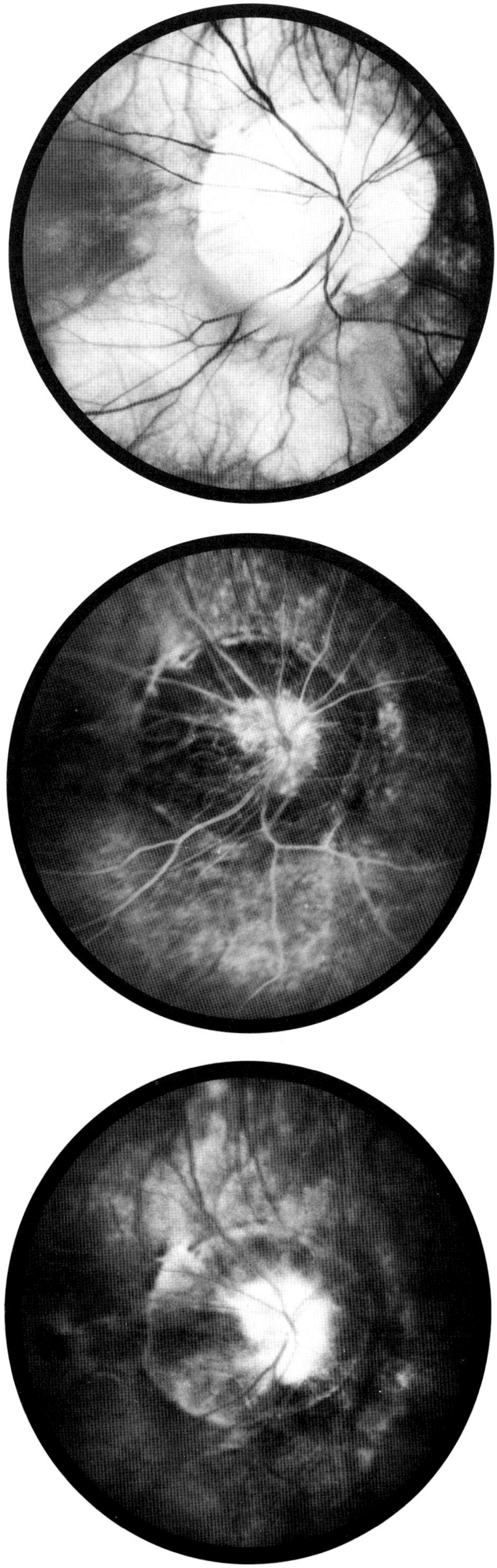

Figure 19.2. Fluorescein angiography in myopia with myopic crescent. *A*, ophthalmoscopic photograph. Note the large myopic scleral crescent encircling the disc. Widespread thinning and atrophy of the retinal pigment epithelium is evident elsewhere in the fundus, making medium-sized and large choroidal vessels visible. *B*, early venous phase fluorescein angiogram. The peripapillary myopic crescent is noted to be dark except for the presence of medium-sized and large choroidal vessels coursing through it. In spite of absent pigment epithelium, there is no transmitted fluorescence because the choriocapillaris is absent or markedly reduced. *C*, late phase fluorescein angiogram. Note the rim of late hyperfluorescence at the margins and within the myopic crescent. This late hyperfluorescence corresponds to staining of the sclera originating predominantly from the intact choriocapillaris present at the margins of the crescent. A fuzzy late hyperfluorescence also surrounds the disc, corresponding to staining of peripapillary visible sclera. The large choroidal vessels appear to silhouette in relief against staining sclera.

Eversion Of The Inner Aspect Of The Optic Nerve

This is of particular interest and importance because it is seen in those cases in which the optic nerve is completely involved within the borders of the posterior staphyloma. In such cases the inner aspect of the posterior scleral foramen distends and the lamina cribrosa is displaced anteriorly by an average of 0.33 mm [3]. This is significant because it can limit the degree of optic nerve cupping in cases of coexistent glaucoma. Another consequence of this eversion is the frequent visualization of about 0.5 mm of the distal segment of the central artery and vein. These are seen with their bifurcations resting on the disc surface, usually temporally, the central vessel and bifurcation roughly forming the letter T (the T sign) (Fig. 19.3).

Straightening Of The Retinal Vessels

The distention of the posterior pole also produces the effect of straightening the course of the retinal arterioles and venules. The normal tortuosity is absent whenever there is any degree of generalized scleral ectasia (Fig. 19.3).

RETINAL PIGMENT EPITHELIUM-BRUCH'S MEMBRANE-CHORIOCAPILLARIS COMPLEX

The retinal pigment epithelium (RPE) is in intimate anatomic and functional association with both Bruch's membrane and the choriocapillaris. The changes, especially biomechanical, that affect the retinal pigment epithelium can involve these other tissues as well.

Pallor of Ectatic Areas of the Fundus

In high myopia this pallor is especially striking because of the usual normal pigmentation of the surrounding fundus. Generalized pallor of the fundus is always a basis for the suspicion of albinism. In pathologic myopia, however, the pallor is clearly confined to the area of the posterior staphyloma, whereas the surrounding fundus reveals normal pigmentation (Fig. 19.4).

Tessellation

Invariably associated with some degree of pallor, tessellation represents nothing more than the increased visibility of the choroidal pigment and vessels through the thinned retinal pigment epithelium (Fig. 19.4). As with pallor, it is only significant when localized to one area of the fundus.

Hyperpigmentation of the Macula

Macular hyperpigmentation is not infrequently encountered in the examination of the younger myopes. It has been described in association with nystagmus and some congenital myopia pedigrees [4]. It is not uncommonly found in early pathologic myopia without associated ocular findings. The cause of this phenomenon is unknown. It may constitute a developmental anomaly, or be a reaction to the unusual distention of the posterior segment or, in fact, the normal macula pigmentation, which becomes more noticeable in contrast to surrounding fundus pallor.

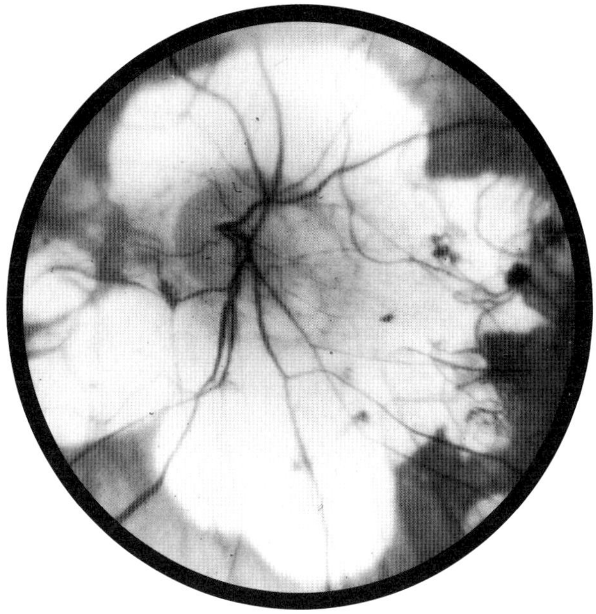

Figure 19.4. Ophthalmoscopic photograph of a myopic fundus with developmental changes. Note the widespread pigment epithelial atrophy surrounding the peripapillary area. Tessellation or an increase in the visibility of the choroidal pigment and vessels through the thin pigment epithelium is evident as are patchy areas of hyperpigmentation. These changes are all part of the developmental abnormalities seen in myopia.

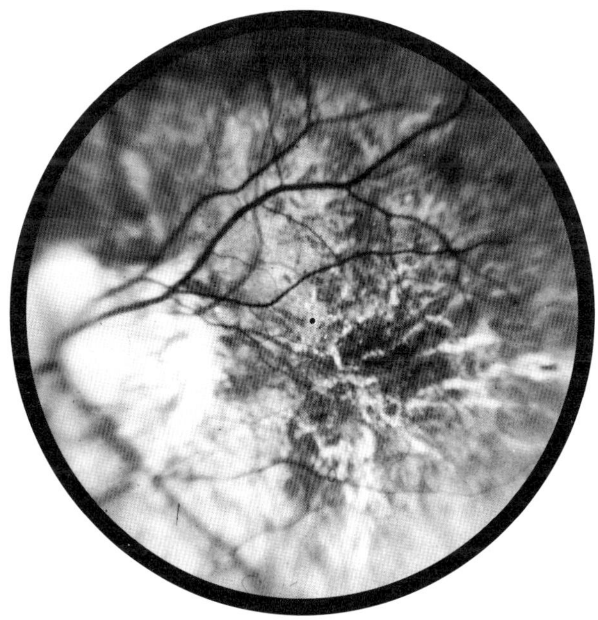

Figure 19.5. Ophthalmoscopic photograph of myopic fundus with lacquer cracks. Note the multiple fine, irregular, yellowish-white lines radiating from the macular region. An associated posterior staphyloma is evident by the poor focusing and ill-defined details at the margins of the photo. Lacquer cracks probably represent small fissures in the retinal pigment epithelium-Bruch's membrane-choriocapillaris complex.

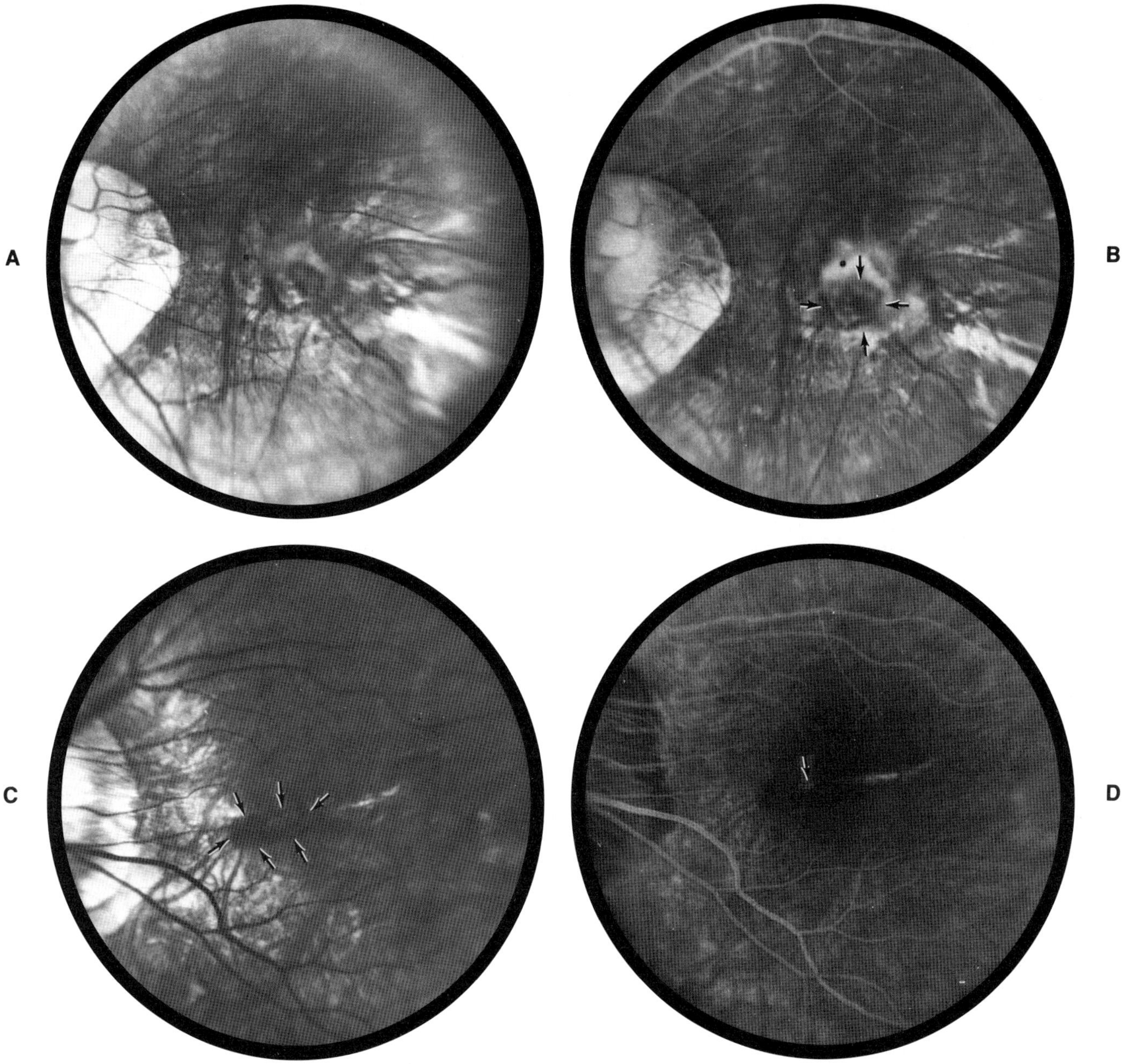

Figure 19.6. Myopic fundus with lacquer cracks and subretinal neovascularization. *A*, ophthalmoscopic photograph. Note the converging linear lacquer cracks radiating from the temporal position towards a subretinal pigment ring present in the juxtafoveal region subretinally. *B*, late venous phase fluorescein angiogram. Lacy hyperfluorescence is seen within the pigment ring centrally (*arrows*), indicative of subretinal neovascularization or a so-called Fuchs' spot. Note the medium-sized and large choroidal vessels coursing through the lacquer cracks, indicating that this defect is at the site of the pigment epithelium-Bruch's membrane-choriocapillaris junction with relative preservation of the outer vascular layers of the choroid. The *black dot* below the membrane is a photographic artifact. *C*, ophthalmoscopic photograph. Note the lacquer crack with subretinal hemorrhage (*arrows*) evident at its nasal aspect. The widespread tessellation with visible choroidal vessels and the peripapillary crescent are additional signs of myopic change. *D*, late venous phase fluorescein angiogram. Late hyperfluorescence at the nasal aspect of a lacquer crack corresponds to a fine fibrovascular membrane or Fuchs' spot (*arrow*). The hypofluorescence surrounding the Fuchs' spot is due to subretinal hemorrhage. Lacquer cracks resemble histopathologically angioid streaks and traumatic ruptures of the choroid. It is, therefore, not unreasonable to expect the possibility of subretinal neovascularization originating in association with lacquer cracks.

Lacquer Cracks

One of the most unusual fundus changes noted in high myopia is the "lacquer crack" which is seen from the second to the fifth decade of life (Fig. 19.5). These fine, irregular, yellow-white lines are usually found at the posterior pole and lying at the level of Bruch's membrane. They probably represent small fissures in the retinal pigment epithelium-Bruch's membrane-choriocapillaris complex. Because of the high incidence of associated posterior staphyloma, there can be a significant visual reduction in these eyes. This visual loss is more attributable to the functional deficiency of the myopic eye than to the lacquer crack itself. These lesions rarely demonstrate the visual field changes. Myopic eyes with macular lacquer cracks carry a guarded prognosis for the retention of central vision in the later years of life. Eventually these lesions become lost in large geographic areas of chorioretinal degeneration. Lacquer cracks are seen virtually always in eyes with posterior staphyloma.

The fluorescein angiogram in lacquer cracks often reveals the presence of larger choroidal vessels crossing through them indicating a split or absence in the choriocapillaris at the site of a crack. Late staining of visible sclera is also evident. While these cracks do not seem to have a definite predilection for the development of fibrovascular membranes, because of their histopathologic and clinical similarities to angioid streaks and traumatic ruptures of the choroid, it is reasonable to expect the possibility of subretinal neovascularization originating at their sites (Fig. 19.6).

CHOROID-SCLERA

Posterior Staphyloma

There is no early change in the myopic fundus of greater importance than the presence of posterior staphyloma. This finding immediately classifies the myopia as pathologic. It consists of a localized ectasia of the posterior wall of the eye, and therefore involves supportive (scleral), vascular (choroidal), and neuro (retinal) tissues (Fig. 19.7). Posterior staphyloma are variable in location, area, and depth. Within its ectasia, the localized pallor and tessellation of the optic fundus are seen. When it also involves the macular area, as do lacquer cracks, it also imparts a guarded prognosis for the later retention of central vision. Among eyes of patients 40-years-old and over that exhibit staphyloma involving the macula, 43% have vision of 20/200 or less. At age 60 and above, this percentage rises to 53% [6]. The location, size, and depth of the staphyloma has a direct effect upon macular function. In eyes with staphylomas that do not involve the macula, normal vision can often be obtained. With macular involvement, there is often some degree of visual acuity reduction. This can be attributed to the spreading of neuroepithelial elements as well as to a derangement of their orientation with the visual axis, as they lie on the sloping walls of the staphyloma (Stiles-Crawford effect). As a general rule, the larger the staphyloma and the greater its depth, the more impact it has upon the function of the retina in both the early and the late stages of its development.

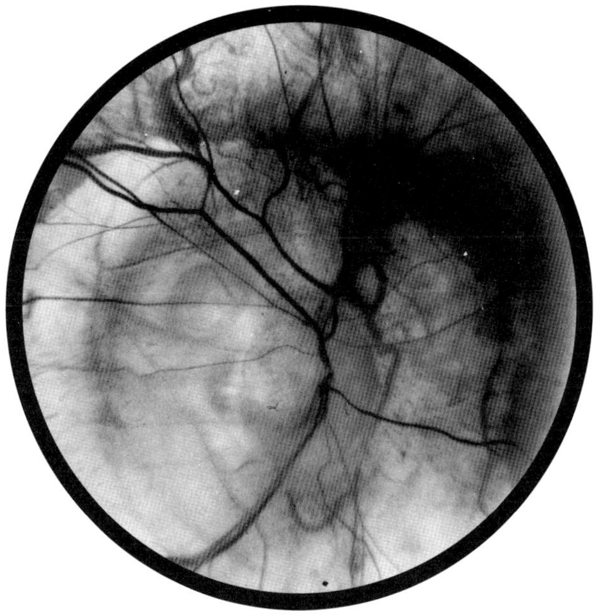

Figure 19.7. Ophthalmoscopic photograph of a myopic fundus with a posterior staphyloma. The presence of a posterior staphyloma immediately classifies the myopia as pathologic. Posterior staphylomas are variable in location, area, depth, and effect on macular function.

Choroid

The stretching and thinning of the ocular tissues involved in the staphyloma are of particular importance in the choroid. Here the anatomic distortion and increased intrawall stress combine to produce elongation, shearing, and compression of the choroidal vessels. Any one of these forces is capable of producing a significant derangement in the normal hemodynamics of this delicate tissue.

Degenerative Fundus Changes

The pathogenesis of the later chorioretinal degenerative changes of the myopic fundus are unknown. There are two schools of thought concerning their pathogenesis, the developmental and the abiotrophic. In the former, the degenerative changes are seen to be a result of age, superimposed on the unique mechanical and vascular changes produced in the choroid and retina by the marked distention of the posterior segment of the myopic eye. The opposing theory, the abiotrophic, holds that these changes are genetic, abiotrophic effects and that the areas of chorioretinal atrophy characteristic of pathologic myopia may, therefore, occur independent of scleral distention. The scleral weakness is thought to be the effect of an abnormal retinal pigment epithelium which, in embryonic ontogenesis, produces a defective choroid as well as sclera. As in most disagreements of this nature, there is probably some truth in both views.

The degenerative changes of the fundus in pathologic myopia are largely vascular in nature. The sensory retina, the retinal pigment epithelium-Bruch's membrane-choriocapillaris complex, and the choroidal vessels are all involved in the myopic degenerative process.

SENSORY RETINA

The greater incidence and early onset of posterior vitreous detachments in myopic eyes adds a considerable note of gravity to the problem of macular cyst and hole formation. The normal vitreous attachments at the posterior pole are especially strong at the macula and surrounding the optic nerve head. Traction is produced at these points during the posterior vitreous detachment process, and this can produce superficial as well as deep retinal hemorrhages [7]. Retinal breaks may also occur at these same locations. Furthermore, highly myopic eyes have an increased prevalence of macular hole formation and, in the presence of posterior vitreous detachment, conditions are conducive to retinal detachment at the posterior pole.

Macular hole formation is characteristically associated with diminished visual acuity. Some degree of surrounding retinal elevation is found in 86% of the cases and the average vision is reduced to the level of 20/200 [8]. The diagnosis of macular hole or cyst can be made with ophthalmoscopy or monochromatic photography, but the detailed study of these lesions is best accomplished by slit-lamp biomicroscopy with the Goldmann lens. With this technique stereopsis and oblique illumination with the slit beam yield considerably more diagnostic information.

Fluorescein angiography in a posterior retinal detachment secondary to a myopic hole reveals no late hyperfluorescence or leak (Fig. 19.8). Early hyperfluorescence secondary to choroidal transmitted fluorescence or a pigment epithelial window defect in the region of the retinal pigment epithelial atrophy may, however, be seen occasionally. The absence of a leak from the level of the pigment epithelium, with pooling into the subsensory retinal space, differentiates this form of macular detachment from that of central serous chorioretinopathy.

When a small, progressing posterior detachment is noted in association with a macular hole, the sensory retinal separation can rarely be "walled off" with very minimal photocoagulation utilizing argon laser, thereby preventing a full-scale rhegmatogenous detachment and the technical difficulties for reattachment that it presents. The photocoagulation treatment, unfortunately, does nothing to improve the central vision.

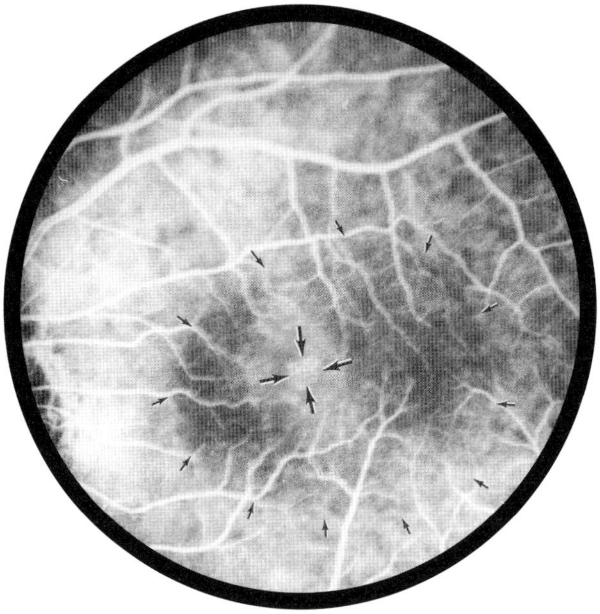

Figure 19.8. Fluorescein angiogram of a macular hole with posterior retinal detachment in myopia. Note the central macular hole (*large arrows*) revealing choroidal transmitted fluorescence from atrophy in the retinal pigment epithelium. A circumscribed area of relative hypofluorescence corresponds to the posterior retinal detachment and its blockage of the choroidal circulation (*small arrows*). Unlike degenerative holes, macular holes in high myopia may be full thickness and predispose to retinal detachment. Macular hole formation, along with subretinal neovascularization, represent the two principal histopathologic developments in the macula associated with sudden diminished visual acuity in myopia.

RETINAL PIGMENT EPITHELIUM-BRUCH'S MEMBRANE-CHORIOCAPILLARIS COMPLEX

The prevalence of punched-out, depressed, circumscribed areas of focal atrophy seen in myopia increases with age and with increased axial length of the eye [2]. The sites of predilection for these lesions are the margins of the crescent, notably the temporal, and at the posterior pole, especially in or near lacquer cracks. Any area within a posterior staphyloma of the posterior pole can be involved, however, and it is not unusual to see these lesions near or actually on the edge of the staphyloma. All eyes with posterior staphylomas in patients beyond the age of 40 tend to show some degree of chorioretinal atrophy [2]. In the early stages, small, isolated, focal areas of atrophy occur. These later become confluent to form eventually large, oddly shaped geographic areas of degeneration (Fig. 19.3 and Fig. 19.4). Pigment proliferation at the margins of these lesions can occur, and islands of pigment surrounded by large areas of atrophy may be the only indication of the prior presence of smaller areas of degeneration. Scotomata can be plotted in those parts of the visual field that correspond to these changes. In the late stages of the disease, only peninsulas and bridges of somewhat normal tissue are seen overlying what has come to be known as "bare sclera."

Fluorescein angiography has made an enormous contribution to our understanding of the pathogenesis of the myopic fundus. This has been in the area of subretinal neovascularization (SRN). The earliest clinical manifestation of SRN in myopia is the presence of subretinal red spots in the fundus, heretofore attributed to small "choroidal" hemorrhages. Their persistent presence in many cases causes them to be labeled as dilated capillary tufts, and it remained for fluorescein angiography to reveal the exact nature of the subretinal vascularized networks responsible for their presence. As in other macular diseases associated with subretinal neovascularization, the pathologic myopic eye commonly develops breaks in Bruch's membrane predisposing to subpigment epithelial fibrovascular ingrowth from the choroid. Secondary to these breaks and the primary ischemic factors related to them, there is a proliferation of new vessels in the space between Bruch's membrane and the pigment epithelium, the subpigment epithelial space [9]. It may be that these vessels, at least for a time, have a

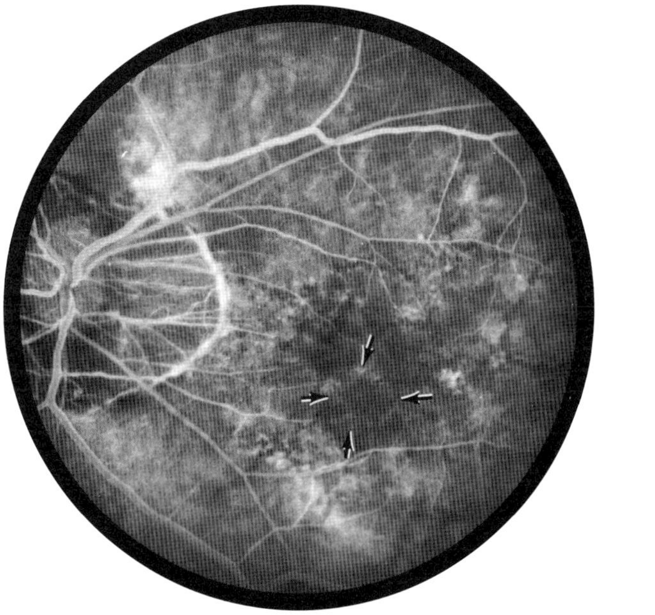

Figure 19.9. Myopia with subretinal neovascularization. (Fuchs' spot). Early venous phase fluorescein angiogram shows the lacy hyperfluorescence in the central macula (*arrows*), which corresponds to a fibrovascular ingrowth from the choroidal circulation into the subpigment epithelial space.

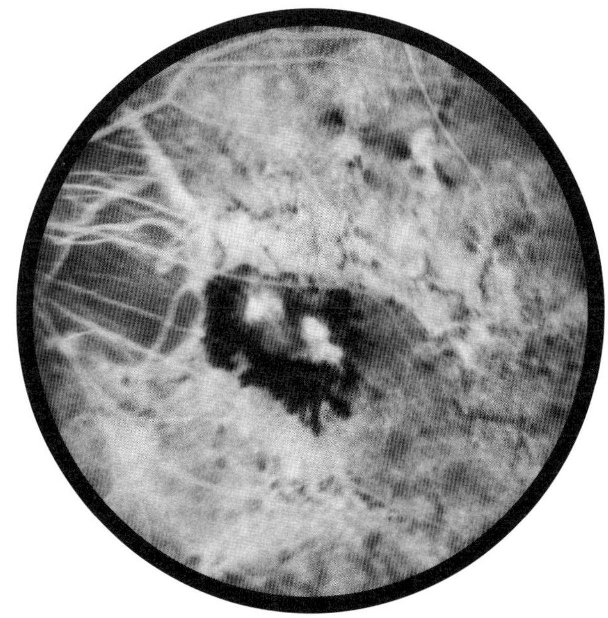

Figure 19.10. Late venous phase fluorescein angiogram in myopia with subretinal hemorrhage and neovascularization (Fuchs' spot). Note the hyperfluorescence beneath the sensory retina in the macular region associated with a dark zone which, in this case, represents subretinal hemorrhage with characteristic "drip lines."

beneficial effect and nourish some areas of the outer retina in which the choriocapillaris is deficient (Fig. 19.9). It is now fully recognized, however, that these new thin-walled vessels predispose to subretinal hemorrhage and serous exudation under the pigment epithelium and/or sensory retina which can evolve into the later fibrotic stages of the disciform process (Fig. 19.10). In the macular region of the myopic eye the transudation from these fibrovascular membranes, often with accompanying hemorrhages, produces the classic Fuchs' spot [10]. This typically round, elevated lesion varies greatly in color, depending on the degree of retinal pigment epithelial proliferation that accompanies it and on the extent of the lesion. Lesions with transudation confined essentially to the subpigment epithelial space are dark with well defined margins. Other lesions, in which the subretinal transudation has extended through the pigment epithelium to accumulate beneath the sensory retina tend to be larger, irregular in shape, and lighter in color. Colors vary, therefore, from light gray to jet black, and rarely, green. The color green may be an effect of the degeneration of pigment granules (lipofuscin and melanin) and blood cells and their products although there is no exact pathologic counterpart.

The most reliable ophthalmoscopic findings for the presence of a Fuchs' spot are subretinal hemorrhage or a pigment ring with an exudative detachment of the pigment epithelium or sensory retina. These manifestations are virtually pathognomonic of a Fuchs' spot. The Fuchs' spot usually has its onset during the fourth to sixth decades of life and is associated in the vast majority of cases with loss of central vision. In younger patients, the spot tends to be small, but unfortunately proximal to the fovea (Fig. 19.11). It frequently has a benign course. In older patients the

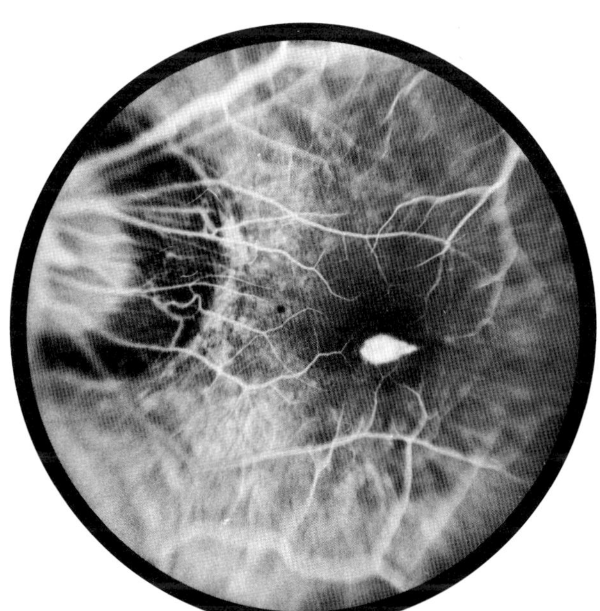

Figure 19.11. Late venous phase angiogram in myopia with subretinal neovascularization (Fuchs' spot) in a young patient. Note the late hyperfluorescence centrally in the macula from pooling beneath the subpigment epithelial space.

lesions are often larger, perhaps representing the combined effects of myopia with involutional changes (Fig. 19.12). As time passes, these lesions lose their disciform shape and become flattened, with well defined edges, and are frequently surrounded by a large geographic area of atrophy with pigment dispersion (Fig. 19.13). Some Fuchs' spots may show an increase in size of the vascularized complex (Fig. 19.14).

At its inception, the Fuchs' spot can be occasionally associated with a lacquer crack. In this situation, the neovascularization resembles the vascular membranes that develop at the site of an angioid streak or a traumatic choroidal rupture which are histopathologically similar to lacquer cracks.

The fluorescein angiogram is typical of focal subretinal neovascularization from any cause with an irregular lacy hyperfluorescence at the site of the neovascularization evident early on the angiogram, and a late hyperfluorescence

A

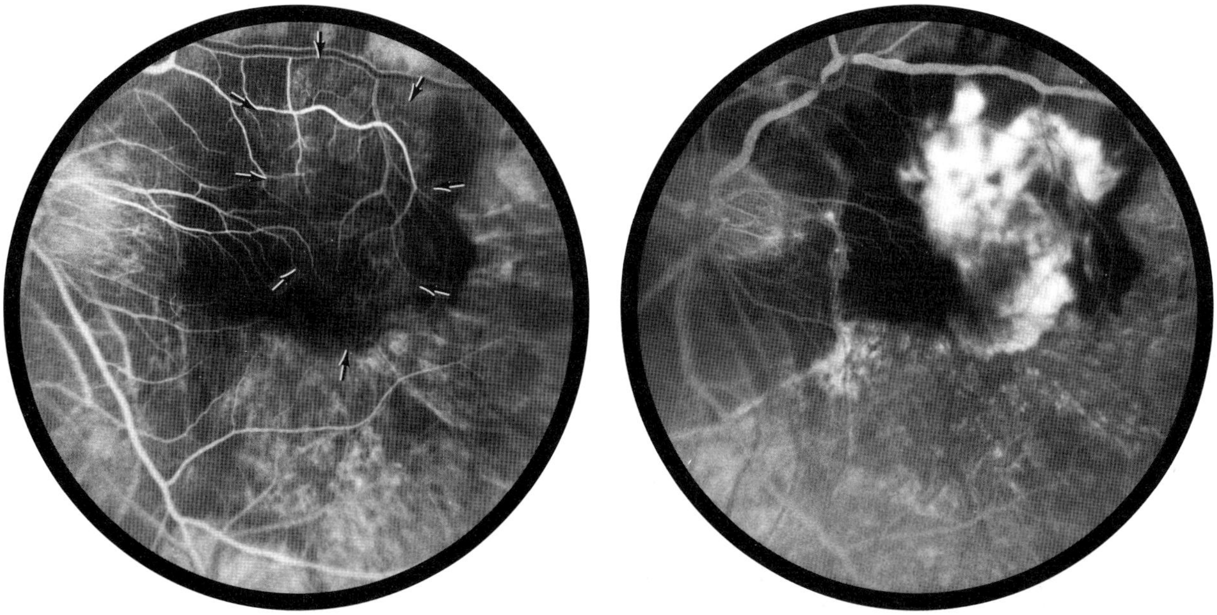

B

Figure 19.12. Myopia with subretinal neovascularization in an elderly patient. *A*, arteriovenous phase fluorescein angiogram. Note the large faint area of lacy hyperfluorescence beneath the sensory retina in the macula region (*arrows*), produced by a subretinal neovascularized membrane obscured partially by blood. *B*, late venous phase fluorescein angiogram. Late hyperfluorescence is present from pooling into the associated subsensory retinal space. The hypofluorescence is due largely to the presence of blood. In elderly myopes, subretinal neovascularization (Fuchs' spot) tends to be more extensive perhaps representing the combined effects of myopia and involutional degeneration.

A

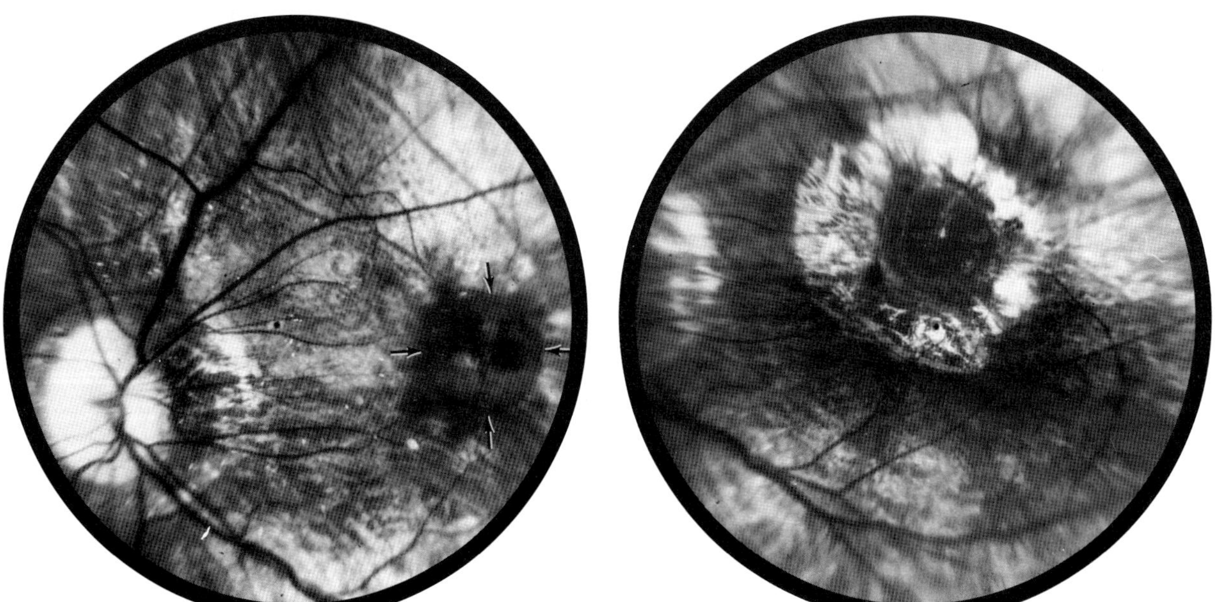

B

Figure 19.13. Evolution of a Fuchs' spot. *A*, ophthalmoscopic photograph. Note the fresh Fuchs' spot with subretinal hemorrhage (*arrows*). *B*, ophthalmoscopic photograph of the same patient, one year later. There was increased pigmentation and flattening of the Fuchs' spot centrally and a surrounding large geographic area of atrophy.

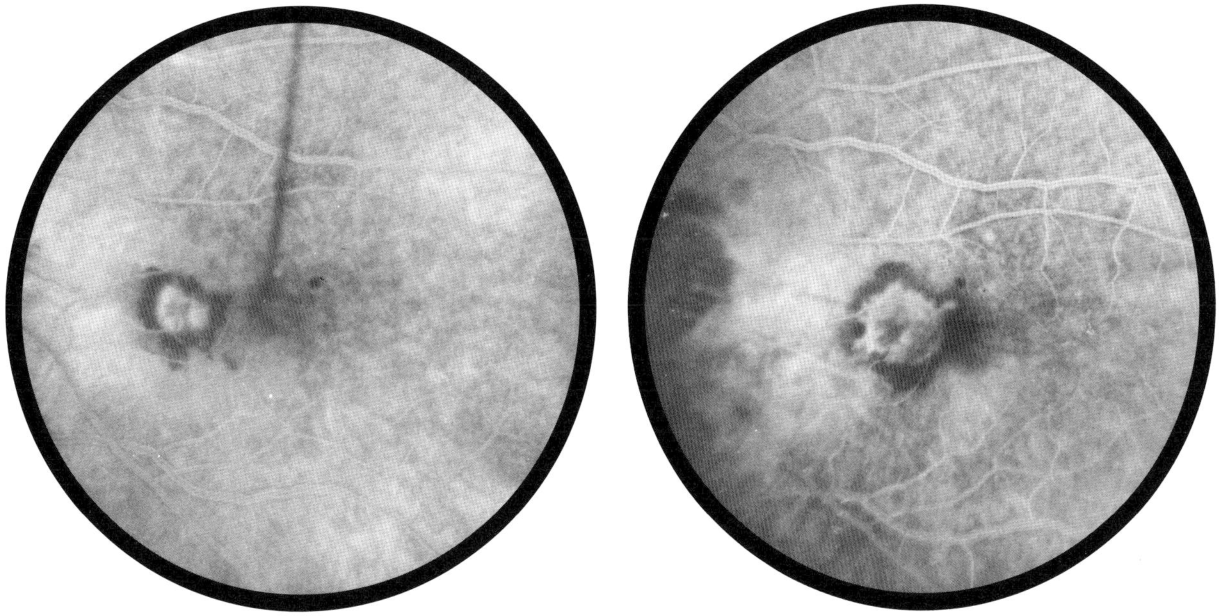

Figure 19.14. Evolution of a Fuchs' spot. *A*, late venous phase fluorescein angiogram. Note the subretinal hyperfluorescence surrounded by a dark zone in the macula of this myope (Fuchs' spot), located just nasal to the perifoveal capillary free zone. *B*, venous phase fluorescein angiogram, 3 weeks later, shows an increase in the size of the subretinal neovascular membrane with proliferation to the juxtafoveal region.

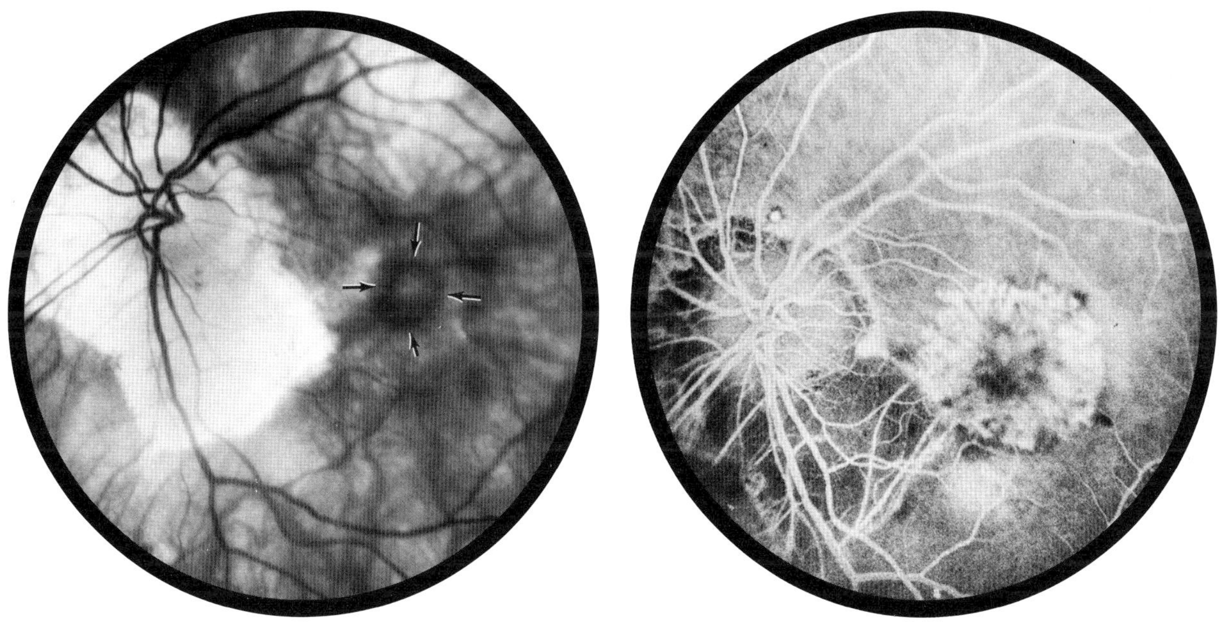

Figure 19.15. Fluorescein angiogram in Fuchs' spot. *A*, in this ophthalmoscopic photograph of a myopic eye, note the presence of a subretinal "pigment ring" with an overlying exudative detachment (*arrows*). *B*, late venous phase fluorescein angiogram. Note the large area of lacy hyperfluorescence which extends beyond the area of the "pigment ring" due to subretinal neovascularization Fuchs' spot. While the presence of a subretinal pigment ring is virtually pathognomonic of the presence of underlying neovascularization, the full extent of the vascular proliferation can only be appreciated with fluorescein angiography.

or leak from the permeable neovascularized membrane. A dark zone usually encircles the fibrovascular membrane, and the primitive vascular channels contained within it on occasion show a nodular type of fluorescence as the dye diffuses from the most immature capillary buds within the membrane. Late pooling into the subsensory retinal space produces a diffuse or fuzzy appearance overlying the membrane, while the Fuchs' spot indicates subretinal neovascularization, the full extent of the vascularity can only be determined by the fluorescein angiogram which often reveals more extensive vascular proliferation than suspected clinically (Fig. 19.15).

Photocoagulation treatment of subretinal neovascularization in myopia is a hazardous procedure because of the usual proximity of these membranes to the fovea. Hemorrhage and fertilization of the membrane exist as potential complications of inadequate treatment resulting from incomplete thermal obliteration of the membrane. In the unusual instance of macular involvement due to the transudation from extramacular neovascularization, photocoagulation may prove to be of value. However, the potential value of this modality must be weighed against its intrinsic risks and the distinct tendency for the Fuchs' spot to stabilize and remain relatively small with little expansion in a significant percentage of patients, particularly younger ones.

CHOROID

"Choroidal sclerosis" involving the larger choroidal vessels is a frequent accompaniment of the myopic degenerative process. With thinning or loss of the overlying retinal pigment epithelium and choriocapillaris, the larger choroidal vessels become visible and, with age, the arteriosclerotic changes affecting these vessels become apparent.

In summary, the posterior fundus changes of pathologic myopia can be separated into two distinct types: developmental and degenerative. The former are an effect of the unique distention of the posterior segment of the eye, which, when localized, presents as the posterior staphyloma. These changes can be compatible with good visual function. The degenerative changes occur later and are for the most part vascular in nature. The more serious of these, chorioretinal atrophy, macular holes, and the Fuchs' spot primarily involve the posterior pole and are responsible for the high prevalence of blindness in this disease. Characteristic changes of each stage of the disease can be seen with careful ophthalmoscopic examination. Fluorescein angiography, with its ability to detect subretinal neovascularization, gives an added dimension to the evaluation of these eyes.

References

1. Blach, R.K.: The nature of degenerative myopia, Thesis, University of Cambridge, 1964, p. 73.
2. Curtin, B.J., and Karlin, D.B.: Axial length measurements and fundus changes of the myopic eye. *Am J Ophthalmol, 71:* 42, 1971.
3. Goldmann, H.: The glaucoma problem. *In* Glaucoma: Transactions of the Second Conference, 1956, ed. by F. Newell, Madison Printing Co., Madison, N.J., 1957, p. 161.
4. Brückner, A., and Franceschetti, A.: Myopie im Kindesalter. *Arch Augenheilkd, 105:* 1, 1931.
5. Klein, R.M., and Curtin, B.J.: Lacquer crack lesions in pathologic myopia. *Am J Ophthalmol, 79:* 386, 1975.
6. Curtin, B.J.: Visual acuity in myopia. *In* Clinical Low Vision, ed. by E. Faye, Little, Brown & Co., Boston, 1976, p. 295.
7. Cibis, G.W., Watzke, R.C., and Chua, J.: Retinal hemorrhages in posterior vitreous detachment. *Am J Ophthalmol, 80:* 1043, 1975.
8. Aaberg, T.M., Blair, C.J., and Gass, J.D.M.: Macular holes. *Am J Ophthalmol, 69:* 555, 1970.
9. Goldberg, M.F.: Bruch's membrane and vascular growth. *Invest Ophthalmol, 15:* 443, 1976.
10. Levy, J.H., Pollack, H.M., and Curtin, B.J.: The Fuchs' spot: an ophthalmoscopic and fluorescein angiographic study. *Ann Ophthalmol,* in press.

CHAPTER 20

Choroidal Folds

Charles R. Beyrer, M.D.

The finding of choroidal folds should alert the clinician to initiate the appropriate investigation of the most commonly associated ocular disorders. The table lists the most commonly associated causative lesions. The earlier literature emphasized retinal folds or striae. Later histologic studies demonstrated that choroid, Bruch's membrane, and pigment epithelium are also folded [1]. Norton [2] first coined the term "choroidal folds" during the Lang lecture in 1968, by pointing out the importance of fluorescein angiography in delineating choroidal folds as a separate entity, differentiating them from retinal folds or striae.

Clinical Features

Choroidal folds appear clinically as alternating dark and light lines or grooves in the posterior fundus (Fig. 20.1). The lines may be horizontally, vertically, or concentrically oriented. Typically, the lighter lines are broader than the darker ones. They are always observed in the deeper aspect of the fundus, i.e., retinal pigment epithelium-Bruch's membrane-choroidal complex, and can best be observed employing stereoscopic methods of examination, such as indirect ophthalmoscopy or slit-lamp biomicroscopy. The findings on fluorescein angiography are consistent and pathognomonic and consist of alternating hypo- and hyperfluorescent lines or grooves appearing in the initial phase of the choroidal background flush, which disappear late without staining.

Monochromatic ophthalmoscopy can be extremely useful in the detection of choroidal folds. This technique makes use of the fact that the choroid and deeper layers of the retina are best seen utilizing monochromatic light at longer wavelengths. Choroidal folds rarely appear as an isolated entity, i.e., in the absence of associated intra- or extraocular disease processes [3].

I have recently examined a patient who developed choroidal folds and cystoid macular edema following scleral buckling surgery for rhegmatogenous retinal detachment (Fig. 20.2), a phenomenon previously unreported.

Retinal and choroidal folds in typical cases are associated with a change in refraction toward hyperopia. The folds however, usually do not interfere with good visual function [4].

Although it has been stated that folds secondary to an orbital mass usually disappear when pressure on the sclera is removed, most investigators noted that folds persist postoperatively and remain evident at subsequent follow-up examinations. Kroll and Norton [1], however, reported three cases, documented by fluorescein angiography, in which appropriate therapy of the patient's underlying disease process led to regression of the folds.

HISTOPATHOLOGY

Histopathologic specimens of eyes harboring choroidal folds are rare. Yanoff [4] stated that choroidal folds are commonly noted in histopathology of eyes enucleated after severe traumatic lacerations.

Wolter [5] described the histopathology of choroidal folds in two cases of severe exophthalmos due to malignant orbital neoplasms (Fig. 20.3). The major histologic findings were distinct choroidal folds (valleys) and more extensive crests involving Bruch's membrane and pigment epithelium with thickening and congestion of the choroid. The folds appeared to involve Bruch's membrane primarily with a secondary "piling up and thickening" of the pigment epithelium in the valleys of each fold. These valleys were 0.2–0.5 mm apart. The crests of the folds were long and smooth with no visible changes in structure of the pigment epithelium.

Histopathologic examination of a case studied by fluorescein angiography has been carried out only once [2]. In

TABLE 20.1. Underlying Etiology of Choroidal Folds

Congenital
Exophthalmos
Orbital cellulitis
Orbital tumor
Malignant melanoma of the choroid
Scleral buckling
Ocular trauma
Stationary or progressive hypermetropia
Papilledema due to intracranial hypertension
Macular disciform degeneration
Metastatic carcinoma of the choroid
Idiopathic

A

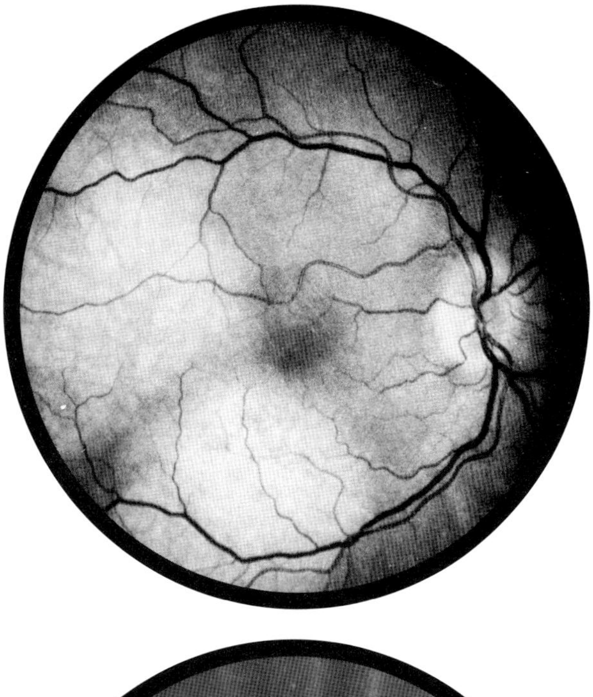

B

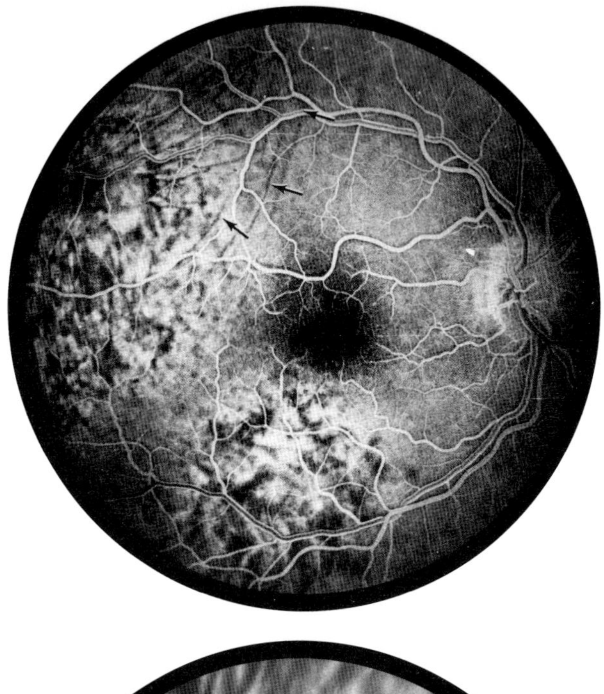

C

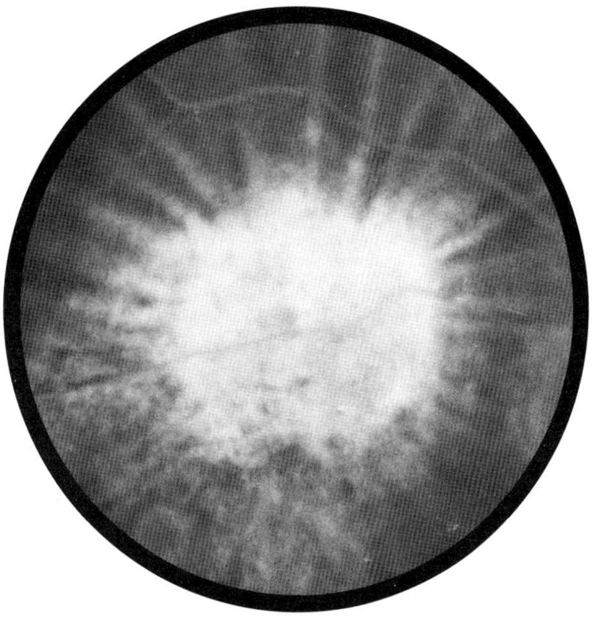

D

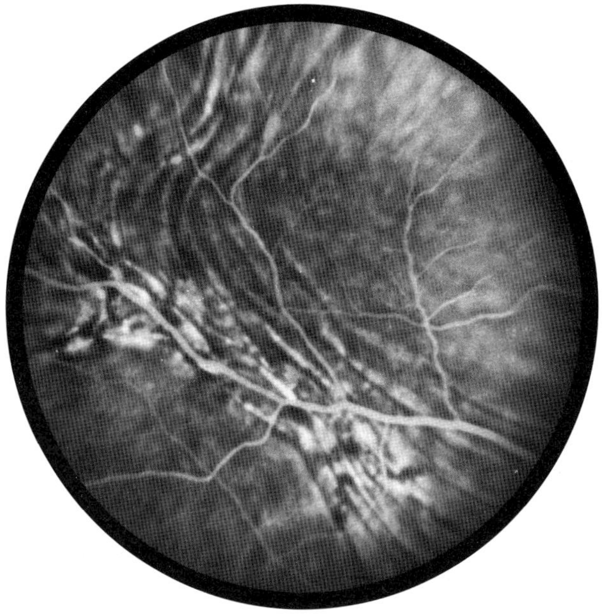

E

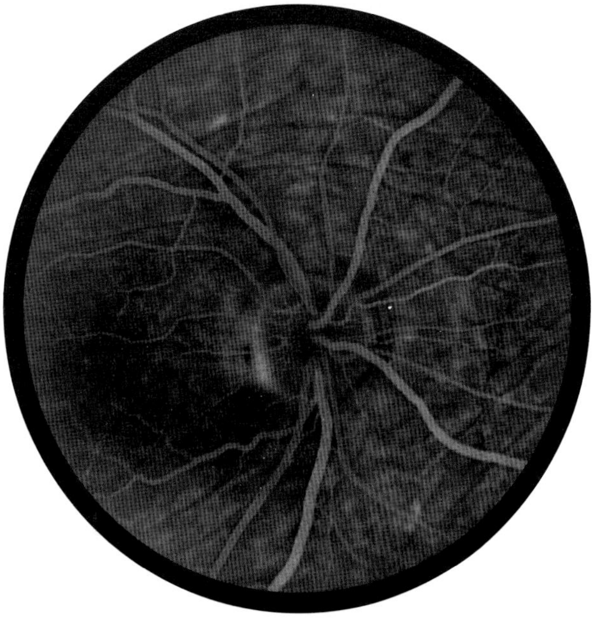

Figure 20.1. Choroidal folds—metastatic carcinoma of the posterior fundus. *A*, ophthalmoscopic photograph showing two dome-shaped amelanotic solid tumors of the choroid. *B*, arteriovenous phase angiogram showing hyperfluorescence of the two metastatic lesions and concentrically oriented choroidal folds (*arrows*) temporal to the macula. (Courtesy of Emanuel Rosen, M.D.). *C*, late phase angiogram of an eye with disciform degeneration showing choroidal folds radiating in all directions. *D*, venous phase angiogram of idiopathic choroidal folds temporal to the macula seen as hypo- and hyperfluorescent lines. *E*, venous phase angiogram of eye with an orbital tumor compressing the posterior globe. The choroidal folds are clearly seen surrounding the disc.

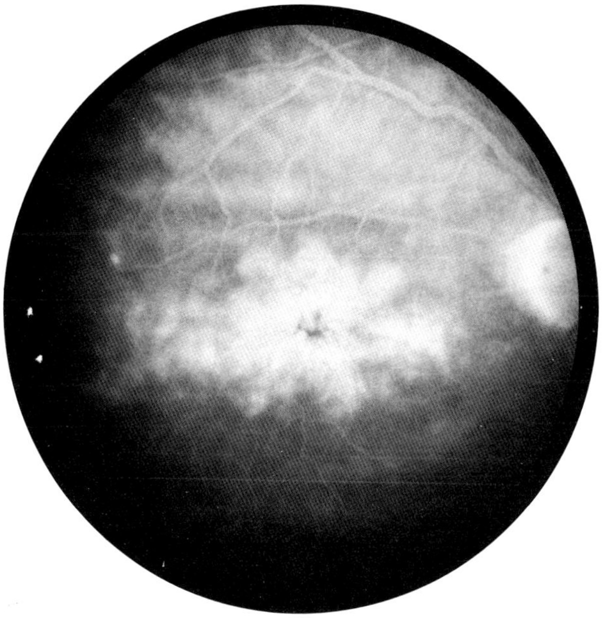

Figure 20.2. Venous phase angiogram of a patient with choroidal folds, postbuckling procedure. Cystoid macular edema and horizontal lines in the superior macula of hypo- and hyperfluorescence, indicative of the choroidal folds.

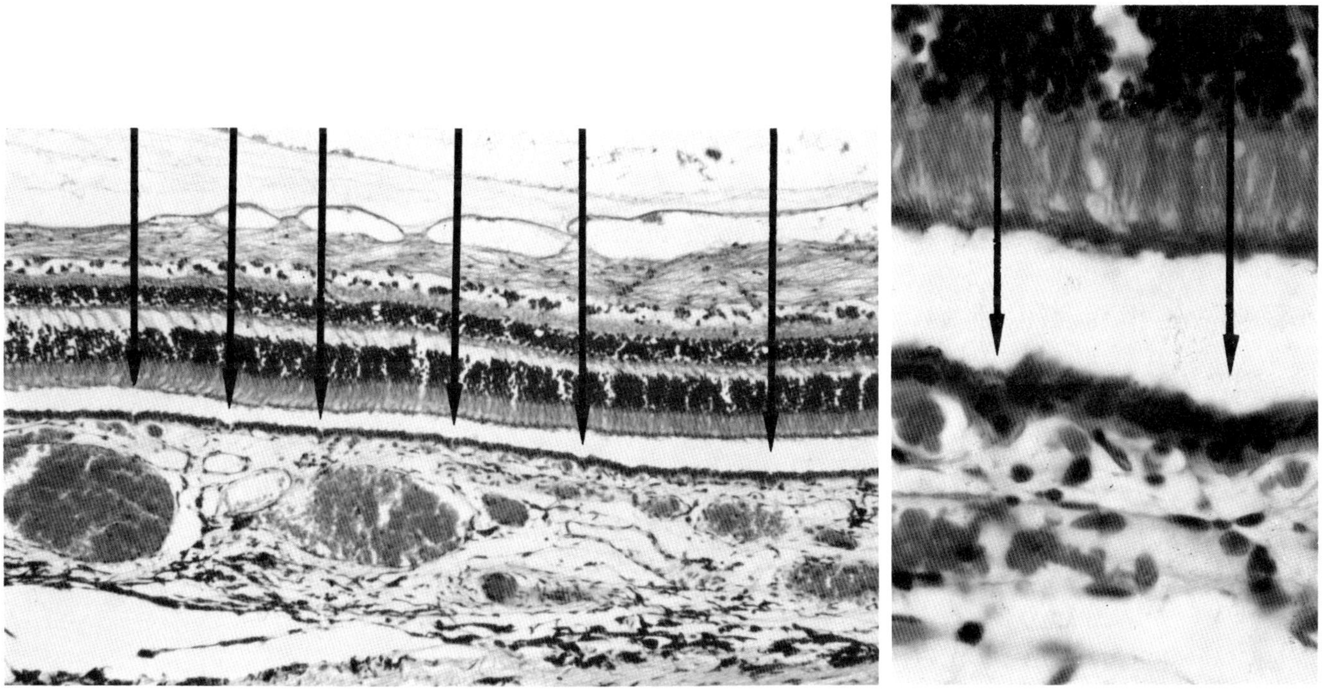

Figure 20.3. *A*, vertical section of retina and choroid in an area between disc and fovea showing six distinct wrinkles of pigment epithelium and Bruch's membrane (*arrows*) representing the narrow valleys of choroidal folds. The choroid is thickened and its blood vessels are congested. Paraffin section. Hematoxylin and eosin. ×100. *B*, sharp valley (*arrows*) between two crests of choroidal folding in the same case. Pigment cells are piled up in the valley. Paraffin section. Hematoxylin and eosin. ×600. (Courtesy of J.R. Wolter, M.D. from *Am J Ophthalmol, 77:* 669, 1974; reprinted with permission.)

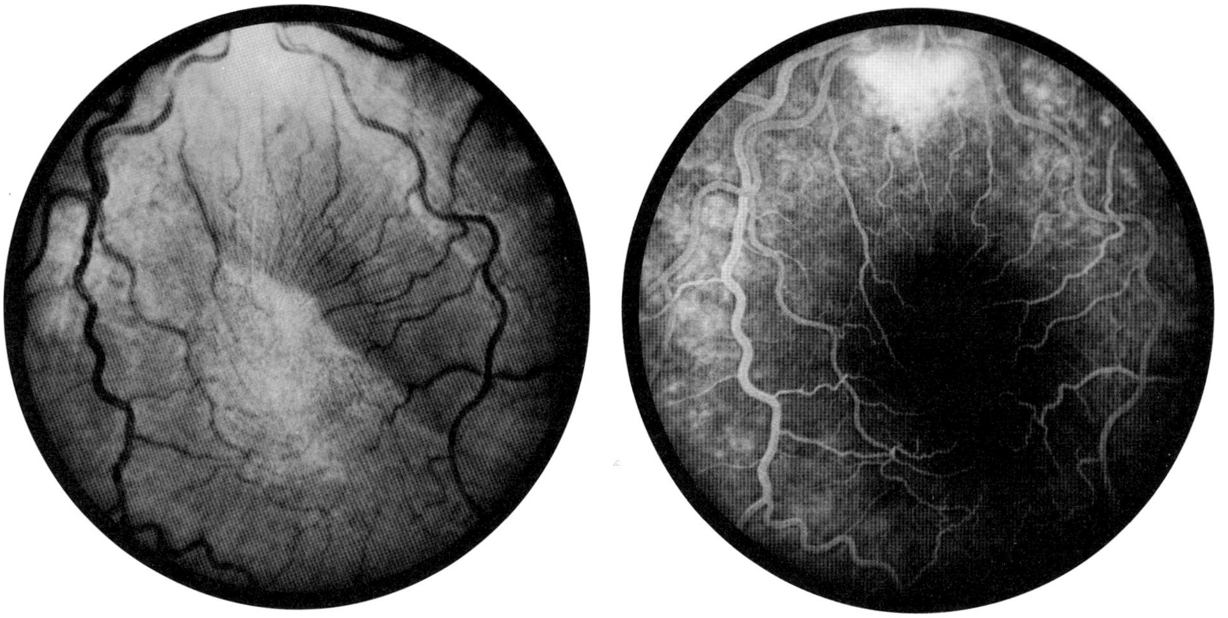

Figure 20.4. Retinal folds. *A*, monochromatic photograph, 560 nm (green). Note the fibrosis in the macula associated with radiating parallel folds. *B*, late venous phase angiogram. Note that these folds are not evident on the fluorescein angiogram. Unlike choroidal folds, retinal folds produce abnormal fluorescence. Their presence is accentuated on monochromatic red-free photography.

this case, the folds as described above, were indeed observed. The choroid was congested. The pigment epithelium on the crests of the fold appeared normal but was thickened in the valleys.

According to Norton and Kroll [1], the histopathology of choroidal folds appears to correlate well with the typical findings on fluorescein angiography. The light portions of the folds correspond to the crests and transmit the choroidal fluorescence brilliantly, while the dark portions correspond to the valleys and transmit the choroidal fluorescence poorly due to their inclination and poor light reflectivity.

Differential Diagnosis

Choroidal folds can usually be diagnosed by clinical appearance and typical pattern observed on fluorescein angiography. They may, on occasion, be confused with retinal folds or striae. Although folds in the inner retina, presumably the internal limiting membrane, are found occasionally in eyes with choroidal folds, these folds alone do not provide the fluorescein pattern of alternating dark and light lines. Similarly, wrinkling of the inner retina in eyes with preretinal membrane formation (epiretinal membrane) do not produce these fluorescein patterns (Fig. 20.4).

References

1. Kroll, A.J., and Norton, E.W.D.: Regression of choroidal folds. *Trans Am Acad Ophthalmol Otolaryngol, 74:* 515, 1970.
2. Norton, E.W.D.: A characteristic fluorescein angiographic pattern in choroidal folds. *Proc Roy Soc Med, 62:* 119, 1969.
3. von Winning, S.H.O.M.: Fluorography of choroidal folds. Proceedings of the Netherlands Ophthalmol Society, 165th Meeting, The Hague, 1970.
4. Yanoff, M.: Personal communication.
5. Wolter, J.R.: Parallel horizontal choroidal folds secondary to an orbital tumor. *Am J Ophthalmol, 77:* 669, 1974.

CHAPTER 21

Inflammation of the Pigment Epithelium and Choriocapillaris

Howard Schatz, M.D., Kurt A. Gitter, M.D., and Lawrence A. Yannuzzi, M.D.

A number of inflammatory conditions affect the pigment epithelium and choriocapillaris. Among these are:

(1) Acute multifocal posterior placoid pigment epitheliopathy (AMPPPE)
(2) Retinal pigment epitheliitis
(3) Geographic helicoid peripapillary choroidopathy (GHPC)

Each of these conditions may cause visual reduction if the fovea is severely affected. This chapter will review and discuss these disorders.

AMPPPE

This disorder is a bilateral acute inflammation of the retinal pigment epithelium and choriocapillaris. It affects young patients more frequently than old, and females more frequently than males. There is often a history of recent viral illness, especially upper respiratory infection (URI), or a flu-like syndrome, preceding the onset of these symptoms. One report has shown evidence of an adenoviral infection, another of a cerebral vasculitis with inflammatory cells in the cerebrospinal fluid, and another of associated thyroiditis.

Affected patients usually notice an acute loss of vision in one or both eyes. The ophthalmoscopic examination is usually normal except for the fundi which demonstrate yellowish-white multifocal placoid lesions in the posterior pole, at the level of the pigment epithelium and choriocapillaris (Figs. 21.1 and 21.2). The lesions are gray, flat, and either round or irregular. The overlying retina appears normal on slit-lamp contact lens examination. Occasionally, vitreous cells can be seen. In some cases the optic nerve is moderately edematous and other patients have been reported to demonstrate episcleritis or iridocyclitis. Further evidence of inflammation may be indicated by retinal perivascular sheathing, seen in some cases. A sensory retinal detachment has been observed in one patient, and a focal area of subretinal neovascularization developed at the margin of a subacute lesion in another patient.

The characteristic fluorescein angiogram of AMPPPE demonstrates that in the acute stage of the disorder the yellowish-white lesions hypofluoresce in the early phase. Later in the angiogram moderate hyperfluorescence can be seen, indicating fluorescein staining of the lesion.

In one or two weeks following the acute stage of the disease, the flat pigment epithelial lesions appear to fade. Eventually the lesions become both irregularly pigmented and depigmented, demonstrating pigment clumping (Fig. 21.2). Some new lesions may appear as older lesions begin to resolve. The final stages of the disease may continue for 2–3 months and show irregular pigment epithelial hyper- and hypopigmentation (Fig. 21.3). Recurrence is rare.

Although the central visual acuity usually returns, vision may not be fully recovered if the central macula is severely involved. Fluorescein angiography in the later stages of the disease demonstrates irregular hyper- and hypofluorescence, depending on the degree of pigmentation. The histopathology is not known but presumably there is a thickening or swelling of the pigment epithelium with a cellular infiltration at the level of the choriocapillaris. Later as the acute inflammatory stage of the disease resolves, the pigment epithelium probably undergoes a variable change with some hypertrophy and hyperplasia and in other areas, atrophy. This is now fluorescein angiographic evidence suggestive of nonperfusion of the choriocapillaris with normal perfusion of the intermediate and larger choroidal vessels. These filling defects may have been caused by acute occlusion of the precapillary arterioles of the choroid, induced initially by inflammation.

Since the natural history of AMPPPE usually leads to resolution and complete return of central vision, the treatment is still uncertain and difficult to evaluate. However, some feel that steroids are helpful in this inflammatory disorder.

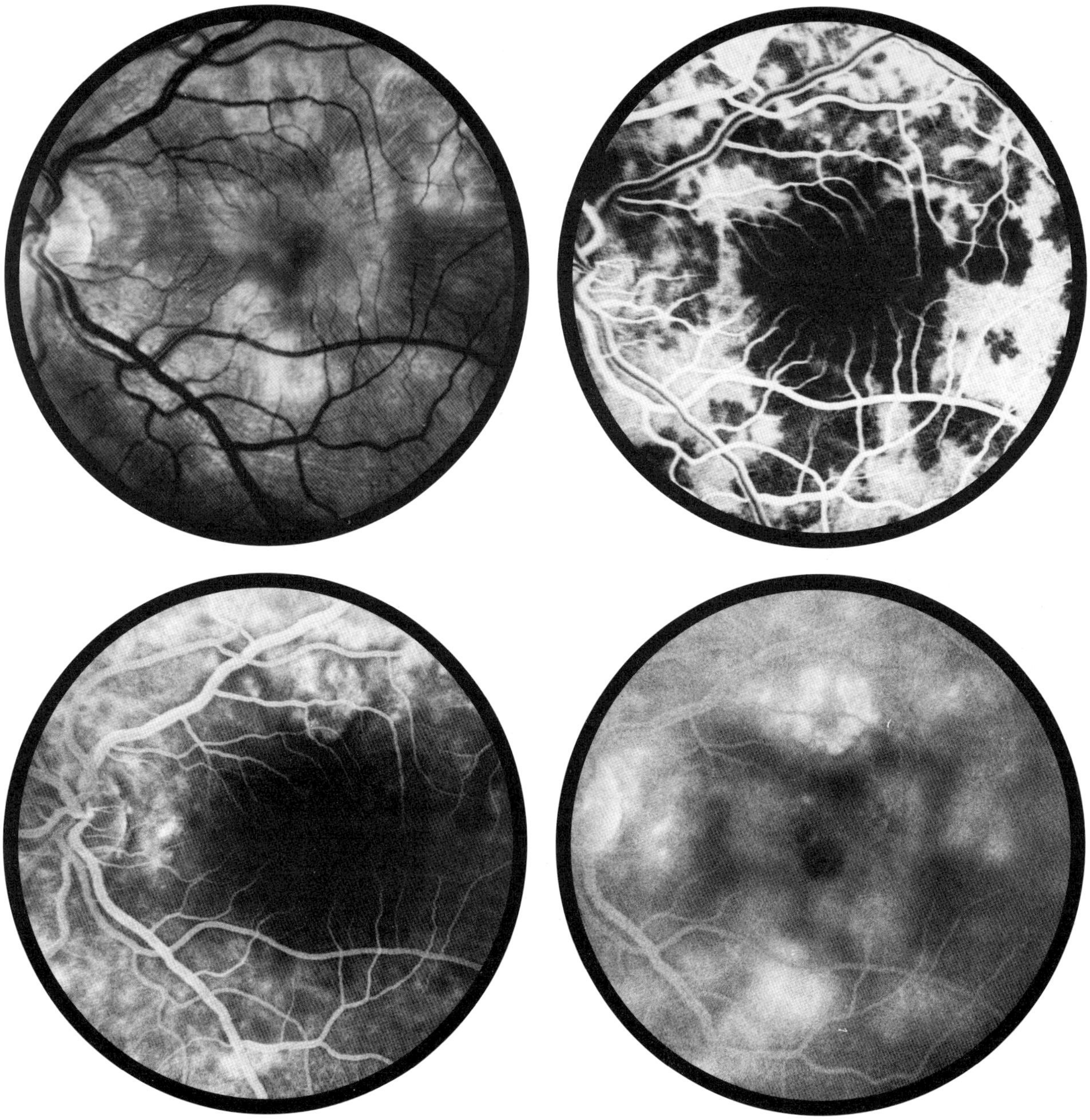

Figure 21.1. AMPPPE. *A*, ophthalmoscopic photograph of the macula showing numerous pale, round, flat lesions scattered over the posterior pole. *B*, arteriovenous phase angiogram demonstrating that the lesions are hypofluorescent at this stage in the study. *C*, in the late venous phase angiogram, the lesions being to hyperfluoresce. *D*, in the late phase angiogram, the lesions stain showing fuzzy hyperfluorescence. (From H. Schatz, T. Burton, L. Yannuzzi, and M. Rabb: Interpretation of Fundus Fluorescein Angiography, © C. V. Mosby Co., 1978; all reprinted with permission.)

Figure 21.2. AMPPPE. *A*, ophthalmoscopic photograph showing pigment clumping in the center of the macula and two fuzzy pigment epithelial lesions, one above and one below the fovea. *B*, early venous phase angiogram showing hypofluorescence of the lesions. Choroidal transmission hyperfluorescence (pigment epithelial window defect) is apparent around the margins of the pigmentary lesion in the center of the macula (*arrows*). *C*, late phase angiogram showing marked staining of the lesion, above and below the macula. The central lesion demonstrates hypofluorescence with staining of sclera around its edges. In this case, lesions of variable age or stage are evident. The central lesion is an older, resolved one showing pigment clumping. The lesions above and below the macula are more acute and demonstrate active inflammatory activity as indicated by fuzzy leakage of fluorescein. (From H. Schatz, T. Burton, L. Yannuzzi, and M. Rabb: Interpretation of Fundus Fluorescein Angiography, © C. V. Mosby Co., 1978; all reprinted with permission.)

Figure 21.3. AMPPPE, healed. *A*, ophthalmoscopic photograph of the left macula showing irregular multifocal lesions associated with pigment clumping and atrophy in a widespread distribution in the posterior pole. *B*, early venous phase angiogram showing hyperfluorescence of the scattered atrophic focal lesions mixed with hypofluorescence in regions of pigment clumping. *C*, late phase angiogram showing stainings of the pigment epithelial lesions and visible sclera. There is no fuzzy hyperfluorescence seen in acute lesions, indicating an absence of fluid in these lesions which have become scars.

A

B

C

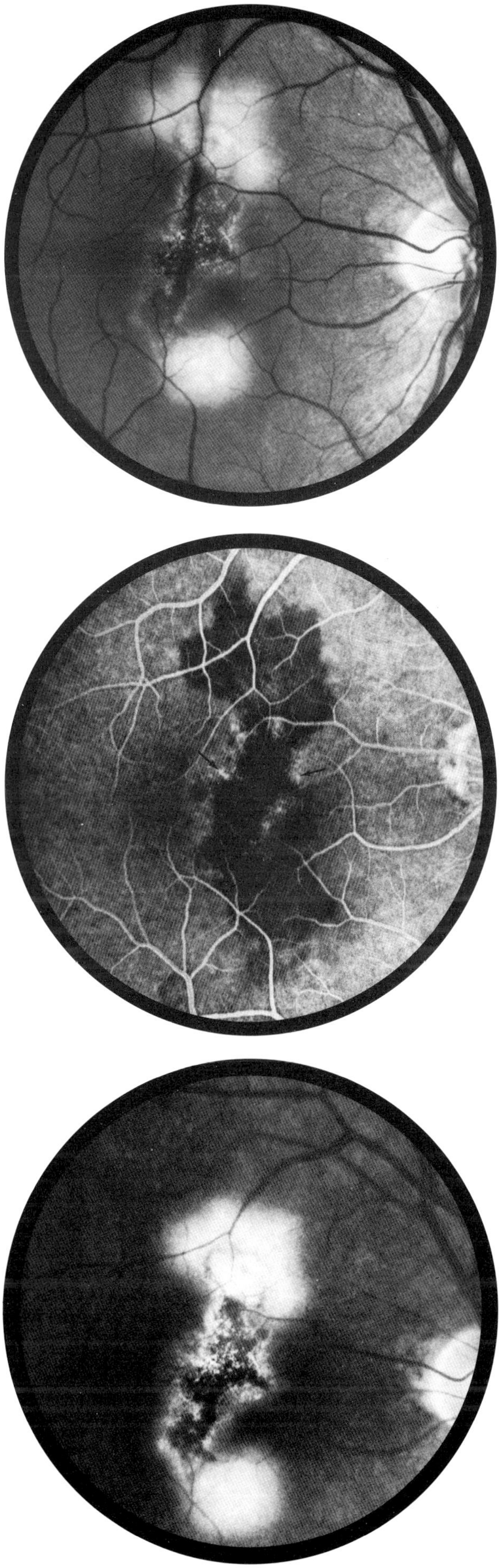

Figure 21.2.

A

B

C

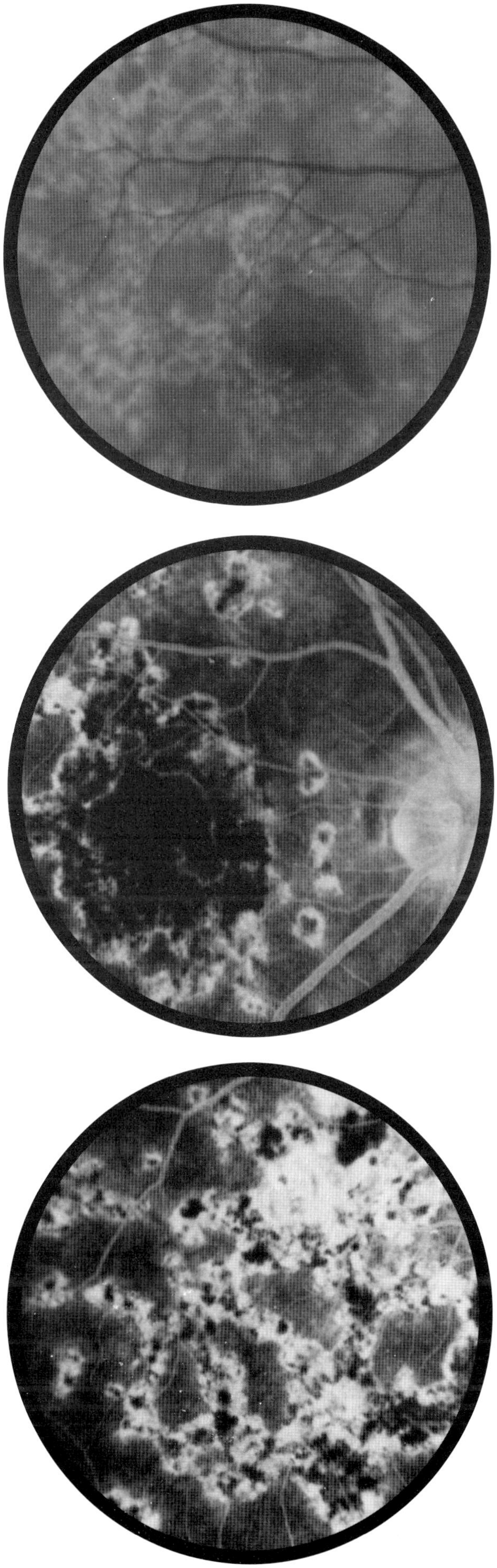

Figure 21.3.

Acute Retinal Pigment Epitheliitis

Acute retinal pigment epitheliitis is a condition affecting both young and middle-aged patients who experience an acute temporary reduction of central vision in one or both eyes, followed by a complete return of vision within 2–3 months.

The acute lesions, located in the macula at the level of the pigment epithelium, are approximately 300–500 μ in size (Figs. 21.4 and 21.5), much smaller than those seen in AMPPPE. They are multifocal and hyperpigmented with rings of depigmentation. The vision is reduced when the lesions are foveal.

On fluorescein angiography, spotty choroidal transmitted fluorescence (pigment epithelial window defects) are frequently noted. In some cases, a ring of hyperfluorescence is present around the hyperpigmented hypofluorescent center of the lesions. If a lesion affects the central macular area, the angiogram may be entirely normal because of the darker pigment epithelium in the macula. When the lesions resolve, a small hyperpigmented spot may be seen ophthalmoscopically. The treatment for this condition is not known.

Retinal pigment epitheliitis differs from AMPPPE in that the lesions are usually fewer in number, smaller in size, and appear different angiographically. However, some feel that this condition is a forme fruste or less severe form of AMPPPE because of its multifocal nature and its clinical course.

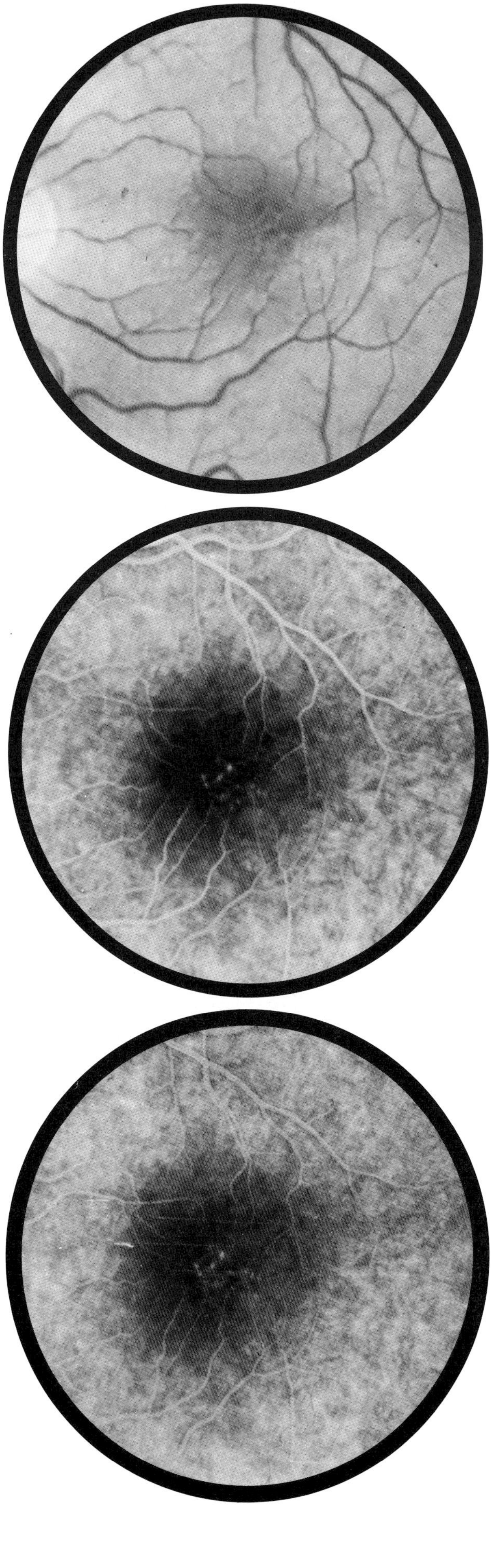

Figure 21.4. Acute retinal pigment epitheliitis. *A*, ophthalmoscopic photograph of the macula, showing fine pigment clumping and patchy atrophy. *B*, arteriovenous phase angiogram. Note the hyperfluorescent ring around the small pigment epithelial lesions. The center of the lesions are dark. *C*, late phase angiogram showing staining of the ring around the lesions.

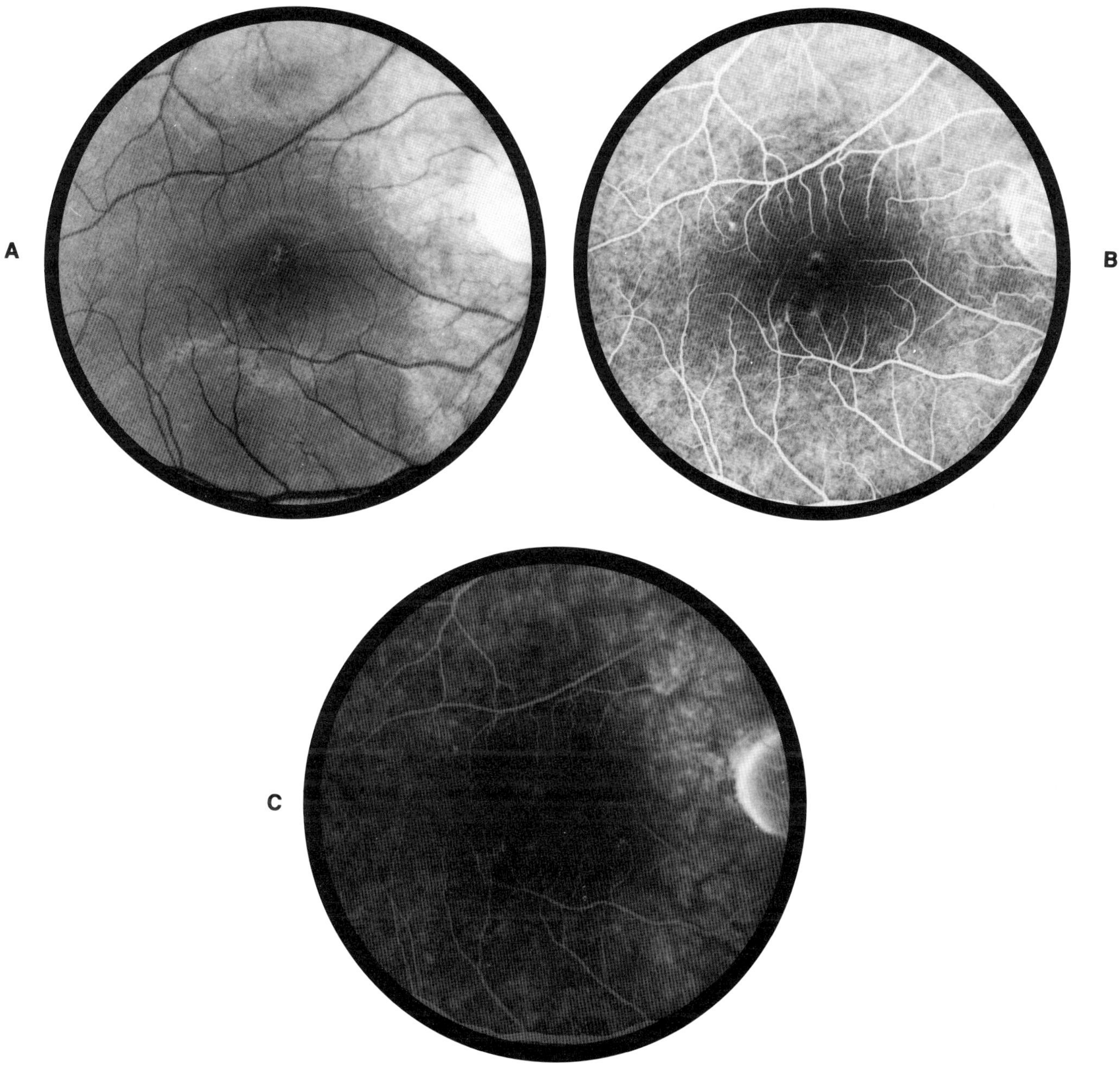

Figure 21.5. Acute retinal pigment epithelium. *A*, ophthalmoscopic photograph. Note the small pigment epithelial disturbance in the center of the fovea, and in the inferior and superior temporal macula. *B*, early venous phase angiogram showing a central pigment epithelial lesion which is hypofluorescent, surrounded by an irregular hyperfluorescent ring. A few smaller lesions are evident elsewhere in the macula. *C*, late phase angiogram showing fading of the hyperfluorescence.

GHPC

GHPC, also known as serpiginous choroidopathy, is a disorder of the peripapillary pigment epithelium, choriocapillaris, and choroid.

The condition is primary and progressive, extending out from the disc (Fig. 21.6), and in many instances, advancing into the macula, thereby reducing central visual acuity. The advancing edges of the primary lesion resemble pseudopods (Fig. 21.7). The disease is manifested in stages with an initial acute phase preceding chronic recurrent attacks adjacent to and continuous with old scans, or, less commonly as separate focal areas elsewhere in the fundus. A progressive course results in widespread geographic atrophy of the pigment epithelium and choriocapillaris (Fig. 21.8). There is also a forme fruste of the disorder: a small stationary lesion of the pigment epithelium adjacent to the optic nerve

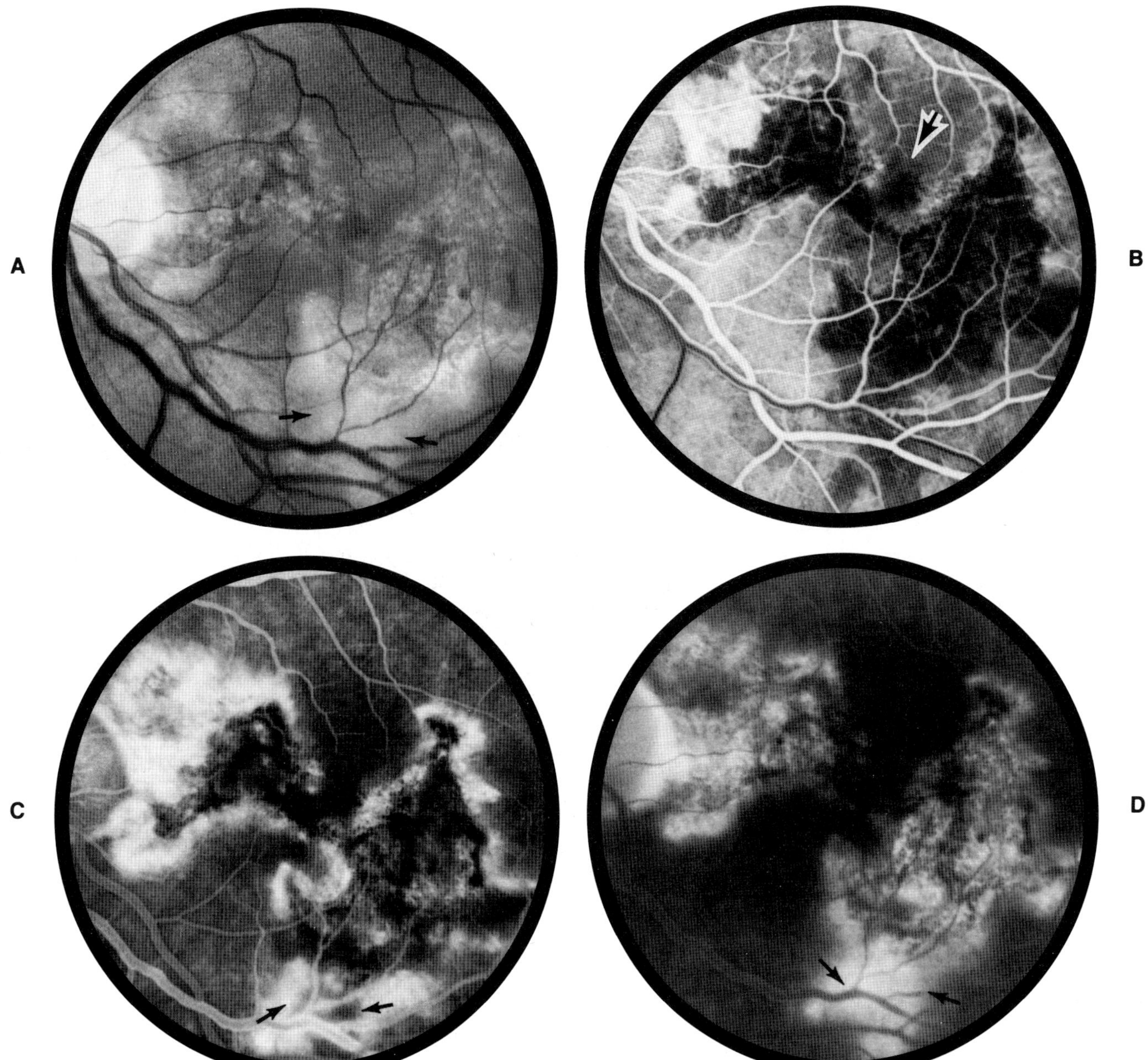

Figure 21.6. GHPC. *A*, ophthalmoscopic photograph of the fundus, showing irregular, geographic subretinal lesions with scattered pigmentation occupying the papillomacular bundle and macula. In the inferior macula, there is some subretinal whitening of the margin of one of the lesions (*arrows*). *B*, arteriovenous phase angiogram. Note the lesions are largely hypofluorescent except for some hyperfluorescence around the edges. The fovea (*arrow*) is spared. *C*, late venous phase angiogram. The margins are more hyperfluorescent. At the inferior aspect of the large macular lesion, fuzzy hyperfluorescence is now evident (*arrows*). The overlying retinal vessel also shows some perivascular leakage. *D*, late phase angiogram showing that most of the lesions are hyperfluorescent from staining of the subretinal scar and sclera. Fuzzy hyperfluorescence is present only at the inferior aspect of the large macular lesion (*arrows*) indicative of active inflammation. This case represents a recurrence at the margin of an old lesion. Because the fovea was spared, the vision was still 20/20.

head which may at some later date change into an acutely progressive lesion.

The condition affects equally both males and females. Most patients are between 40 and 60 years of age, although the disease has been reported in younger patients.

There is no known systemic disease associated with this condition. The medical history is usually negative, although a few patients have been reported to have had mild upper respiratory illnesses preceding the disorder.

Other than the complaint of recently reduced vision in those patients whose macula has been affected, there is no history of eye disease, pain, trauma, or infection. If the fovea is involved, central vision will be reduced; otherwise, the vision is usually excellent.

During the initial acute stage of the disease, the pale gray lesions appear as well circumscribed areas extending out from the optic nerve head. The slightly elevated and inflamed surrounding margins appear to be pigment epithelial

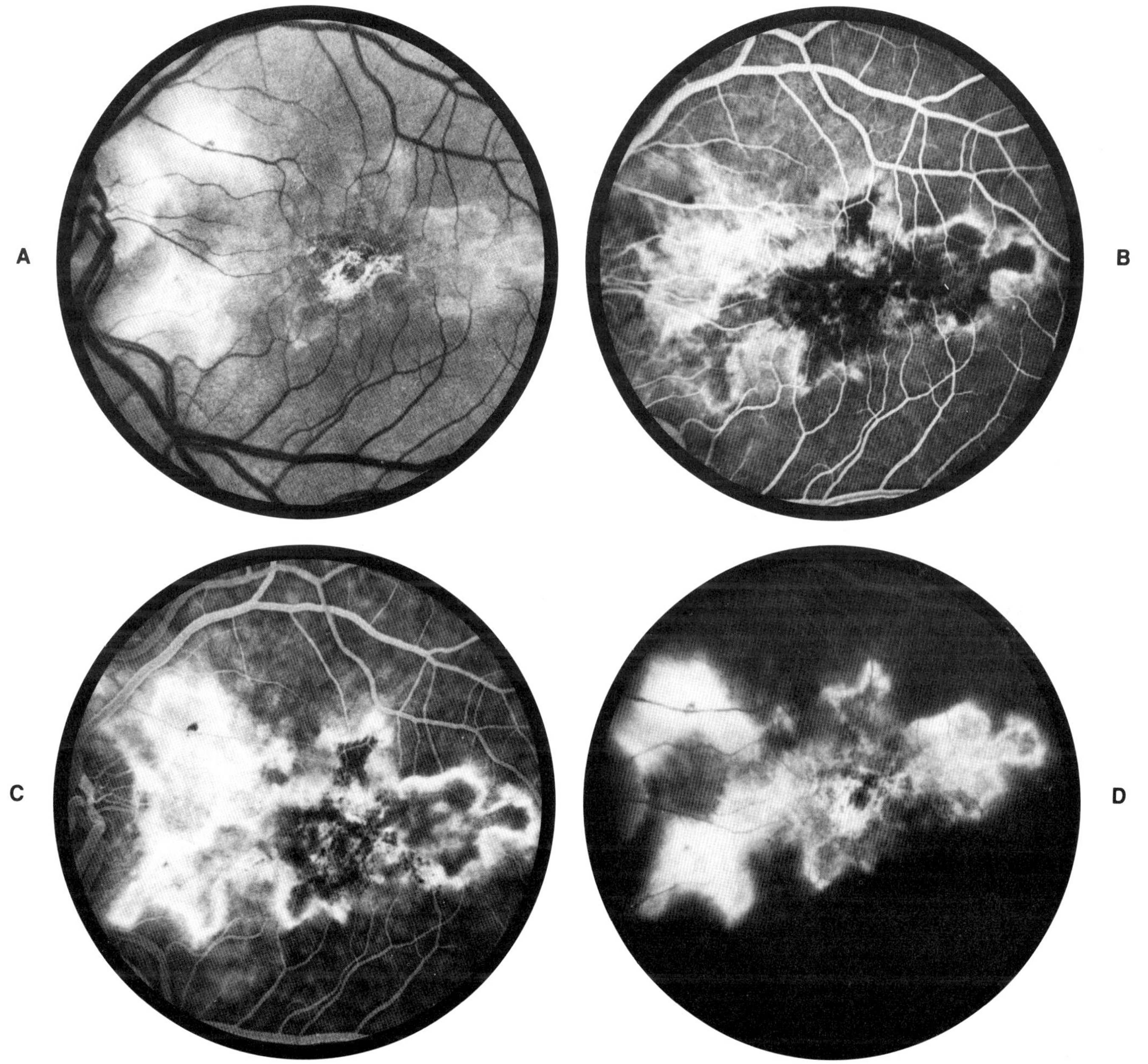

Figure 21.7. GHPC. *A*, ophthalmoscopic photograph of the disc and macula, showing an irregular geographic lesion emanating from the optic nerve head and coursing through and temporal to the macula. There is scarring adjacent to the disc, and irregular pigment clumping in the center of the fovea. *B*, arteriovenous phase angiogram showing that much of the lesion is hypofluorescent with hyperfluorescent borders. The portion of the lesion adjacent to the optic nerve head is also hyperfluorescent. *C*, late venous phase angiogram. Note that the hyperfluorescent border around the lesion has increased. *D*, late phase angiogram showing irregular hyperfluorescence of the lesion with some hypofluorescence in areas of pigmentation. The fuzzy, homogeneous hyperfluorescence in the portion of the lesion just supra- and infratemporal to the disc is suggestive of recent inflammation at these sites. The advancing edges of the lesion resemble pseudopods or protrusions from the primary sites. (From H. Schatz, T. Burton, L. Yannuzzi, and M. Rabb: Interpretation of Fundus Fluorescein Angiography, © C. V. Mosby Co., 1978; all reprinted with permission.)

A B C D

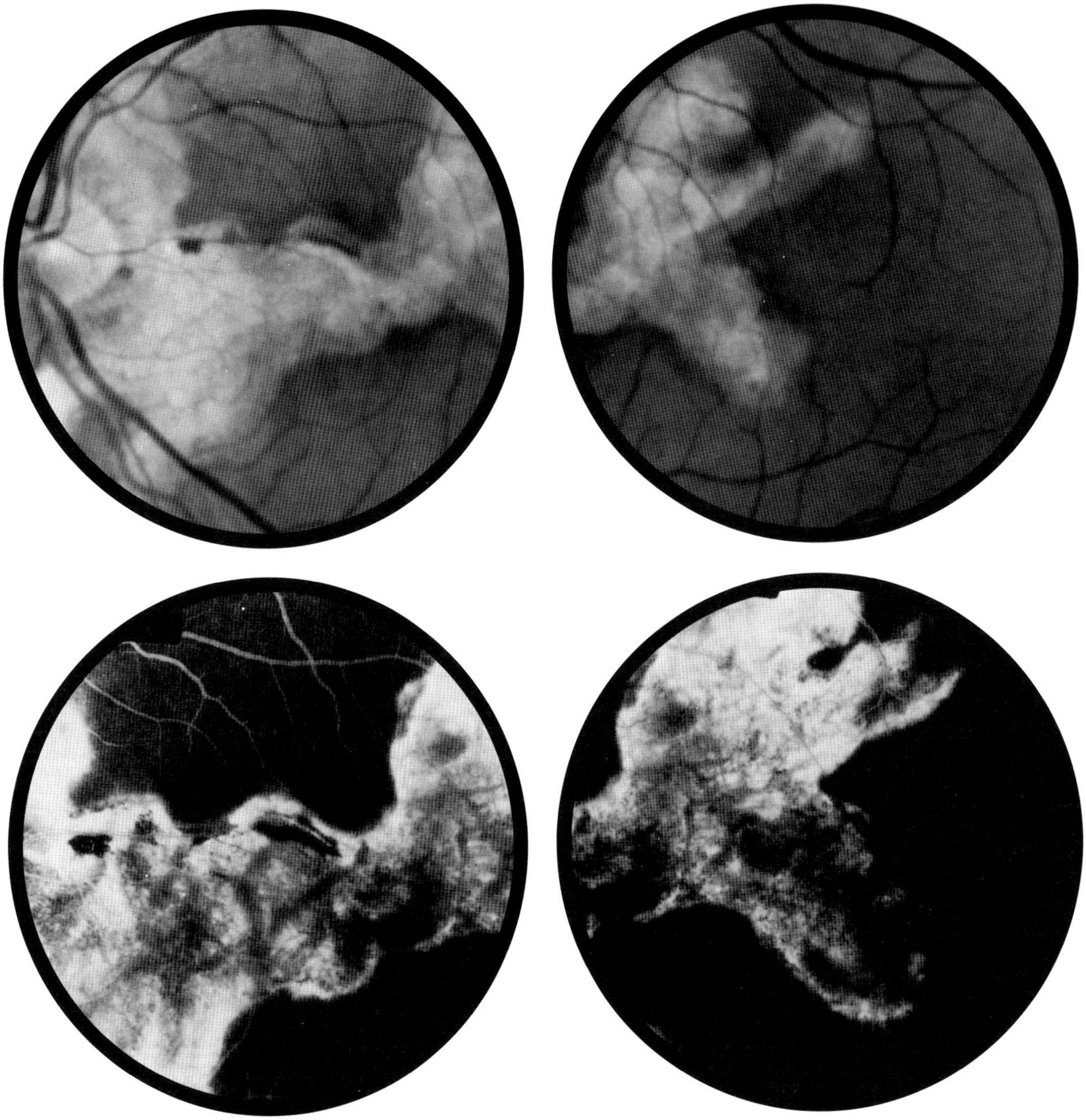

Figure 21.8. GHPC. *A* and *B*, ophthalmoscopic photographs of the left disc and macula. A geographic lesion is apparent coursing through the macula from the disc. Its temporal margins show pseudopod formation. *C* and *D*, late venous phase of the angiogram, the lesion appears to be hyperfluorescent with the exception of hypofluorescence in the areas of pigmentation. The subretinal hyperfluorescence is due, in part, to staining of scar but principally to staining of visible sclera as dark choroidal vessels can be seen to overly the more posterior fluorescence. There is no late fuzzy hyperfluorescence. This is an old, "burned out" lesion, showing atrophy with no evidence of any active inflammatory activity.

swelling. The lesions do not necessarily connect with the optic nerve head as "skip" areas of normal retina can be seen between lesions in some cases. Some lesions can involve a very broad area adjacent to the disc.

The sensory retina is usually flat although, occasionally, serous detachment may be present. Hemorrhages or exudates are not typically seen although subretinal neovascularization has been present in a few cases.

Although the lesion may be active in both eyes, it is usually at a different stage in each eye. Occasionally, the fellow eye has no involvement other than a very tiny peripapillary pigment epithelial scar area of depigmentation, which is possibly a forme fruste of the condition.

Over a period of one or two months the acute, pale gray lesions demonstrate irregular hyper- and hypopigmentation. The advancing edge of the lesion may continue to grow and to appear acute. The older lesions may eventually undergo severe atrophy affecting the choriocapillaris so that the large choroidal vessels and sclera become visible. Large areas of choroidal vascular atrophy have been seen in some cases. In some cases subretinal scarring may be present; this is probably a fibrous metaplasia of the pigment epithelium. An occasional patient may have retinal vascular leakage on fluorescein angiography indicating a perivasculitis of the overlying retinal vessels. A few patients will have acute lesions which are not connected to the primary peripapillary scar (skip lesions).

Recurrent episodes of activity may occur over a period of 1 or more years. When the lesion avoids the fovea, central vision is not affected but when the fovea is involved central vision will be poor. The central visual fields usually demonstrate a scotoma corresponding closely to the ophthalmoscopic pattern of the lesion. The scotoma indicates that the lesion involves the visual elements in the affected areas but does not include the nerve fiber bundle.

The fluorescein angiogram of this lesion is pathognomonic: in the early phases of the angiogram, the main part of the lesion is dark and has a hyperfluorescent border; it is not until later in the angiogram that the lesion shows spotty hyperfluorescence. The older portions of the lesion (adjacent to the disc) show hyperfluorescent staining caused by subretinal scarring. After the lesion has "burned out," atrophy of pigment epithelium and choriocapillaris is apparent so that the large choroidal vessels are visible within the lesion.

This condition differs from AMPPPE although the fluorescein pattern of the early hypofluorescent lesions with later staining may be quite similar. GHPC is a condition that is usually peripapillary with connected lesions, whereas in AMPPPE the lesions are multifocal, affecting mainly the macula and sometimes a greater portion of the posterior pole. The acute stage of GHPC may recur continually for many months or even years and when the lesion affects the fovea, visual acuity may be poor. In AMPPPE the acute stage lasts only a few weeks, recurrences are rare, and vision usually recovers.

There has been no definite histopathologic material of GHPC available for study. It is our opinion that this lesion is an inflammation and may possibly be controlled by steroids when the fovea and central vision are threatened. If the fovea and central vision are not threatened the lesion should be carefully watched for possible progression into the fovea. We have used systemic or retrobulbar steroids with good results in some, but not all, patients. After such treatment, the patient should be followed very carefully for recurrence. The prognosis in this disease is quite uncertain, since the macula may suddenly become involved in many cases, resulting in reduction in vision.

Suggested Readings

Azar, P., Jr., Gohd, R.S., Waltman, D., and Gitter, K.A.: Acute posterior multifocal placoid pigment epitheliopathy associated with an adenotype V virus. *Am J Ophthalmol, 80:* 1003, 1975.

Deutman, F.D., and Lion, F.: Choriocapillaris nonperfusion in acute multifocal placoid pigment epitheliopathy. *Am J Ophthalmol, 84:* 652, 1977.

Gass, J.D.M.: Acute multifocal posterior placoid pigment epitheliopathy. *Arch Ophthalmol, 80:* 173, 1968.

Hamilton, A.M., and Bird, A.C.: Geographical choroidopathy. *Brit J Ophthalmol, 58:* 784, 1974.

Krill, A. E., and Deutman, A F : Acute retinal pigment epitheliitis. *Am J Ophthalmol, 74:* 193, 1972.

Schatz, H.: Other retinal pigment epithelial diseases *Int Ophthalmol Clin, 15:* 181, 1975.

Schatz, H.: Fundus Fluorescein Angiography: A Composite Slide Collection, Appleton-Century-Crofts, New York, 1975.

Schatz, H., Maumenee, A.E., and Patz, A.: Geographic helicoid peripapillary choroidopathy (GHPC). *Trans Am Acad Ophthalmol Otolaryngol, 78:* 33, 1974.

Schatz, H., Burton, T., Yannuzzi, L., and Rabb, M.: Interpretation of Fundus Fluorescein Angiography, C.V. Mosby Co., St. Louis, 1978.

PART IV

Miscellaneous Diseases

CHAPTER 22

Cystoid Macular Edema, Preretinal Membrane Formation and Macular Holes

James R. Brinkley, Jr., M.D., and Stephen J. Ryan, M.D.

Cystoid Macular Edema

The misuse of the term "macular edema" to cover a host of morphologic appearances, ranging from serous detachment of the sensory retina to intracellular cloudy swelling characteristic of central retinal artery occlusion, has been the source of much confusion. Fluorescein angiography and improved methods of clinical examination have allowed us to be more specific and to use the term "edema" to refer to extracellular fluid accumulation.

Cystoid macular edema or cystoid maculopathy is the accumulation of extracellular fluid (from leaking macular capillaries) in an anatomic pattern conforming to Henle's layer (the outer plexiform layer) of the macula [1]. Although the fluid accumulates most extensively in Henle's fiber layer, it also extends into the inner nuclear layer [2]. Clinically, one can visualize the intraretinal cystoid spaces in a concentric pattern around the fovea by using the slit lamp with a Hruby or fundus contact lens.

The importance of cystoid maculopathy rests with the fact that it can lead to the loss of central vision, although the degree of reduction in visual acuity does not always correlate with the visible edema [3].

A variety of intraocular diseases, originating from the vitreous, retina or choroid, may be the underlying basis for cystoid macular edema [4] (Table 22.1). Vitreous inflammation (vitritis or chronic cyclitis), preretinal membrane formation, topical epinephrine, and involvement of the retinal vasculature from diabetes, hypertension, radiation, telangiectasia, venous occlusive disease, vasculitis, retinitis pigmentosa, macroaneurysm formation, and postcataract surgery (Irvine-Gass syndrome) are common causes of cystoid macular edema. In addition, subretinal disorders such as choroidal inflammation, tumors, and neovascularization may also predispose to this manifestation.

In the case of retinitis pigmentosa, a cystoid appearance may exist in the macula without true leakage evident on fluorescein angiography. This form of "cystoid appearing" maculopathy without leakage resembles the macular findings in juvenile retinoschisis, some preretinal membranes, and eyes with previously active leakage and irreversible intraretinal structural damage. Other causes of a cystoid-appearing maculopathy without fluorescein leakage are listed in Table 22.2.

IRVINE-GASS SYNDROME

Cystoid macular edema after cataract extraction (Irvine-Gass syndrome) has been more thoroughly studied than cystoid maculopathy from any other condition and this will be considered first [2, 5]. The incidence of rupture of the

Table 22.1. Cystoid macular edema

- Vitreous
  - Preretinal membrane formation
  - Inflammation (vitritis, chronic cyclitis)
- Retina
  - Venous occlusive disease
    - Diabetic
    - Nondiabetic (branch and central)
  - Hypertension
  - Macroaneurysm
  - Tumors
  - Telangiectasia
  - Hereditary disease (retinitis pigmentosa)
  - Epinephrine toxicity
  - Inflammations
    - Phlebitis
    - Arteritis
    - Papillophlebitis
    - Post intraocular surgery (Irvine-Gass syndrome)
- Choroid
  - Tumors
  - Subretinal neovascularization
  - Inflammation

Table 22.2. Cystoid-appearing maculopathy (no leakage)

- Vitreous
  - Preretinal membrane formation
- Retina
  - Resolved cystoid macular edema with irreversible retinal structural change
  - Degenerative cystic change
    - Involutional cyst formation
    - Resolved sensory retinal detachment
  - Hereditary diseases
    - Retinitis pigmentosa
    - Juvenile retinoschisis
    - Goldmann-Favre disease
- Retinal pigment epithelium
  - Nicotinic acid toxicity

anterior hyaloid face, mild intraocular inflammation, and macular edema occuring in the postoperative cataract patient with a resultant loss of vision (after an initial good visual result) was originally estimated to be approximately 2% [5]. Subsequently, a prospective study has shown the incidence to be as high as 50% [3] in those patients examined at the time of highest incidence [6]. It should be noted that when fluorescein angiographic criteria are employed for the diagnosis of Irvine-Gass syndrome, a much higher incidence is reported since many patients with cystoid do not have significant visual symptoms. The incidence of cystoid macular edema in patients with visual decline in this period is most probably 10–15%. It is very uncommon to see cystoid edema in the 1st week following cataract surgery [7].

Both sexes are affected equally in this condition and the age of the patient at the time of cataract extraction is not a factor [3, 8]. Although a higher incidence of cystoid macular edema has been observed in Caucasians than in Negroes, the importance of racial factors cannot be discussed with certainty [8].

The clinical presentation of patients with the Irvine-Gass syndrome follows a typical pattern. Usually, patients have a good visual result immediately following cataract extraction; but later during the postoperative course (usually 1–4 months) they begin to experience a decrease in visual acuity often accompanied by irritation of the eye and photophobia [2]. This drop in visual acuity may not be appreciated by the patient if he has not been fitted with an aphakic correction. Although the syndrome most frequently occurs from 4–12 weeks postoperatively [2], it may occur up to 20 years later [9]. However, 50% of cases occur within 3 months of the time of surgery and 75% occur within 6 months [8].

The clinical findings and fluorescein angiographic picture have been described in detail in the classic article of Gass and Norton [2]. Visual acuity is usually reduced to the range of 20/50 to 20/100. Strands of vitreous to the cataract incision and/or peaking of the pupil are observed in approximately 50% of the cases and there is often mild circumlimbal injection and a small number of vitreous cells. Examination of the macular region with the slit lamp and Hruby or fundus contact lens frequently reveals prominent intraretinal cystoid spaces of variable size in a concentric pattern around the fovea. Occasionally, a small amount of subretinal fluid is present in addition to the intraretinal cystoid edema.

The fluorescein angiographic findings typically show leakage from the deep perifoveal capillaries in a circular or wreath-like pattern [2] which progresses centrally and peripherally (at a variable rate). Eventually (usually within 15 minutes) a stellate figure is apparent which conforms to the oblique orientation of the outer plexiform fibers in the macular region. The outer margins of the area of dye leakage are irregular and superficial. Macular vessels can be seen to pass over the dye (Fig. 22.1).

Histopathologically, the retina is thickened and extensive cystoid spaces are seen in the outer plexiform and inner nuclear layers. The larger of these spaces are seen in the outer plexiform (Henle's layer). These spaces contain an eosinophilic exudate which displaces the rod and cone nuclei and the receptor cell axons. It is the ability of these cells to be displaced that allows such a large fluid accumulation in this layer. If the fluid remains for a long period, degenerative changes may lead to irreversible loss of nerve tissue and resultant permanent cystoid spaces, which persist even after the integrity of the perifoveal capillaries is restored and may lead to permanent decrease in vision. However, cases have been documented in which visual acuity of 20/30 or better was maintained despite persistent cystoid macular edema present for more than 1 year [2, 3]. While the possible etiologic role of direct vitreous traction has been proposed, most authors dismiss this cause as insignificant in the pathogenesis of cystoid macular edema [1, 8, 9]. Gass and Norton found no evidence of vitreoretinal traction on the macula in their pathologic studies [2].

The course of cystoid macular edema following cataract extraction is quite variable [3, 8]. The majority of cases resolve either completely or partially without treatment (70–75%) whereas a few remain unchanged or become worse. Although it is not possible to correlate the degree of reduction in visual acuity with the amount of edema present clinically or on fluorescein angiography, it is sometimes possible to predict the course of the patient's visual acuity based on an increase or decrease of edema [3]. There do not appear to be specific factors in the initial history, clinical examination, or angiographic studies which enable one to predict the course of this condition in any given patient [2, 3, 8]. However Gass and Norton [8] demonstrated that patients with vitreous to the wound were more likely to have persistent cystoid macular edema and reduction in vision [8].

Although the etiology of cystoid macular edema following cataract extraction is unknown, certain predisposing factors do exist [2, 3, 8]. These include some forms of systemic vascular disease; the most frequent are hypertension, diabetes, and other cardiovascular disease, in that order [8]. Hitchings, *et al.* [3] felt that intraocular inflammatory disease might be a significant contributing factor, although in most cases he attributed the condition to the trauma of lens removal and postoperative iritis.

Patients who have developed cystoid macular edema after cataract extraction in their first eye seem to have a tendency to develop cystoid in the second eye as well, although the exact incidence of this occurrence is not known. It is the clinical impression of some that cystoid macular edema is less frequent in extracapsular cataract extraction as compared with intracapsular. Some cataract surgeons who favor implantation of intraocular lenses have argued that the incidence of macular edema is lower in patients with implants than in patients without implants and particularly lower when an extracapsular extraction is performed. A recent study by Allen and Jaffe [10] does suggest that both the preceding statements may have some merit. However, it must be emphasized that this was an interim report in an ongoing study, that the follow-up time was short, and the number of patients was relatively small when their report was issued.

It has also been the clinical impression of some surgeons that the incidence of cystoid macular edema is less in patients who have undergone phacoemulsification as compared with more traditional methods of cataract extraction.

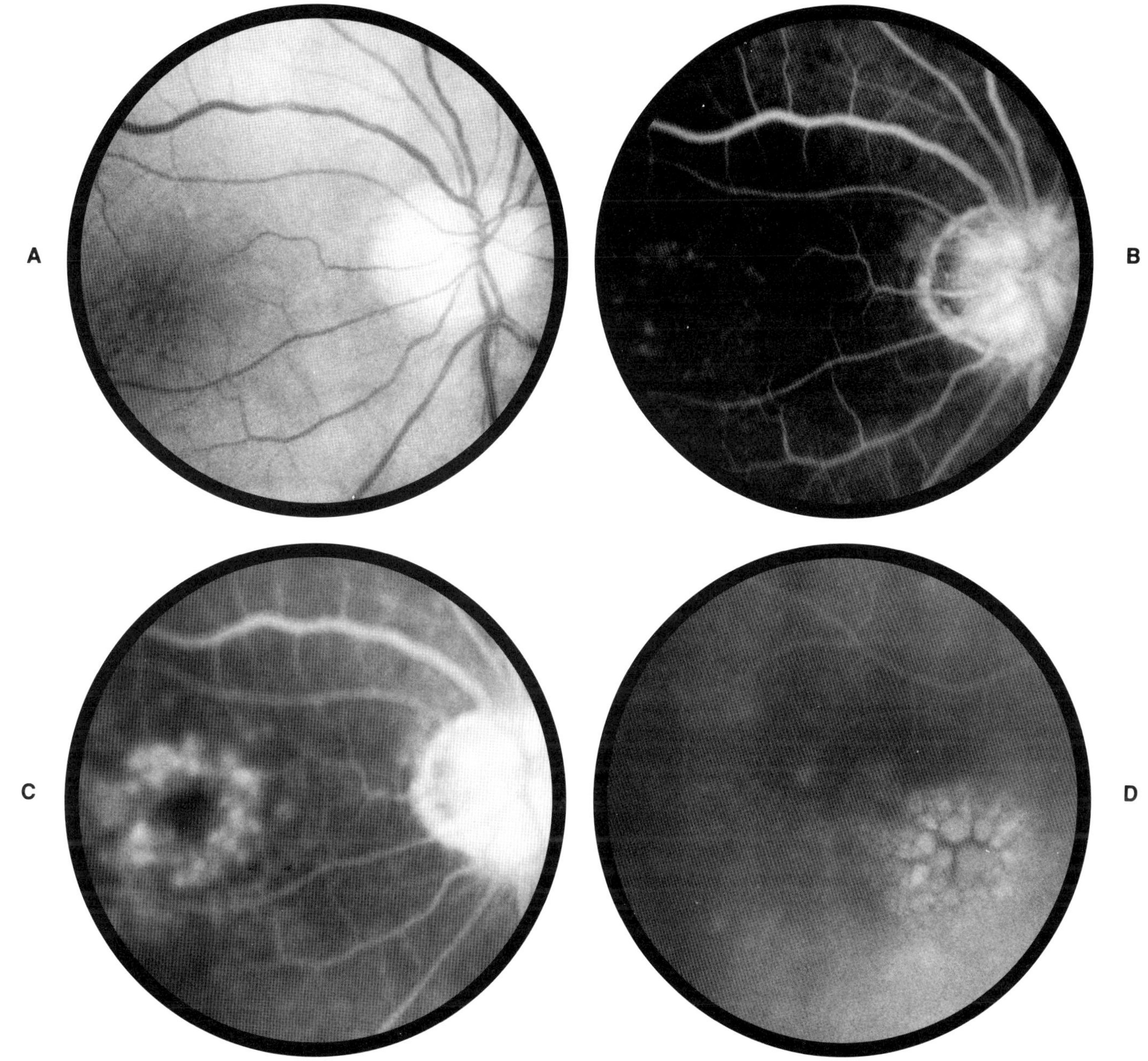

Figure 22.1. Cystoid macular edema after cataract extraction. *A*, red-free photograph. Note the intraretinal cystoid spaces in the macula. *B*, venous phase angiogram; note the dye leaking from perifoveal capillaries. *C*, venous phase angiogram; note the dye diffusing both inward and outward. *D*, late phase angiogram. A dark stellate pattern is seen against a white background of dye in cystoid spaces. Note the irregular outer margins of accumulated dye.

However, no well controlled series has been reported to substantiate this.

To date, there is no satisfactory treatment for aphakic cystoid macular edema. Photocoagulation appears to serve no useful purpose. While there is a rationale for treatment of cystoid macular edema with an antiprostaglandin such as indomethacin, one controlled study failed to show any value to this form of therapy [11]. The same authors have had encouraging experience with oral indomethacin used prophylactically, commencing the first day of cataract surgery, in the reduction of the incidence of cystoid edema when compared to a controlled untreated group. Some patients seem to respond favorably to systemic or subconjunctival steroids but often experience visual decline following its discontinuation. Finally, pars plana vitrectomy with revision of the anterior segment has been employed by some, but there is still no definite evidence that this is a reliable and safe means of therapy.

CYSTOID MACULAR EDEMA FOLLOWING OCULAR SURGERY OTHER THAN CATARACT EXTRACTION

Although cystoid macular edema has long been known as a complication of retinal detachment, it has not traditionally been considered a complication of retinal detachment surgery. It has now been demonstrated that cystoid macular edema may occur as a complication of retinal surgery in phakic patients whose maculas were attached preoperatively [9]. Thus, it would seem that some cases of cystoid macular edema occurring after retinal reattachment procedures (in aphakic patients) in whom the macula was attached preoperatively might also be the result of the retinal surgery itself rather than a late occurring Irvine-Gass syndrome.

Cystoid macular edema may also follow combined penetrating keratoplasty and cataract extraction as well as penetrating keratoplasty alone in previously aphakic patients. In one series, it occurred in over 50% of the patients [12]. A number of additional patients, after these procedures, showed diffuse or patchy macular edema, not present in the typical cystoid pattern. Most of the patients with cystoid macular edema or macular edema in other patterns following the surgical procedures had some vitreous manipulation during surgery or vitreous to the wound postoperatively. However, all eight patients in this series who underwent surgery without vitreous manipulation and who had no vitreous to the wound postoperatively, nonetheless developed cystoid macular edema or diffuse macular edema.

Maumenee [9] has observed the development of cystoid macular edema in phakic patients following filtering surgery for glaucoma, and Michels and Ryan [13] noted this condition following pars plana vitrectomy in both phakic and aphakic patients.

RETINAL VASCULAR AND INFLAMMATORY DISORDERS CAUSING CYSTOID MACULAR EDEMA

Cystoid macular edema may occur as a complication of diabetic retinopathy, hypertensive retinopathy, central retinal vein obstruction, branch retinal vein obstruction, retinal telangiectasia, and radiation therapy [14]. In both central and branch retinal venous obstruction of a low-grade chronic type, the degree of visual loss does correlate with the amount of edema in the macula. In addition to the typical stellate pattern about the fovea on the angiogram, the other angiographic findings of the venous obstruction are present.

In hypertensive retinopathy, the cystoid edema may be accompanied by preretinal membrane formation which may play a role in the reduction of perifoveal capillary integrity. However, cystoid maculopathy alone may account for the decreased vision. In diabetic retinopathy, the earliest angiographic findings are alterations in capillary permeability and development of microaneurysms. However, findings of cystoid macular edema in diabetics are not uncommon (Fig. 22.2). Cystoid macular edema may also occur in patients with retinal telangiectasia and Coats' disease [14].

Gass [14] reported that triad of chronic iridocyclitis, cystoid macular edema, and papilledema in a number of conditions, including pars planitis, the Irvine-Gass syndrome, mild intraocular inflammation of unknown etiology in older patients, and peripheral retinitis due to toxoplasmosis. The fluorescein angiographic findings in these patients is identical with all other conditions previously discussed. Cystoid macular edema may also occur in Behçet's syndrome, acute nongranulomatous iridocyclitis, nodular cyclitis, and nematode endophthalmitis [4].

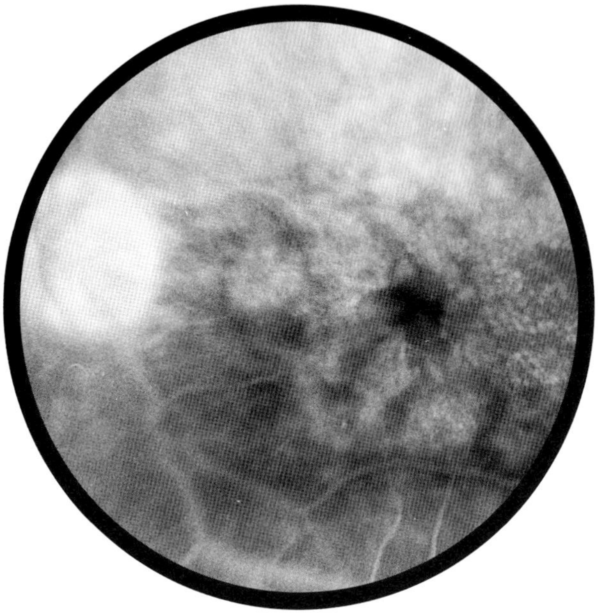

Figure 22.2. Cystoid macular edema in a diabetic. Venous phase; 2 minutes. Note the more diffuse leakage of dye than that seen in cystoid macular edema after cataract extraction (compare with Fig. 22.1).

EPINEPHRINE MACULOPATHY

Cystoid maculopathy due to topically administered epinephrine in aphakic patients and reversible on cessation of the epinephrine was initially noted by Kolker and Becker [15]. The reduction in visual acuity is quite variable in these patients, and the time required for restoration of vision after discontinuing epinephrine therapy ranges from 1–6 months and occasionally longer. There are also those patients who do not respond to the withdrawal of epinephrine.

A recent study, describing the angiographic findings in this condition as being typical of cystoid macular edema, demonstrated decreases in the cystoid edema when epinephrine was withdrawn and recurrences when it was reinstituted [4].

SUBRETINAL CAUSES OF CYSTOID MACULAR EDEMA

There are essentially three general causes of cystoid macular edema originating from subretinal factors. These are: choroidal inflammation, subretinal neovascularization, and choroidal tumors. The choroidal neovascularization which predisposes to cystoid edema may be from any of the many causes of choroidal membranes. While choroidal hemangiomas are typically associated with overlying cystoid retinal edema, any other choroidal tumor may lead to this change in the retina.

Preretinal Membrane Formation

Preretinal membrane formation is a condition characterized by the formation of a preretinal membrane in the macular area with fair to good preservation of visual acuity.

Other names, or more appropriately divisions of this disorder, according to severity, include: cellophane maculopathy, wrinkling of the internal limiting membrane, epiretinal membrane, macular pucker surface wrinkling maculopathy, preretinal fibrosis, and preretinal gliosis [16].

INCIDENCE AND CLINICAL FINDINGS

Wise followed 150 cases of preretinal membrane formation which he referred to as idiopathic preretinal macular fibrosis [16]. Twenty percent of his cases were bilateral and the average age of onset was 65. Wise pointed out that there are no symptoms early in the evolution of these membranes. As the fovea became involved, the patient experienced some metamorphopsia and ultimately a decrease in visual acuity.

Examination of a patient with an early preretinal membrane reveals a glinting light reflex. Later, retinal folds or traction lines appear and eventually a band or membrane over the retina is seen. This can sometimes partially detach and spontaneously pull off into the vitreous. Posterior vitreous detachment is usually present when the diagnosis is made. However, it has been shown that only a very small number of patients with posterior vitreous detachment develop cellophane-like macular changes [17].

The progression of the condition is slow. After development of folds in the retina, a characteristic tortuosity of the perimacular vessels is seen [18] with the superior and inferior retinal vessels pulled closer together than in the normal eye [1].

Fluorescein findings range from no leakage [1] to spotty and irregular leakage from the perifoveal capillaries or small veins about the macula [14]. Adhesions between the preretinal membrane and the detached posterior vitreous are usually not seen [1, 16]. Maumenee has noted that these membranes may rarely peel off spontaneously leading to a return of a normal visual acuity [1]. Infrequently, cystoid edema may occur and the contracting membrane may then cause rupture of the cysts leading to a lamellar macular hole [16]. Recently, Allen and Gass [19] have reported four cases in which holes in preretinal membranes simulated macular holes (Fig. 22.3). A similar finding had previously been reported by Maumenee [1].

The importance of red-free photographs to document the presence of inner retinal changes in conditions such as lamellar holes and preretinal membranes should be noted. Often the fluorescein angiogram and color photographs are relatively normal but the red-free photographs are diagnostic (Fig. 22.4).

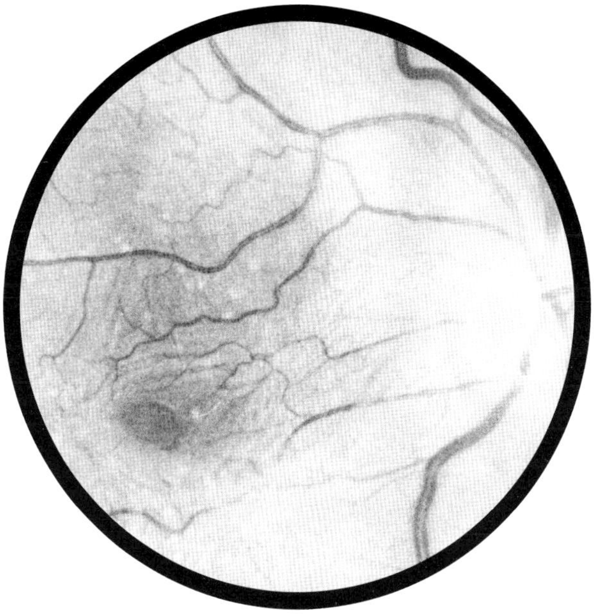

Figure 22.3. Preretinal membrane formation. Note the pseudohole which has formed in the membrane over the macular area.

ETIOLOGY

Although the exact etiology of preretinal membrane disease is unknown, it is associated with a number of ocular conditions, including postvascular occlusion, macular pucker after retinal detachment surgery, postphotocoagulation, posttrauma, postinflammation, and as a proliferative reaction after venous obstruction [16]. In Wise's series, the only associated ocular finding was retinal arteriosclerosis, and no systemic disease was found in association with this cellophane change [16].

Maumenee [1], in 1967, suggested three possible causes for preretinal membrane formation. The first was condensation and contraction of the vitreous on the surface of the retina. The second was splitting of the internal limiting membrane with proliferation of vitreous cells on the vitreous part of the internal limiting membrane leading to contraction of the internal surface of the retina (documented histologically in one case). The third possibility was contraction of the internal limiting membrane alone.

Jaffe [18] postulated that wrinkling or contraction of the internal limiting membrane of the retina occurs as a late complication of vitreoretinal traction. In some cases of posterior vitreous detachment, residual vitreous remains on the retina after separation, which then leads to contraction of the inner retinal layers. While this may be the mechanism in some cases, Bellhorn and associates [20] have shown that the cause of these membranes is glial cell proliferation on the surface of the retina. They described a single layer of astrocytic glial cells that had migrated through a break in the internal limiting membrane and proliferated on the surface of the retina in an eye which clinically had a glinting reflex. In a second case in which the patient was seen clinically to have retinal folds and a malignant melanoma in the periphery, a glial cell membrane (composed primarily of astrocytic glial cells, but also of Müller-like cells and perivascular glial cells) was found on the surface of the retina histologically. This case was studied by electron microscopy and there were noted to be intercellular desmosomes within the membrane as well as attachments of the glial cell membrane to the internal limiting membrane of the retina. The nerve fiber layer was not involved. It was thus postulated that when the surface cells in the membrane contracted, the superficial layers, including the glial cell membrane and the inner limiting membrane of the retina, could slide along the uninvolved nerve fiber layer and lead to retinal folds without reducing visual acuity. No vitreoretinal lesions were seen in these cases. This work suggests

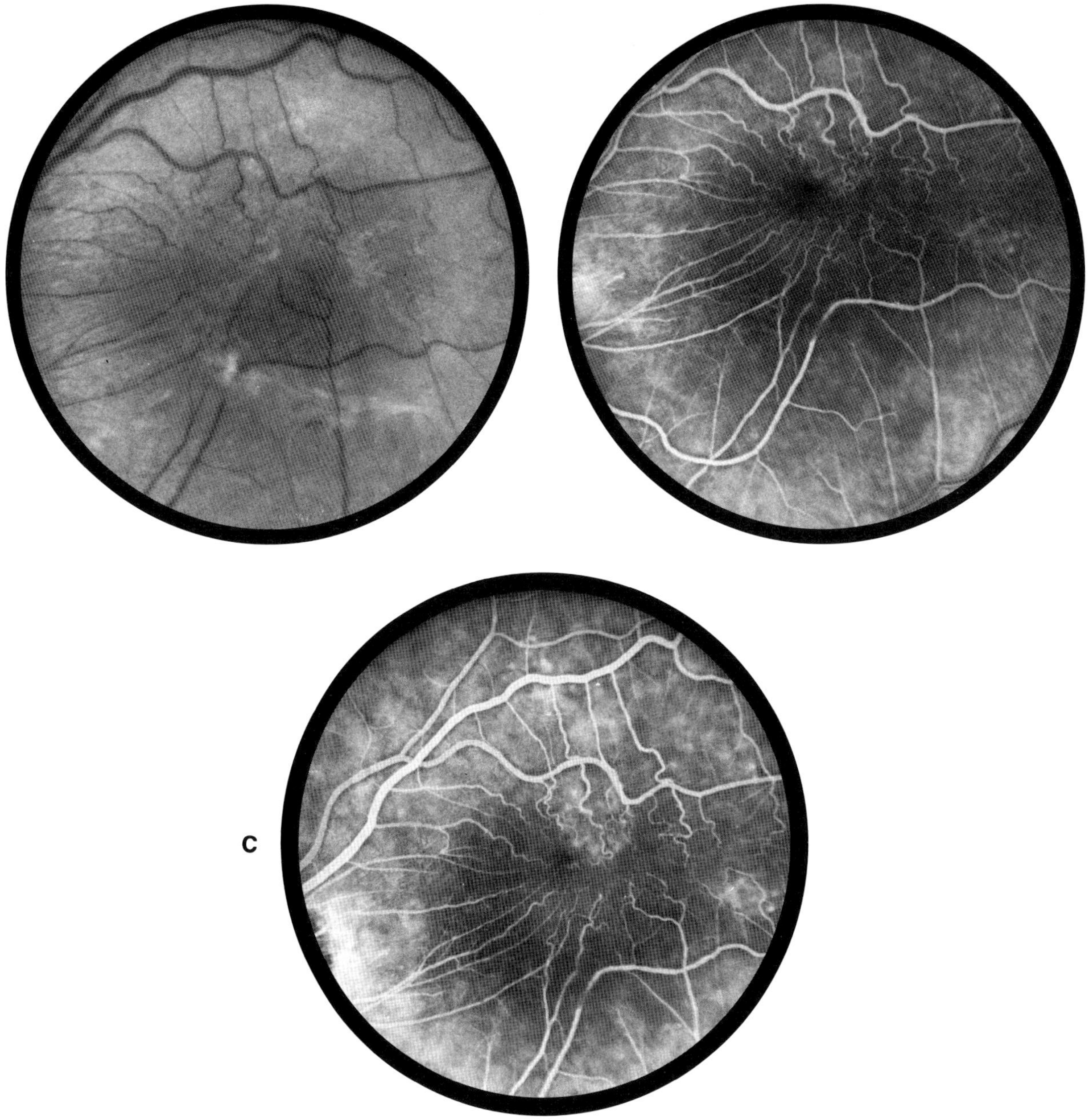

Figure 22.4. *A*, ophthalmoscopic photograph of preretinal membrane formation, showing contraction and pucker of the macula with increased tortuosity of the paramacular retinal vasculature. *B* and *C*, fluorescein angiograms documenting retinovascular tortuosity and vascular dye leakage seen in these eyes.

that the origin of the preretinal membranes is from retinal glial, which migrate through defects in the internal limiting membrane and then proliferate on the retinal surface [20]. At this stage, clinical examination of the patient would reveal only a glinting retinal reflex. When the cells of this preretinal membrane contract, the retinal folds seen clinically are then produced in the manner just described. Previous authors have felt that the cells comprising this membrane might have been epithelial, mesenchymal, retinal pigment epithelial, retinal vessel adventitial, or vitreal [19]. Evidence in support of this has now been described by Clarkson and his associates [21]. Glial, fibrous, cortical vitreous, retinal pigment epithelial, and combinations of these elements most commonly formed membranes in selected cases studied by electron microscopy. Glial membranes resulted from defects in the internal limiting membrane (such as retinal pits or holes) or from the disc in association with posterior vitreous detachments; fibrous membranes were seen in eyes with proliferative retinopathies and long-standing detachments; cortical vitreous membranes were seen in eyes with no other pathology, and pigment epithelial membranes were found in eyes with rhegmatogenous retinal detachments.

PROGNOSIS

Many of these patients retain stable vision throughout their course [1]. Progression of the disease is slow and even when vision decreases, subsequent spontaneous peeling off of the membrane from the surface of the retina may lead to a return of good vision [1, 19].

Macular Holes

The etiology of macular holes most often remains obscure. Classically, atrophic degeneration, breakdown of cystoid macular edema, and trauma are considered the leading causes [22].

Other rare causes for macular hole formation include foveomacular retinitis, solar burns, severe intraocular inflammation, and high myopia. Macular hole formation in high myopia can result in retinal detachment even in the absence of peripheral retinal holes.

INCIDENCE AND CLINICAL FINDINGS

Aaberg [22] analyzed 90 consecutive cases of macular holes with regard to vitreous and retinal abnormalities, excluding those unusual cases in which hole formation was caused by one of the conditions listed above. In this series, only 10% of cases were due to trauma. The nontraumatic cases were analyzed for data that might be helpful in discerning an etiology but the cause remained unknown. It was found that 90% of the patients were women, 39% were hypertensive, and 9% were aphakic. Hole formation was bilateral in 17% of the patients and the average vision in these eyes was 20/200.

The majority of macular holes are ¼–⅓ disc diameter in size. Often, white opacities remain at the floor of the hole, which are most likely residual retinal tissue, macrophages, or exudate [22, 23]. There is often a fine cystoid edema surrounding the hole. Eighty-five percent of eyes have posterior vitreous detachments and an operculum is seen in one-quarter of the cases. It is rare, however, to find actual vitreous strands to the edge of the hole or operculum [1, 22, 23].

ANGIOGRAPHIC FINDINGS

Although there is no clinical or photographic method to absolutely differentiate between lamellar and full thickness holes, fluorescein angiography is sometimes helpful. A full thickness hole usually will show an increase in the background or transmitted fluorescence in the area of the hole, possibly due to loss of normal xanthochromic pigment [23] (Fig. 22.5). Also contributing to this increased background fluorescence is pigment loss from the underlying pigment epithelium [24]. Lamellar macular holes, on the other hand, do not stain and instead remain dark, appearing as normal macula. This is because the underlying pigment epithelium is intact and enough xanthochromic pigment remains to make the fluorescein appearance normal. When a patient with cystoid macular edema develops a lamellar hole, the dye which was leaking into the cysts freely diffuses through the ruptured inner wall into the vitreous cavity. It, therefore, does not concentrate and the area appears dark on the angiogram. This finding is obviously of prognostic significance, since patients with cystoid macular edema might be expected to recover good vision (should the edema resolve), whereas, those patients who have gone on to develop a lamellar hole will have permanent visual loss.

ETIOLOGY

The etiology of senile macular holes is unknown. Certainly, some cases are due to trauma and some cases are

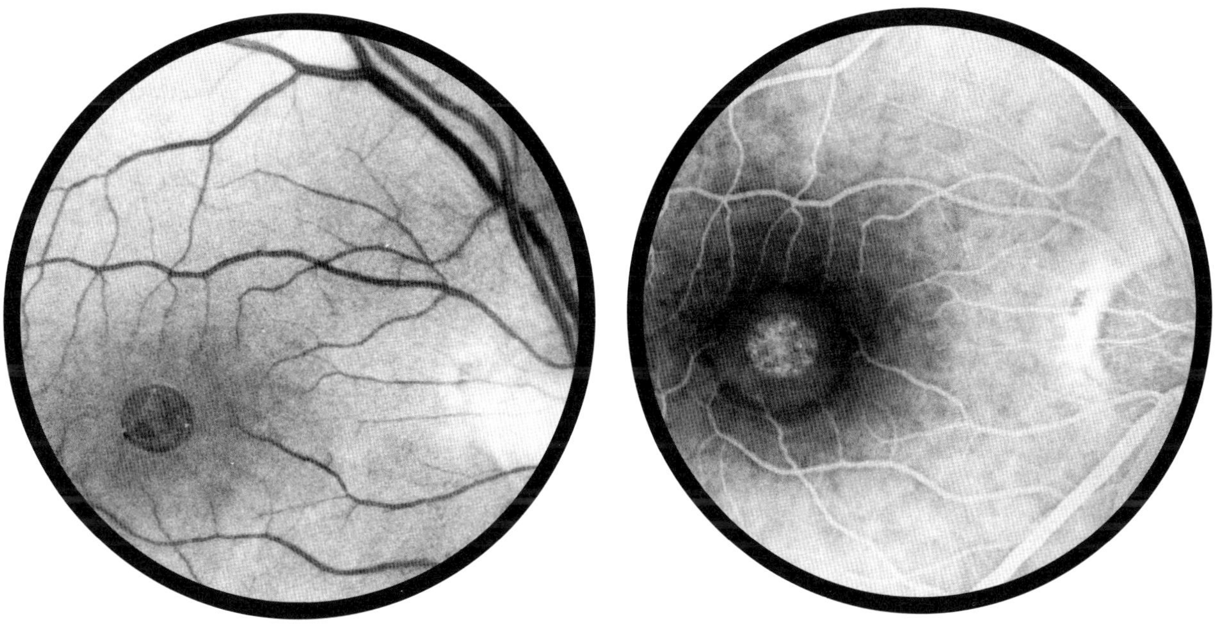

A B

Figure 22.5. Full thickness macular hole. *A*, monochromatic photograph. Note the small area of retinal detachment surrounding the hole. *B*, venous phase angiogram. Note the increased transmission of fluorescence through the hole. The surrounding detachment stains lightly.

due to rupture of the inner wall of a cyst in cystoid macular edema. However, this still leaves the majority of cases unexplained. Some authors, notably Maumenee and Reese [1], have implicated vitreomacular traction as an etiologic factor in selected cases. Gass [2, 23, 24] failed to demonstrate any evidence of vitreous strands causing traction on the edge of the hole or the operculum. In Aaberg's series [22], this was also true, but 37% of the patients did have vitreoretinal interface change; i.e., a preretinal membrane.

A high percentage of Aaberg's patients were hypertensive. However, a review of a series of 59 branch vein occlusions by the same author [22] failed to reveal any cases in which macular holes developed. In Gass' histopathologic studies [23], no abnormalities of the retinal blood vessels were found.

With rupture of the inner wall of the cyst in cystoid macular edema, there is retraction of retinal tissue which forms an inner lamellar hole with rounded edges [23]. Histologically, there is undercutting of the edges of the hole and thinning of the ganglion cell layer near the edge of the hole, suggesting that spontaneous rupture of the cyst wall occurs at the fovea. This wall is so thin that it can be detected only with electron microscopy [23].

DIFFERENTIAL DIAGNOSIS

One must differentiate between full thickness macular holes, lamellar macular holes, macular cysts, and pseudomacular holes in preretinal membranes.

Clinically, a lamellar macular hole presents with a sharply outlined area visible with the slit-lamp beam and Hruby or fundus contact lens. There is a bright sheen or reflex at the base of the hole, suggesting the presence of a layer of transparent retinal tissue. In addition, there is absence of a surrounding halo of retinal detachment and no yellowish deposits are seen on the surface of the retinal pigment epithelium; these latter two findings are characteristic of full thickness macular holes [23].

Also characteristic of full thickness macular holes is the presence of an operculum and the absence of a light reflex as the slit beam is carried across the base of the hole [23].

References

1. Maumenee, A.E.: Further advances in the study of the macula. *Arch Ophthalmol, 78:* 151, 1967.
2. Gass, J.D.M., and Norton, E.W.D.: Cystoid macular edema and papilledema following cataract extraction: a fluorescein funduscopic and angiographic study. *Arch Ophthalmol, 76:* 646, 1966.
3. Hitchings, R.A., Chisholm, I.H., and Bird, A.C.: Aphakic macular edema: incidence and pathogenesis. *Invest Ophthalmol, 14:* 68, 1975.
4. Michels, R.G., and Maumenee, A.E.: Cystoid macular edema associated with topically applied epinephrine in aphakic eyes. *Am J Ophthalmol, 80:* 379, 1975.
5. Irvine, S.: A newly defined vitreous syndrome following cataract surgery. *Am J Ophthalmol, 36:* 599, 1953.
6. Irvine, A.R., *et al.*: Macular edema after cataract extraction. *Ann Ophthalmol, 3:* 1234, 1971.
7. Klein, R.M., and Yannuzzi, L.: Cystoid macular edema in the first week after cataract extraction. *Am J Ophthal, 81:* 614, 1976.
8. Gass, J.D.M., and Norton, E.W.D.: Follow-up study of cystoid macular edema following cataract extraction. *Trans Am Acad Ophthalmol Otolaryngol, 73:* 665, 1969.
9. Ryan, S.J., Jr.: Cystoid maculopathy in phakic retinal detachment procedures. *Am J Ophthalmol, 76:*519, 1973.
10. Allen, A., and Jaffe, N.S.: Cystoid macular edema: a preliminary study. *Trans Am Acad Ophthalmol Otolaryngol, 81:* 133, 1976.
11. Yannuzzi, L.A., Klein, R., Wallyn, R., Cohen, N., and Katz, I.: Ineffectiveness of indomethacin treatment in chronic cystoid macular edema. *Am J Ophthalmol, 84:* 517, 1977.
12. West, C.E., Fitzgerald, C.R., and Sewell, J.H.: Cystoid macular edema following aphakic keratoplasty. *Am J Ophthalmol, 75:* 77, 1973.
13. Michels, R.G., and Ryan, S.J.: Results and complications of 100 consecutive cases of pars plana vitrectomy. *Am J Ophthalmol, 80:* 24, 1975.
14. Gass, J.D.M.: A fluorescein angiographic study of macular dysfunction secondary to retinal vascular disease. Parts I–VI, *Arch Ophthalmol, 80:* 535, 1968.
15. Kolker, A.E., and Becker, B.: Epinephrine maculopathy. *Arch Ophthalmol, 79:* 552, 1968.
16. Wise, G.N.: Clinical features of idiopathic preretinal macular fibrosis. *Am J Ophthalmol, 79:* 349, 1975.
17. Wise, G.N.: Relationship of idiopathic preretinal macular fibrosis to posterior vitreous detachment. *Am J Ophthalmol, 79:* 358, 1975.
18. Jaffe, N.S.: Macular retinopathy after separation of vitreoretinal adherence. *Arch Ophthalmol, 78:* 585, 1967.
19. Allen, A., and Gass, J.D.M.: Contraction of perifoveal epiretinal membrane simulating a macular hole. *Am J Ophthalmol,* in preparation.
20. Bellhorn, M.B., Friedman, A.H., Wise, G.N., and Henkind, D.: Ultrastructure and clinicopathologic correlation of idiopathic preretinal macular fibrosis. *Am J Ophthalmol, 79:* 366, 1975.
21. Clarkson, J.G., Green, W.R., and Massof, D.: A histopathologic review of 168 cases of preretinal membrane. *Am J Ophthalmol, 84:* 1, 1977.
22. Aaberg, T.M., Blair, C.J., and Gass, J.D.M.: Macular holes. *Am J Ophthalmol, 69:* 555, 1970.
23. Gass, J.D.M.: Lamellar macular hole: a complication of cystoid macular edema after cataract extraction: a clinicopathologic case report. *Trans Am Ophthalmol Soc, 73:* 231, 1975.
24. Gass, J.D.M.: Stereoscopic Atlas of Macular Diseases: a Funduscopic and Angiographic Presentation, C.V. Mosby, St. Louis, 1970, pp. 193–199.

CHAPTER 23

Hereditary Diseases of the Macula

Maurice F. Rabb, M.D.

Certain hereditary disorders of the fundus involve principally the macular region. Early recognition of the various features of hereditary macular disease is important in order that the true nature of the abnormality be determined and appropriate genetic counseling be instituted. These disorders vary widely in mode of transmission, histopathologic manifestations, clinical features, electrophysiologic abnormalities, and fluorescein angiographic findings (Table). In this chapter a number of well known hereditary diseases of the macula will be reviewed with respect to these characteristics.

X-Linked Juvenile Retinoschisis

X-linked juvenile retinoschisis is classified under the vitreal retinal dystrophies. The pattern of transmission is sex-linked and its frequency today is felt to be more common than was originally reported [1]. It involves primarily the nerve fiber layer of the retina and affects males. The primary ophthalmoscopic finding is foveal cysts which are best seen on slit-lamp biomicroscopic exam with red-free light [2–3]. The vision may range anywhere from 20/20 to 20/100, but marked visual reduction may not be recognized until the patient is in the early teens. Many individuals have repeated refractions without satisfactory correction prior to discovery of the correct diagnosis. The foveal changes are almost always present but the peripheral retinoschisis is evident in only about half the cases [4]. The macular changes consist of a cystic change in the fovea with an optically clear zone between the two retinal layers (Fig. 23.1*A*). The macular involvement is usually bilateral, and the cysts may become less apparent with increasing age. Other ophthalmoscopic findings may include perivascular cuffing, peripheral retinoschisis, vitreous veils, pseudoneuritis of the optic disc, changes in the vitreous structure, and posterior vitreous detachment [5–7] (Fig. 23.1*B*). Fluorescein angiograms in many cases are normal with no changes evident in the macular region. Some cases are associated

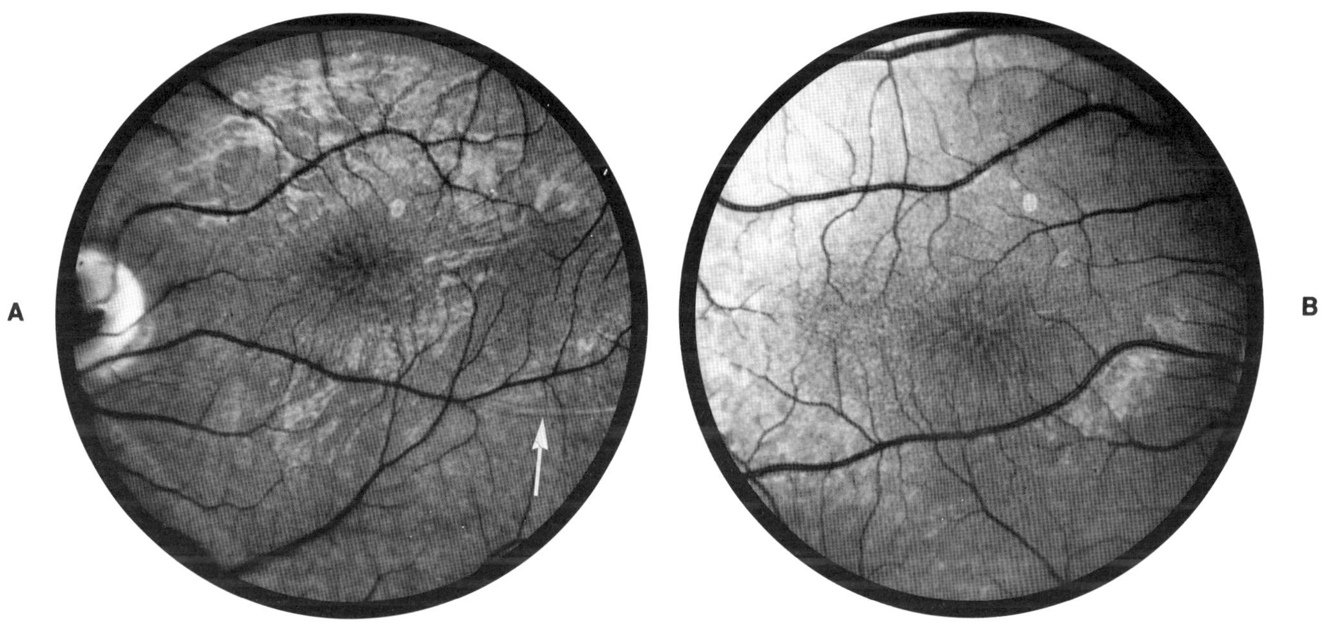

Figure 23.1. *A*, ophthalmoscopic photograph of X-linked juvenile retinoschisis of right eye. Note cystic changes and the eccentric elevation of the macula. *B*, ophthalmoscopic photograph of the left eye. Note cystic changes and the eccentricity of the macula. Also note a vitreous veil (*arrow*).

with areas of hypopigmentation in the macula that show focal window defect patterns [8] (Fig. 23.2). Some have suggested a sluggish blood flow through the retinal vessels in this condition. An interesting phenomenon noted in three patients is bilateral eccentricity of the fovea above the median raphe in a superotemporal direction from the disc (Fig. 23.1) associated with nasal dragging of the retinal vessels over the disc. To be considered in the differential diagnosis are Goldmann-Favre's disease, Wagner's vitreal dystrophy, Stargardt's disease, Eales' disease, senile retinoschisis, and sickle cell disease.

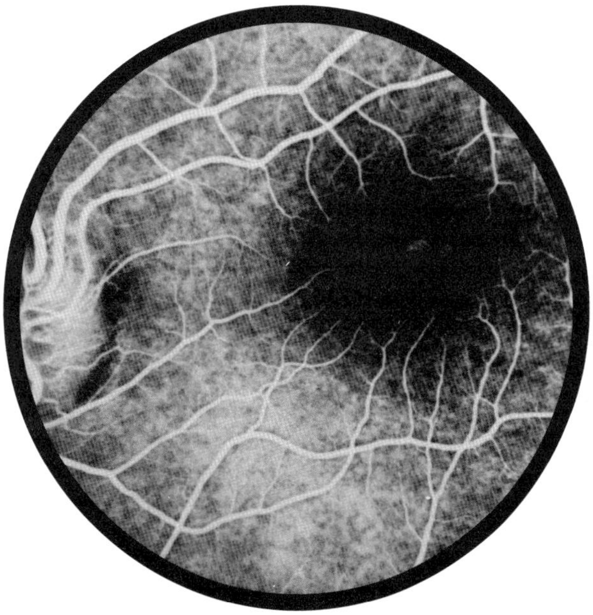

Figure 23.2. Fluorescein angiogram of X-linked juvenile retinoschisis. Note the choroidal transmitted fluorescence (pigment epithelial window defect in the macula).

The ERG is abnormal in severe cases; in mild cases the EOG may be normal but such patients can later become more severely affected [3].

FUNDUS FLAVIMACULATUS

In 1953, Francheschetti [9] described an unusual fundus picture that could not be classified among known retinal dystrophies. It consisted of fuzzy yellowish spots in the deep portion of the retina in the posterior pole. In 1963 he described several cases characterized by yellowish-white spots in the deeper retinal layers, calling the condition fundus flavimaculatus [10]. Confusion arose because Stargardt [11], in 1909, reported similar changes in a number of patients who also had atrophic macular disturbances. It now appears that Stargardt's cases were actually fundus flavimaculatus associated with atrophic macular degeneration, possibly a later stage of the disease Francheschetti described in 1963 [10]. As they are now generally considered different manifestations of the same autosomal recessive disease [12–15], they will be covered under fundus flavimaculatus. Deutman [3] in 1971, delineated the two stages of fundus flavimaculatus as follows: that with no or late macular involvement, usually occurring in adults; that with atrophic macular involvement in juveniles (Stargardt's disease). Individuals with the pure form who have no macular involvement may have normal vision until actual macular changes become apparent. These changes may have the typical appearance of atrophic beaded metal, and/or accumulated flecks surrounding the foveal area.

Ophthalmoscopy reveals diffuse, pisciform, yellowish spots in the deeper retinal layers (Fig. 23.3*A*). The lesions may also be circular, semi-circular or linear and located temporal to the macula, nasal to the disc, or may completely

A

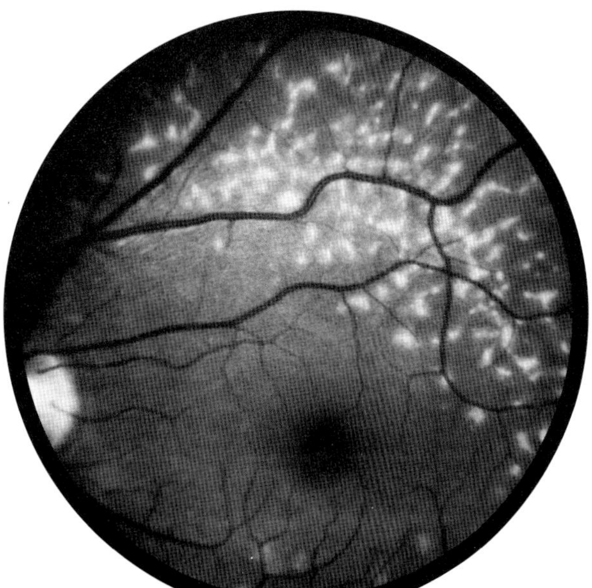

B

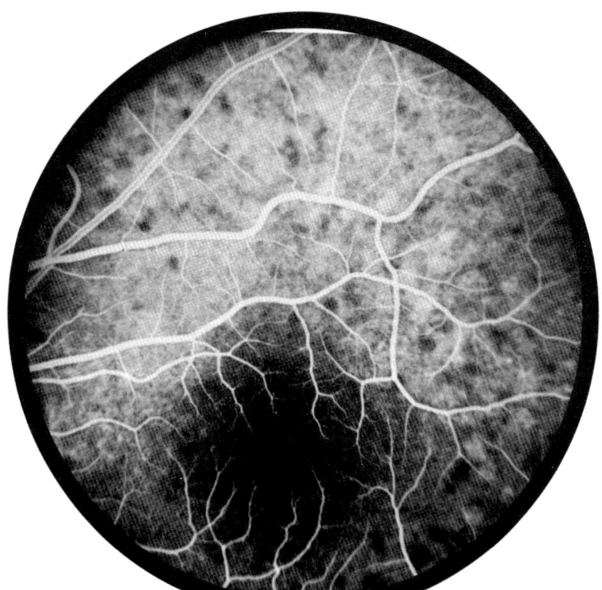

Figure 23.3. *A*, ophthalmoscopic photograph of fundus flavimaculatus, showing pisciform flecks in the midperiphery with no macular involvement. The vision in this patient was normal. *B*, arteriovenous phase fluorescein angiogram demonstrating hypo- and hyperfluorescence of the lesions.

surround the macular area. They are only rarely seen peripheral to the equator. The flecks may become less obvious with time; as new flecks appear, old ones may disappear. The important clinical finding is symmetric involvement of both posterior poles. Fluorescein angiography shows many flecks not observed ophthalmoscopically. The newer flecks tend to be hypofluorescent while the older ones are hyperfluorescent due to atrophy of the pigment epithelium (Fig. 23.3*B*). No flecks may be apparent clinically but on fluorescein angiography pigment epithelial areas become visible, demonstrating pisciform hypofluorescent spots [3]. When yellowish flecks appear early, atrophic changes may occur later in the macula with or without such flecks in the parafoveal region. The foveal area may eventually have a slimy configuration like that of varnish. A zone of pigmentary atrophy up to 12 disc diameters in size may develop later in the macular region (Fig. 23.4). Flecks usually noted in a large ring around the macula may eventually coalesce. The pigment epithelium in the macular region may show atrophy along with the choriocapillaris in the late stages of the disease, leading to a condition sometimes known as central areolar choroidal degeneration [14] (Fig. 23.5). The mid-peripheral retina may eventually develop small clumps of pigment surrounded by white halos, resembling a salt and pepper appearance due to the presence of hypo- and hyperpigmentation (Fig. 23.6). Fluorescein angiography at this stage often shows early hypofluorescence in the central zone of pigment epithelial atrophy because of concomitant atrophy of the choriocapillaris. The small pisciform hazy flecks tend to often hyperfluoresce in the late venous stage but with no leakage of dye from these lesions. Both forms of fundus flavimaculatus have the autosomal recessive type of inheritance. Electrophysiologic testing is usually normal except in widespread disease.

VITELLIFORM DYSTROPHY

Vitelliform dystrophy of the macula or Best's disease, reported by Best [15] in 1905, is also known as vitelline dystrophy or vitelliruptive degeneration. In some cases there are obvious macular changes but in others the macular region appears essentially normal, often precluding early diagnosis or resulting in misdiagnosis in the late stage because of the peculiar clinical picture. Vitelliform dystro-

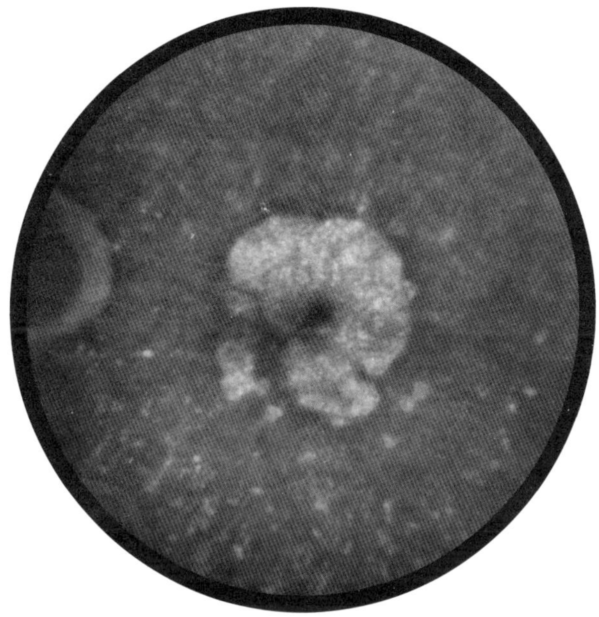

Figure 23.5. Fundus flavimaculatus. Late phase fluorescein angiogram with atrophy of the macular pigment epithelium.

A

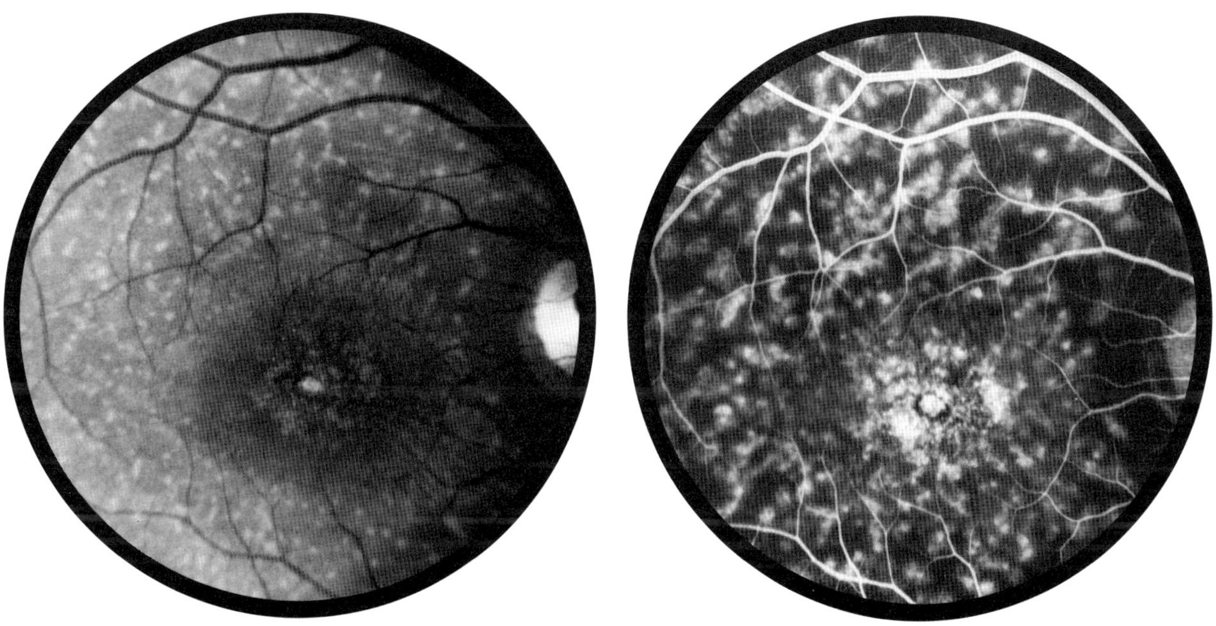

B

Figure 23.4. Fundus flavimaculatus with macular involvement. *A*, ophthalmoscopic photograph. Note the flecks along the vascular arcades and the atrophic and pigmentary changes in the macula. *B*, arteriovenous phase fluorescein angiogram of same eye demonstrating choroidal transmission fluorescence secondary to retina pigment epithelium atrophy in the macula.

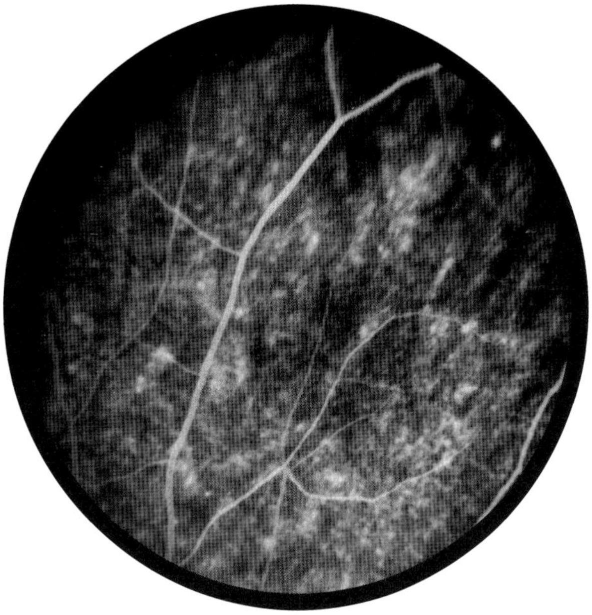

Figure 23.6. Fundus flavimaculatus. Venous phase angiogram demonstrating midperipheral irregular hyper- and hypofluorescence.

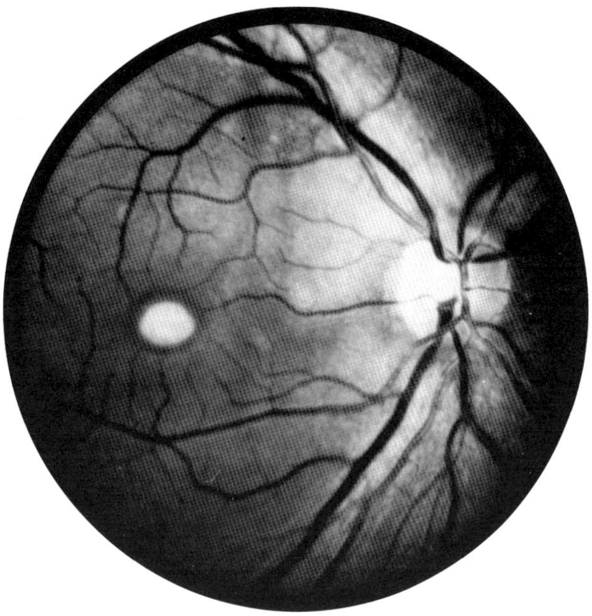

Figure 23.7. Vitelliform dystrophy. Ophthalmoscopic photograph demonstrating a small egg-yolk lesion in the macula.

phy is essentially a bilateral dominantly inherited disease although the macular change may rarely be unilateral. Vision may be markedly or minimally affected, or even normal for years in which case early diagnosis is difficult. Hyperopia or astigmatism is associated with this macular disorder, which frequently affects the 10- to 25-year age group but has been noted as late as age 40 [3].

The classic vitelliform lesion has an "egg yolk" appearance (Fig 23.7). The overlying retina is undisturbed, and the vasculature is normal. All patients do not have the dramatic egg yolk effect, but may have instead only a small foveal lesion (Fig. 23.8*A*). The lesion varies from ½–3 disc diameters in size, and is sometimes located eccentric to the macular region. Multiple and eccentric vitelliform lesions may be found either superotemporal to the disc or temporal or superior to the macular region [15]. Fluorescein angiography is helpful in delineating these lesions (Fig. 23.8, *B* and *C*). The peripheral retina and the optic nerve head do not appear to be involved. Various stages of vitelliform dystrophy have been described by Deutman as follows [3]:

(1) Normal fovea
(2) Previtelliform stage
(3) Vitelliform stage
(4) "Scrambled egg" or disruptive stage
(5) Cyst stage
(6) Pseudohypopyon stage
(7) Round chorioretinal atrophy stage.

Fluorescein angiography is not particularly helpful in the early diagnosis as angiograms are normal in the normal or previtelliform stages. However, the lesion in the vitelliform stage tends to block fluorescence of the normal choroid causing a round classic area of hypofluorescence. The egg

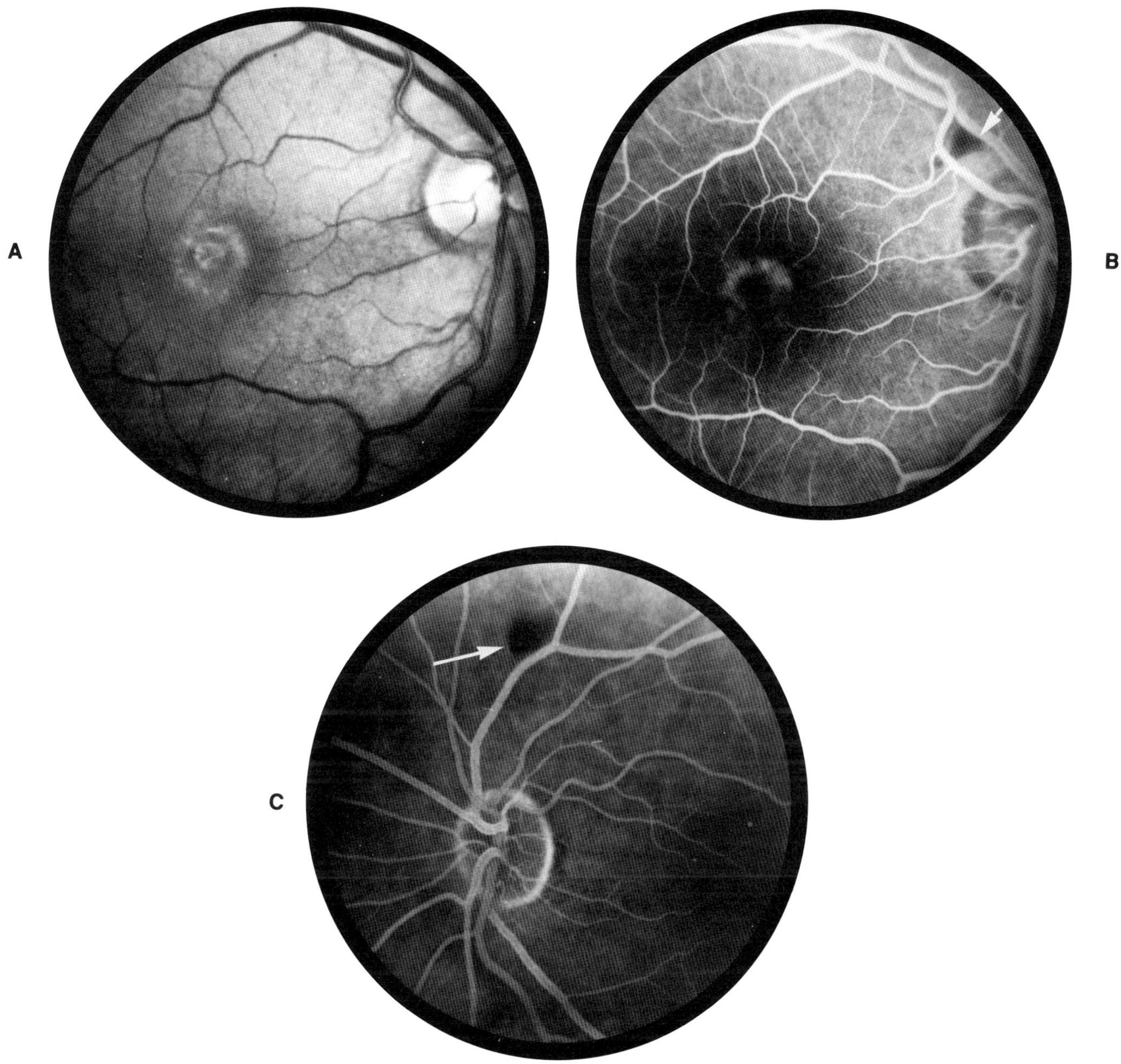

Figure 23.8. Vitelliform dystrophy. *A*, ophthalmoscopic photograph. Note the macular lesion. *B*, venous phase angiogram of same eye. Note hyperfluorescence of macular lesion. There is a hyperfluorescent extramacular lesion (*arrow*). *C*, venous phase angiogram of opposite eye also showing a similar extramacular lesion (*arrow*).

yolk lesion may then become disrupted and enter a scrambled egg stage (Fig. 23.9*A*). A pseudohypopyon stage may also occur and may be associated with subretinal neovascularization [17] (Fig. 23.9, *B* and *C*).

Because of its varied appearance, vitelliform dystrophy has been confused with a number of other macular diseases. The differential diagnosis includes serous detachment of the retinal pigment epithelium, central serous chorioretinopathy, toxoplasmosis, macula coloboma, and any macular disease associated with subretinal neovascularization. Electrical studies show a normal ERG, but the EOG is virtually always subnormal. Carriers, whose clinical findings may be normal, may also have a subnormal EOG which helps to determine the hereditary pattern of this disease.

DOMINANT DRUSEN

Dominant drusen of the central retina is a bilateral condition which involves Bruch's membrane and affects both sexes equally. The lesions usually develop in the 25- to 35-year-old age group and are strikingly symmetric in both eyes. They are multiple, round, fairly discrete, whitish

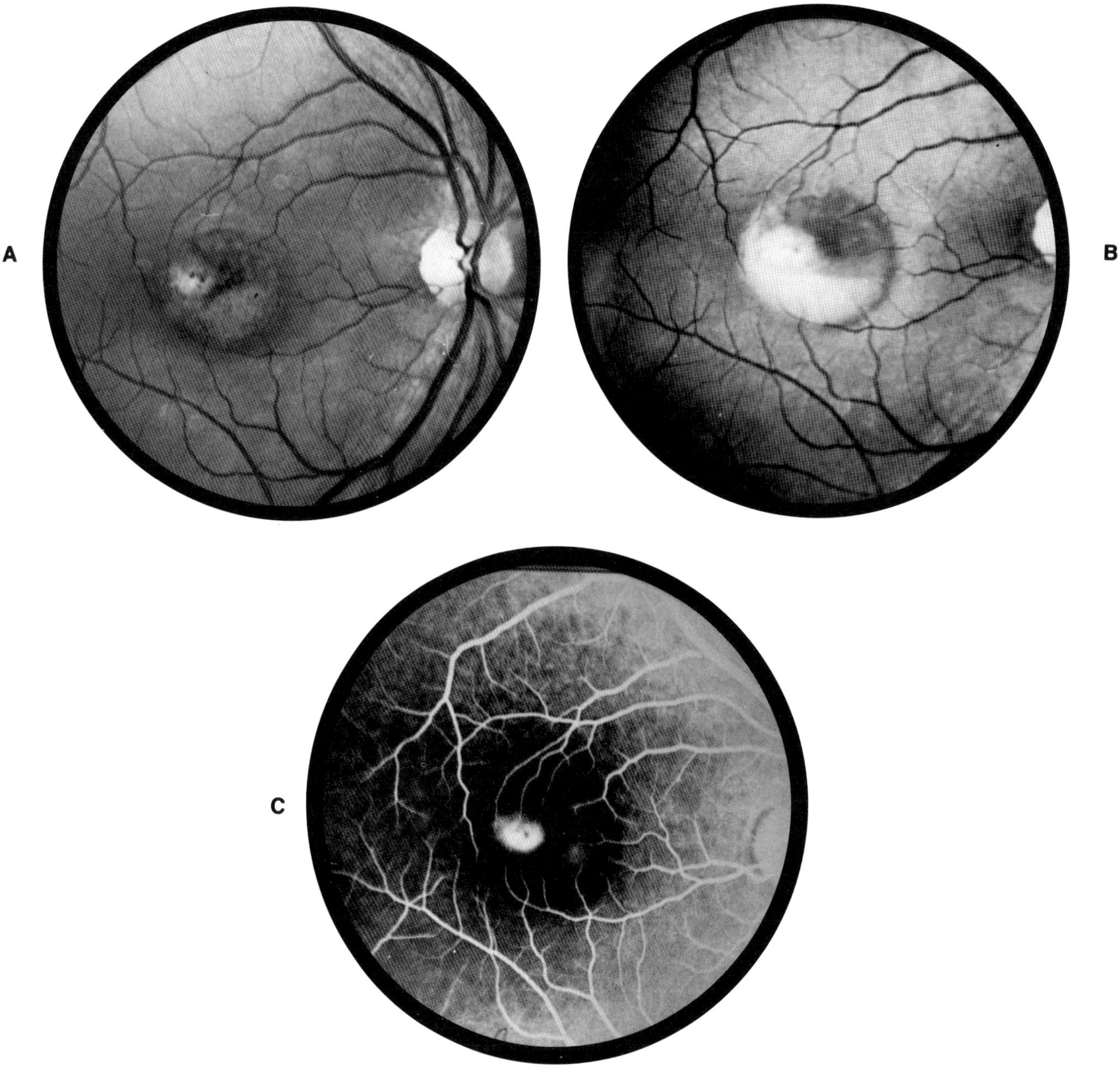

Figure 23.9. Vitelliform dystrophy, "scrambled egg" stage. *A*, ophthalmoscopic photograph. Note lesion in the macula. *B*, ophthalmoscopic photograph. Same eye, 6 months later shows progression to a "pseudohypopyon" stage. *C*, venous phase angiogram in same eye showing hyperfluorescence in macular area, secondary to subretinal neovascularization, and a hypofluorescence corresponding to the pseudohypopyon.

to yellowish in color, present at the level of the pigment epithelium, particularly in the posterior pole [18]. The dots in rare cases form a honeycomb or mosaic appearance referred to as Doyne's honeycomb retinopathy. The drusen are usually discrete and round in contrast to the diffuse pisciform lesions found in fundus flavimaculatus. In the later stages the drusen may coalesce resembling small pigment epithelial detachments in the macular and perimacular regions (Fig. 23.10). Areas of hypo- and hyperpigmentation due to proliferative and atrophic changes in the retinal pigment epithelium are sometimes present. As these drusen disappear, atrophic areas may remain, leading to marked disorganization of the macula in the late stages.

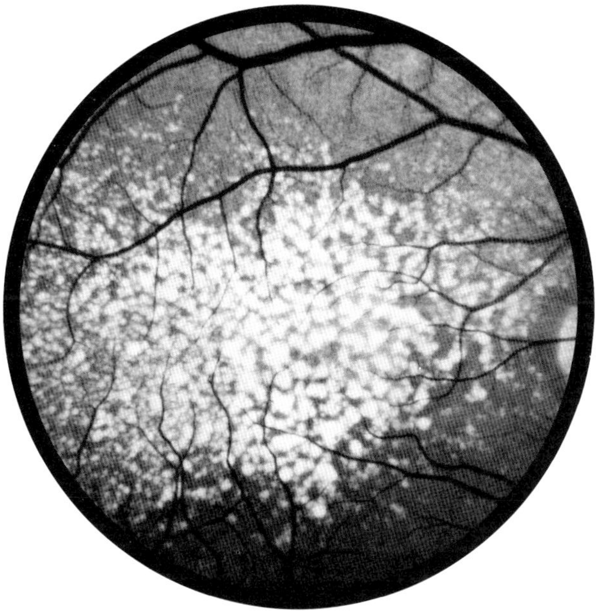

Figure 23.10. Dominant drusen, ophthalmoscopic photograph. Note the multiple drusen.

The peripheral retinal as well as the retinal vessels and optic disc are usually normal. In the early arterial and arteriovenous phase, fluorescein angiography shows early hyperfluorescence of the drusen as a result of choroidal transmission or pigment epithelial window defects. As the drusen become older and larger, late hyperfluorescence or leak from pooling of dye beneath the involved pigment epithelium is the rule. When leakage in or around areas of drusen is profuse, the possibility of subretinal neovascularization beneath the lesions must be considered. The differential diagnosis of dominant drusen includes the fleck retina syndrome [19] (fundus flavimaculatus, fundus albipunctatus, and involutional macular degeneration). The mode of inheritance is autosomal dominant. The ERG and EOG are both normal.

CONE DYSTROPHY

Autosomal dominant inherited cone dystrophy ranges from mild to severe even among members within the same family [20–24]. Visual loss and secondary photophobia are the most important findings. Defective color vision is an early manifestation. Fluorescein angiography is particularly helpful in the diagnosis because it reveals obvious hypofluorescence due to pigment epithelial atrophy. In its most common presentation there is a bull's eye appearance in the macula consisting of a zone of pigment epithelial atrophy surrounding the normal dark central fovea (Fig. 23.11, *A* and *B*). This fluorescent bull's eye pattern resembles the macular changes seen in chloroquine retinopathy. The differential diagnosis includes resolved central serous chorioretinopathy, involutional macular degeneration, and ret-

A

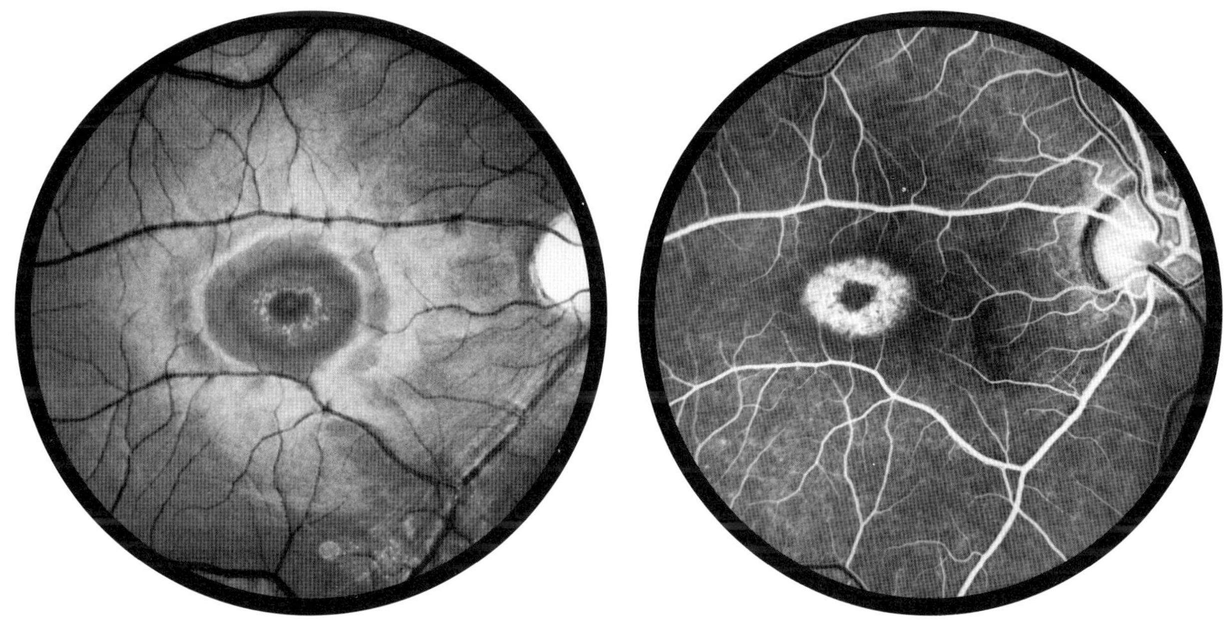

B

Figure 23.11. Cone dystrophy. *A*, ophthalmoscopic photograph. Note the "bull's-eye" appearance in the macula. *B*, arteriovenous phase angiogram. Note the patchy hyperfluorescence encircling the hypofluorescent fovea.

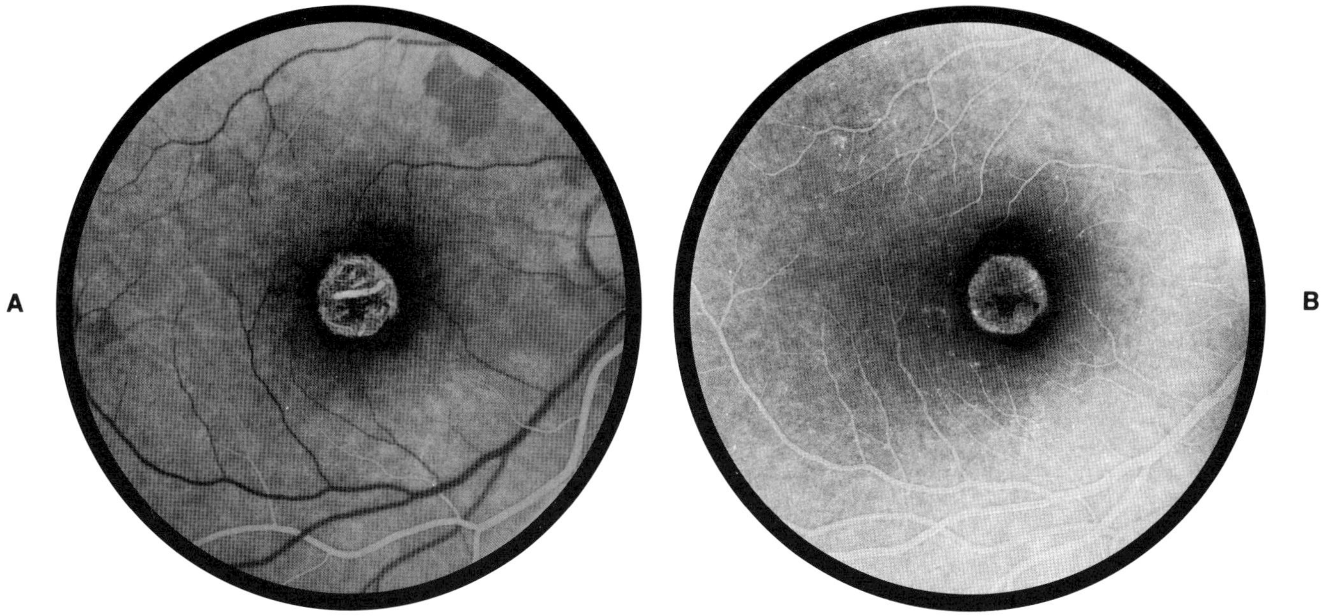

Figure 23.12. Central areolar choroidal dystrophy. *A*, arteriovenous phase angiogram. Note the large choroidal vessels in the macula. *B*, late venous phase angiogram. Note the circumscribed area of hyperfluorescence in the macula corresponding to staining of the visible sclera from adjacent choriocapillaris. (Courtesy of Kenneth G. Noble, M.D.).

initis pigmentosa, as well as chloroquine retinopathy [25] and Stargardt's disease. The ERG is generally abnormal and the EOG is normal in early mild cases. In severe cases the EOG is subnormal.

CENTRAL AREOLAR CHOROIDAL DYSTROPHY

For over 100 years clinical investigators reported cases of a disorder called central areolar choroidal atrophy in the central posterior pole of the eye. In 1939, Sorsby [26] noted its dominant hereditary nature and proposed the term central areolar choroidal sclerosis. "Sclerosis" was based only on the ophthalmoscopic finding which was not confirmed histopathologically. In 1953, Ashton [27] demonstrated that the choroidal vessel pattern was due to atrophy rather than sclerosis. In 1961, Waardenburg [28] first suggested the term "dystrophy" in preference to "atrophy." Carr [29] and Deutman [3] accepted this terminology because of the hereditary nature of this entity. It is characterized by a sharply circumscribed area in the macular region with obvious atrophy of the retinal pigment epithelium and choriocapillaris. The typical "punched-out" lesion leaves the underlying atrophic choroid and sclera exposed [29]. The fluorescein angiogram reveals the presence of large chorodial vessels through the atrophic pigment epithelium and, because of the absence of the choriocapillaris, late staining of visible sclera originating from adjacent normal choriocapillaris (Fig. 23.12, *A* and *B*). The early absence of the choriocapillaris in this disease differentiates it from Stargardt's disease and the cone dystrophies. The mode of inheritance is autosomal dominant. The ERG and EOG are usually normal.

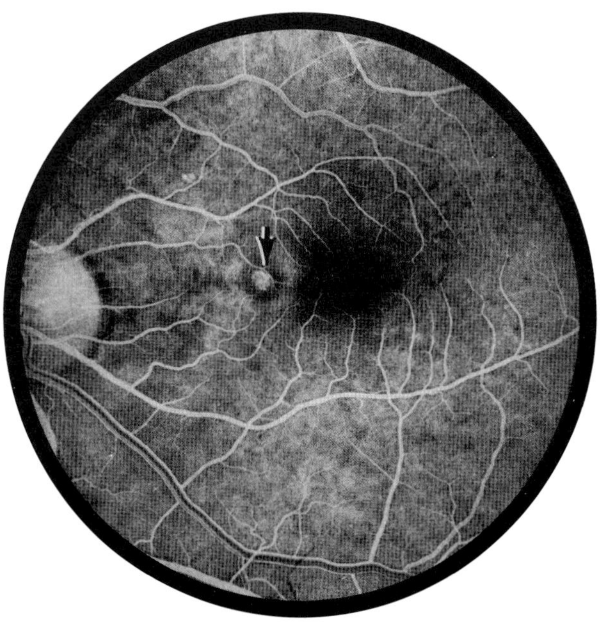

Figure 23.13. Sorsby's pseudoinflammatory dystrophy. Arteriovenous phase angiogram showing a focal area of subretinal neovascularization nasal to the fovea (*arrow*). (Courtesy of Kenneth G. Noble, M.D.)

RARE HEREDITARY MACULAR DISORDERS

A few extremely rare hereditary macular disorders have been described, among them butterfly dystrophy, Sorsby's pseudoinflammatory dystrophy, and dominant cystoid macular edema.

Two pedigrees of *butterfly dystrophy*, which have an autosomal dominant mode of transmission, have been reported, the first by Deutman and associates [30]. The lesion appears to be confined to the retinal pigment epithelium. Clinically, the linear pigmented, butterfly-shaped configurations crossing over the involved pigment epithelial area resemble the changes seen in long-standing serous detachments of the pigment epithelium. The ERG is normal, but the EOG is reduced, presumably by dysfunction at the level of the pigment epithelium.

Sorsby's pseudoinflammatory dystrophy (Fig. 23.13), also autosomal dominant, appears at about age 40. The principal histopathologic abnormality appears to be subretinal neovascularization and its sequelae including subretinal hemorrhage, serous detachment of the sensory retina and pigment epithelium, and, ultimately, disciform scarring resembling that seen in involutional macular degeneration. Two of Sorsby's original patients were examined histopathologically in their early 70's, establishing the presence of subretinal neovascularization. Problems in the exact identification of this disorder arise largely because of difficulties inherent in attempts to establish an autosomal dominant pattern that begins at the age of 40, questionable significance in relating subretinal neovascularization as a primary histopathologic mechanism when evidence of its existence was related to 70-year-old individuals who frequently exhibit these changes, and to the scarcity of pedigrees. The ERG is normal, and the EOG is not known.

Five pedigrees of *dominant cystoid macular edema* have been reported by Deutman *et al.* [31]. In this autosomal dominant disorder, which appears at about age 20, the intraretinal edema is confined to the outer plexiform layer of the sensory retina. There are a few opacities in the posterior vitreous but no inflammatory cells at the pars plana. The ERG is normal in these eyes, and the EOG tends to be abnormal.

HEREDITARY DISEASE OF THE MACULA

DISORDERS	TRANSMISSION	AGE OF ONSET	HISTOPATHOLOGY	ELECTROPHYSIOLOGY
Vitreo-Retinal Disorders				
Juvenile Retinoschisis	X-linked recessive	4-8	Vitreous membranes. Cleavage nerve fiber layer. Macula cystoid appearance (100%) of cases. Peripheral retinoschisis (50%) of cases.	ERG-Subnormal B-wave EOG-Normal
Wagner's Disease	Autosomal dominant	20+	Lens opacities. Vitreous syneresis but optically clear. Inner retinal abnormalities (presumed). Peripheral retinoschisis, lattice degeneration and detachment. Atrophy of RPE and choriocapillaris.	ERG-Normal or subnormal EOG-Normal
Goldman-Favre	Autosomal recessive	4-8	Vitreous degeneration. Inner retinal abnormalities (presumed). Macular cystoid appearance. Peripheral retinoschisis and lattice degeneration. Tapetoretinal pigmentary changes resembling retinitis pigmentosa.	ERG-Abnormal EOG-Normal
Dominant Cystoid Macular Edema	Autosomal dominant	20	Cystoid edema of macula	ERG-Normal EOG-Abnormal
Cone Dystrophies	Autosomal dominant	6-50	Selective enzyme disorder involving the cones (hypothesized).	ERG-Abnormal cone EOG-Normal
Stargardt's Disease-Fundus Flavimaculatus	Autosomal recessive	6-20	Complete disappearance of visual elements and RPE in macula. Flecks in macula and/or periphery. Choriocapillaris atrophy (late).	ERG-Normal in central form EOG-Normal in central form
Central Areolar Choroidal Dystrophy	Irregular autosomal dominant	20-50	Atrophy of choriocapillaris, RPE and outer layer of neuroepithelium.	ERG-Normal EOG-Normal or subnormal
Butterfly Dystrophy	Autosomal dominant	10	Probably RPE	ERG-Normal EOG-Abnormal
Vitelliform Dystrophy (Best's Disease)	Autosomal dominant	Birth -15	Probably RPE Subretinal neovascularization (SRN).	ERG-Normal EOG-Abnormal
Dominant Drusen	Autosomal dominant	20-30	Hyaline accumulation beneath RPE. Breaks in Bruch's membrane. Subretinal neovascularization (SRN). Disciform scar.	ERG-Normal EOG-Normal early
Sorsby's Pseudoinflammatory Dystrophy	Autosomal dominant	40+	Breaks in Bruch's membrane. Subretinal neovascularization (SRN) Disciform scar.	ERG-Normal early EOG-Unknown

References

1. Yanoff, M., Rahn, E.K., and Zimmerman, L.E.: Histopathology of juvenile retinoschisis. *Arch Ophthalmol, 79:* 49, 1968.
2. Krill, A.E., and Deutman, A.F.: The various categories of juvenile macular degeneration. *Trans Am Ophthalmol Soc, 70:* 220, 1972.
3. Deutman, A.F.: The Hereditary Dystrophies of the Posterior Pole of the Eye. Charles C Thomas, Springfield, Ill., 1971, p. 48.
4. Tasman, W.: Macular changes in congenital retinoschisis. *Mod Prob Ophthalmol, 15:* 40, 1975.
5. Sheehan, B.: Congenital vascular veils in the vitreous. *Trans Ophthalmol Soc U K, 72:* 623, 1952.
6. MacRae, A.: Congenital vascular veils in the vitreous. *Trans Ophthalmol Soc U K, 74:* 187, 1954.
7. Condon, R.A., and Somerville-Large, L.B.: Vitreous veils and associated conditions in five brothers. *Trans Ophthalmol Soc U K, 75:* 709, 1955.
8. Krause, U., Vainio-Mattila, B., Eriksson, A., and Forsius, H.: Fluorescein angiographic studies on X-chromosomal retinoschisis. *Acta Ophthalmol, 48:* 794, 1970.
9. Franceschetti, A.: Über tapeto-retinale Degenerationen im Kindesalter. *In* Entwicklung und Fortschritt in der Augenheilkunde, Enke, Stuttgart, 1953, p. 107.
10. Franceschetti, A., Francois, J., and Babel, J.: Les Hérédodégénérescences chorio-rétiniennes (Dégénérescences Tapétorétiniennes). Masson & Cie, Paris, 1963.
11. Stargardt, K.: Über familiäre, progressive Degeneration in der Makula-gegend des Auges. *Albrecht von Graefes Arch Klin Ophthalmol, 71:* 534, 1909.
12. Klein, B.A., and Krill, A.E.: Fundus flavimaculatus: clinical, functional and histopathologic observations. *Am J Ophthalmol, 64:* 3, 1967.
13. Deutman, A.F.: Macular dystrophies. *In* Genetic and Metabolic Eye Diseases, ed. by M. F. Goldberg, Little, Brown & Co., Boston, 1974, pp. 380–385.
14. Fishman, G.A.: Fundus flavimaculatus. *Arch Ophthalmol, 94:* 2061, 1976.
15. Best, F.: Über eine hereditare Maculaaffektion: Beitrage zur Vererbungslehre. *Z Augenheilkd, 13:* 199, 1905.
16. Deutman, A.F.: Electro-oculography in families with vitelliform dystrophy of the fovea: detection of the carrier state. *Arch Ophthalmol, 81:* 305, 1969.
17. Miller, S.A., Bresnick, G.H., and Chandra, S.R.: Choroidal neovascular membrane in Best's vitelliform macular dystrophy. *Am J Ophthalmol, 82:* 252, 1976.
18. Deutman, A.F., and Jansen, L.M.A.A.: Dominantly inherited drusen of Bruch's membrane. *Brit J Ophthalmol, 54:* 373, 1970.
19. Krill, A.E., and Klien, B.A.: Flecked retina syndrome. *Arch Ophthalmol, 74:* 496, 1965.
20. Sorsby, A., and Davey, J.B.: Dominant macular dystrophy. *Brit J Ophthalmol, 39:* 385, 1955.
21. Goodman, G., Ripps, H., and Siegel, I.M.: Cone dysfunction syndromes. *Arch Ophthalmol, 70:* 214, 1963.
22. Berson, E.L., Gouras, P., and Gunkel, R.D.: Progressive cone-rod degeneration. *Arch Ophthalmol, 80:* 68, 1968.
23. Krill, A.E., and Deutman, A.F.: Dominant macular degenerations: the cone dystrophies. *Am J Ophthalmol, 73:* 352, 1972.
24. Fishman, G.A.: Progressive human cone-rod dysfunction (dystrophy). *Trans Am Acad Ophthalmol Otolaryngol, 81:* 716, 1976.
25. Weise, E.E., and Yannuzzi, L.A.: Ring maculopathies mimicking chloroquine retinopathy. *Am J Ophthalmol, 78:* 204, 1974.
26. Sorsby, A.: Choroidal angiosclerosis with special reference to its hereditary character. *Brit J Ophthalmol, 23:* 433, 1939.
27. Ashton, N.: Central areolar choroidal sclerosis: a histopathological study. *Brit J Ophthalmol, 37:* 140, 1953.
28. Waardenburg, P.J., Franceschetti, A., and Klein, D.: Genetics and Ophthalmology, Charles C Thomas, Springfield, Ill., 1961.
29. Carr, R.E.: Central areolar choroidal dystrophy. *Arch Ophthalmol, 73:* 32, 1965.
30. Deutman, A.F., van Blommestein, J.D.A., Henkes, H.E., Waardenburg, P.J., and Solleveld-van Driest, E.: Butterfly-shaped pigment dystrophy of the fovea. *Arch Ophthalmol, 83:* 558, 1970.
31. Deutman, A.F., Pinckers, A.J.L.G., and Aan de Kerk, A.L.: Dominantly inherited cystoid macular edema. *Am J Ophthalmol, 82:* 540, 1976.

CHAPTER 24

Optic Nerve

Lawrence A. Yannuzzi, M.D., Kurt A. Gitter, M.D., Howard Schatz, M.D., and William M. Haining, M.D.

In evaluating the posterior segment of the eye, the optic nerve, and macula are invariably considered as alternative possibilities for visual decline. Certain clinical situations, such as ischemic optic neuropathy, some primary tumors of the optic nerve, and papillitis clearly involve the optic nerve as the sole site of pathology. In most instances, however, optic nerve disorders have either combined optic nerve and macular histopathologic changes or secondary manifestations in the macula. This chapter deals predominantly with those optic nerve disorders which have combined or secondary effects in the macula. These macular changes include: preretinal membrane formation, lipid and serous intraretinal exudation, sensory retinal detachment, pigment epithelial atrophy and subretinal peripapillary neovascularization.

The use of fluorescein angiography has introduced an important dimension in the anatomic, physiologic, and clinical study of the optic nerve in its normal and abnormal state. Rapid sequential stereo fundus photography provides a means for both spatial and temporal analysis of optic nerve fluorescein angiograms that demonstrate the perfusion and permeability characteristics of the superficial as well as the deeper intrapapillary vasculature. Alterations in normal perfusion and permeability of these circulations reveal the pathophysiologic mechanisms in a number of primary optic disorders as well as those that are responsible for changes in the macula. It is essential, therefore, to briefly review the normal anatomy of the optic nerve and the fluorescein angiographic findings in the normal and abnormal states.

ANATOMIC CONSIDERATIONS

The microvasculature of the optic nerve may be conveniently divided into three primary planes as suggested by Hayreh (Fig. 24.1).

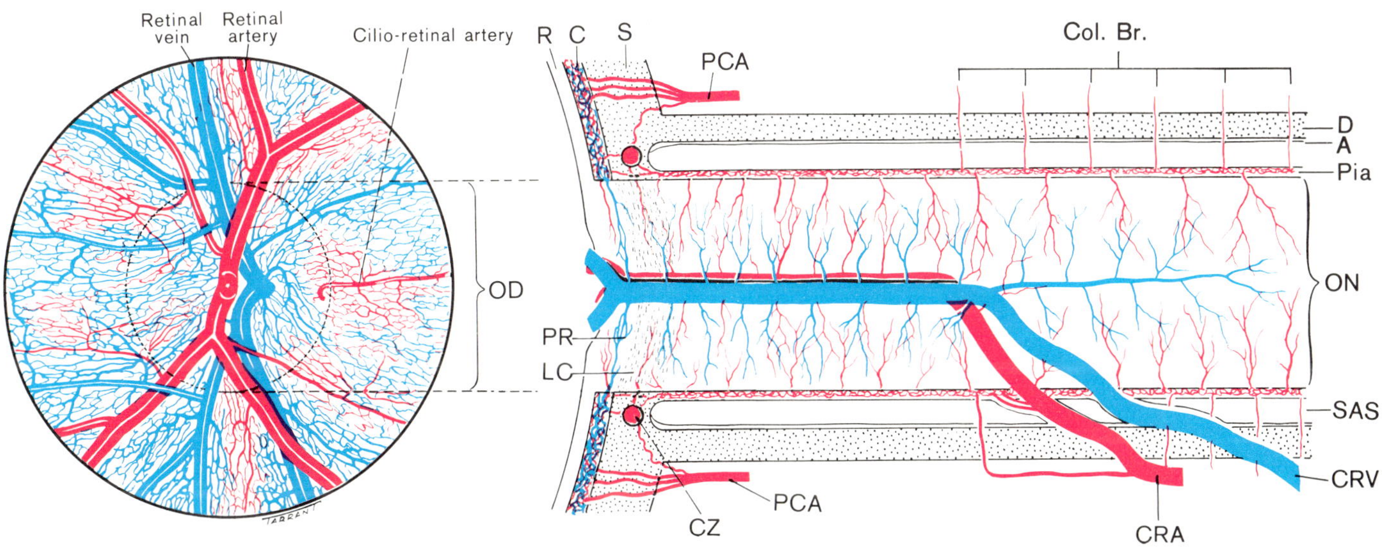

Figure 24.1. Diagrammatic representation of the blood supply to the optic nerve. *ON*, optic nerve; *OD*, optic disc; *CRA*, central retinal artery; *CRV*, central retinal vein; *PCA*, short posterior ciliary artery; *CZ*, circle of Zinn; *LC*, lamina cribrosa; *PR*, prelaminar region; *SAS*, subarachnoid spaces; *D*, dura; *A*, arachnoid; *S*, sclera; *C*, choroid; *R*, retina; *Col. Br.*, collateral branches of ophthalmic artery. (Modified from S. S. Hayreh: *Trans Am Acad Ophthalmol Otolaryngol, 78:* 240, © 1974; with permission.)

(1) Retrolaminar area

This region is supplied predominantly by branches of the pial vessels, which are derived from the peripapillary choroid and, in some instances, from direct branches of the posterior ciliary artery.

(2) Superficial intrapapillary layer including the lamina cribrosa

This region of the lamina cribrosa is supplied entirely by branches of the short posterior ciliary arteries. The prelaminar region is nourished mainly by branches of the peripapillary choroidal vessels.

(3) Superficial papillary capillary plexus

This plexus of capillaries is derived from the central retinal artery and its branches and from recurrent fine contributions from the superficial radial peripapillary plexus. This latter plexus appears to be either a venous collector capillary network or, in conditions of altered hemodynamics, a shunt system. The intrapapillary vessels contribute directly toward forming part of the superficial plexus via a cilioretinal artery when it is present.

The central retinal artery supplies only the superficial papillary capillary plexus. This component can be detected in normal and abnormal eyes in unusual cases when the central retinal artery filling precedes choroidal or cilioretinal artery perfusion.

Beginning at the prelaminar region at the level of the choroid, the blood supply of the optic nerve is derived mainly from scleral branches of the short posterior ciliary vessels and to a lesser degree from the centripetal branches from the circumpapillary choroid [2]. The retrolaminar area is supplied principally by centripetal and longitudinal vessels of pial origin. Axial continuity of small vessels extending from the retrolaminar nerve to the retinal surface have been observed forming a continuous vasculature [2, 3]. This longitudinal system freely anastomoses with three transverse systems: (1) from the short posterior ciliary arteries in the sclera to the lamina cribrosa, (2) from smaller short posterior ciliary branches and choroidal capillaries to the prelaminar portion, and (3) from the central retinal artery in and around the disc [2]. These histopathologic observations on the ciliary origin of the blood flow to the optic disc have been supported by studies involving the central retinal and posterior ciliary arteries in which occlusions were produced experimentally and subsequently studied by fluorescein angiography [4, 5]. The intrapapillary layers combine with the retrolaminar circulation to produce the pink or flashy ophthalmoscopic appearance of the optic disc. The three circulations share a common drainage system in the central retinal vein [2].

FLUORESCEIN ANGIOGRAPHY

There are four fluorescein angiographic stages in the study of the normal optic nerve.

(1) Retrolaminar filling

Filling of the retrolaminar circulation may appear as the first manifestation following intravenous fluorescein in the prechoroidal filling phase as the capillary plexus in and posterior to the lamina cribrosa fills with fluorescein. This event is rarely witnessed on fluorescein angiograms because individual capillaries are seldom identified at this level except when there is an unusually large and deep physiologic cup with a highly resolved and rapidly sequential series of photographs. The clinical significance of alterations in the filling of this microcirculation is not known because they have rarely been documented and studied.

(2) Superficial intrapapillary filling (prelaminar)

This microcirculation fills in a heterogeneous fashion simultaneously with patchy choroidal filling, prior to filling of the retinal arterioles (Fig. 24.2). The filling of the superficial intrapapillary vessels resemble, and in some cases correspond to the adjacent choroidal filling in the juxtapapillary choroid. A perfusion delay at the level of this microcirculation can be suspected only after the adjacent choroid has completely filled and the corresponding sector of the disc has not filled. A cilioretinal artery present at the nerve head will also fill at this time, distributing its branches on the nerve head (Fig. 24.3). There is an accentuation to the prelaminar microcirculation filling when there is attenuation of the overlying retinal capillary network on the superficial aspects of the disc in central retinal artery occlusion or retinitis pigmentosa (Fig. 24.4). Once the superficial capillaries on the nerve head begin to fluoresce, the prelaminar circulation can only be poorly discerned in normal and other abnormal states. In atrophy of the optic nerve the prelaminar circulation is reduced and remains hypofluorescent on the fluorescein angiogram (Fig. 24.5).

(3) Superficial retinal capillary filling

While the deep fluorescence of the optic nerve is caused by filling of the microcirculations predominantly at the level of the lamina cribrosa, the fluorescence of the superficial aspects of the disc is derived largely from the central retinal artery. Peripapillary capillaries are apparent on the surface of the disc following filling of the retinal arterioles. As this circulation fills, the prelaminar microvasculature becomes less evident. The more anteriorly situated and radially arranged capillaries on the nerve head (radial peripapillary circulation) become visible angiographically only after the retinal arterioles fill, suggesting that this capillary plexus is predominantly venous in nature serving as drainage channels for vessels in the peripapillary area [6] (see Fig. 24.2*C*). This peripapillary radial vascular network becomes extremely prominent and permeable during retinal vascular inflammatory and occlusive diseases.

A

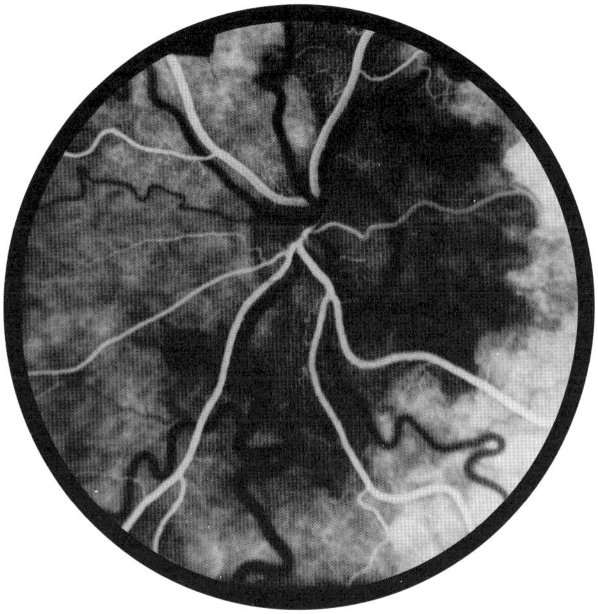

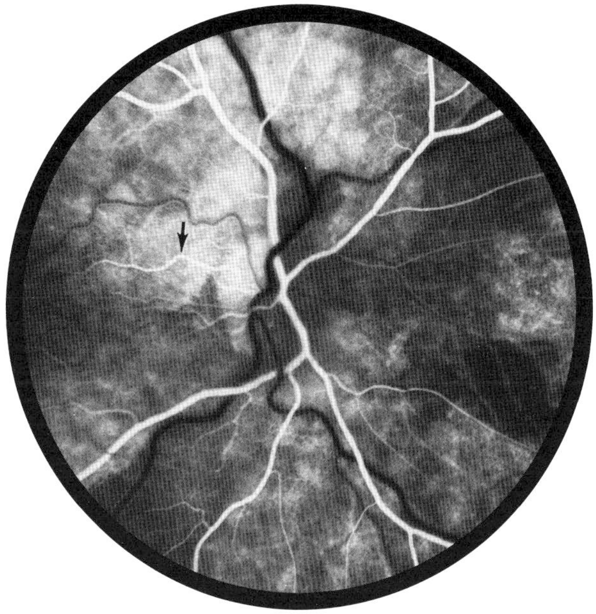

Figure 24.3. Cilioretinal artery, normal eye. Note the complete filling of the cilioretinal artery present at the temporal aspect of the disc (*arrow*). The cilioretinal artery fills at the time simultaneously with the superficial intrapapillary (prelaminar) circulation of the disc and during the patchy choroidal filling prior to perfusion of the retinal arteriolar circulation.

B

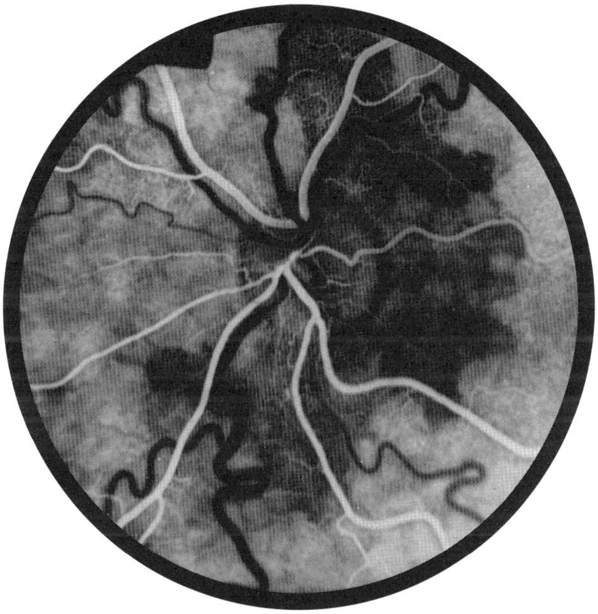

C

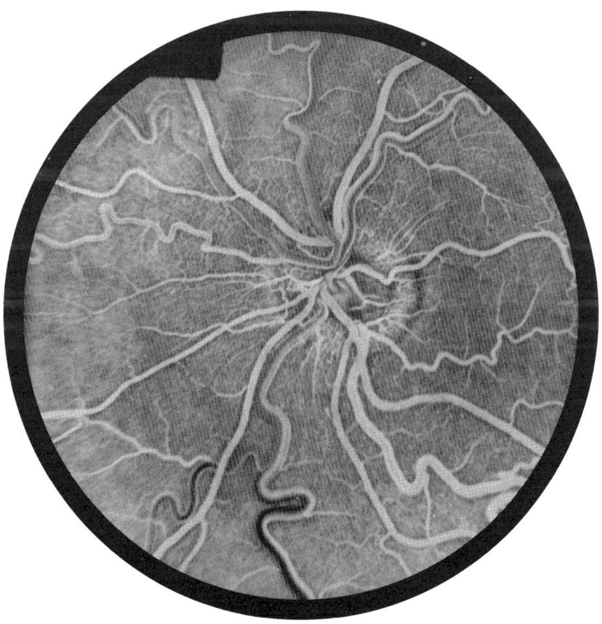

Figure 24.2 Fluorescein angiography of normal optic nerve. *A*, retinal arteriolar phase. Note the patchy, heterogeneous filling of the superficial (prelaminar) intrapapillary circulation and adjacent choroidal circulation. *B*, one second later. Note the gradual increase in perfusion of the prelaminar disc circulation and corresponding juxtapapillary choriocapillaris. *C*, arteriovenous phase. Note the superficial retinal capillary filling with radially arranged capillaries on the nerve head (radial peripapillary circulation). The intrapapillary superficial capillary plexus is no longer evident being obscured by this more superficial anteriorly situated papillary plexus. The juxtapapillary choriocapillaris is now completely perfused with dye.

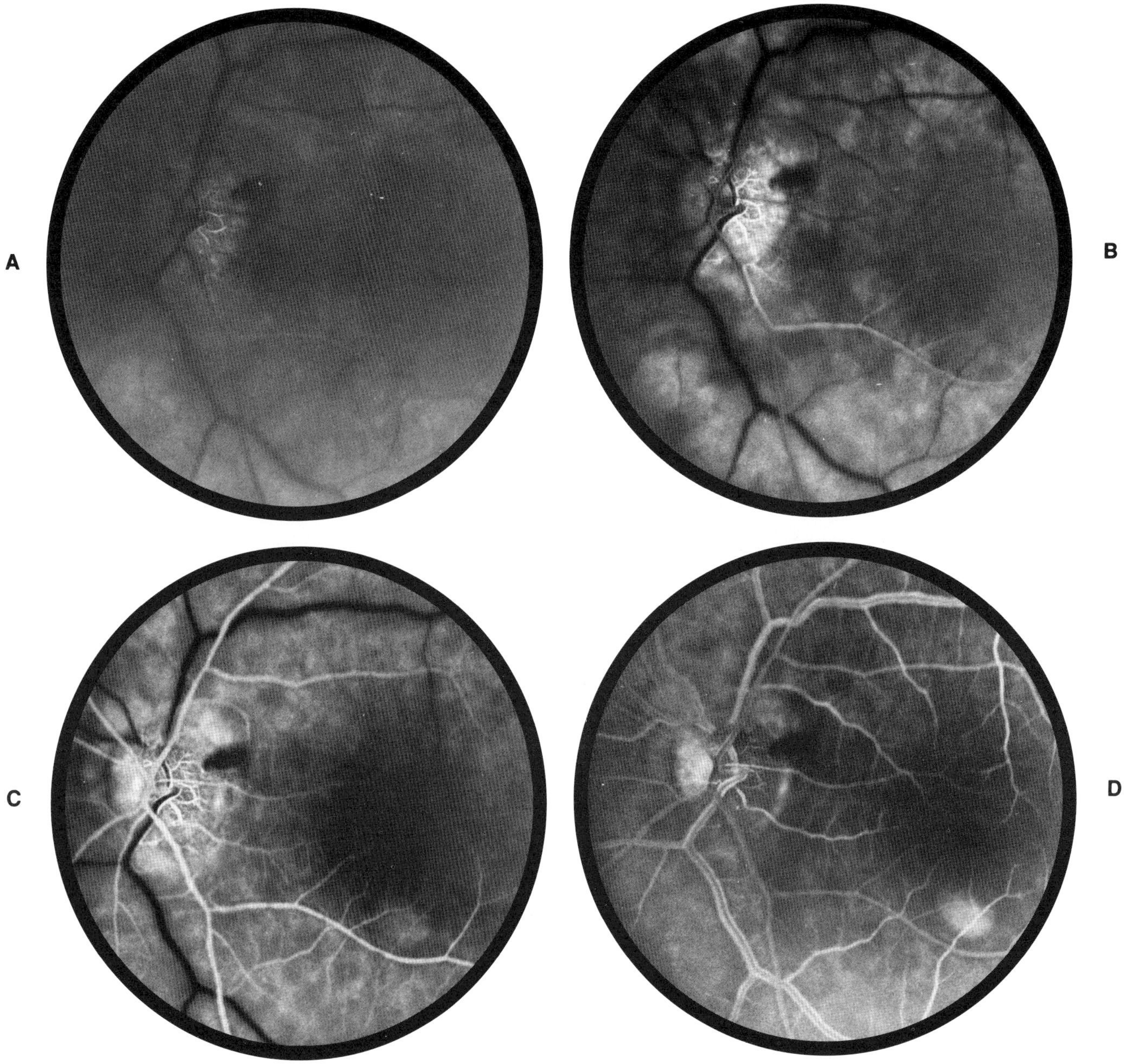

Figure 24.4. Accentuation of the prelaminar microcirculation in central retinal artery occlusion. *A*, superficial intrapapillary (prelaminar) filling. Note the fluorescence of the microcirculation at the level of the lamina cribrosa. A small hemorrhage is also present at the temporal aspect of the disc, producing hypofluorescence. *B*, arteriolar phase fluorescein angiogram. There is marked prominence of the prelaminar circulation with patchy filling of the choroidal circulation, and early slow perfusion of the central retinal artery and its branches. *C*, retinal arteriolar phase, 11 seconds later. The prelaminar circulation remains fluorescent and is not obscured by filling of the overlying superficial papillary circulation. The central retinal artery and its branches are slowly being perfused. *D*, arteriovenous phase fluorescein angiogram. Twenty-two seconds later, dye has finally entered the retinal venous system. Fluorescence has faded from the superficial intrapapillary circulation. The prelaminar vessels were accentuated both because of central retinal artery occlusion and a deep physiologic cup. With marked optic nerve cupping, the deeper circulations of the nerve are more easily seen on the fluorescein angiogram. This is particularly true when the overlying retinal capillary network is attenuated as in central retinal artery occlusion and retinitis pigmentosa.

(4) Late hyperfluorescence (staining) of the optic nerve

When the fluorescein has visibly left the retinal and choroidal circulations in the late phase angiogram, there is peripapillary staining surrounding the margins of the disc as dye diffuses from the adjacent choriocapillaris [7, 8]. Staining also occurs centrally in the nerve head at the site of the lamina cribrosa. When there is a peripapillary crescent, late hyperfluorescence or staining of the visible sclera will also take place as adjacent intact choriocapillaris leaks into the sclera (Fig. 24.6). In the normal eye, there is no leakage from any of the three circulations of the nerve into the nerve head. Unlike the choriocapillaris, which is similarly derived from the posterior ciliary artery and leaks fluorescein profusely, the middle and deep microvascular layers of the disc do not show this permeability characteristic.

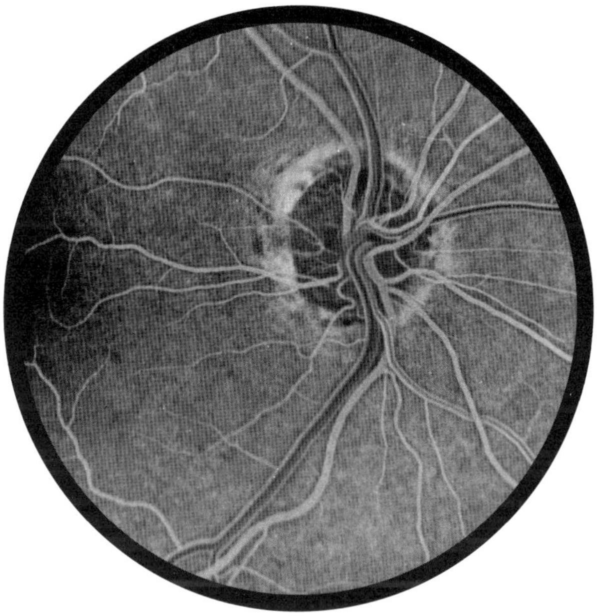

Figure 24.5. Reduced intrapapillary or prelaminar filling in optic atrophy. Note the diffuse hypofluorescence of the optic nerve from reduction of the superficial intrapapillary (prelaminar) circulation. The surrounding choriocapillaris has a normal "ground glass" homogeneous fluorescent pattern.

It has always been somewhat apocryphal to find an absence of any late intrapapillary fluorescence or staining in the normal angiogram despite the presence of arterial inflow from the circumpapillary choroid. The endothelium of the choriocapillaris has a fenestrated basement membrane and porous intracellular junctions which are freely permeable to fluorescein [9, 10]. Glial tissue separates the anterior portion of the sclera and the whole thickness of the choroid from the optic nerve. It continues anteriorly beyond the pigment epithelium to form the so-called intramedullary tissue of Kuhnt. These cells form a ring or partial ring of glial tissue that separate the retina, except for the nerve fibers, from the optic nerve. At a more posterior level, the end loops of the choriocapillaris, which circumscribe the optic nerve, are in direct apposition to the glial cells which form the intervening border between the tissue of Jacoby and the intramedullary tissue of Kuhnt at the retinal level. It is possible that the intervening borders of glial cells, more specifically, the interglial junction zones, provide the only "watertight" barrier between the choriocapillaris and the extracellular compartment of the optic nerve [11]. Further evidence in support of this hypothesis was derived from a study involving the passage of electron dense tracer particles into the optic nerve head in the rhesus monkey [7]. This work suggested that any defect of the glial border tissue would result in a breakdown of this barrier layer with free leakage from the choriocapillaris into the nerve head and possibly into the subretinal space. These histopathologic factors may be implicated in certain optic nerve disorders associated with juxtapapillary sensory retinal detachment.

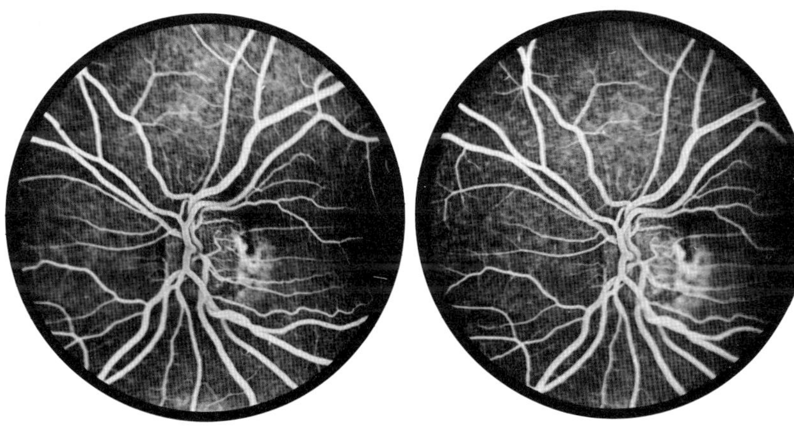

Figure 24.6 Stereo fluorescein angiogram of normal disc with juxtapapillary scleral staining. Note the late hyperfluorescence or staining of the juxtapapillary sclera at the site of a temporal crescent. Peripapillary staining takes place in the normal disc as dye diffuses from the adjacent choriocapillaris: (1) into its margins, (2) at the lamina cribrosa, and (3) at visible juxtapapillary sclera. *Note:* These photos are stereoscopic pairs and can be viewed from a distance of approximately 10 inches by holding +5 spheres close to the eyes.

OPTIC NERVE ABNORMALITIES

Certain congenital anomalies of the discs, most disorders resulting in optic nerve head edema, and a few optic nerve tumors may be associated with concomitant or secondary manifestations in the macula. The histopathologic changes present in the macula include: preretinal membrane formation, intraretinal serous and lipid exudation, hemorrhage, retinal pigment epithelial atrophy and proliferation, subretinal peripapillary neovascularization, and choroidal folds. Stereo fluorescein angiography is extremely useful in the evaluation of these disorders, documenting the pathophysiologic changes in the various microcirculations of these nerve heads, and in some instances such as subretinal neovascularition and intraretinal cystoid edema, establishing the exact pathologic changes present in the macula as well.

Congenital Anomalies

Situs inversus (the anomalous origin of the disc vessels from its temporal aspect), tilting, hypoplasia, megaloplasia, medullation, and persistent hyaloidal vessels are all easily recognized by the experienced ophthalmologist and rarely produce secondary changes in the macular region. Congenital pits or coloboma of the optic nerve, peripapillary staphyloma, and drusen of the optic disc are congenital abnormalities that are frequently associated with macular manifestations.

Congenital pits are crater-like holes in the nerve head generally seen in otherwise normal eyes. When the pits are located temporally or on the nerve head they may become associated with abnormalities in the macula. The pits are usually evident on clinical examination with direct ophthalmoscopy and posterior slit-lamp biomicroscopy. In the vast majority of cases, there is only one pit in the nerve and there is unilateral involvement. The nerve head in the uninvolved eye is usually somewhat smaller in size. The pits themselves vary in size, from 150–500 μ in diameter, or ⅛–⅓ normal disc diameter. There is a temporal predilection with 65% of the pits located infratemporally, 15% supratemporally, and only 20% nasally. Central field defects are associated with the pits, but the principal threat to central vision lies in the development of sensory retinal detachments involving the macula, which clinically resemble those seen in central serous chorioretinopathy. These detachments develop in eyes with temporal pits [12], usually in patients between the ages of 10 and 30 years of age [13]. We have observed macular detachments only in eyes with temporal pits located at the *margins* of the optic nerve head. The sensory retinal detachments always communicate with the disc unlike those seen in central serous chorioretinopathy which are more variable. Juxtapapillary retinal pigment epithelial atrophy and pigment epithelial proliferation as well as macular cystic degeneration may develop as sequelae to detachments [13] (Fig. 24.7). Sensory retinal detachments in the nasal retina, associated with nasal optic nerve head pits have only rarely been observed because the patient tends to be visually asymptomatic and because the pits are infrequently located in the nasal quadrants of the disc.

The pathogenesis of macular detachments associated with optic nerve pits is still unknown. Serous leakage from:(1) the posterior fluid vitreous, (2) the cerebrospinal fluid, (3) the vascular complex at the margins or within the depth of the pit, or (4) via a focal absence of the interglial junction zones between the choriocapillaris and the extracellular compartment of the optic nerve have been suggested as possible mechanisms related to the development of these detachments.

A

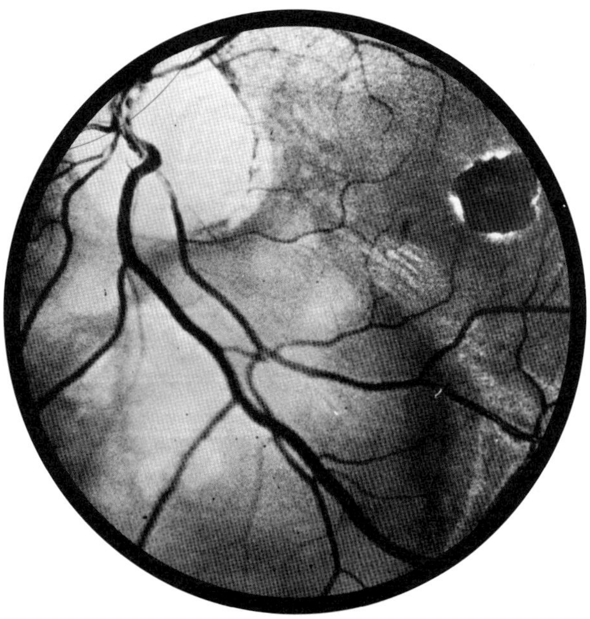

B

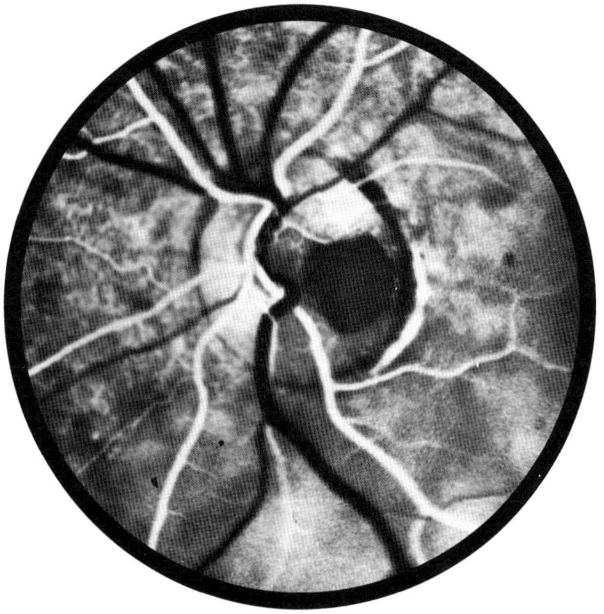

Figure 24.7. Optic pit with serous detachment and cystic degeneration of the macula. *A*, ophthalmoscopic photograph of eye with an optic pit and juxtapapillary sensory retinal detachment which involves the macula. Linear retinal folds radiating from the disc toward the macula and cystic degeneration surrounding the fovea are also evident. *B*, arterial phase angiogram. Note the characteristic early hypofluorescence at the site of a large optic pit.

Fluorescein angiography is sometimes helpful in accentuating the site of a pit that is not absolutely evident clinically (Fig. 24.8). There is a distinct zone of hypofluorescence at the site of the pit early in the angiogram from the absence of glial tissue. Late hyperfluorescence from leakage at the margins and/or from the depth of the pit becomes evident in the late phase of the angiogram (Fig. 24.9). In eyes with juxtapapillary retinal pigment epithelial atrophy, transmitted fluorescence (pigment epithelial window defect) may be present as early hyperfluorescence which gradually fades except for late staining of visible sclera. A clearly, undisputable communication between the late hyperfluorescence originating from the optic pit to the adjoining subsensory retinal space has not yet been documented with fluorescein angiography (Fig. 24.10). This logical mechanism related to the detachment still, however, remains a possibility (Fig. 24.11).

A B

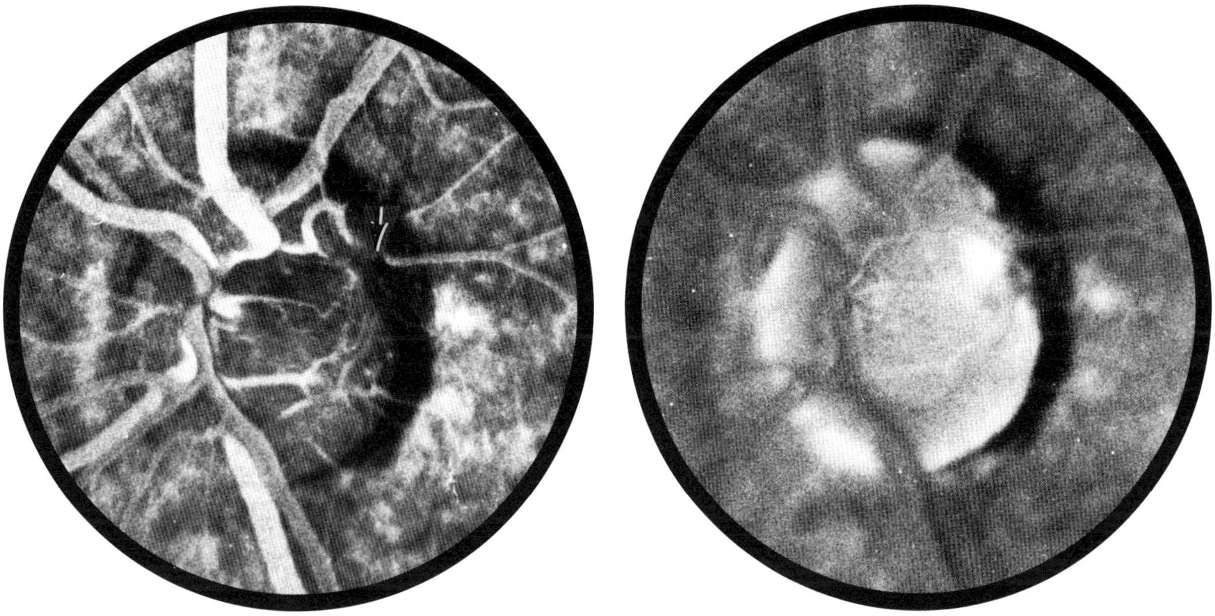

Figure 24.8. Optic nerve pit. *A*, late venous phase angiogram. Note the central cupping in the optic nerve. A small circular zone of hypofluorescence is evident at the temporal margin of the disc at the site of an optic pit (*arrow*). *B*, late phase angiogram. Late hyperfluorescence from pooling has developed at the site of the optic pit.

A B

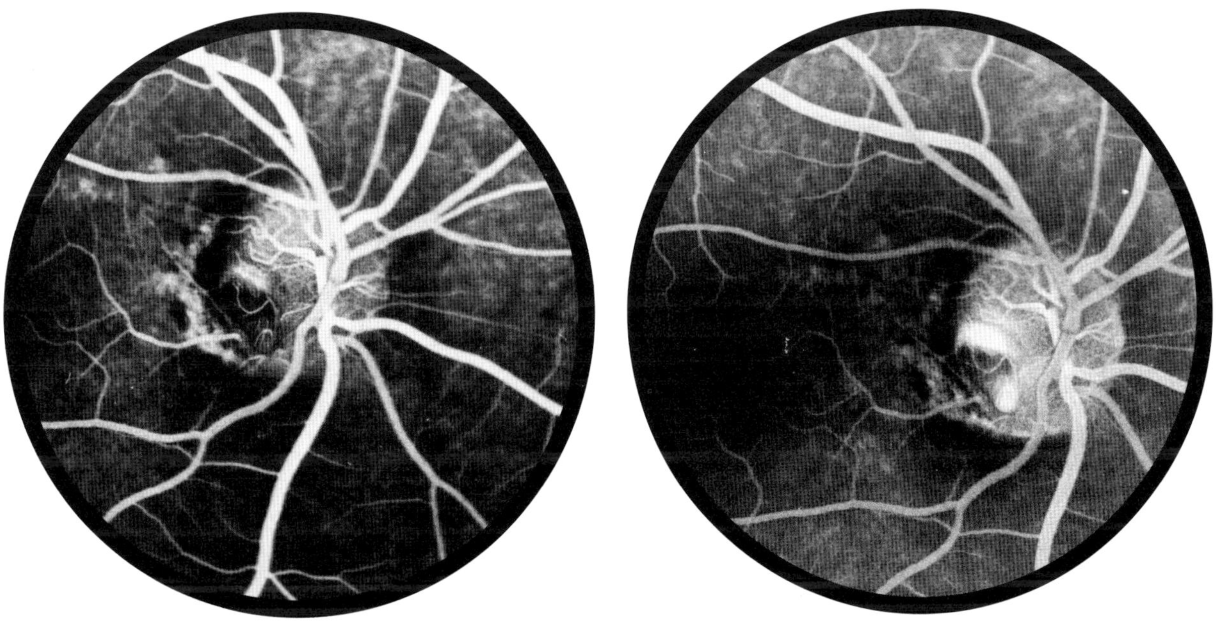

Figure 24.9. Fluorescein angiogram, optic pit. *A*, early venous phase angiogram. Note the circumscribed hypofluorescence at the inferior temporal aspect of the disc at the site of an optic pit. There is also juxtapapillary atrophy producing early hyperfluorescence from choroidal transmission. *B*, late venous phase angiogram. Hyperfluorescence is now noted at the margins of the pit. The characteristic angiographic features of optic pits are early hypofluorescence from an absence of tissue and late hyperfluorescence from leakage at the margins or from the depths of the pit.

A
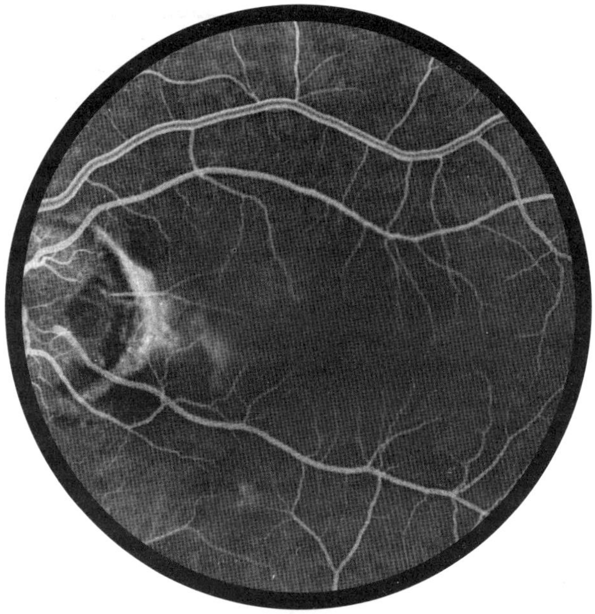

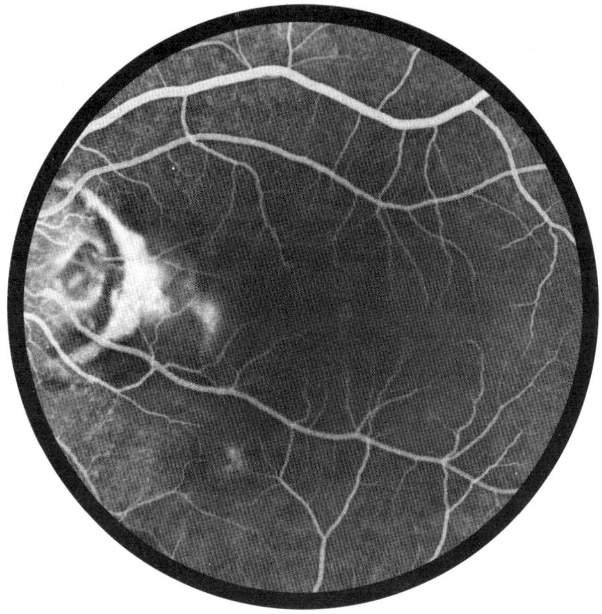
B

C
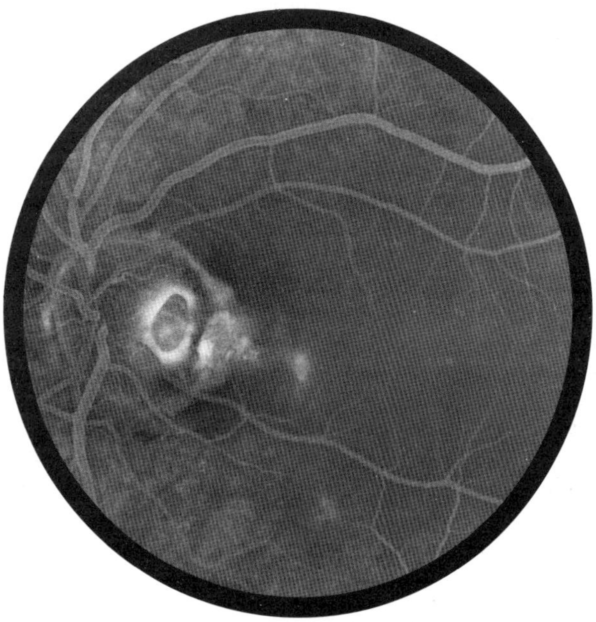

Figure 24.10. Fluorescein angiogram, optic pit with macular detachment. *A*, arteriovenous phase angiogram. Note the hypofluorescence at the site of the optic pit on the temporal aspect of the disc. There is also early hyperfluorescence in the papillomacular bundle at the level of the pigment epithelium secondary to atrophic changes and choroidal transmission. *B*, early venous phase angiogram. Note the hyperfluorescence developing at the margins of the pit and the staining of the scleral crescent. *C*, late phase angiogram. There is marked fuzzy hyperfluorescence at the margins and depth of the optic pit.

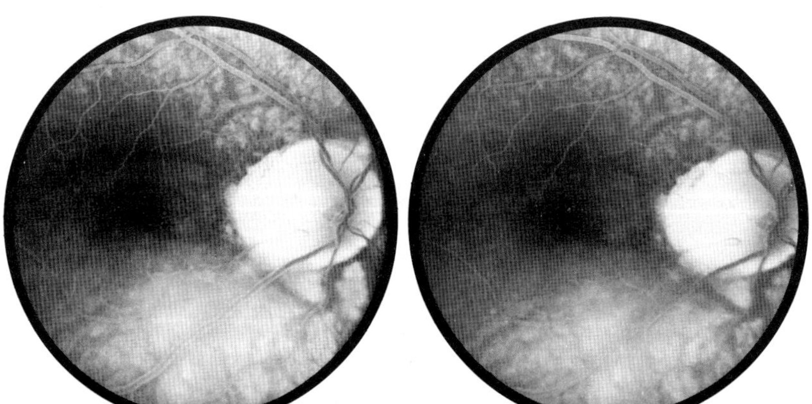

Figure 24.11. Stereo late phase fluorescein angiogram of optic pit with detachment. Note the hyperfluorescence of the optic pit. Late hyperfluorescence is present at the optic pit and beneath the sensory retinal detachment although there is no clear line of communication between the two. *Note:* These photos are stereoscopic pairs and can be viewed from a distance of approximately 10 inches by holding +5 spheres close to the eyes.

A 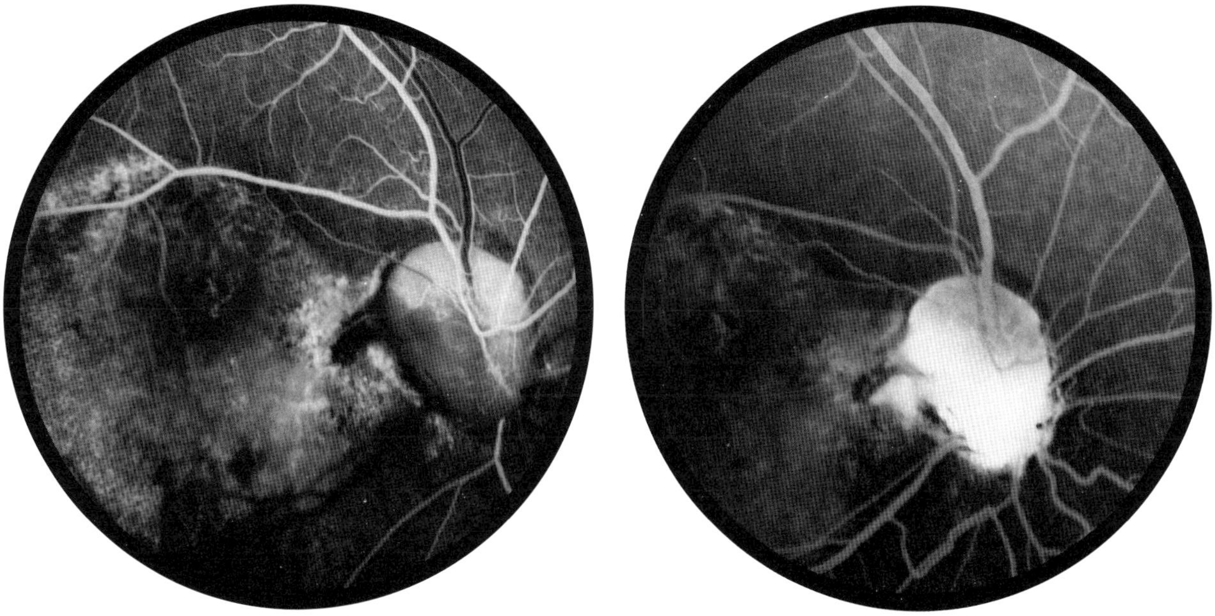 B

Figure 24.12. Coloboma of optic nerve. *A*, arteriovenous phase angiogram. Note the hypofluorescence of a wedge-shaped gap or fissure in the inferior temporal portion of the optic nerve. This is a coloboma associated with a circumscribed area of retinal pigment epithelial atrophy from an associated long-standing sensory retinal detachment. *B*, late phase angiogram. Note the hyperfluorescence in the region of the coloboma. The early transmitted hyperfluorescence in the macula associated with retinal pigment epithelial atrophy has diminished. As in optic pits early hypofluorescence and late hyperfluorescence are the characteristic fluorescein angiographic features of optic nerve coloboma.

The use of photocoagulation to treat detachments associated with optic pits is still controversial. Eyes treated with this modality appear to do no better than comparative untreated cases which ultimately spontaneously resolve with reduced but useful vision in approximately ⅓ of the patients.

Optic nerve coloboma are congenital notches, gaps, or fissures, in the nerve head (Fig. 24.12). They are classically but not exclusively located inferiorly, and vary from simple inferior crescents to more extensive defects which also involve the adjacent retina and choroid. As with pits, juxtapapillary retinal detachments and secondary degenerative changes may develop (Fig. 24.13). Severe forms may be associated with other congenital ocular malformations including microphthalmus and extrabulbar evagination and marked visual impairment.

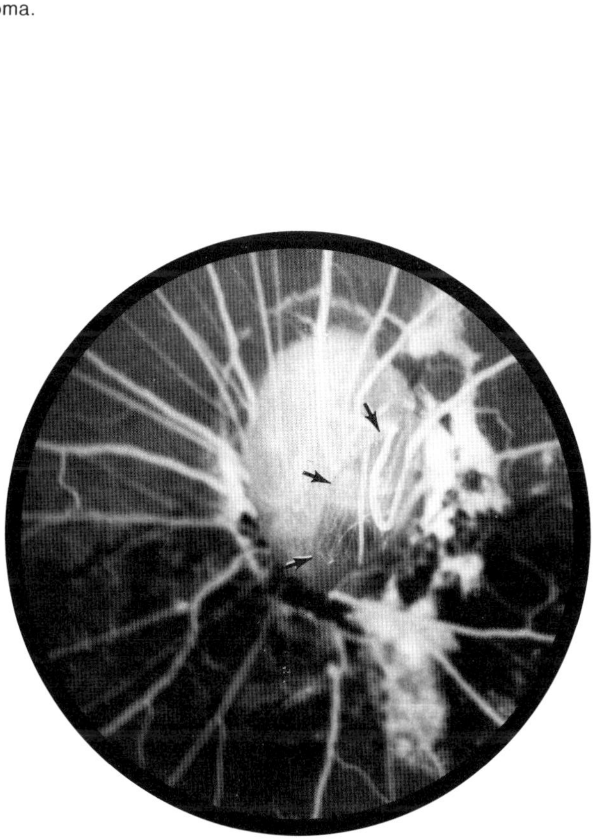

Figure 24.13. Coloboma of the optic nerve with associated retinal and choroidal defects. Early venous phase angiogram. Note the presence of a coloboma at the inferotemporal aspect of the disc (*arrows*) associated with widespread juxtapapillary hypofluorescence associated with a reduction of the choriocapillaris. Severe forms of optic nerve coloboma may also involve adjacent retina and choroid, and be associated with other congenital ocular malformations.

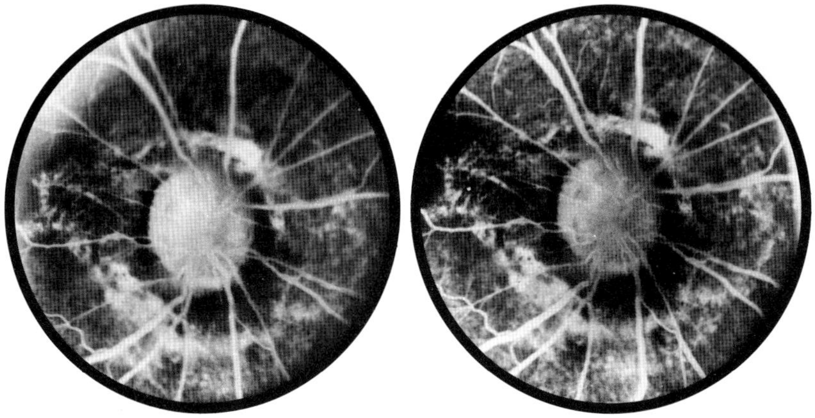

Figure 24.14. Stereo fluorescein angiogram of a peripapillary staphyloma. Note the normal optic nerve head which is displaced posteriorly to the base of a posterior excavation of the sclera. The margins of the disc are well defined, and the peripapillary vessels course posteriorly at a sharp angle. The peripapillary choroid and sclera appear stretched and there is atrophy as well as some pigment proliferation. *Note:* These photos are stereoscopic pairs and can be viewed from a distance of approximately 10 inches by holding +5 spheres close to the eyes.

The optic nerve head, in an eye with a *peripapillary staphyloma* may be normal in appearance but displaced posteriorly at the base of the posterior excavation of the sclera. The margins of the disc are well defined, and the peripapillary vessels are noted to course posteriorly at a rather sharp angle as they approach the disc. The peripapillary choroid and sclera appear stretched and there is usually atrophy of the pigment epithelium and pigment epithelial proliferation. These eyes are usually of normal axial lengths, and the posterior displacement of the optic nerve head is variable [14]. Fluorescein angiography reveals the presence of second-order retinal arterioles at the margins of the staphyloma (Fig. 24.14). The vascularity of the nerve head itself may be obscured because of poor camera resolution due to the marked refractive difference or by blockage from disorganized neuro or retinal tissue in front of the displaced lamina cribrosa [15].

The principal congenital anomaly of the optic nerve which causes elevation of the disc is *optic nerve head drusen.* Optic nerve head drusen are transmitted in families as an irregular dominant and are seen principally in Caucasians. A diagnosis of optic nerve head drusen may be difficult to establish particularly in children because of its resemblance to papilledema. Particularly troublesome are subpapillary drusen which usually become evident within the first or second decades of life. They first appear as irregular, slight elevations in the disc with nodular or feathery margins. In childhood, they are the principal cause of pseudopapilledema, presenting more diagnostic difficulties than all other forms of pseudopapilledema combined, including high hyperopia, persistent hyaloidal tissue, myelinated nerve fibers, and the like. At any age drusen may be associated with papillary vascular proliferation and peripapillary subretinal neovascularization which may result in juxtapapillary hemorrhage, exudate, and retinal detachment. New vessels, which originate from the drusen may course around Bruch's membrane in the juxtapapillary region to emerge in the adjacent macula to become associated with hemorrhagic detachments and disciform scarring. Optic nerve head drusen may also be associated with other vascular aberrations such as arteriovenous tortuosity, premature branching, and multiple cilioretinal vessels [16]. The drusen are usually bilateral but seldom symmetrical.

Fluorescein angiography may be of value in the evaluation of optic nerve head drusen. In the pre-injection phases of the angiogram, the phenomenon of autofluorescence may be observed in some but not all drusen (Fig. 24.15). In these instances, the refractile bodies appear to convert blue light to green light in much the same way that the fluorescein molecule does. In the early filling stages of the angiogram, the retinovascular aberrations characteristic of drusen are seen; however, the vascular engorgement and prominence to the papillary circulation, so evident in papilledema and papillitis, are conspicuously absent in optic nerve head drusen. Also, there is no evidence of retinal vascular stasis such as delayed filling or late staining of perivascular spaces. In the late phase angiogram a nodular type of hyperfluorescence producing a scalloped disc margin from leakage at the site of the drusen is evident (Fig. 24.16). The absence of dilation and leakage of disc capillaries at all levels, and a characteristic late nodular staining of the nerve head, seem to differentiate optic nerve head drusen from true papilledema (Fig. 24.17).

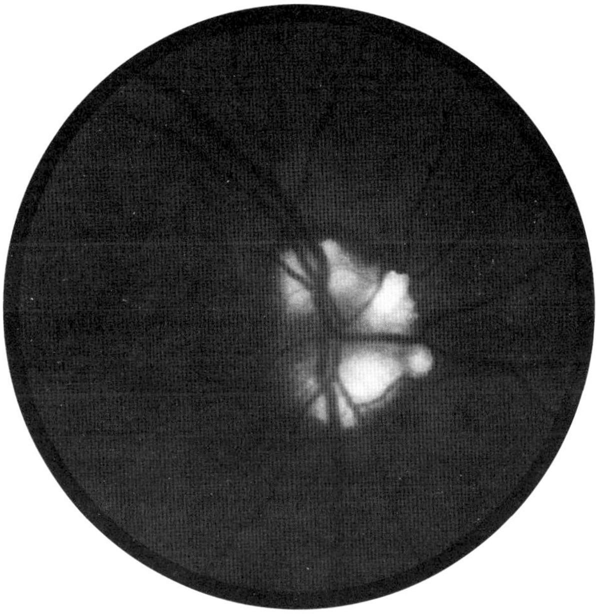

Figure 24.15. Optic nerve drusen demonstrating autofluorescence. This preinjection photo was taken with ideal or mutually exclusive filters. Excitatory blue light was nonetheless converted to fluorescing green light and then recorded on the control photograph demonstrating autofluorescence. Some, but not all, papillary drusen demonstrate this phenomenon.

A

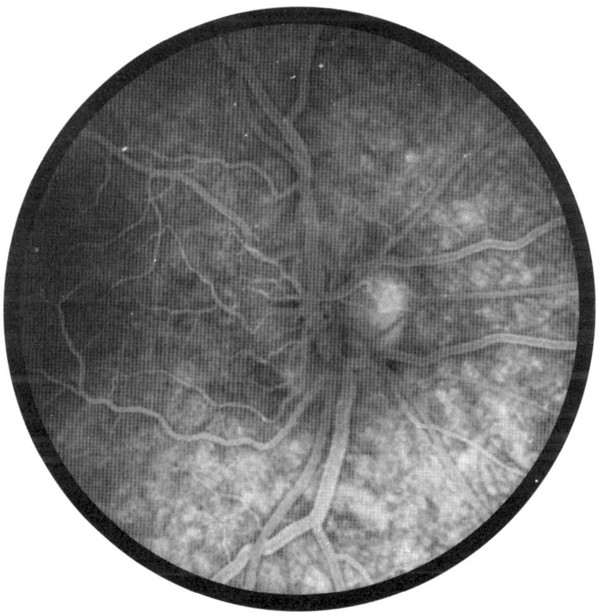

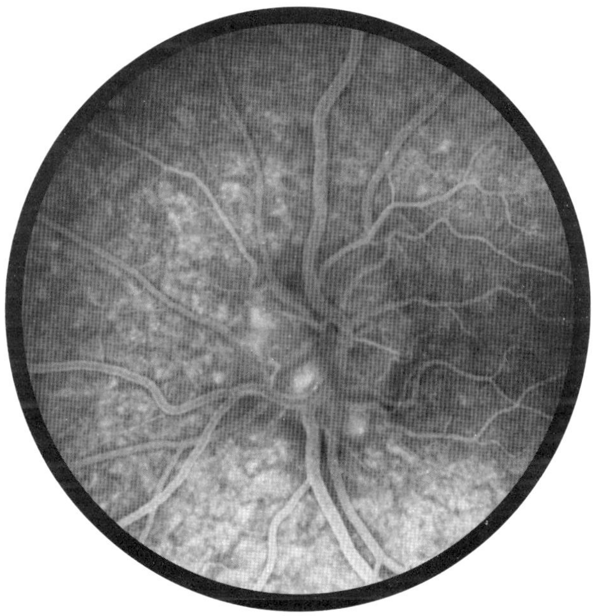

B

Figure 24.16. Optic nerve drusen with late nodular staining. Note the nodular staining of the nasal aspect of the disc *A*, and the multinodular staining with scalloped margins *B*, in these eyes with subpapillary drusen. The absence of disc capillary leakage and the presence of late nodular staining of the nerve head are characteristic of optic nerve drusen.

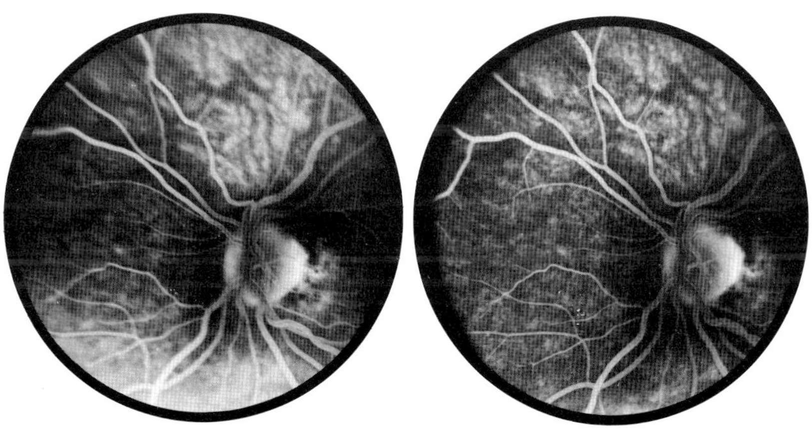

Figure 24.17. Stereo angiogram of late staining of optic nerve drusen. Note the deep staining of the optic nerve in this eye with subpapillary drusen. Dilation and leakage of the superficial disc circulations are conspicuously absent, differentiating this staining from that induced by true papilledema. *Note:* These photos are stereoscopic pairs and can be viewed from a distance of approximately 10 inches by holding +5 spheres close to the eyes.

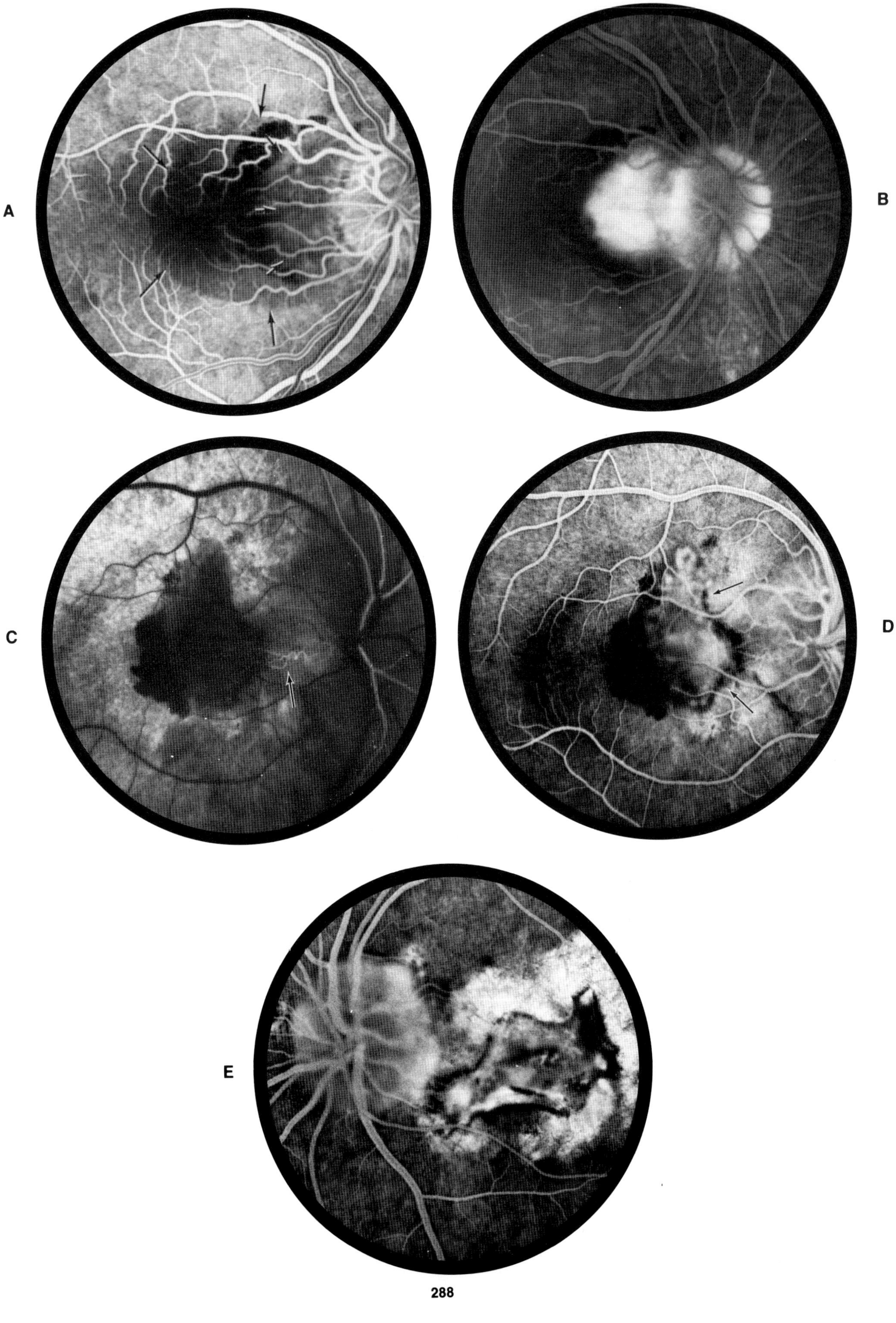
A
B
C
D
E

In cases in which subretinal neovascularization is associated with optic nerve head drusen, the fluorescein angiogram reveals early lacy hyperfluorescence of the subretinal vessels and late hyperfluorescence from pooling into the overlying subsensory retinal space (Fig. 24.18). Occasionally the vessels can be traced on a fluorescein angiogram from their originating peripapillary location, but most often they are obscured by intervening retinal pigment epithelium, exudate, and blood on papillary tissue (Fig. 24.19).

Peripapillary Subretinal Neovascularization

Proliferation of blood vessels from the papillary circulation with extension around Bruch's membrane to emerge as a subpigment epithelial fibrovascular complex may develop in a variety of disorders including: optic nerve head drusen, angioid streaks, myopia, involutional macular degeneration, presumed ocular histoplasmosis. As in optic nerve head drusen, the origin of the vessels is frequently obscured by the tissue densities associated with the exudative response. Early lacy hyperfluorescence of the vascular network and late hyperfluorescence from staining of scar tissue or pooling into the subsensory retinal space are the fluorescein angiographic features of the neovascularization.

A

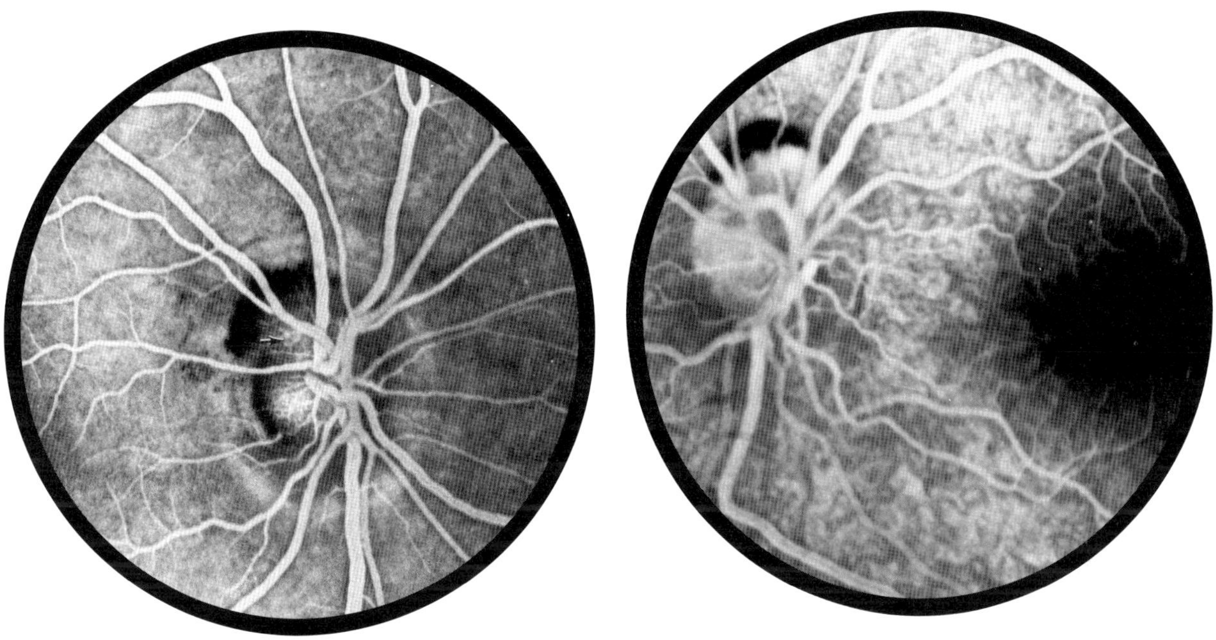

B

Figure 24.19. Optic nerve head drusen with peripapillary crescent-shaped hemorrhage. *A*, late venous phase angiogram with peripapillary hemorrhage secondary to vascular proliferation on the nerve (*arrow*). *B*, peripapillary hemorrhage in another patient with optic nerve head drusen but without evident vascular proliferation. Fluorescein angiography often demonstrates the neovascularization in optic nerve drusen associated with peripapillary hemorrhage, but sometimes the vessels are obscured by intervening retinal pigment epithelium, exudate, blood or even the papillary tissue, itself.

Figure 24.18. Subretinal neovascularization associated with drusen of the optic nerve. *A*, arteriovenous phase angiogram. In this eye with optic nerve drusen, note the notched appearance to the margins of the disc, the crescent-shaped area of subretinal hyperfluorescence corresponding to a fibrovascular membrane at the temporal aspect of the disc (*small arrows*), a margin of intense hypofluorescence from blood between the fovea and the membrane, and the large circumscribed area of macular hypofluorescence induced by the turbid subretinal fluid (*large arrows*). *B*, late phase angiogram. Note the hyperfluorescence produced by pooling into the subsensory retinal space by the peripapillary subretinal membrane and the nodular hyperfluorescence of the disc at the site of optic nerve drusen. *C*, choroidal phase of a fluorescein angiogram of an 11-year-old with optic nerve drusen. Note the peripapillary vessels (arrow) from the prelaminar circulation coursing around Bruch's membrane into a subretinal membrane. *D*, early venous phase angiogram showing the subretinal peripapillary membrane (arrows). *E*, late phase angiogram in the opposite eye of same patient showing an old disciform scar from subretinal neovascularization secondary to optic nerve head drusen. While these membranes often regress without growth into the perifoveal area, occasionally they will extend into the fovea as in this case.

Optic Nerve Head Edema

Edema of the optic nerve head may occur from a number of primary and secondary disorders of the optic nerve. In some instances the nerve head edema occurs as an isolated phenomenon, but invariably there are concomitant or secondary manifestations in the adjacent peripapillary retina and choroid, and less frequently in the macula. In addition, there are certain primary diseases of the macula and a few generalized chorioretinal diseases that are associated with optic nerve head edema that is usually subclinical and evident only on fluorescein angiography.

Papilledema is a form of disc swelling that results from increased intracranial pressure. In severe forms there may be juxtapapillary hemorrhages and exudates, and peripapillary sensory retinal detachment. Full appreciation of the microcirculatory abnormalities associated with papilledema, at all levels of the disc capillaries, are best appreciated utilizing stereo-fluorescein angiography (Fig. 24.20). The fluorescein angiogram demonstrates characteristic changes which include pronounced dilation and leakage of the superficial and intrapapillary disc capillaries and late staining of the disc. In some instances pooling may occur into an adjacent peripapillary subsensory retinal space, threatening or affecting the macula (Fig. 24.21). There is no reliable means of differentiating papilledema from optic neuritis by fluorescein angiography alone. Visual function studies, as well as ophthalmoscopic and slit-lamp biomicroscopic examination utilizing a Goldmann lens are more valuable to the clinical ophthalmologist in making this differentiation. Fluorescein angiography is also of no definite value in diagnosing retrobulbar neuritis, although there have been reports of sectorial or diffuse minimal staining of the disc in the late phase angiogram in association with this disease. In a series of well documented cases of retrobulbar neuritis in eyes without clinically visible ophthalmoscopic changes, the fluorescein angiogram failed to reveal any late hyperfluorescence or staining of the optic nerve head [17].

A

B

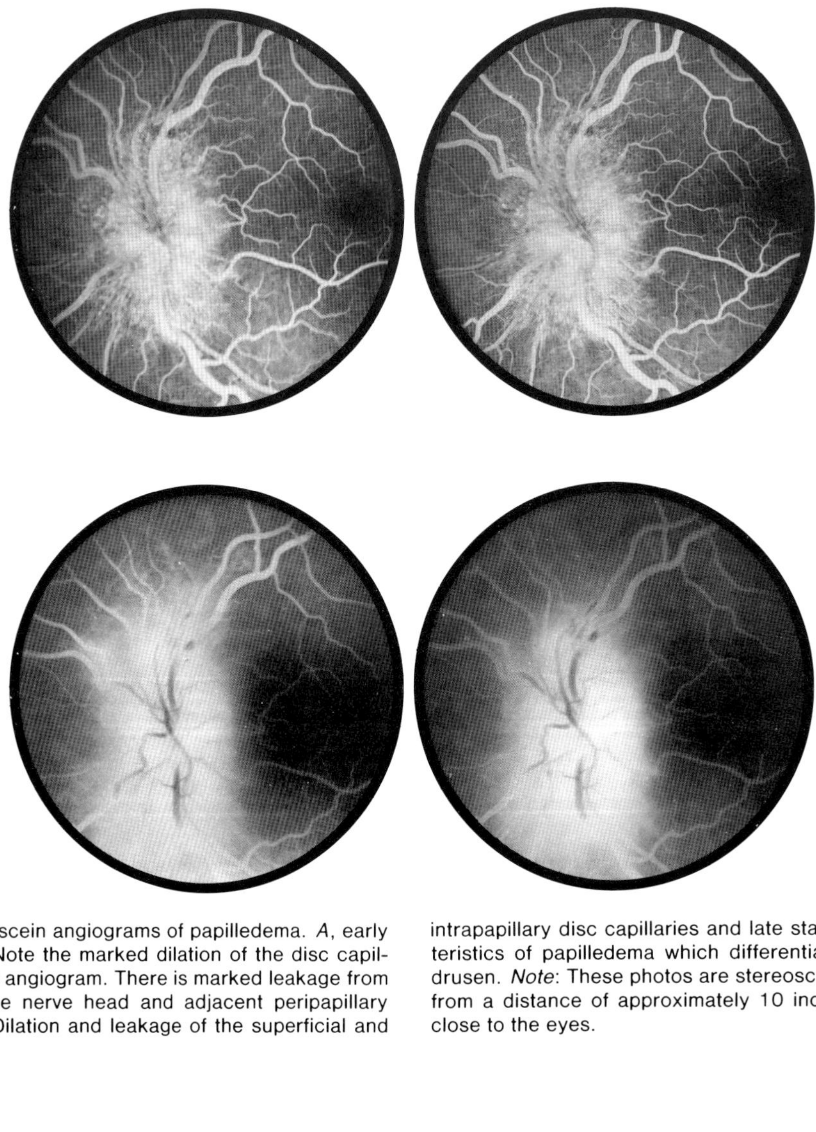

Figure 24.20. Stereo fluorescein angiograms of papilledema. *A*, early venous phase angiogram. Note the marked dilation of the disc capillaries. *B*, late venous phase angiogram. There is marked leakage from the disc circulation into the nerve head and adjacent peripapillary subsensory retinal space. Dilation and leakage of the superficial and intrapapillary disc capillaries and late staining of the disc are characteristics of papilledema which differentiate it from optic nerve head drusen. *Note*: These photos are stereoscopic pairs and can be viewed from a distance of approximately 10 inches by holding +5 spheres close to the eyes.

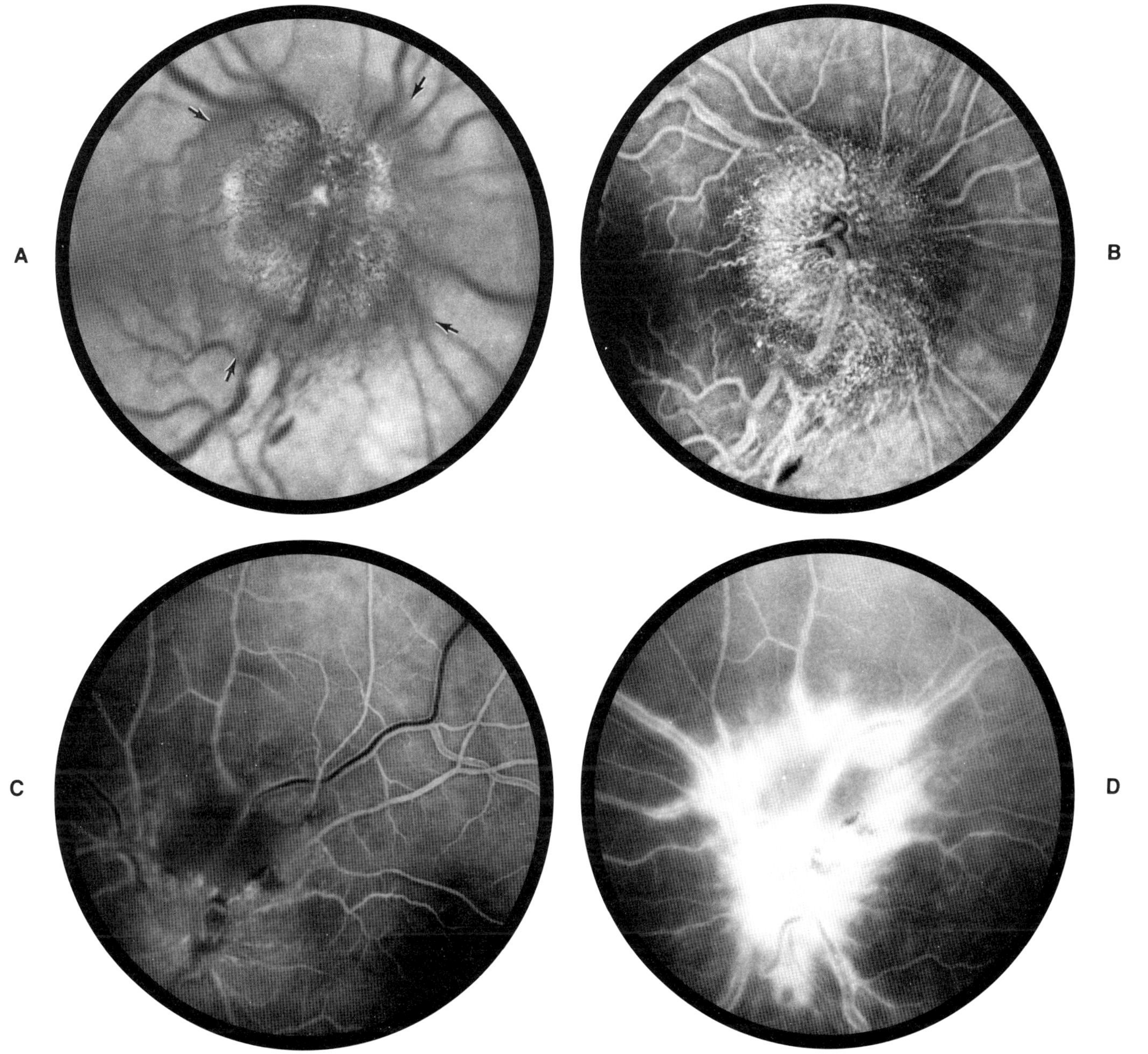

Figure 24.21. Optic nerve head edema with peripapillary sensory retinal detachment. *A*, ophthalmoscopic photograph. Note the elevated disc with markedly dilated superficial and intrapapillary capillaries in this eye with papilledema. There is also a peripapillary sensory retinal detachment encircling the disc (*arrows*). *B*, arteriovenous phase angiogram. The dilated and tortuous superficial and intrapapillary capillaries are accentuated. A ring of hypofluorescence which blocks the underlying choroidal fluorescence, surrounds the peripapillary area corresponds to the subsensory retinal fluid. *C*, arteriovenous phase angiogram of papillophlebitis and associated neurosensory detachment. Note the superficial and intrapapillary dilation of nerve vasculature and the hypofluorescence on the superior aspect of the disc at the site of the exudate. A marked peripapillary detachment encircled the optic nerve and involved the macula. *D*, late phase angiogram. Note the massive staining of optic nerve and retinal vessels and pooling into the peripapillary subsensory retinal space. Neurosensory detachments of the macula and peripapillary space may accompany any type of optic nerve edema. These fluorescein angiographic findings can be similar in optic neuritis and papilledema.

Optic nerve head edema may also be associated with intraocular inflammation including posterior uveitis, pars planitis or chronic cyclitis, papillophlebitis, retinal vasculitis, retinochoroiditis, uveal-meningeal syndromes, acute multifocal posterior placoid pigment epitheliopathy, geographic helicoid peripapillary choroidopathy (serpiginous choroidopathy), and generalized chorioretinal and primarily macular hereditary diseases. In addition to the usual clinical and fluorescein angiographic findings in the macula in these diseases, late hyperfluorescence or staining of the optic nerve may be present, usually in the late stages of the angiogram. In some instances, such as toxoplasmosis or Harada's disease, optic nerve head edema may be the first manifestation to appear and the last to disappear, as the most sensitive indicator of inflammatory activity. Localized subclinical disc inflammation, a toxicity-induced irritability or perhaps an immune response, may be the mechanism producing disc leakage in some of the hereditary conditions such as Stargardt's disease, retinitis pigmentosa, or cone dystrophy (Fig. 24.22).

Optic nerve head edema frequently accompanies retinal vascular disturbances such as collagen, vascular disease, malignant hypertension, toxemia of pregnancy, and uremia. Central retinal vein obstruction may often cause optic nerve head edema. The spectacular appearance of the retinal vasculature with preretinal, widespread intraretinal, and subretinal hemorrhages usually eliminates any diagnostic confusion. Fluorescein angiography is helpful in demonstrating the delayed filling of the central retinal vein, areas of capillary nonperfusion, concomitant arteriolar insufficiency when present, compensatory collateralization, and variable degrees of macular edema. The patency of the prelaminar circulation controls the degree of edema of the nerve head and leads to compensatory retinociliary collateralization (retinal venous to ciliary venous collaterals) most obvious following evidence of the venous obstruction. Sometimes these vessels, which clinically resemble neovascularization, are the only remaining evidence of antecedent central retinal vein thrombosis.

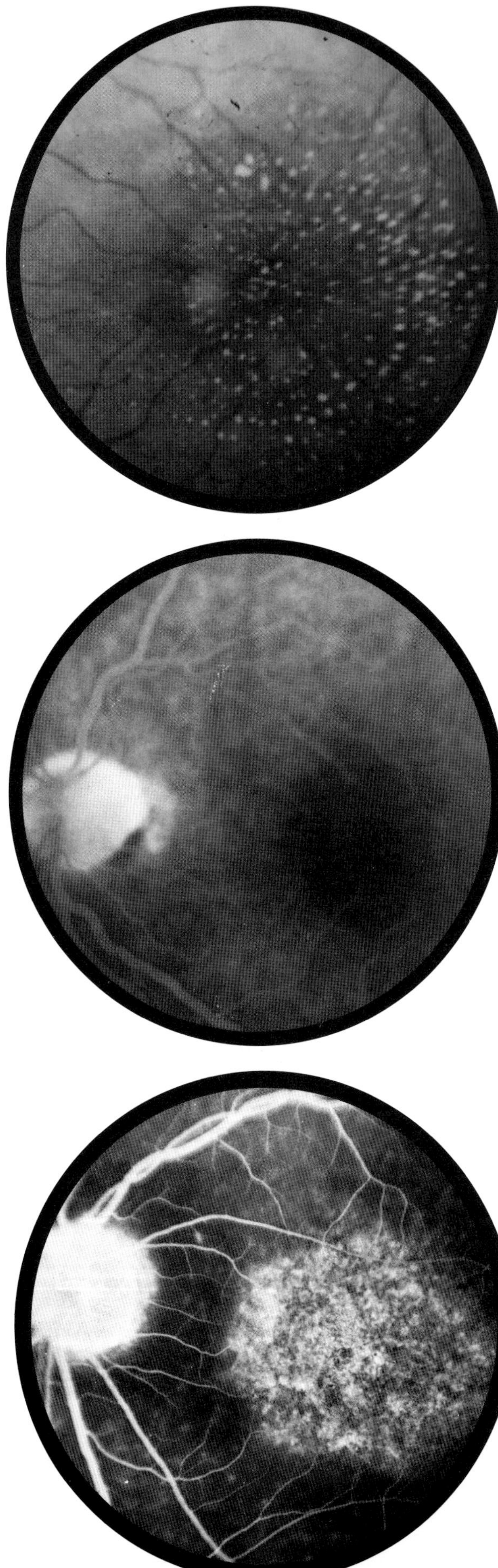

A

B

C

Figure 24.22. Disc leakage in chorioretinal inflammatory and hereditary diseases. *A*, ophthalmoscopic photograph. Note the exudate in the macula of this 26-year-old patient who had reduced vision following an upper respiratory infection. *B*, late phase angiogram reveals mild papillophlebitis with staining of the disc. *C*, late venous phase angiogram in a patient with Stargardt's disease. Note the staining of the optic disc. Disc leakage may be associated with a number of intraocular inflammatory and hereditary diseases.

In *ischemic optic neuropathy*, optic nerve head swelling may occur in association with sudden visual loss in a sector, altitudinal, or complete fashion secondary to peripapillary vascular occlusive disease. The edema is frequently accompanied by one or more superficial flame-shaped hemorrhages on or near the disc. The fluorescein angiogram typically reveals delayed or incomplete filling of the ciliary circumpapillary capillaries, and late hyperfluorescence or staining of the optic nerve in a fashion which corresponds to an induced field defect [18]. In the acute phase, there is a marked delay and incomplete filling of the choroid by the posterior ciliary arteries, perfusing the peripapillary region (Fig. 24.23). If the process is sectorial, defects in the choroid and peripapillary choroid are seen only in the involved sector (Fig. 24.24). Perfusion of the choroidal and peripapillary circulation is usually improved by the 2nd week following onset of the disease and is unimpaired after approximately 2 months. The retinal circulation is usually normal, although a cilioretinal artery occlusion may be evident, and a combined central retinal artery occlusion may rarely be present if it arises from a common trunk with the posterior ciliary artery [5].

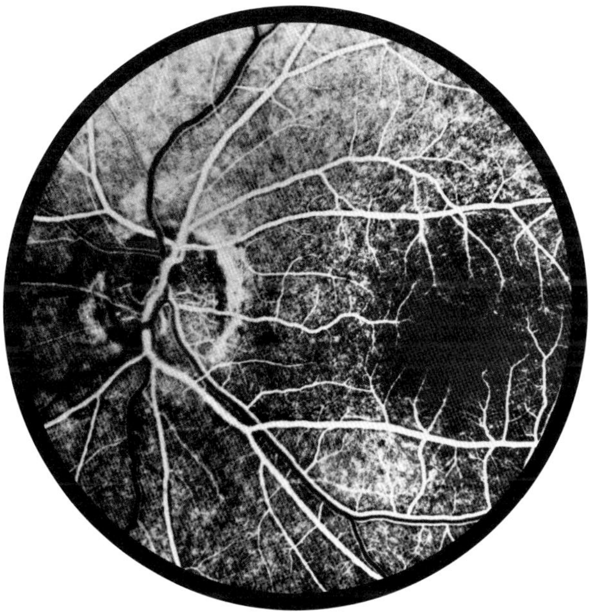

Figure 24.24. Ischemic optic neuropathy with sectorial involvement. Note the hypofluorescence at the superonasal aspect of the disc. Compare the hypofluorescence to the normal vascularity of the inferotemporal aspect of the disc.

A

B

C

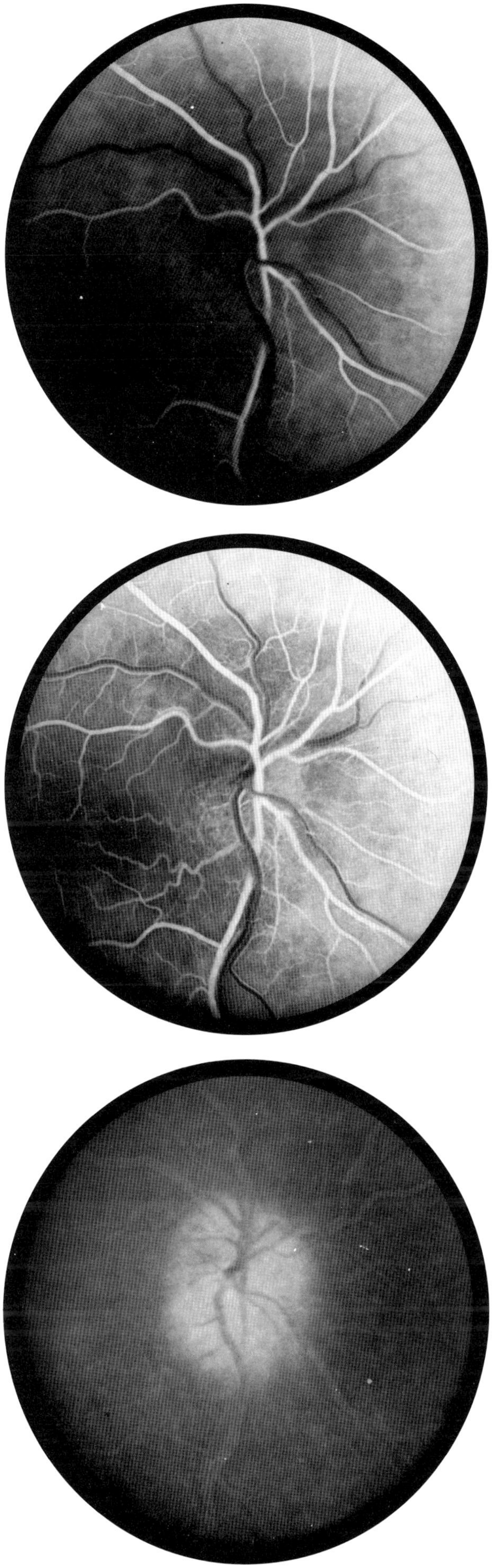

Figure 24.23. Ischemic optic neuropathy with delayed intrapapillary perfusion. *A*, arterial phase angiogram. Note the filling of the retinal arterioles in this eye with an edematous optic nerve and a juxtapapillary flame-shaped hemorrhage. Although there is a background choroidal fluorescence at this stage, there is no evident perfusion of the superficial intrapapillary vessels. *B*, late phase angiogram. The intrapapillary or prelaminar vessels are still not evident, although there is now fluorescence of the superficial papillary vascular network derived from the retinal artery as evidenced by the small fluorescing capillaries anterior to the deeper juxtapapillary hemorrhage. *C*, late phase angiogram. Note the diffuse hyperfluorescence from staining of the optic nerve head.

Neovascularization of the disc may sometimes be confused with edema of the optic nerve. Disc neovascularization is most commonly seen secondary to retinal vascular occlusive disease such as diabetes mellitus and branch retinal vein occlusion. Other retinal vascular ischemic disorders, as well as intraocular inflammation, are known to cause disc neovascularization although with less frequency [19] (Fig. 24.25). The diagnosis of disc neovascularization is readily documented on fluorescein angiography. Early lacy hyperfluorescence overlying the disc with marked leakage resulting in vitreous hyperfluorescence that has "cotton ball" appearance are the usual angiographic findings. The late leakage into the vitreous and the sharply outlined disc margins differentiate this neovascularization from retinociliary collaterals and disc edema, respectively.

Ocular hypotony may also lead to disc edema. Marked disc swelling associated with a peripapillary sensory retinal detachment and choroidal folds or in an eye with reduced intraocular pressure are the usual clinical findings. The primary disturbance appears to be in the relationship between the hydrostatic and intraocular pressures in this disorder. The fluorescein angiogram usually reveals marked dilatation and tortuosity of the retinal vessels and late staining of the optic nerve head (Fig. 24.26). The choroidal folds reveal linear areas of alternating hypo- and hyperfluorescence corresponding to the valleys and domes of the folds themselves.

The optic nerve and nerve head may be invaded secondarily by *intraocular tumors* resulting in optic nerve head edema. Certain primary tumors with an endophytic growth such as retinoblastoma may shed cells into the vitreous cavity and seed the nerve or nerve head [20]. Malignant melanomas may rarely spread in this way as well, particularly if they erode through the retina into the vitreous cavity. Peripapillary malignant melanomas, however, most often produce compression or distortion of the nerve head with little or no appreciable spread into the optic nerve itself, which is relatively resistant to invasion. On the other hand, metastatic choroidal carcinoma may invade the optic nerve head frequently causing edema and profound reduction in vision. Similarly leukemic infiltration of the optic nerve may produce pale, cloudy swelling of the nerve head with extension into the adjacent retina and vitreous. Marked improvement with restoration to normal anatomic configuration may occur during periods of remission [21]. In metastatic disease to the optic nerve head, with associated optic nerve head edema, the fluorescein angiogram reveals a nonspecific late hyperfluorescence or staining of the disc.

A

B

C

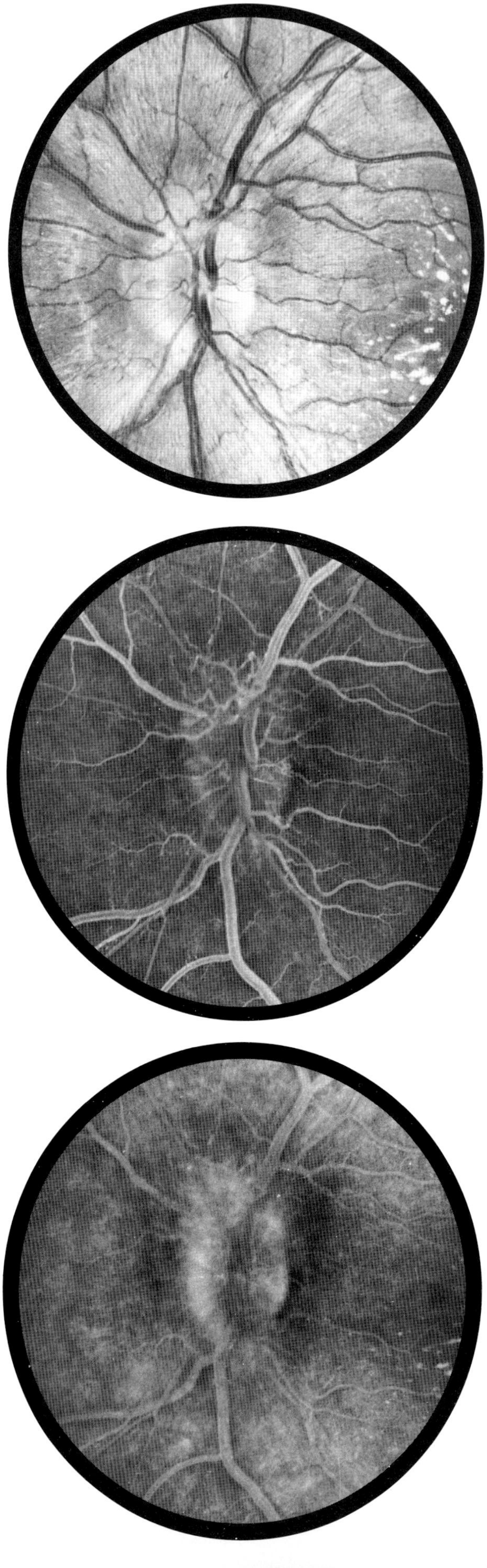

Figure 24.25. Optic nerve edema and neovascularization in chronic uveitis with macular exudation. *A*, ophthalmoscopic photograph. Note the edematous optic nerve associated with vascular proliferation at its superior aspect and exudate in the macula. *B*, early venous phase angiogram. The dilated and tortuous vessels on the nerve head are accentuated and the new vessel growth on the disc shows early leakage. *C*, late phase angiogram. The disc neovascularization shows leakage into the vitreous.

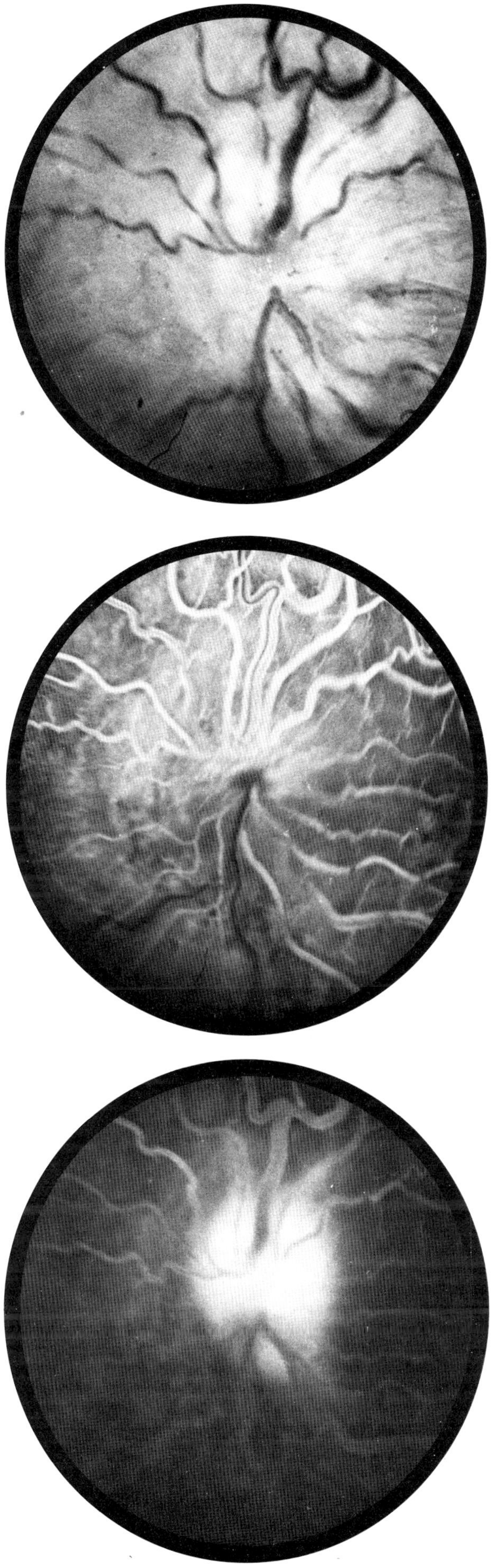

A

B

C

Figure 24.26. Hypotony. *A*, ophthalmoscopic photograph. Note the edematous optic nerve head with retinal vascular dilatation and tortuosity and a peripapillary sensory retinal detachment. *B*, arteriovenous phase angiogram. The dilated and tortuous vessels are accentuated on the angiogram. *C*, late phase angiogram. There is late hyperfluorescence from staining of the optic nerve and pooling into peripapillary subsensory retinal space. There is no leakage in the macula.

Primary Optic Nerve Head Tumors

Certain optic nerve head tumors may extend into the adjacent peripapillary choroid or retina, threatening or involving the macula. In some instances secondary manifestations such as lipid exudation, preretinal membrane formation, or subretinal neovascularization develop in the macula. Because of the absence of an intervening pigment epithelial layer barrier, optic nerve head tumors reveal their histopathologic character on the fluorescein angiogram more readily than their subpigment epithelial counterparts elsewhere in the fundus. The fluorescein angiographic findings reflect largely the degree of pigmentation of the tumor and their vascular components.

Melanocytoma of the optic nerve is a densely pigmented tumor of variable size which originates from the melanocytes in the region of the lamina cribrosa. The tumor may be limited to the nerve or extend beyond it into the adjacent choroid. When it involves the temporal aspect of the disc, secondary manifestations such as pigment epithelial atrophy or proliferation may be seen in the macula. The fluorescein angiogram typically demonstrates hypofluorescence from blockage of the tumor's vascularity by the dense pigmentation. In the late phase angiogram, there is often a "halo" of hyperfluorescence from pooling into the overlying vitreous (vitreohyperfluorescence). Occasionally, the vascularity of the tumor is superficial or prominent and visible on the fluorescein angiogram (Fig. 24.27). One large melanocytoma, followed by the authors, became associated with subretinal neovascularization and a localized detachment at a point where it extended into the adjacent juxtapapillary nasal choroid.

Papillary and juxtapapillary endophytic and exophytic angiomas may occur at the disc in ocular angiomatosis. Endophytic tumors obscure the superficial retinal vascular network; whereas, the exophytic ones develop deeper in the retina and are more likely to be associated with intraretinal and subretinal exudation that may extend into the macula (Fig. 24.28). On fluorescein angiography, the highly vascularized capillary network of the tumor reveals a lacy type of hyperfluorescence early and marked late hyperfluorescence or leakage late. The authors have noted a case of telangiectasia of the disc which resembled an angioma clinically. The fluorescein angiographic findings, however, revealed the characteristic changes of capillary telangiectasia, capillary nonperfusion, aneurysmal dilatation, and leakage (Fig. 24.28).

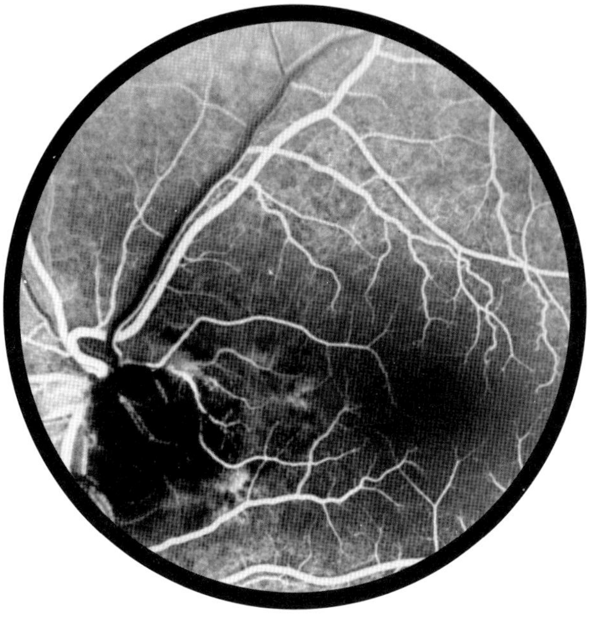

Figure 24.27. Melanocytoma of optic nerve with secondary changes in the macula. Note the densely pigmented tumor of the optic nerve which extends into the juxtapapillary choroid at its temporal aspect. Part of the vascularity of the tumor is superficial. Early hyperfluorescence is also noted in the adjacent macula from atrophy of the retinal pigment epithelium.

Figure 24.28. Juxtapapillary exophytic angioma with lipid exudation into the macula. *A*, ophthalmoscopic photograph. Note the elevation at the temporal aspect of the optic nerve with dilated tortuous capillaries. Lipid exudation surrounds the lesion and extends into the macula. *B*, arterial phase angiogram. Note the lacy-like hyperfluorescence originating from the deep retinal capillary network and the normal overlying superficial retinal vessels. Pseudofluorescence at the site of the lipid exudation is present because of poorly matched filters. Papillary and juxtapapillary angiomas, particularly exophytic ones, may develop at the disc, and be associated with lipid deposition in the macula. *C*, ophthalmoscopic photograph of a patient with telangiectasia of the optic nerve. Note the optic nerve head edema associated with dilated disc vessels, lipid exudation, subretinal hemorrhage, peripapillary sensory retinal detachment, and cystic degeneration of the macula. *D*, arterial phase angiogram. Note the dilated telangiectatic vessels, the capillary nonperfusion, and the aneurysmal changes. *E*, venous phase angiogram. Note the early leakage from the involved vasculature. *F*, late phase angiogram. Note the extensive vitreous and papillary subretinal and intraretinal leakage. This case clinically resembled an angioma, but the fluorescein angiographic findings were more compatible with telangiectasia.

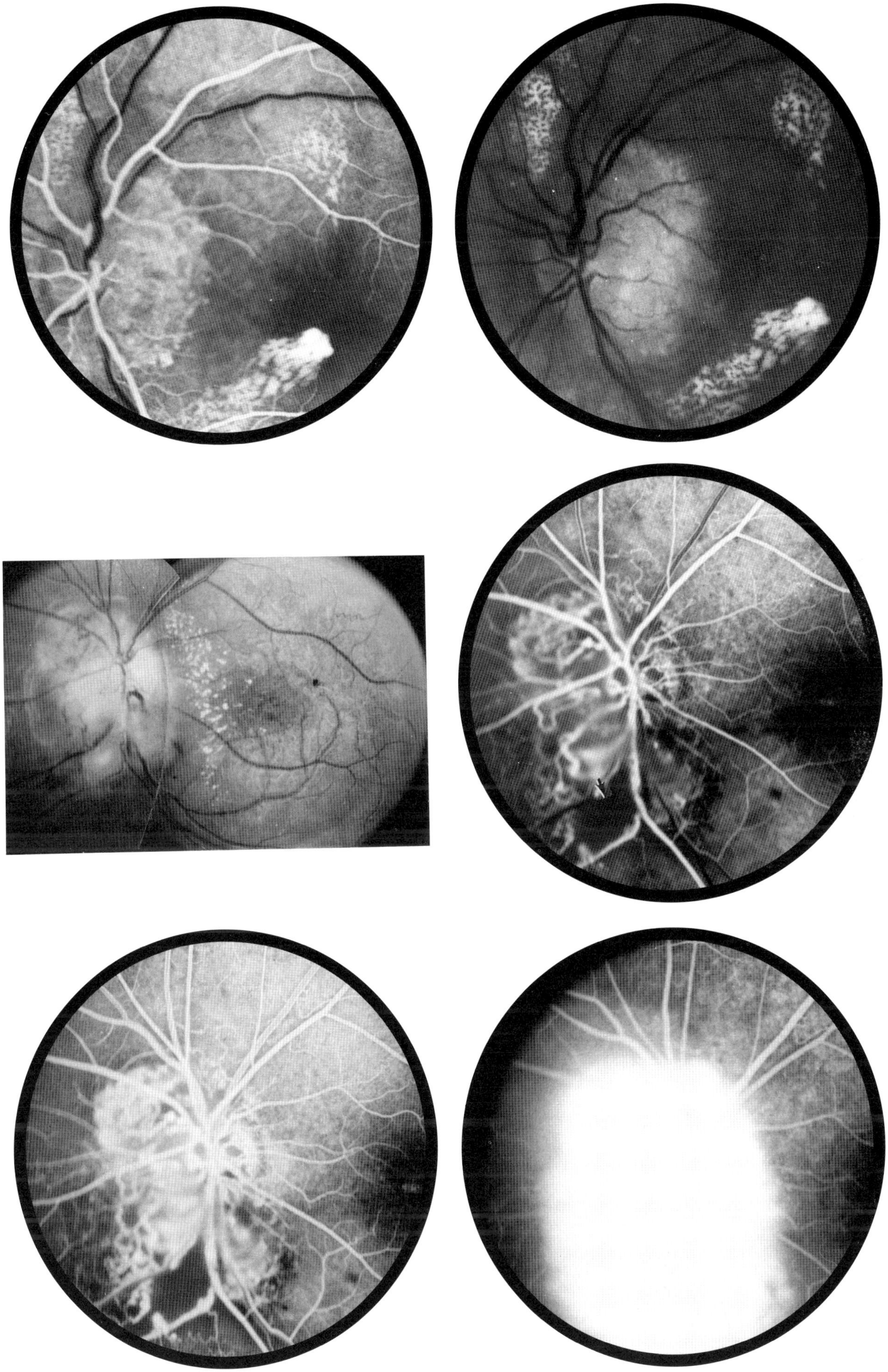

A B C D E F

Hamartomas of the retinal pigment epithelium and retina occur most frequently at the nerve head; they also may be found in the macula or peripheral retina as well. Those at the nerve head are associated with a vitreal retinal interface disturbance with retinal folds coursing toward and into the macula. They are also associated with heavy pigmentation secondary to duplication of the pigment epithelium and proliferation of retinal pigment epithelial, glial and vascular elements. Fluorescein angiography reveals a marked vascular hyperfluorescence from the capillaries within the tumor (Fig. 24.29). These vessels also leak, producing late hyperfluorescence or staining of the tumor. Subretinal or choroidal neovascularization has been observed to develop in one of these tumors (Fig. 24.30). The presence of accompanying histopathologic changes in the macula are fully recognized only through fluorescein stereoangiography, which reveals the nature and location of the tumor's vascular components and the exact location of leakage (Fig. 24.31).

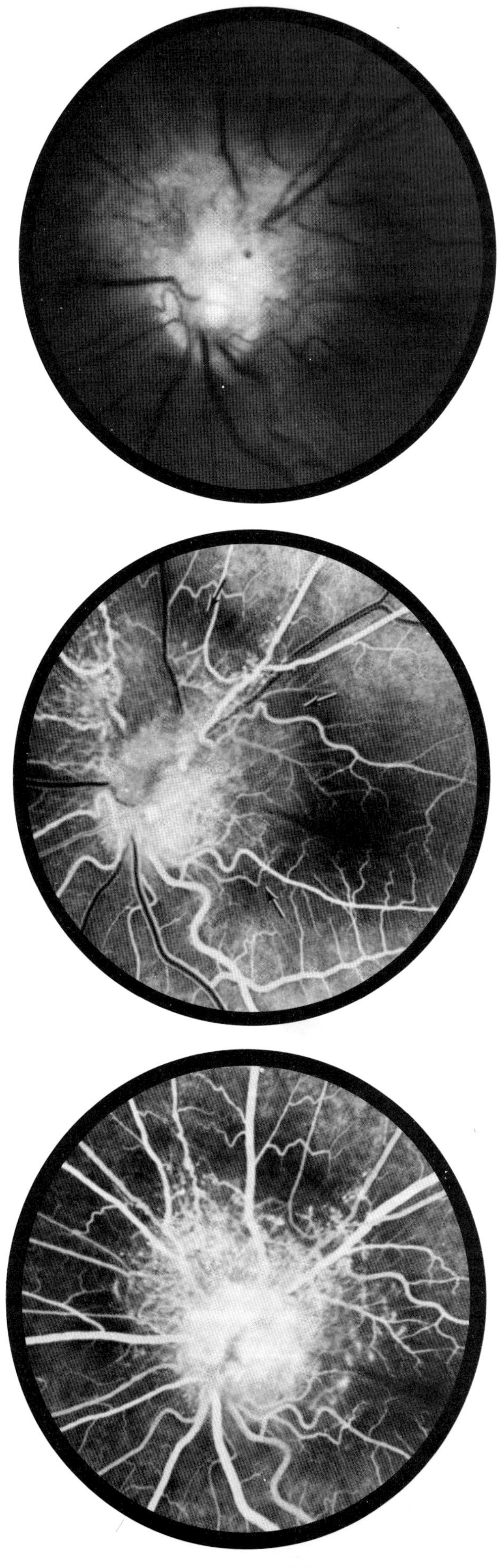

A

B

C

Figure 24.29. Hamartoma of the retinal pigment epithelium and retina. *A*, ophthalmoscopic photograph. Note the elevation and distortion at the site of the optic nerve associated with vascular prominence, dilation and tortuosity and a vitreoretinal interface disturbance with radiating retinal folds coursing from the lesion toward the macula. *B*, arteriovenous phase. The fluorescein angiogram accentuates the retinal vascular components of this tumor. There is a zone of hypofluorescence (*arrows*) corresponding to pigment proliferation and retinal pigment epithelial hyperplasia. *C*, late venous phase angiogram. Note the late hyperfluorescence from leakage of these abnormal capillaries.

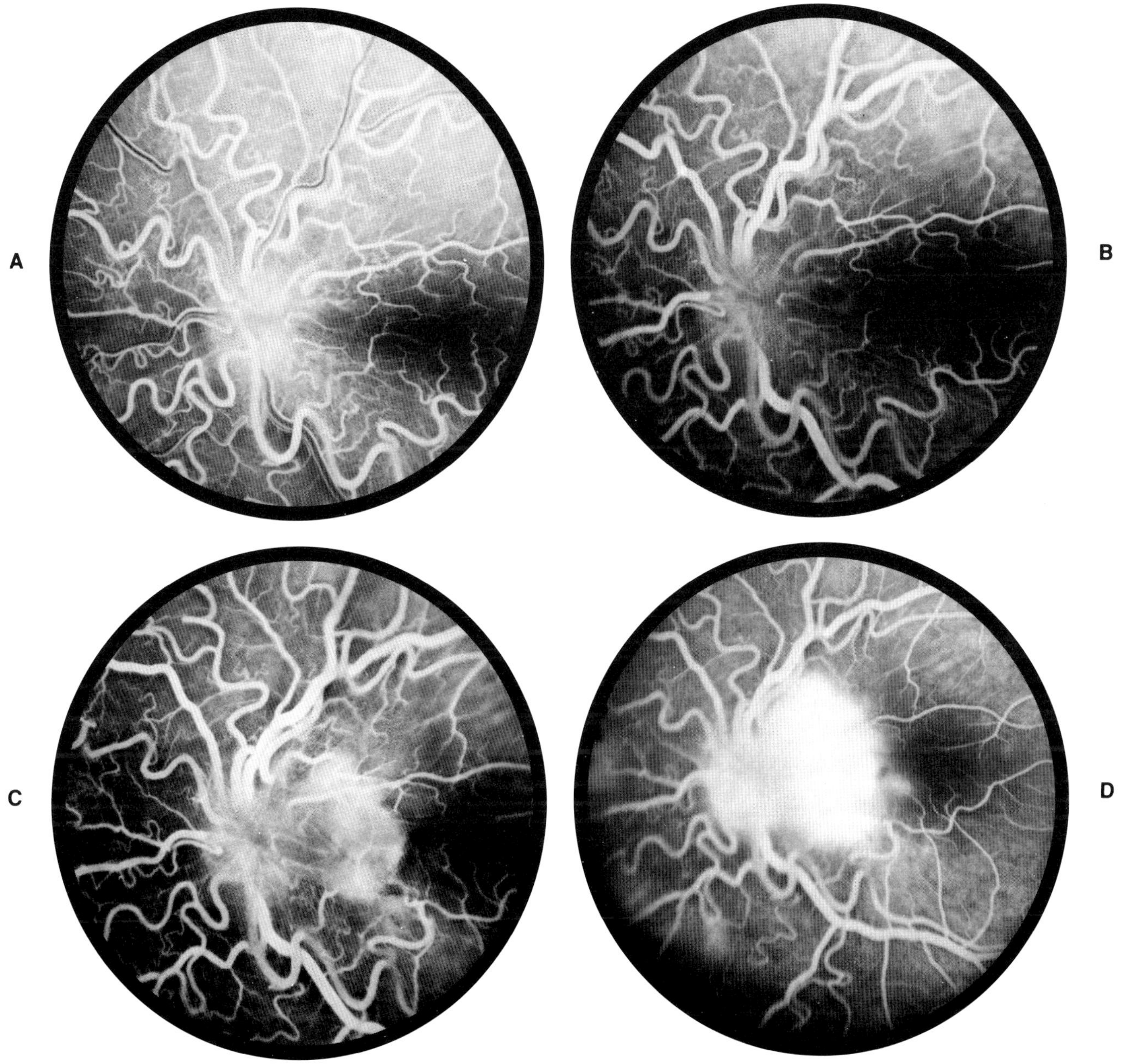

Figure 24.30. Hamartoma of the retinal pigment epithelium and retina associated with subretinal neovascularization. *A*, arteriovenous phase angiogram. Note the marked tortuosity and prominence of the retinal vasculature surrounding the optic nerve. Numerous arteriovenous shunts are evident. *B*, late phase angiogram. The tumor vessels are relatively impermeable to fluorescein with minimal late leakage. *C* and *D*, same eye, 2 years later. Note the development of a localized area of subretinal hyperfluorescence corresponding to a fibrovascular network at the temporal peripapillary area. More superficial retinal and tumor vessels are seen to course over the subretinal hyperfluorescence without evidence of leakage (*C*). In the late stage angiogram (*D*), a diffuse late hyperfluorescence is evident from pooling into the accompanying subsensory macular detachment.

In summary, diseases of the optic nerve are commonly associated with combined or secondary manifestations in the macula. Certain congenital anomalies, a number of disorders resulting in optic nerve head edema, and a few primary tumors of the optic nerve may be associated with intraretinal serous and lipid exudation, peripapillary sensory retinal detachment, retinal pigment epithelial atrophy and retinal pigment epithelial proliferation, peripapillary subretinal neovascularization, and choroidal folds, which extend into the adjacent choroid and retina to threaten or involve the macula. The pathophysiologic alterations associated with these diseases are best demonstrated and understood through a knowledge of the unique microcirculations of the optic nerve head and the use of stereo fluorescein angiography. Originating from the central retinal artery, the superficial papillary capillary plexus extends posteriorly to the intrapapillary or prelaminar circulation which is derived predominantly from the peripapillary choroidal circulation and the posterior ciliary arteries. Ultimately, this longitudinal, freely anastomosing circulation blends more posteriorly with the postlaminar capillary network formed largely from contributions from the pial vessels. Despite the dual origin to this continuous circulation (retinal and ciliary), the microcirculations throughout maintain an impermeable state to fluorescein in the normal eye. Fluorescein angiography is extremely useful in ascertaining the histopathologic alterations in the microcirculations of the disc in disorders of the optic nerve, particularly those with secondary manifestations in the macula.

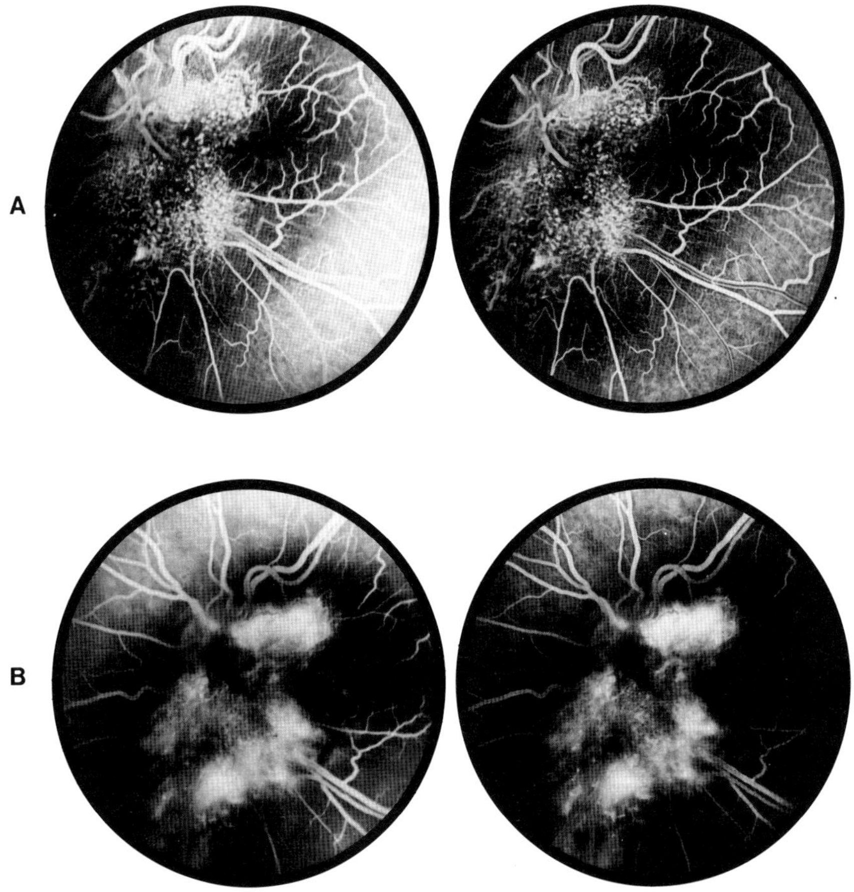

Figure 24.31. Stereo angiograms of hamartoma of the retinal pigment epithelium and retina. *A*, arteriovenous phase angiogram. Note the vascular components of this tumor which originate from the deep capillary plexus just temporal to the disc and from the more superficial retinal vascular circulation just inferotemporal to the disc. The larger nontumor vessels are obscured in areas where there is superficial vascular tumor ingrowth. The macula itself is elevated, and there is a vitreoretinal membranous change as well as a circumscribed area of pigment epithelial proliferation. *B*, late phase angiogram. Dye leakage can be isolated stereoscopically to its exact location beneath the sensory retina superotemporal to the disc within and above the retina inferiorly. Note the deep retinal edema in the macular region. *Note:* These photos are stereoscopic pairs and can be viewed from a distance of approximately 10 inches by holding +5 spheres close to the eyes.

References

1. Hayreh, S.S.: Anatomy and physiology of the optic nerve head. *Trans Am Acad Ophthalmol Otolaryngol, 78:* 240, 1974.
2. Lieberman, M.F., Maumenee, A.E., and Green, W.R.: Histologic studies of the vasculature of the anterior optic nerve. *Am J Ophthalmol, 82:* 405, 1976.
3. Anderson, D.R., and Braverman, S.: Reevaluation of the optic disc vasculature. *Am J Ophthalmol, 82:* 165, 1976.
4. Hayreh, S.S.: Pathogenesis of visual field defects: role of ciliary circulation. *Brit J Ophthalmol, 54:* 289, 1970.
5. Hayreh, S.S.: Anterior Ischemic Optic Neuropathy, Springer-Verlag, New York, 1975, pp. 1–14.
6. Shimizu, K.: Fluorescein Microangiography of the Ocular Fundus, Williams & Wilkins, Baltimore, 1973, pp. 79–90.
7. Ben Sira, I., and Riva, C.E.: Fluorescein diffusion in the human optic disc. *Invest Ophthalmol, 14:* 205, 1975.
8. Tso, M.O.M., Shih, C.-Y., and McLean, I.W.: Is there a blood-brain barrier at the optic nerve? *Arch Ophthalmol, 93:* 815, 1975.
9. Bernstein, M.H., and Hollenberg, M.J.: Fine structure of the chorio-capillaris and retinal capillaries. *Invest Ophthalmol, 14:* 1016, 1975.
10. Spitznas, M., and Reale, E.: Fracture faces of fenestrations and junctions of endothelial cells in human choroidal vessels. *Invest Ophthalmol, 14:* 98, 1975.
11. Grayson, M.C., and Laties, A.M.: Ocular localization of sodium fluorescein: effects of administration in rabbit and monkey. *Arch Ophthalmol, 85:* 600, 1971.
12. Sugar, H.S.: Congenital pits in the optic disc with acquired macular pathology. *Am J Ophthalmol, 53:* 307, 1962.
13. Ferry, A.P.: Macular detachment associated with congenital pit of the optic nerve head: pathologic findings in 2 cases simulating malignant melanoma of the choroid. *Arch Ophthalmol, 70:* 346, 1963.
14. Wise, J.B., McLean, A.L., and Gass, J.D.M.: Contractile peripapillary staphyloma. *Arch Ophthalmol, 75:* 626, 1965.
15. Walsh, F., and Hoyt, W.F.: Clinical Neuroophthalmology, vol. 1, Williams & Wilkins, Baltimore, 1969, p. 675.
16. Erkkilä, H.: Clinical appearance of the optic disc drusen in childhood. *Albrecht von Graefe's Arch Klin Ophthalmol, 193:* 1, 1975.
17. Yannuzzi, L.A.: Unpublished observations.
18. Follis, W.S.: Ischemic optic neuropathy. *In* Proceedings of the William MacKenzie Centenary Symposium on the Ocular Circulation in Health and Disease, ed. by J.S. Cant, C. V. Mosby, St. Louis, 1969.
19. Shorb, S.R., Irvine, A.R., Kimura, S.J., and Morris, B.W.: Optic disc neovascularization associated with chronic uveitis. *Am J Ophthalmol, 82:* 175, 1976.
20. Spencer, W.: Optic nerve extension of intraocular tumors. *Am J Ophthalmol, 80:* 465, 1975.
21. Gass, J.D.M.: Differential Diagnosis of Intraocular Tumors. C.V. Mosby, St. Louis, 1974.

CHAPTER 25

Intraocular Tumors

Jay L. Federman, M.D., Jerry A. Shields, M.D., and Terrance L. Tomer

A thorough knowledge of intraocular pathology with clinical examinations utilizing the indirect ophthalmoscope and the slit-lamp biomicroscope are the principal means for accurately diagnosing intraocular tumors. In recent years, other more sophisticated diagnostic tools have become available such as ultrasonography, radioactive P^{32} uptake studies, fundus photography, and fluorescein angiography. These modalities, particularly the latter, have aided immensely in the documentation and proper diagnosis of these lesions. This chapter reviews the clinical and fluorescein angiographic features of the more common intraocular tumors, all of which can affect the macula.

Choroidal Tumors

CHOROIDAL NEVI

Choroidal nevi are benign tumors which are seen with increasing freqeuncy in the latter decades of life. They occur in approximately 10% of the population. While they most frequently occur somewhere in the posterior pole, they may be found anywhere in the fundus. These tumors vary in size to several disc diameters; in degree of pigmentation from brown to slate gray; in shape from round to oval, usually with irregular but evident margins. Some choroidal nevi may demonstrate a slight growth potential assuming a clinical appearance indistinguishable from early stage melanomas.

Overlying degenerative changes can occur, the most common being drusen and retinal pigment epithelial atrophy. Less commonly, serous and hemorrhagic detachments of the retinal pigment epithelium, sensory retinal detachments originating from focal leaks resembling central serous chorioretinopathy and subretinal neovascularization may occur. Histopathologically, these tumors are composed of tightly packed nevus cells which usually involve the outer ⅔ of the choroid, but may involve the full thickness of the choroid from the sclera through the choriocapillaris (Fig. 25.1).

Choroidal nevi show three different fluorescein angiographic patterns which are explained by their histopathology (Table 25.1). The majority of choroidal nevi are hypofluorescent during the very early phases of the fluorescein study (Fig. 25.1*C*). As the intravascular and extravascular filling phases of the choroid develop, the area corresponding to the pigmented nevus seen clinically is relatively hypofluorescent (Fig. 25.1*C*). This hypofluorescence is most pronounced when the nevus cells fill the entire thickness of the choroid taking up the extravascular space where the fluorescein would normally be present. The pigment within the nevus may also contribute to the hypofluorescence by absorbing the fluorescent light that would normally be transmitted to the camera. With the complete filling of the extravascular layers of the choroid, the nevus still shows a relative hypofluorescence. This continuing state of hypofluorescence is explained by the same mechanisms (Fig. 25.1*D*). In the very late phases of the study, when most of the fluorescein has been drained from the extravascular layers of the choroid, the nevus still shows a relative hypofluorescence (Fig. 25.1*E*). Again, the explanation is the same because of absorption of light from the pigmented nevus cells and because of a lack of fluorescein in the area of the nevus (Fig. 25.1*E*).

Figure 25.1. *A*, color photo of choroidal nerves which most likely occupies the full-thickness of the choroid. *B*, schematic drawing showing nevus cells (*black*) involving the full thickness of the choroid. Note the nevus cells hugging the base of the choriocapillaris and extending to the inner scleral layers. *C*, arteriovenous phase angiogram showing an area of hypofluorescence (*arrows*) just superior and nasal to the disc. This corresponds to the nevus seen clinically. The hypofluorescence is a result of the fluorescein not diffusing into the area occupied by the nevus cells. *D*, early venous phase angiogram showing a more intense area of hypofluorescence because there is a greater concentration of fluorescein in the surrounding extravascular space of the choroid. *E*, late phase angiogram of the study showing the extravascular fluorescence from the deeper layers of the choroid. The area of hypofluorescence corresponding the nevus is due to the presence of nevus cells in the outer layers causing blockage of the fluorescence and also filling the space where the fluorescein molecules would normally be at this phase of the study.

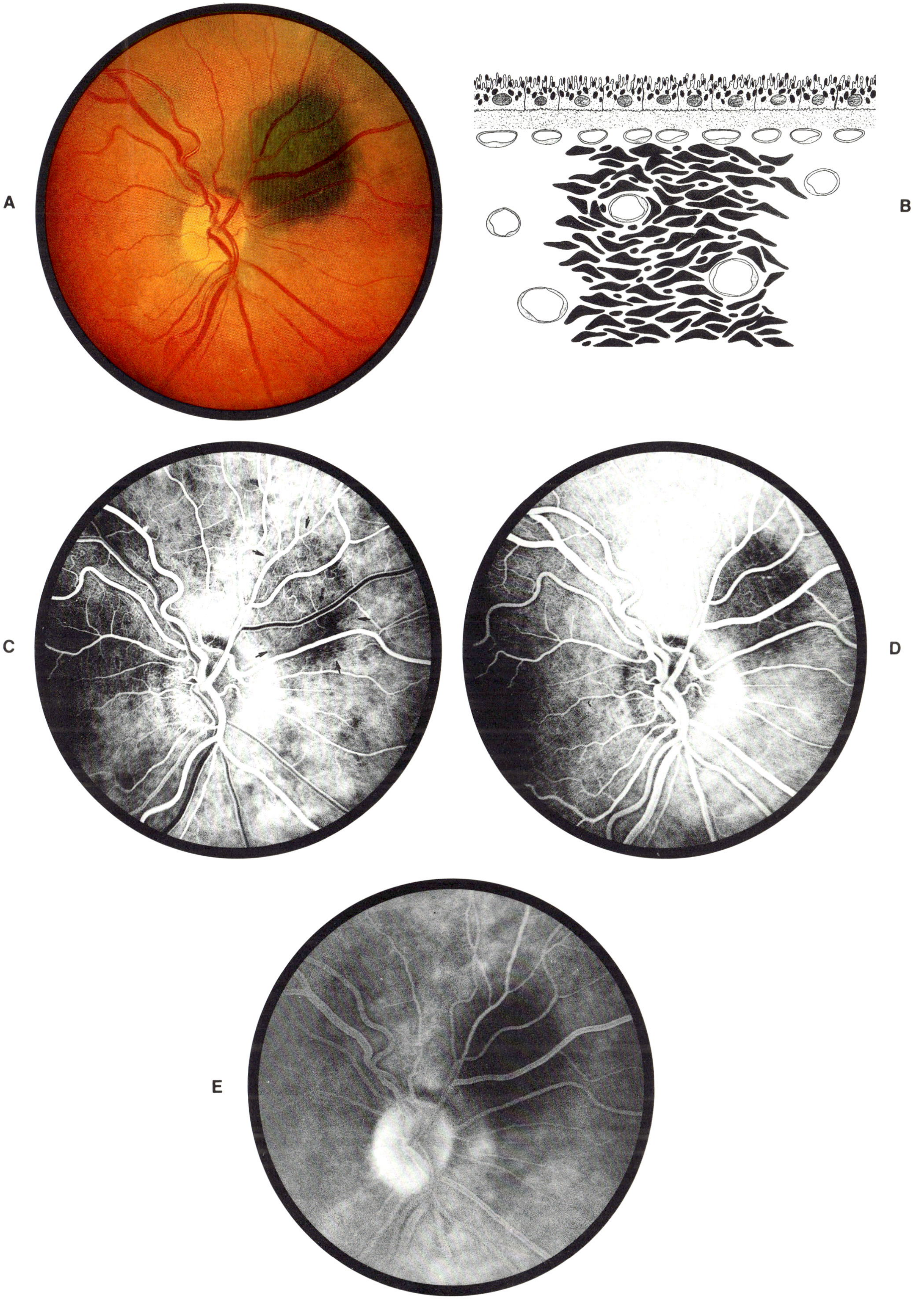
A
B
C
D
E

A second angiographic pattern is seen with a small percentage of choroidal nevi that occupy only the outer third or less of the choroid (Fig. 25.2). There is a normal background choroidal fluorescence during the early phases of the study corresponding to the area of the nevus (Fig. 25.2*B*). In the very late phases of the study, a subtle hypofluorescence develops (Fig. 25.2*D*). This pattern is present when the choroidal nevus occupies the outer layers of the choroid. During the early phases of the study, a normal background fluorescence is seen because the choriocapillaris and inner extravascular layers of the choroid fill in a normal manner. Since there are no nevus cells present in the inner layers of the choroid, the background choroidal fluorescence shows a normal diffuse fluorescence throughout the entire area (Fig. 25.2*C*). The subtle hypofluorescence seen in the late phases of the study results from the tightly packed nevus cells occupying the space in the choroid where the fluorescein would normally be present at this time in the study (Fig. 25.2*D*). This is exaggerated by the presence of the pigment, which also absorbs some of the fluorescent light.

Table 25.1. Fluorescence of choroidal nevi

Type	Early	Late
⅔ choroidal or full thickness	Hypofluorescent	Hypofluorescent
Outer ½ or ⅓ of choroid	Normal background fluorescence	Hypofluorescence
Overlying drusen, pigment epithelial or sensory retired detachment, or subretinal neovascularization	Hyperfluorescent	Hyperfluorescent

Figure 25.2. *A,* color photo of a choroidal nevus which most likely occupies only the outer layers of the choroid. *B,* schematic drawing showing nevus cells (*black*) occupying only the outer layers of the choroid. Note the inner layers of extravascular space and choriocapillaris are not involved; thus, fluorescein can diffuse freely in this area. *C,* arteriovenous phase angiogram of a nevus which represents cells in the outer layers of the choroid. In this study, note that the area corresponding to the nevus shows a normal background choroidal fluorescence (*arrows*) because the fluorescein freely diffuses through the extravascular space of the choroid over the nevus. *D,* late phase angiogram showing a relative area of hypofluorescence (*arrows*) because the extravascular diffusion of dye is now in the outer layers of the choroid and the nevus cells occupy this space.

A

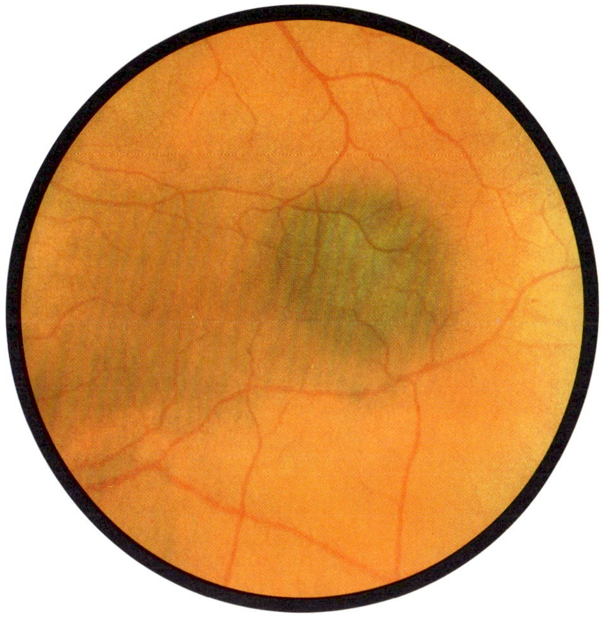

B

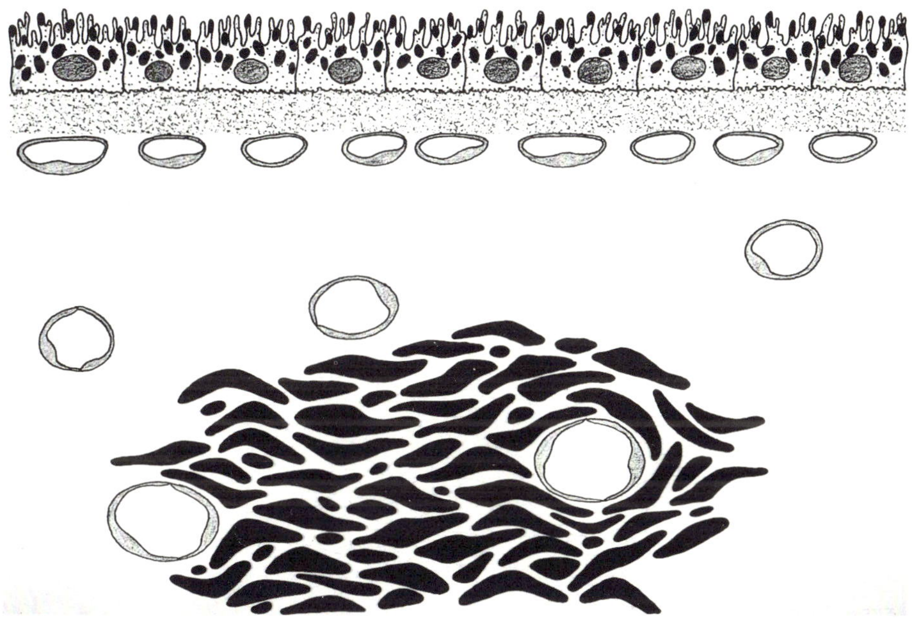

C

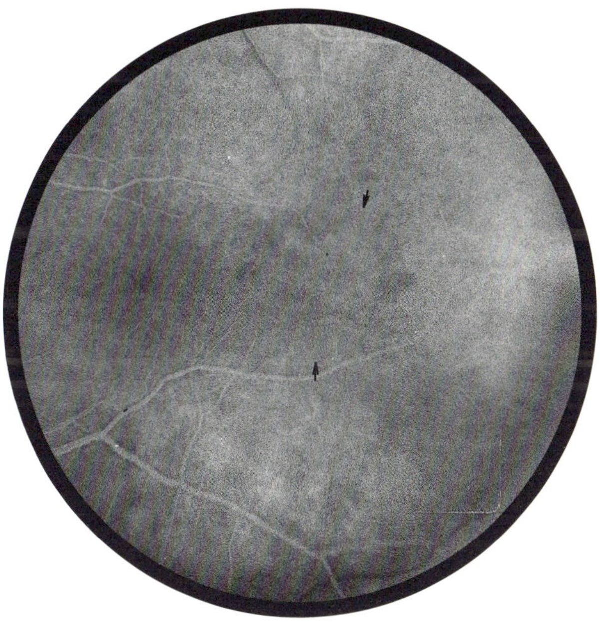

D

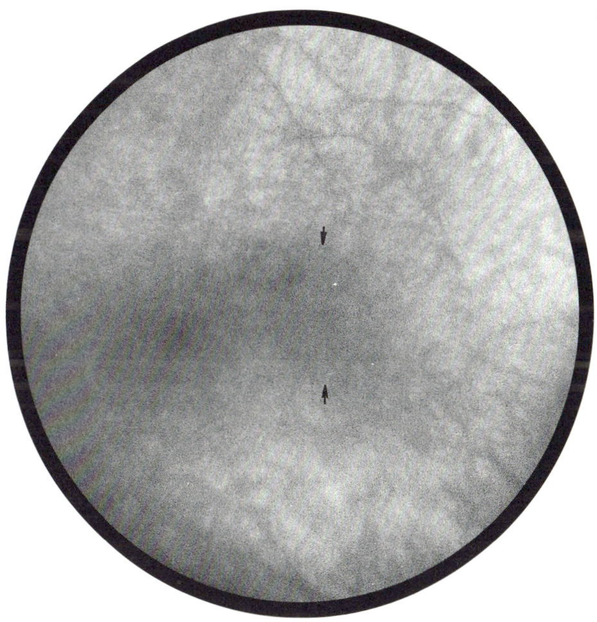

A third fluorescein pattern occurs in those nevi which have overlying drusen (Fig. 25.3). In the early fluorescein sequence, focal hyperfluorescent spots develop which correspond to the drusen seen clinically. During the intra- and extravascular filling phases, the drusen begin to take up fluorescein, and the fluorescent light is transmitted through the overlying thin pigment epithelium (Fig. 25.3*C*). Since the concentration of fluorescein is greater in the area of the drusen than the surrounding Bruch's membrane, these areas retain the fluorescein for a longer period of time. This results in the hyperfluorescence from the drusen persisting into the late phases of the study (Fig. 25.3*D*). The total area corresponding to the nevus shows a relative hypofluorescence throughout the complete study even though the overlying drusen are hyperfluorescent.

When exudative changes develop over a nevus, the fluorescein angiogram will reveal later hyperfluorescence from leakage. In subretinal neovascularization complicating long-standing nevi, the fluorescein angiogram shows the characteristic lacy hyperfluorescence early and leakage of the new vessels (Fig. 25.3, *E* and *F*).

Figure 25.3. *A*, color photo of a choroidal nevus with overlying drusen. *B*, schematic drawing showing nevus cells (*black*) occupying full thickness of choroid with overlying drusen. The drusen cause the overlying pigment epithelium to thin so that when fluorescein diffuses into Bruch's membrane and the drusen, hyperfluorescence occurs due to transmission. *C*, early venous phase angiogram of a nevus with overlying drusen. Note the pinpoint areas of hyperfluorescence (*arrows*) which represent the drusen. These areas fluoresce because of the presence of fluorescein dye and transmission through the overlying thin pigment epithelium. *D*, late phase angiogram showing hyperfluorescence of the larger drusen due to dye retention by the dursen. Note the very subtle surrounding hypofluorescence in the area which the nevus cells occupy. *E*, ophthalmoscopic photograph of subretinal neovascularization overlying a choroidal nevus. Note the pigmented nevus with an overlying exudative detachment of the macula. *F*, venous phase angiogram. Note the lacy hyperfluorescence of the subretinal neovascularization surrounded by a dark zone (*arrows*). Widespread hyperfluorescence overlying the rest of the nevus corresponds to retinal pigment epithelial atrophic changes.

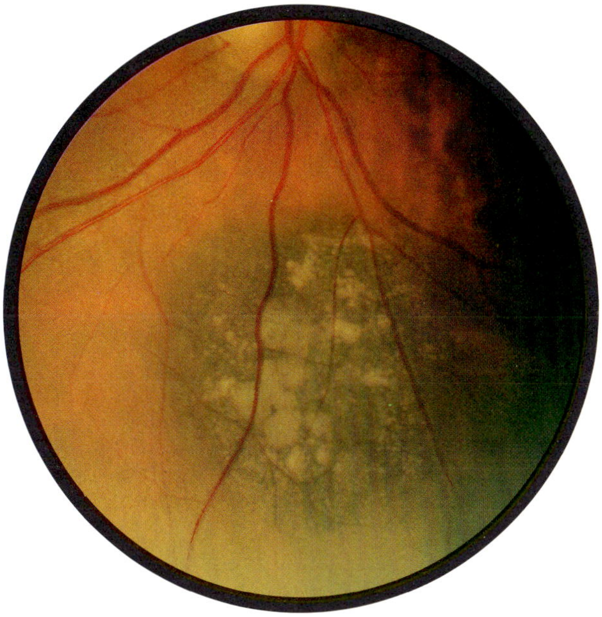

A

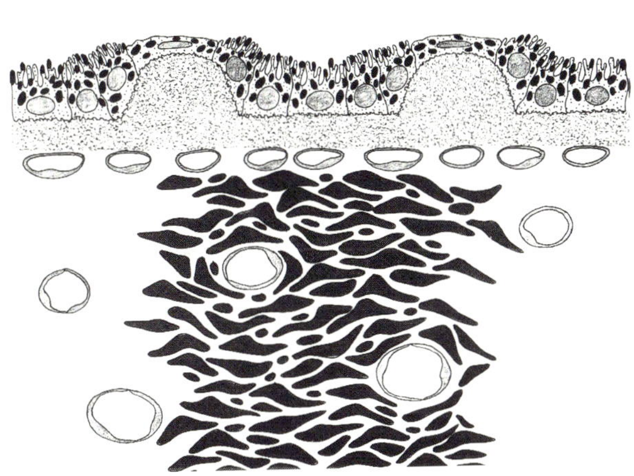

B

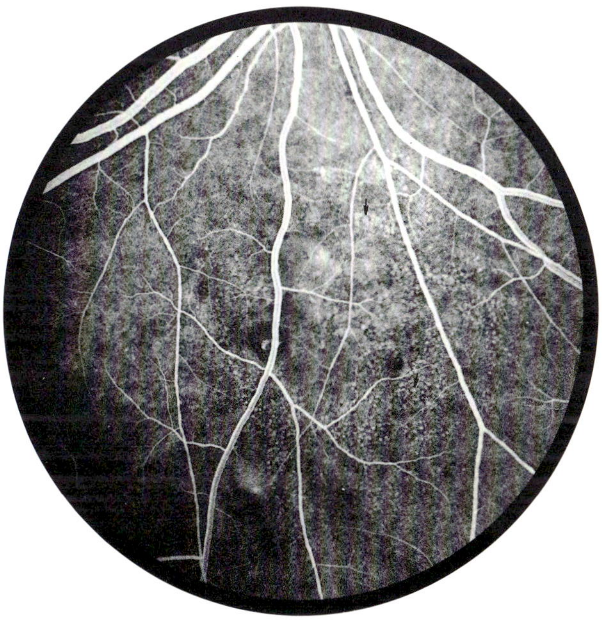

C

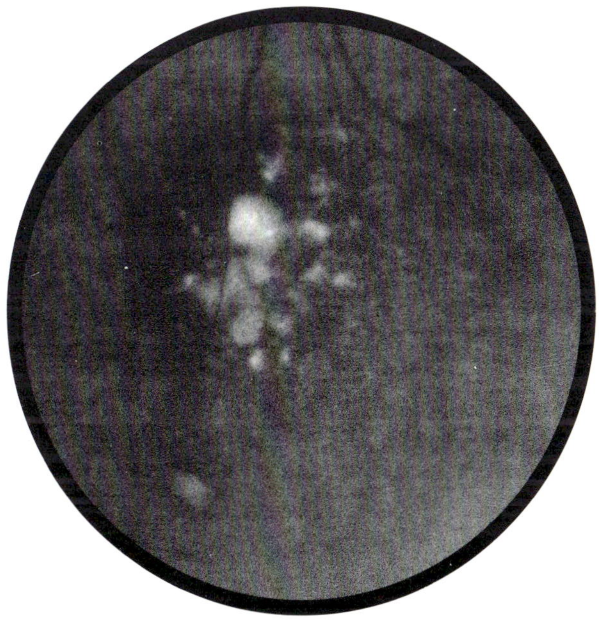

D

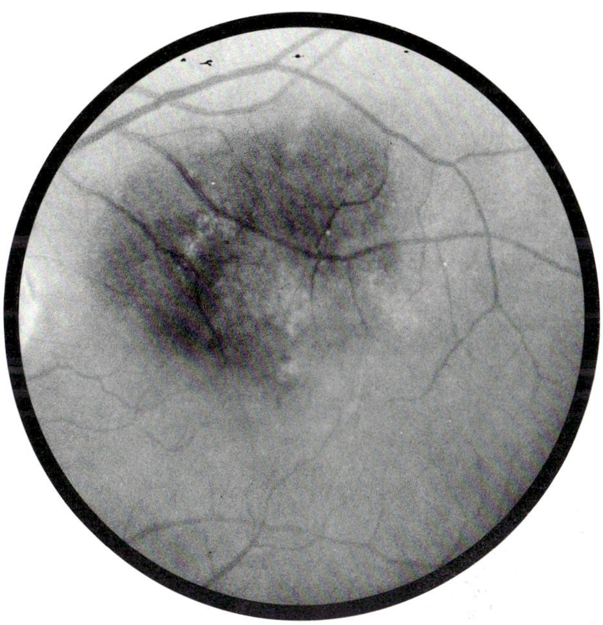

E

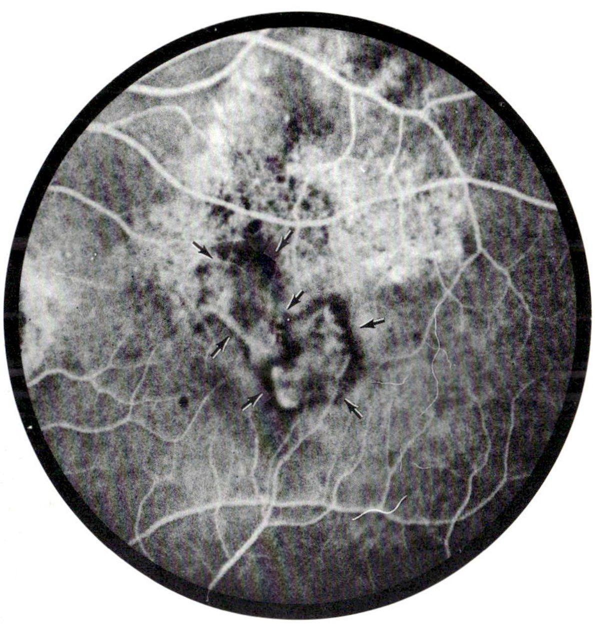

F

MALIGNANT MELANOMAS OF THE CHOROID

Malignant melanomas of the choroid occur infrequently (in 0.02–0.06% of all eyes), most commonly in Caucasians in the fifth to sixth decades of life. It usually grows as a localized globular mass protruding toward the vitreous cavity. Occasionally, it will grow as a diffuse, flat lesion. As the tumor grows it may become associated with widespread changes in the overlying pigment epithelium including: atrophy and degeneration, serous pigment epithelial detachment, sensory retinal detachment, sensory retinal infiltration or erosion, cystoid retinal edema, and occasionally hemorrhage. Metastatic spread of this solid tumor occurs primarily by the intravascular route, although extraocular extension may occur via growth through intrascleral channels. A number of factors affect the overall prognosis including the age of the patient, the size of the tumor (diameter and height), the degree of pigmentation, the state of Bruch's membrane, and the location of the tumor, particularly its anterior border. Histopathologically, these tumors are composed of spindle cells, epitheloid cells, or a combination of the two.

Intraocular melanomas, in general, share several interesting fluorescein angiographic features with metastatic tumors of the choroid and choroidal hemangiomas (Table 25.2). There are subtle differences in the fluorescein angiogram which aid to differentiate these solid tumors, but none is pathognomonic.

The usual solid tumor pattern shows hyperfluorescence throughout the entire study. This hyperfluorescence begins in focal areas scattered diffusely throughout the tumor (Fig. 25.4*A*). These areas of hyperfluorescence may not develop until the venous phase of the retinal circulation. This most likely represents the extravascular filling phase of the choroid and the hyperfluorescence results from the leakage of dye into Bruch's membrane with transmission of the fluorescent light through areas of retinal pigment epithelium degeneration (Fig. 25.4*B*). As the extravascular phase of the choroidal perfusion continues, fluorescein begins to leak through the defective retinal pigment epithelium into the outer retinal layers (Fig. 25.4, *C* and *D*). During this phase of the study, the hyperfluorescence becomes more diffuse. In the later phases of the study, the persistent hyperfluorescence is due to dye at the level of the retinal pigment epithelium, in the subretinal space, and from cystoid spaces in the retina overlying the tumor (Fig. 25.4, *E* and *F*). This represents the usual basic tumor pattern that is seen with ocular melanomas, metastatic tumors, and choroidal hemangiomas.

Several interesting fluorescein features can be seen in addition to this basic tumor pattern. Areas of early hypofluorescence can be seen with ocular melanomas for various reasons (Table 25.3):

Table 25.2. Choroidal tumors in general

Tumor	Fluorescence		
	Early	Mid	Late
Melanomas	Hyper	Hyper	Hyper
Metastases	Hyper	Hyper	Hyper
Hemangiomas	Hyper	Hyper	Hyper

Table 25.3. Causes of hypofluorescence in choroidal melanomas

(1) Tumor mass broken through Bruch's membrane
(2) Normal pigment epithelium
(3) Overlying lipofuscin pigment or hemorrhage

Figure 25.4. *A,* arteriovenous phase angiogram of a typical melanoma. This is the early filling phase showing focal areas of hyperfluorescence. These subtle areas of hyperfluorescence are due to extravascular choroidal filling and transmission through overlying areas of degenerating pigment epithelium. The fluorescein at this point is leaking into Bruch's membrane. *B,* schematic drawing of melanoma showing the same phase seen clinically in (*A*). The *black dots* represent the diffusion of the fluorescein. Note the fluorescein is leaving the choriocapillaris, entering Bruch's membrane, and beginning to diffuse into defective areas of the pigment epithelium. *C,* late venous phase angiogram of retinal circulation, showing an increase in fluorescence. The fluorescein has leaked into Bruch's membrane, the pigment epithelium and is beginning to leak into the subretinal space. *D,* schematic representation showing the events seen clinically in (*C*). Note the greater concentration of fluorescein into Bruch's membrane, the pigment epithelium and diffusion into the subretinal space. *E,* late phase angiogram showing a more diffuse subtle hyperfluorescence after the fluorescein has left the retinal circulation with minimal dye present in the extravascular space of the choroid. The hyperfluorescence is now due to fluorescein in the subretinal space and areas of cystic degeneration within the retina (see *F*). *F,* schematic representation of the events seen clinically in (*E*). Note that the fluorescein is now localized in the subretinal space and in the areas of cystic degeneration in the retina.

A

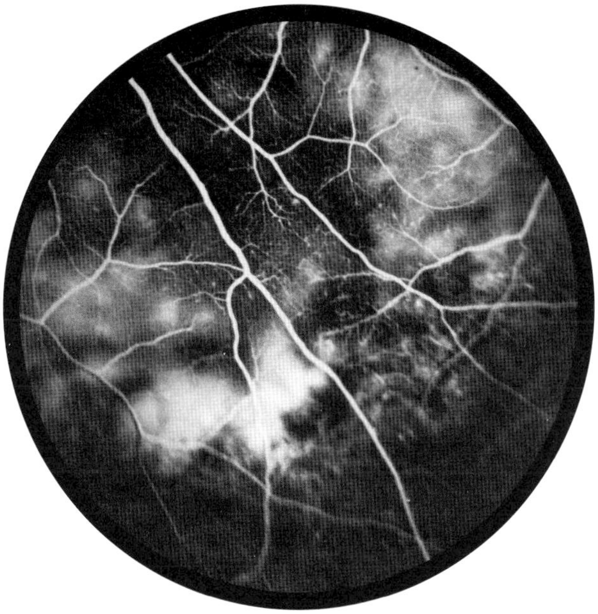

B

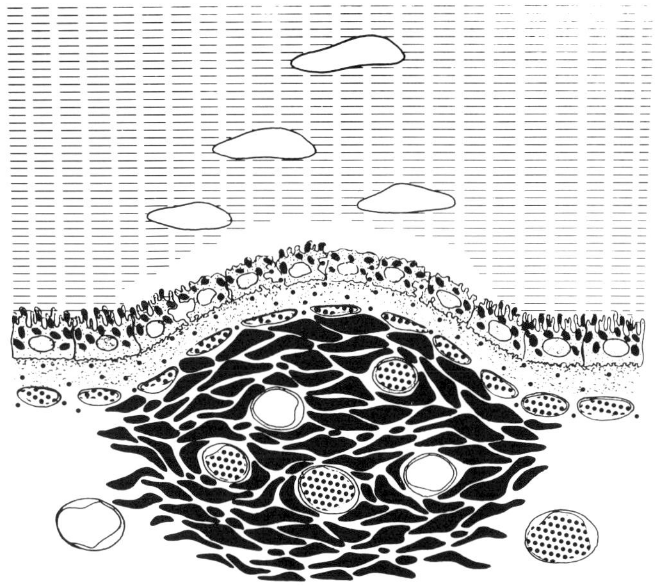

C

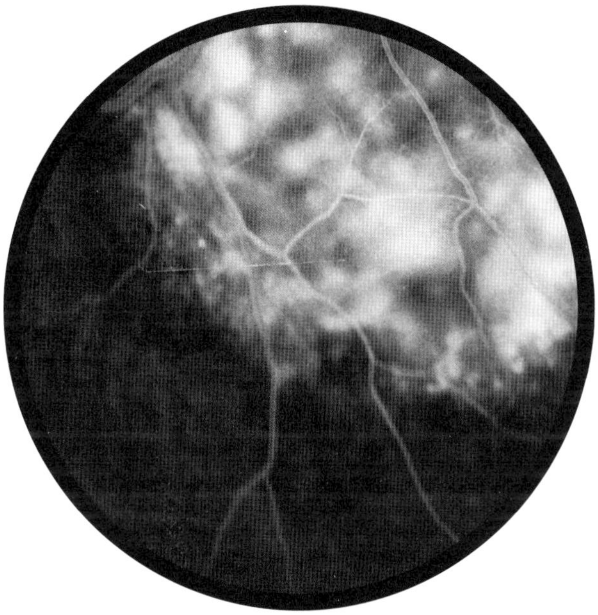

D

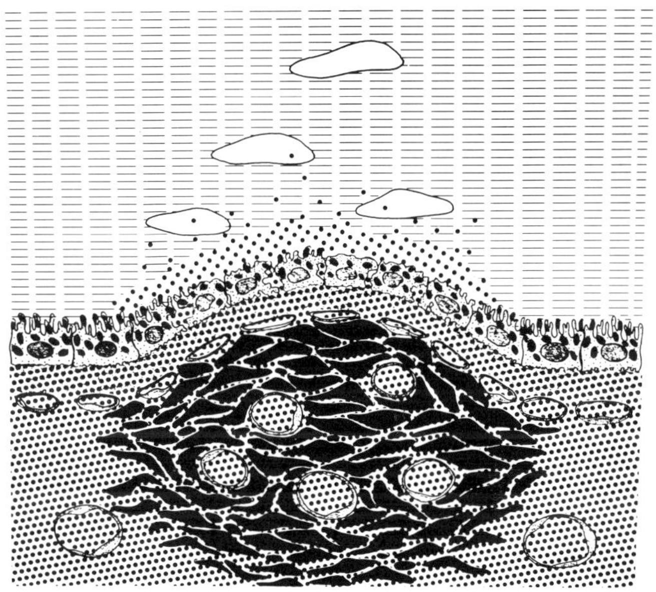

E

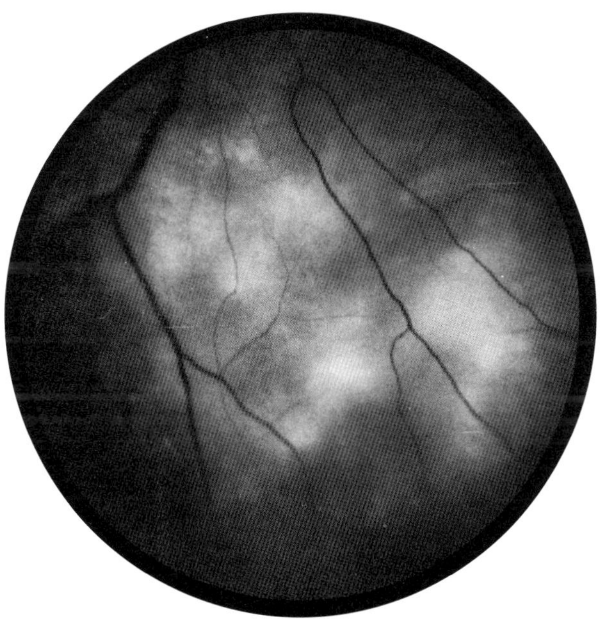

F

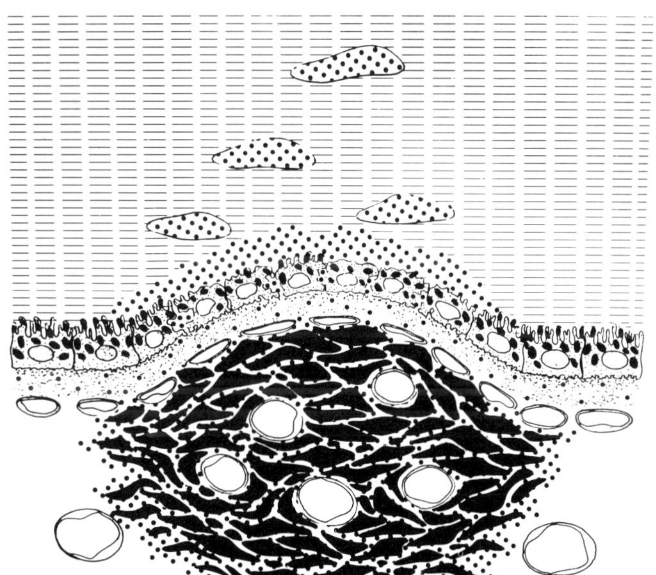

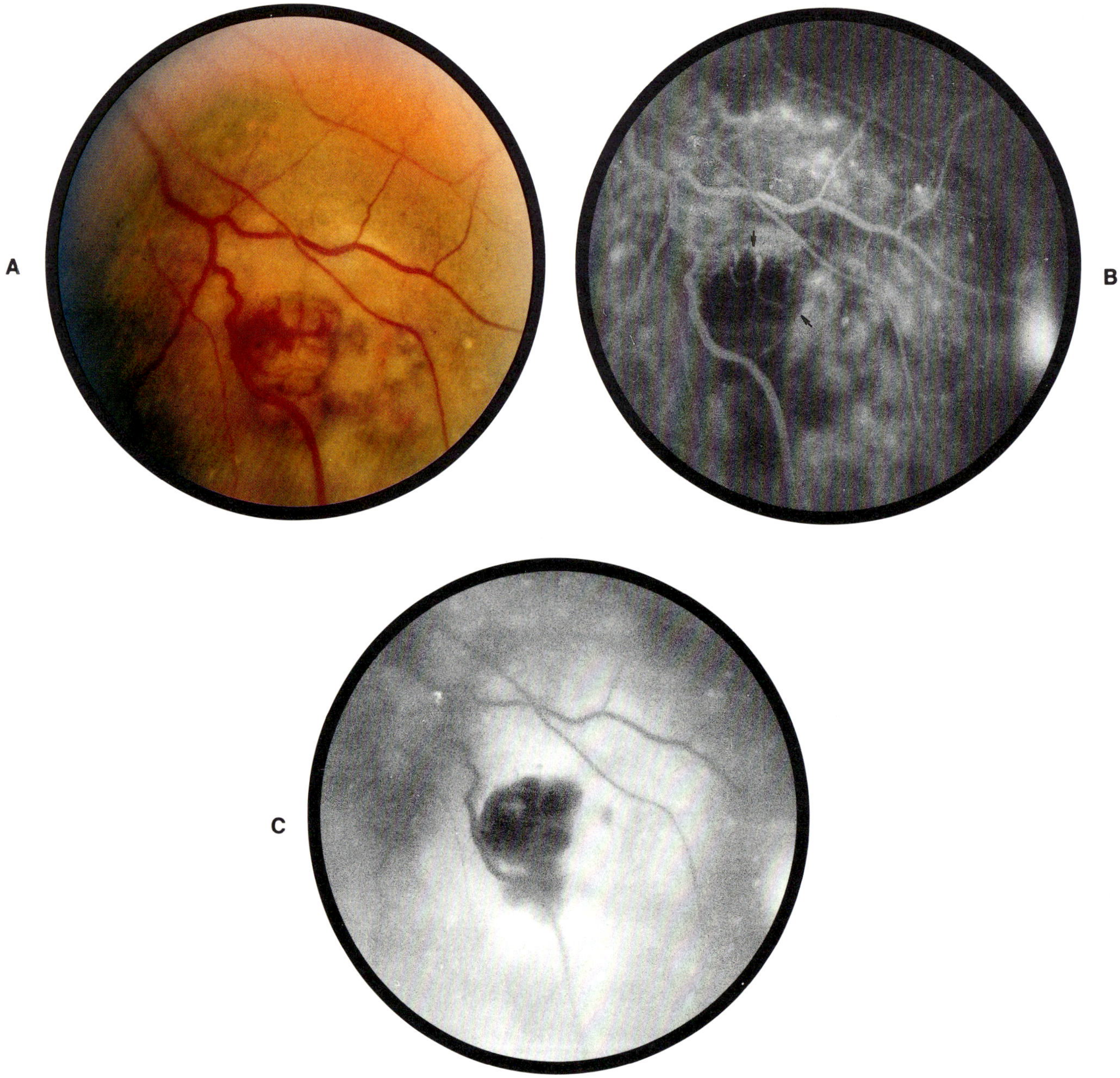

Figure 25.5. *A*, color photo of a large choroidal melanoma with small area which has broken through Bruch's membrane resulting in a collar button (mushroom) appearance. *B*, late venous phase angiogram of melanoma with a collar button (*mushroom*) area. Note the hypofluorescence during this early filling phase of the study (*arrow*). The hypofluorescence is due to a lack of fluorescein within this solid tissue that has broken through Bruch's membrane. One can see the hyperfluorescent retinal vessels coursing over the surface of this area. This solid lesion is also hypofluorescent because it blocks the background fluorescence from the surface of the tumor. *C*, late phase angiogram showing persisting hypofluorescence because the fluorescein has not filled or stained the collar button area of tumor tissue. One can see the late fluorescence over the tumor surrounding this area due to the fluorescein in cystic areas of the retina and subretinal space.

(1) When an area of the tumor breaks through Bruch's membrane, a mushroom-like mass of melanoma cells overhangs Bruch's membrane and the choriocapillaris (Fig. 25.5). This collar button of tumor tissue remains hypofluorescent because there is no overlying choriocapillaris, Bruch's membrane, and pigment epithelium to stain with fluorescein (Fig. 25.5*B*). This protuberance of tumor tissue, therefore, blocks the underlying fluorescence. Any hemorrhage over the collar button will also add to the blockage of the background fluorescence. Blood vessels may persist within the tissue and as they fill, occasionally, they will fluoresce within the hypofluorescent zone.

(2) A small melanoma may have a normal or intact retinal pigment epithelium (Fig. 25.6) which may lead to a relative hypofluorescence or a normal background fluorescence throughout the study (Fig. 25.6*B*). This is because there are no window defects from atrophic RPE to allow transmission of the fluorescent light, and no staining at the level of the RPE. In addition, the mass of tightly packed tumor cells filling the extravascular space of the choroid, most likely does not allow fluorescein leakage into this area.

(3) Another mechanism of the hypofluorescence is due to the accumulation of lipofuscin pigment in macrophages over the surface of the tumor (Fig. 25.7). These macrophages block the underlying fluorescence throughout the angiogram, producing hypofluorescence during the early and late phases of the study (Fig. 25.7 *B* and *C*).

Pin-point hyperfluorescent spots represent another angiographic finding seen with choroidal tumors (Fig. 25.8). These hyperfluorescent spots develop very early in the study during the extravascular filling phase of the choroid (Fig. 25.8, *B* and *C*). They become more prominent as the study progresses, and remain so during the very late phases of the study (Fig. 25.8, *D* through *G*). Occasionally, these spots will enlarge and become blurred. These most likely represent cystic areas of degeneration within the retinal pigment epithelium (Fig. 25.8 *C*, *E*, and *G*). The ones that change and blur in the late phases of the study most likely represent leakage of fluorescein into the subretinal space and outer retinal tissues. During the early phases, as the cystic spaces fill with fluorescein, they are seen as hyperfluorescent spots (Fig. 25.8, *B* through *E*). In the late phases, because they retain the dye longer than other areas, they remain hyperfluorescent (Fig. 25.8, *F* and *G*).

Another fluorescein pattern found with choroidal melanomas has been referred to as a double circulation. In our experience, this finding is rare. Occasionally, when there is a large mushroom-shaped tumor, which has broken through Bruch's membrane, the large vessels coursing near the surface of this tumor may be seen with fluorescein in addition to the overlying retinal vasculature, thus, resulting in a double circulation type of pattern (Fig. 25.9).

A

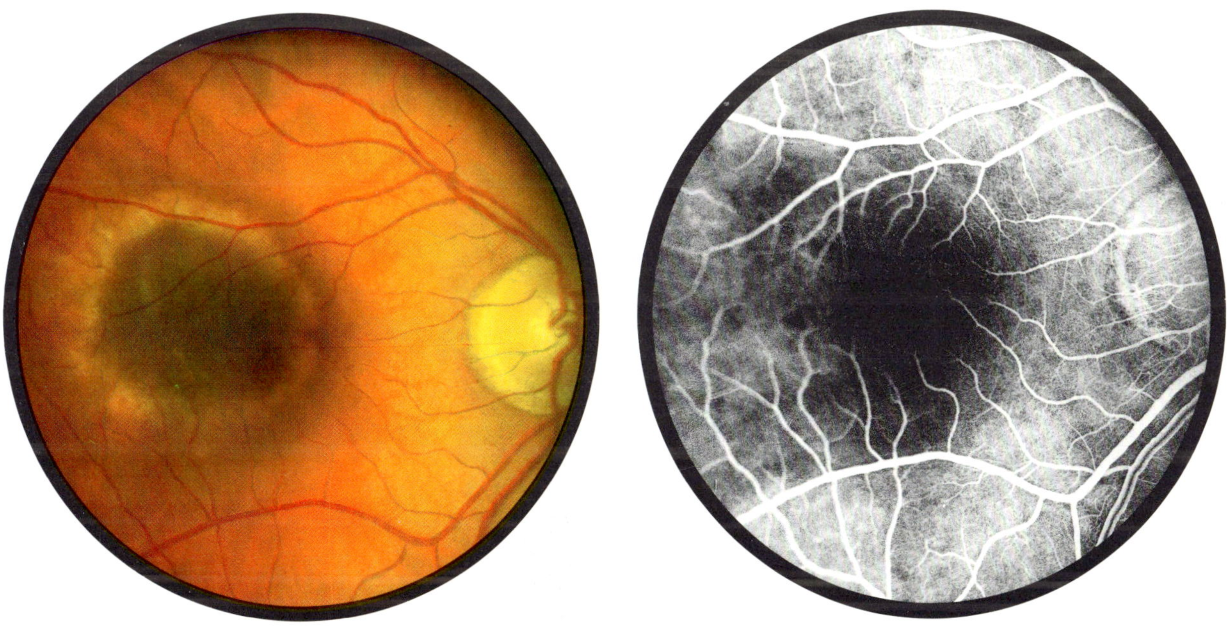

B

Figure 25.6. *A*, color photo of a small melanoma which has not caused defects to occur in the overlying retinal pigment epithelium. *B*, arteriovenous phase angiogram of a small melanoma in the macula that does not show hyperfluorescence. The normal background choroidal fluorescence overlying this lesion is seen. This is explained by the fact that the pigment epithelium overlying the tumor is normal. There has been no cellular breakdown and thus no transmission of the background fluorescence.

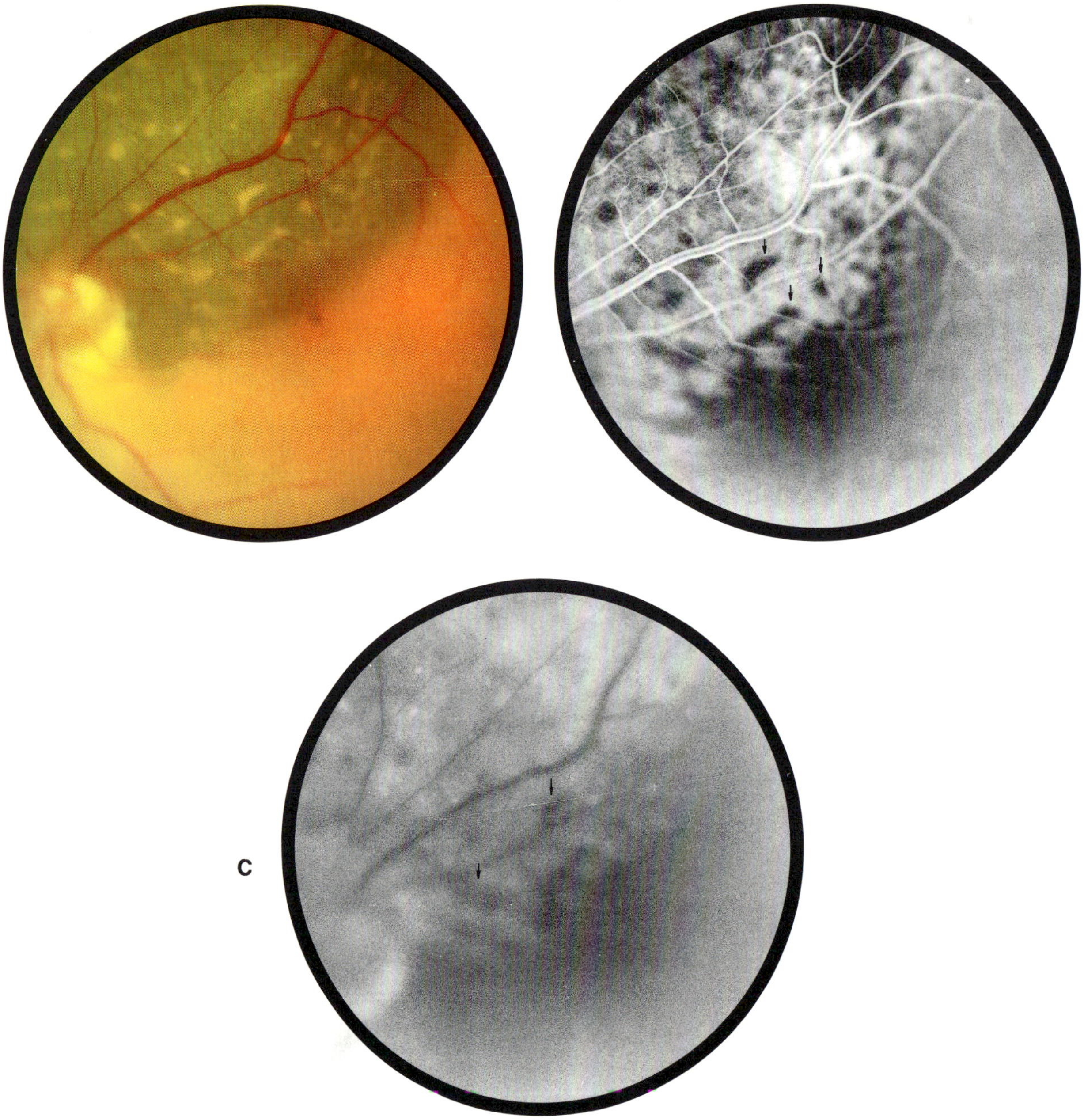

A B C

Figure 25.7. *A*, color photo of a choroidal melanoma with clumps of orange-colored pigment on the surface. *B*, arteriovenous phase angiogram of a melanoma with overlying orange pigment. Note the areas of orange pigment are hypofluorescent during this early filling phase of the study (*arrows*) (see Color Plate 6). *C*, late phase angiogram showing that the areas of orange pigment remain hypofluorescent throughout the study (*arrows*).

Figure 25.8. *A*, color photo of a choroidal melanoma which, when studied with fluorescein angiography, reveals pinpoint hyperfluorescent spots, most likely due to microcystic degeneration of the retinal pigment epithelium. *B*, arteriovenous phase angiogram of a melanoma during the early phase showing the development of pinpoint hyperfluorescent spots (*arrows*). *C*, schematic representation of (*A*) showing the fluorescein leaking from the choriocapillaris into Bruch's membrane and beginning to fill the microcystic areas of degeneration in the retinal pigment epithelium. *D*, venous phase angiogram during the midphases of the study showing the increase in hyperfluorescence of these pinpoint areas (*arrows*). *E*, schematic representation of (*C*) showing an increase in the amount of fluorescein filling the microcystic areas and fluorescein beginning to leak from these areas into the subretinal space. *F*, late phase angiogram showing persistence of the pinpoint hyperfluorescent areas with a more diffuse hyperfluorescence over the melanoma. *G*, schematic representation of (*F*) showing fluorescein persisting in the areas of microcystic degeneration of the retinal pigment epithelium with fluorescein in the subretinal space and areas of cystic degeneration within the retina itself.

A

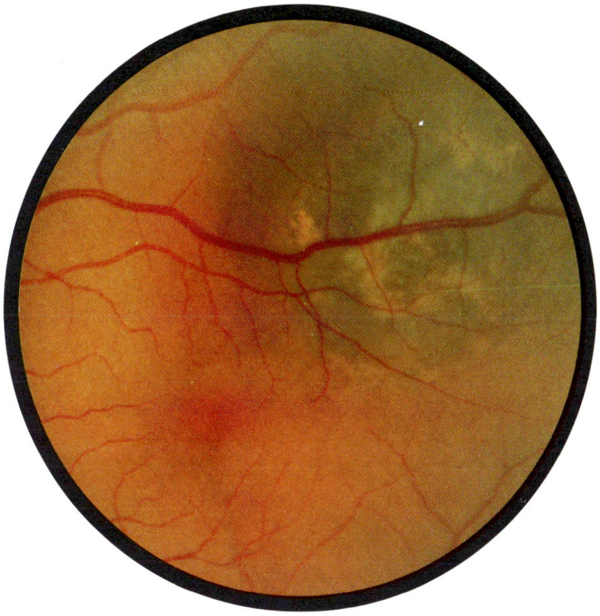

B

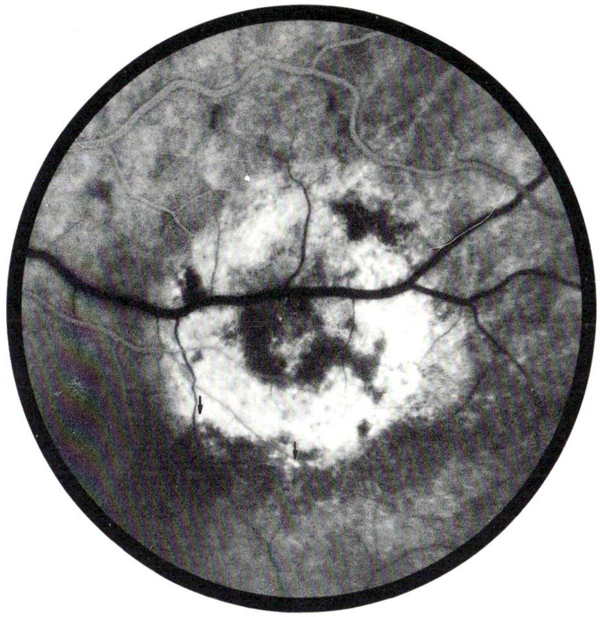

C

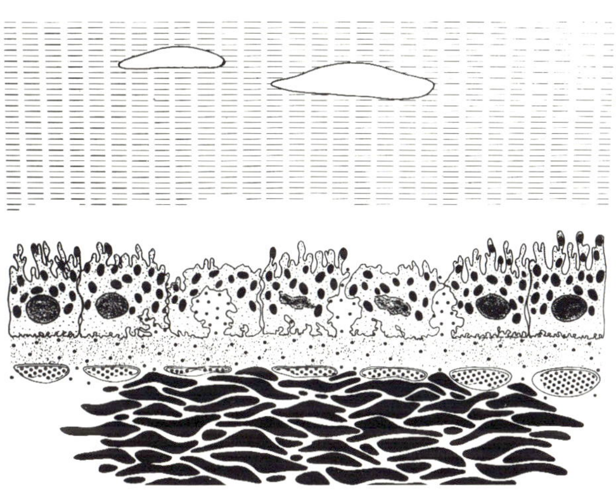

D

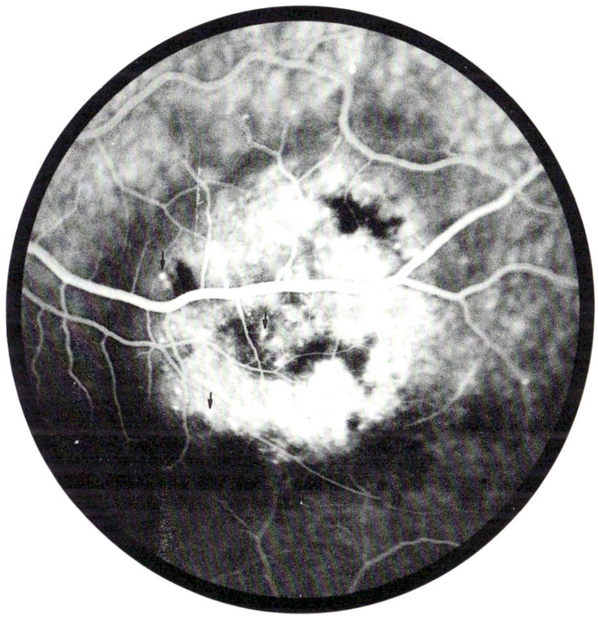

E

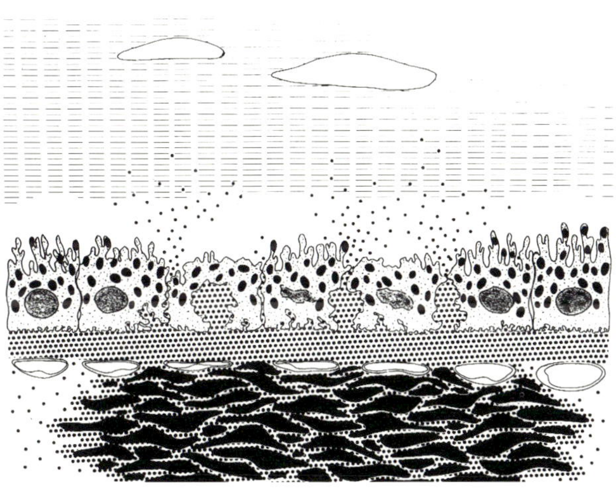

F

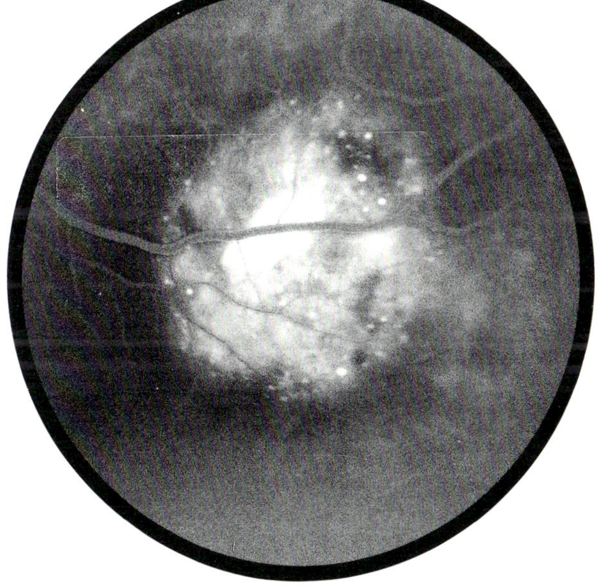

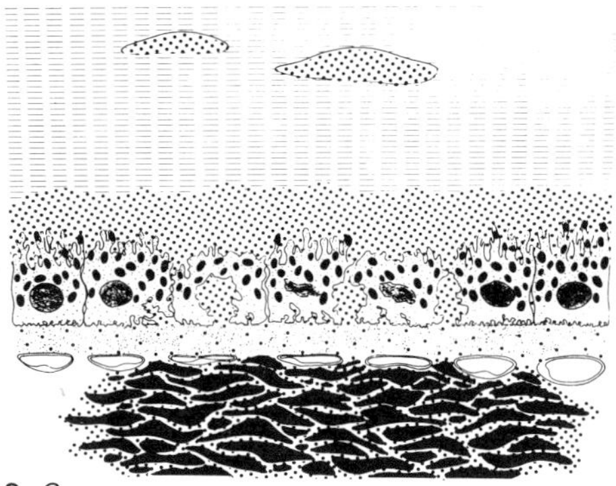

Figure 25.8. *G.*

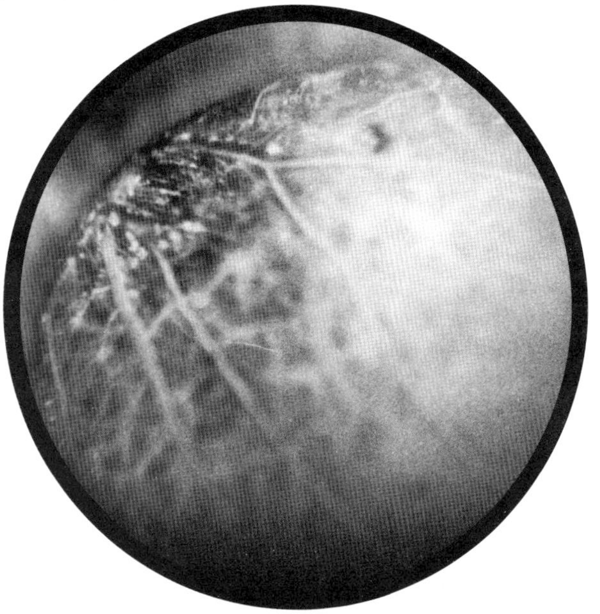

Figure 25.9. Venous phase angiogram of an area of mushrooming over a melanoma showing a double circulation. Note the fluorescein within the retinal circulation plus the fluorescein in the large vessels within the tumor beneath the retina.

METASTATIC TUMORS OF THE CHOROID

Metastatic tumors of the choroid are probably more common than generally realized. They most frequently occur as multicentric choroidal tumors. When seen as a solitary mass, they may resemble other primary tumors of the choroid. They generally appear as flat or slightly elevated amelanotic lesions with poorly discernible margins. Scattered clumps of pigment are often seen throughout the lesion. When they assume a globular growth pattern, their clinical appearance may be indistinguishable from an amelanotic melanoma. Overlying retinal pigment epithelial degenerative changes, bands of pigmentation, sensory retinal detachment, cystic degeneration, and subretinal hemorrhage may accompany these lesions. While they are most commonly found in the posterior pole where they are likely to affect the vision, peripheral lesions are frequently overlooked in the terminally ill patient. The primary sites of pathology are most frequently the breasts and lung. Occasionally the kidney, testicle, prostate, and the GI tract as well as the thyroid will also metastasize to the choroid, with an overall bilateral involvement in approximately 25%.

Metastatic tumors to the choroid may produce fluorescein patterns similar to choroidal melanomas (Figs. 25.10, *A* and *B*). Areas of clumped pigmentation or pigment within macrophages, will cause blockage of the background and surrounding choroidal fluorescence and, thus, result in corresponding areas of focal hypofluorescence. Pin-point hyperfluorescent spots can be seen over metastatic tumors, and are most likely due to microcystic degeneration of the pigment epithelium as with melanomas and hemangiomas. Late hyperfluorescence may be due to leakage through defective areas of the pigment epithelium with staining of the subretinal fluid or cystic degeneration within the retina (Fig. 25.10, *A* and *B*). In general, these tumors fluoresce in the early phases of the study, and remain hyperfluorescent throughout the entire study for the same reasons as other choroidal tumors.

A

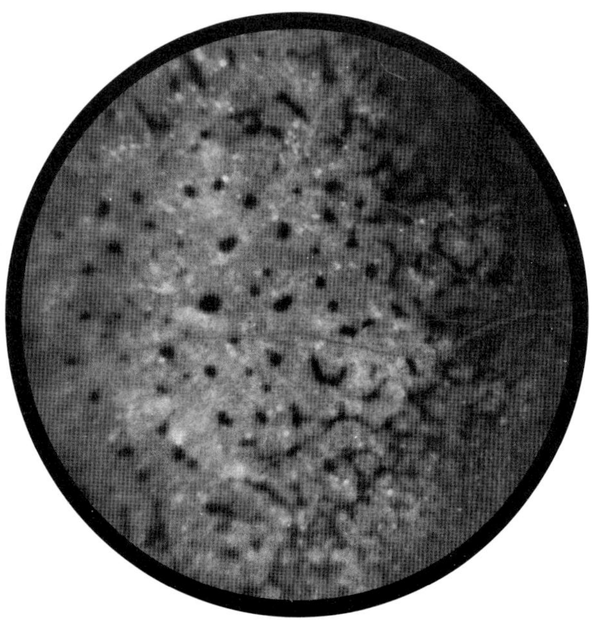

B

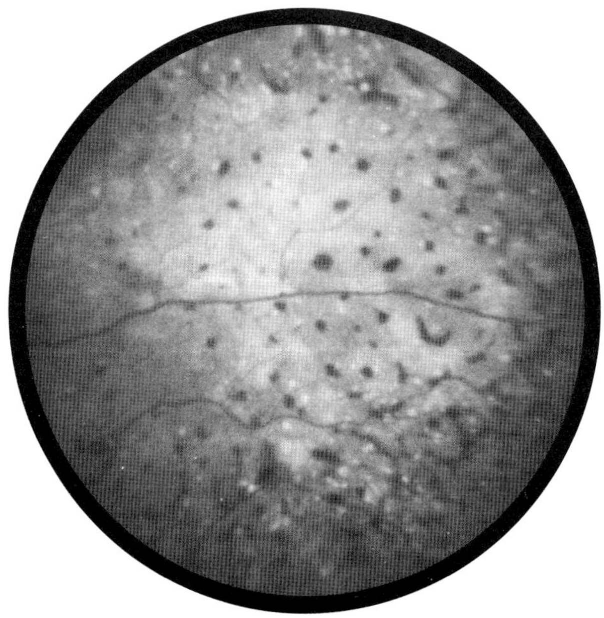

Figure 25.10. *A*, arteriovenous phase angiogram and *B*, late phase angiogram of a metastatic choroidal tumor showing the diffuse hyperfluorescence due to cystic degeneration of the overlying retina and degenerative changes in the pigment epithelium which both stain with fluorescein. Note the focal areas of hypofluorescence due to pigment clumping over the surface of the tumor which blocks the surrounding and background fluorescence.

A B
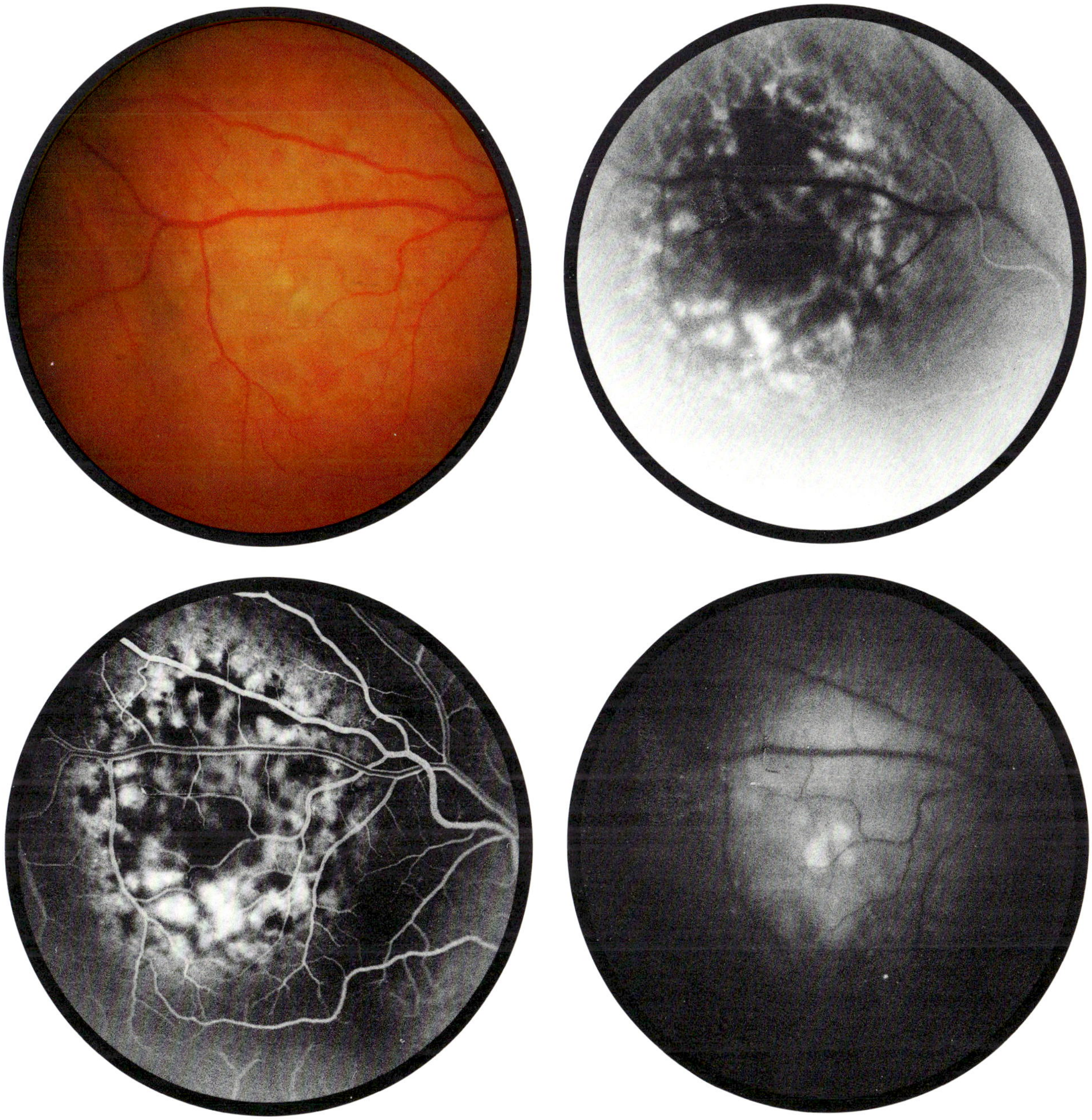
C D

Figure 25.11. *A*, color photo on choroidal hemangioma. *B*, arterial phase angiogram of a choroidal hemangioma. Note the focal areas of hyperfluorescence due to the filling of the large vascular channels within the tumor. This is also due to transmission defects through overlying degenerating pigment epithelium. *C*, arteriovenous phase angiogram showing a more diffuse hyperfluorescence due to transmission through the pigment epithelium and a greater concentration of fluorescein within the vascular channels of the tumor itself. *D*, late phase angiogram of the same lesion, showing hyperfluorescence due to fluorescein within the subretinal tissue and within areas of cystic degeneration of the overlying retina.

CHOROIDAL HEMANGIOMAS

Choroidal hemangiomas are considered hamartomatous lesions and are usually not clinically detectable until the second or third decades of life. The lesions appear typically as round or oval, slightly elevated, pink tumors, with poorly discernible margins. They vary in size from 2 to several disc diameters, usually occurring in the temporal retina or adjacent to the disc. They usually exhibit a slow growth potential in early life and by young adulthood they become associated with atrophic changes in the pigment epithelium, cystoid degeneration of the sensory retina, and sensory retinal detachments. About 25% are diffuse throughout the choroid, and are frequently associated with facial hemangioma (Sturge-Weber disease). Histopathologically they are composed of thin-walled cavernous vascular spaces containing practically no connective tissue stroma.

Choroidal hemangiomas may show all the fluorescein patterns that have previously been discussed for melanomas and metastatic lesions (Fig. 25.11). These vascular tumors of the choroid usually begin to show irregular areas of hyperfluorescence corresponding to the large vessels within the tumor. This occurs earlier during the filling phases of the fluorescein study than with the more solid cellular tumors previously discussed. As the fluorescein leaks into the extravascular space within the tumor, these tumors become markedly hyperfluorescent (Fig. 25.11, *B* and *C*). In addition to the pin-point hyperfluorescent spots that develop during the extravascular phase, fluorescein begins to leak through defective areas of the retinal pigment epithelium to stain the subretinal space and cystic areas of degeneration within the retina (Fig. 25.11*C*). In the very late phases of the study, the hyperfluorescence is partially due to the extravascular fluorescence in the tumor, but more importantly, most probably from fluorescein within the cystoid spaces in the retina overlying the tumor (Fig. 25.11*D*).

Lesions of the Retinal Pigment Epithelium

The lesions affecting the RPE which will be discussed in this section are: (1) congenital hypertrophy of the RPE, (2) reactive hyperplasia of the RPE, (3) hemorrhagic detachment of the RPE, and (4) combined hamartoma of the RPE and retina. In general, these hyperpigmented lesions show hypofluorescence early, due to a relative blockage of the background choroidal fluorescence. Most of the pigmented lesions continue to remain hypofluorescent in the late phases of the study; however, occasionally, some lesions will begin to fluoresce during the mid-phases, and show hyperfluorescence late, due to the presence of dye in the lesion (Table 25.4).

Table 25.4. RPE lesions

Lesion	Fluorescence		
	Early	Mid	Late
Congenital hypertrophy	Hypo	Hypo	Hypo
Reactive hyperplasia	Hypo	Hypo	Hypo
Hemorrhagic detachment	Hypo	Hypo	Hypo
Combined hamartoma	Hypo	Hypo	Hyper

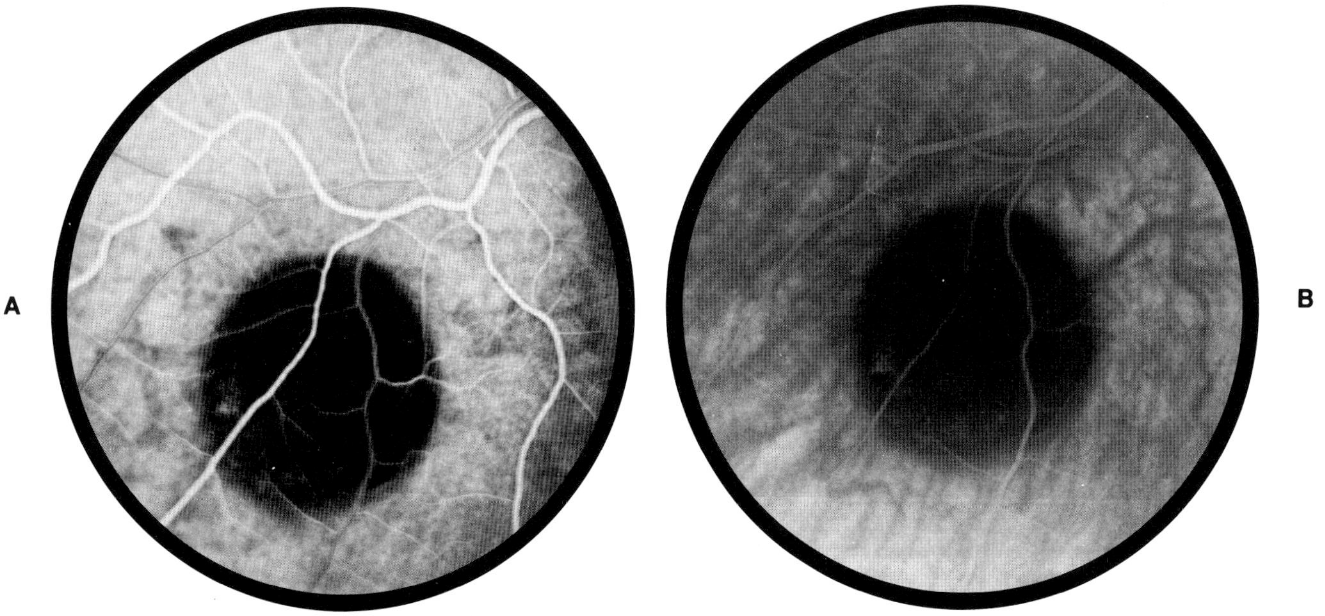

Figure 25.12. *A*, arteriovenous phase angiogram of an area of hypertrophy of the retinal pigment epithelium showing hypofluorescence due to blockage of the background choroidal fluorescence by the pigment. *B*, late phase angiogram showing persistent hypofluorescence due to blockage of the background choroidal fluorescence. During this phase of the study, the fluorescein in the choroid is in the outer layers of the extravascular space.

HYPERTROPHY OF THE RETINAL PIGMENT EPITHELIUM

Hypertrophy of the retinal pigment epithelium is a flat benign heavily pigmented lesion that varies in size from 1 to several disc diameters and may be found anywhere in the fundus. The sharp margins may often be associated with a ring or halo. Patchy areas of hypopigmentation may also occur within the central portion of the lesion. Often, more than one may be seen in an eye and they may occur bilaterally. Rarely, a slight growth potential may be seen. Histopathologically, these lesions represent hypertrophy of the pigment epithelium with large pigment epithelial cells containing round dark pigment granules.

Angiographically, congenital hypertrophy of the RPE shows a marked degree of hypofluorescence during both early and late phases of the study (Fig. 25.12, *A* and *B*). This hypofluorescence is due to blockage of the background choroidal fluorescence by the enlarged, deeply pigmented RPE cells. They may have islands of depigmentation within the lesion which show relative hyperfluorescence due to transmission of the choroidal fluorescence through these areas of defective pigment (Fig. 25.12, *A* and *B*). In addition, there may be a halo of hyperfluorescence due to transmission through the surrounding depigmented rim (Fig. 25.12 *A* and *B*).

REACTIVE HYPERPLASIA

Reactive hyperplasia of the RPE occurs secondary to trauma or inflammation, detachment, or as a phenomenon of aging. These clinically dark hyperplastic areas are hypofluorescent throughout the entire angiographic study (Fig. 25.13, *A* and *B*). This hypofluorescence is due to blockage of the background choroidal fluorescence. Often, there will be an adjacent nonpigmented area that will appear hyperfluorescent because of the transmission of fluorescent light throughout the study (Fig. 25.13, *A* and *B*). Glial tissue is often associated with this lesion and may show some late hyperfluorescence due to the accumulation of fluorescein.

A

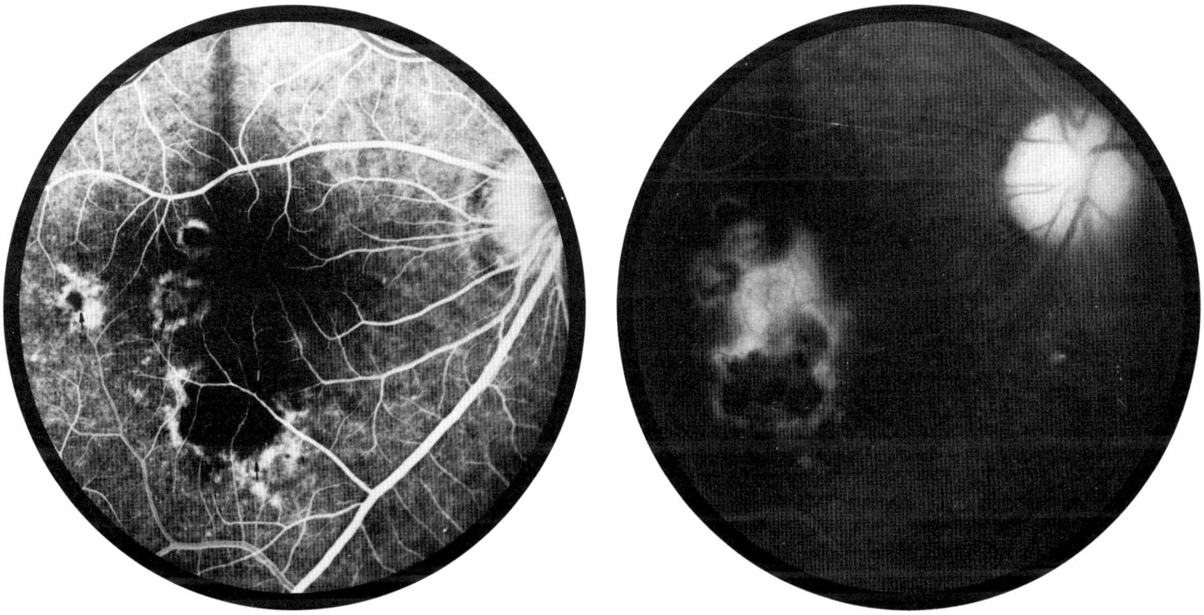

B

Figure 25.13. *A*, arteriovenous phase angiogram of an area of reactive hyperplasia of the pigment epithelium showing hypofluorescence (*arrows*) due to blockage by the hyperpigmented areas with surrounding hyperfluorescence due to transmission through areas of thinned retinal pigment epithelium. *B*, late phase angiogram with persistent hyperfluorescence due to staining at the level of Bruch's membrane and transmission through the thinned pigment epithelium surrounding the areas of hypofluorescence where the pigment is more dense.

HEMORRHAGIC DETACHMENT

Hemorrhagic detachment of the RPE may be associated with tumor, inflammation, trauma, or subretinal neovascularization. The induced hemorrhagic tumefaction may resemble primary or secondary tumors of the choroid. On fluorescein angiography, an area of hypofluorescence is seen corresponding to the sub-RPE hemorrhage. The concentrated hemoglobin pigment produces an area of hypofluorescence which persists throughout the entire phase of the angiographic study (Fig. 25.14, *A* and *B*). This hypofluorescence is due to blockage of background choroidal fluorescence by the increased accumulation of blood pigment.

COMBINED HAMARTOMA OF RETINAL PIGMENT EPITHELIUM AND RETINA

The combined hamartoma of the RPE and retina represents a proliferation of RPE cells along with glial and vascular elements of the retina (Fig. 25.15). It is associated with a vitreoretinal interface disturbance and retinal folds. While most commonly found adjacent to the disc, it may also occur in the macula or mid-periphery. During the early phases of the fluorescein study, there is a relative hypofluorescence because the solid tissue hamartoma blocks the background choroidal fluorescence in the area that corresponds to the lesion seen clinically (Fig. 25.15*B*). With the filling of the retinal circulation, hyperfluorescent spots are seen as the capillaries within the lesion begin to fill (Fig. 25.15*C*). These hyperfluorescent areas gradually become more intense, due to continued leakage of dye from these capillaries into the adjacent surrounding tissue (Fig. 25.15 *D* and *E*). Thus, the early hyperfluorescent lesion gradually becomes hyperfluorescent as the study progresses.

A

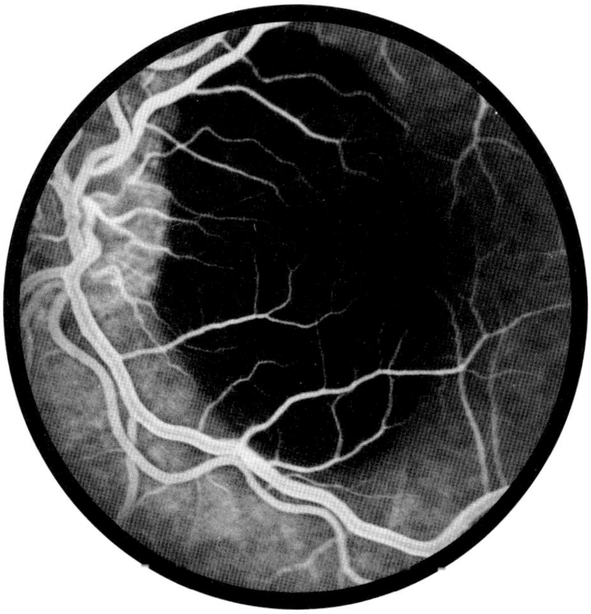

B

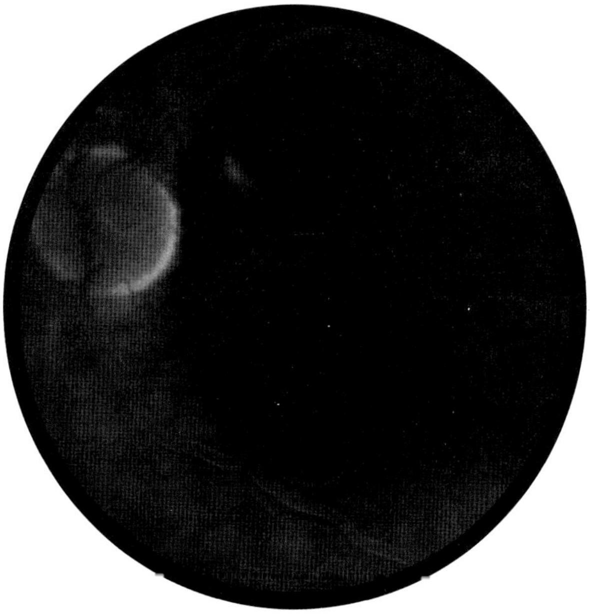

Figure 25.14. *A*, early venous phase angiogram on a patient with subpigment epithelial hemorrhage. Note the large area of marked hypofluorescence due to blockage of the background choroidal fluorescence by the hemorrhage under the retinal pigment epithelium. *B*, late phase angiogram of the same lesion showing persistent hypofluorescence due to blockage.

Figure 25.15. *A*, color photo of a combined hamartoma of the retina and retinal pigment epithelium. *B*, arterial phase angiogram of a combined hamartoma of the retinal pigment epithelium and retina. Very early filling phase showing diffuse hypofluorescence of the lesion except in a few areas where the retinal capillaries fill. *C*, arteriovenous phase angiogram showing a persistent area of hypofluorescence from pigment epithelial proliferation within the central portion of the lesion. There is a subtle hyperfluorescence due to filling of the abnormal capillaries within the lesion itself. There is a deeper hyperfluorescence around the nasal, superior, and inferior portions of the disc due to fluorescence at the level of the retinal pigment epithelium and/or transmission. *D*, late venous phase angiogram showing leakage from the abnormal capillaries within the retina and a more diffuse staining of the underlying retinal pigment epithelium. *E*, late phase angiogram showing persistence of fluorescein within the retinal tissue due to leakage from the capillary system resulting in hyperfluorescence.

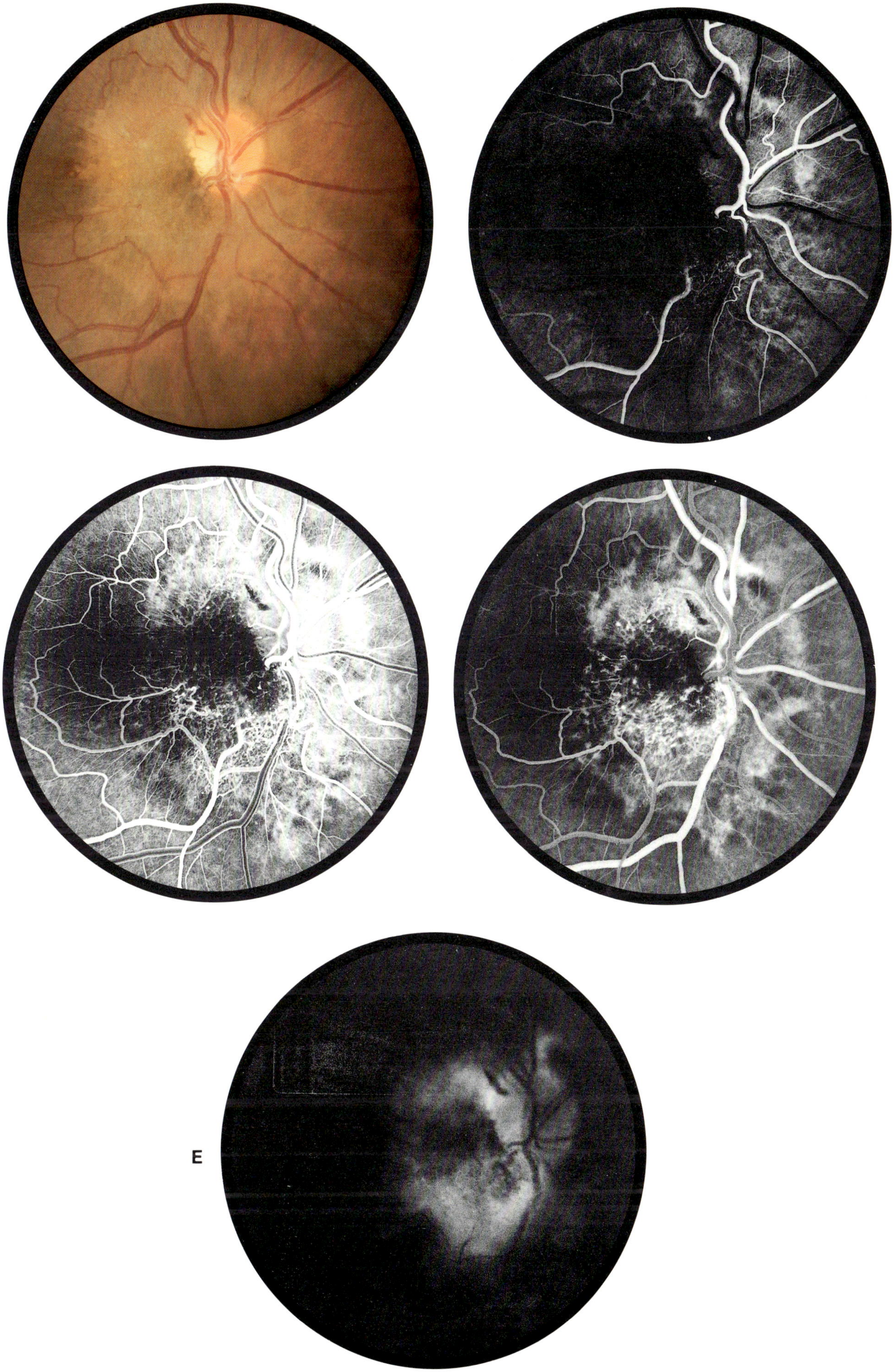
A
B
C
D
E

Tumors of the Retina and Optic Disc

There are essentially six different entities mentioned in this discussion of tumors of the retina and disc: (1) capillary hemangioma, (2) cavernous hemangioma, (3) racemose angioma, (4) astrocytoma, (5) retinoblastoma, and (6) melanocytoma. In general, the tumors involving the optic nerve and retina are hyperfluorescent from the early phases of the study into the late phases (Table 25.5). The melanocytoma, however, is the exception and is hypofluorescent.

CAPILLARY HEMANGIOMA

The capillary hemangioma or angiomatosis retinae (von Hippel's disease) is a hamartoma that may involve the optic nerve and/or retina. These tumors have a dominant hereditary pattern and become clinically apparent in young adulthood. Fifty percent occur bilaterally. When associated with similar lesions of the central nervous system, the syndrome is referred to as von Hippel-Lindau disease. Tumors away from the disc are usually associated with one or more feeding arterioles and draining venules. Lipid exudation in the macula and retinal detachment are possible accompanying manifestions. At the disc the tumor may occur as diffuse (endophytic) or encapsulated (exophytic) juxtapapillary lesions. They appear as reddish-orange tumors of variable size at the disc or in the retina. Intraretinal and subretinal lipid exudation may extend into the macula particularly in the diffuse variety. Histopathologically, these angiograms represent dilated and hyperplastic capillaries with an intravascular network of reticulum. They may originate from the superficial (endophytic) or deep (exophytic) retinal circulation.

With fluorescein angiography these tumors begin to show hyperfluorescence during the arterial filling phase of the retinal circulation (Fig. 25.16*A*). Very shortly the tumor fills with dye, as the fluorescence becomes more intense and outlines the full extent of the tumor and its efferent vessels (Fig. 25.16*B*). Figure 25.16 is an example of a diffuse capillary hemangioma of the retina, and Figure 25.17 is one at the disc. The diffuse peripheral capillary hemangioma shows hyperfluorescence throughout the entire study, but also shows massive leakage of fluorescein into the vitreous cavity during the mid and late phases. The diffuse lesion at the disc begins to fluoresce early and continues to fluoresce in the very late phase of the study with massive leakage into the vitreous cavity. Figures 25.18 and 25.19 are examples of encapsulated tumors. The peripheral encapsulated capillary hemangioma also shows hyperfluorescence throughout all phases of the study, but does not leak into the vitreous cavity late. The encapsulated capillary hemangioma involving the optic nerve shows hyperfluorescence early, and continues to fluoresce in the late phases, but does not leak into the vitreous cavity. Another type of capillary hemangioma is the free-floating diffuse angioma which has been pulled presumably by contracting vitreous from the retinal surface and is suspended in the vitreous cavity (Fig. 25.20).

A

B

C

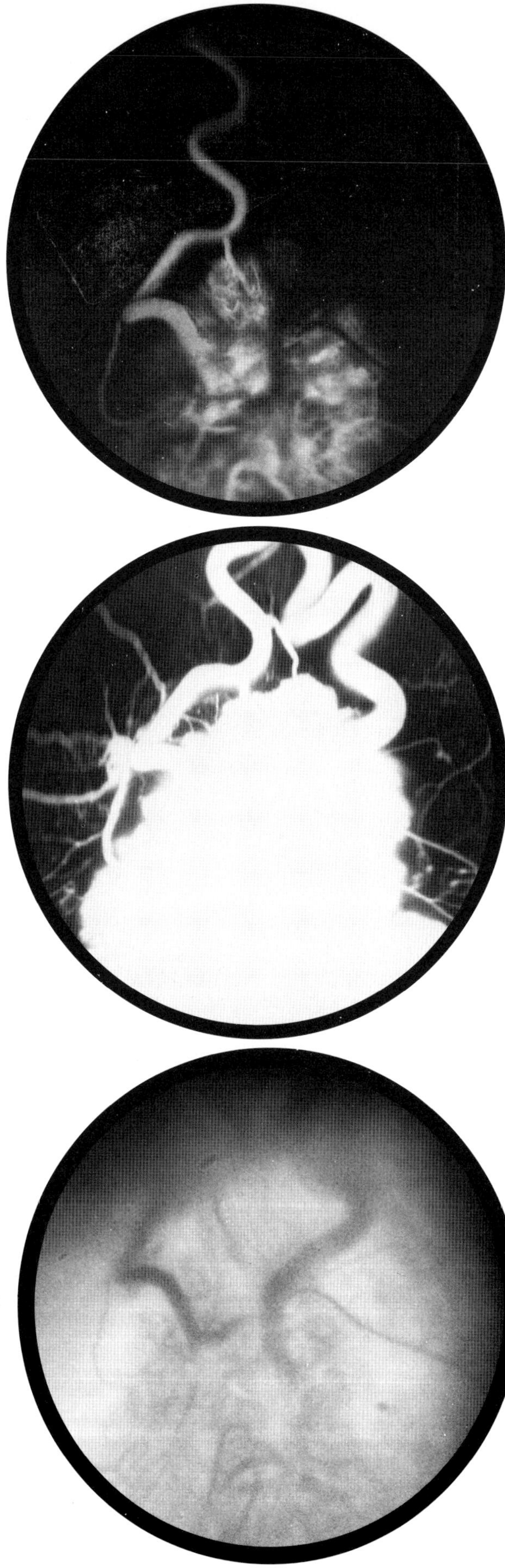

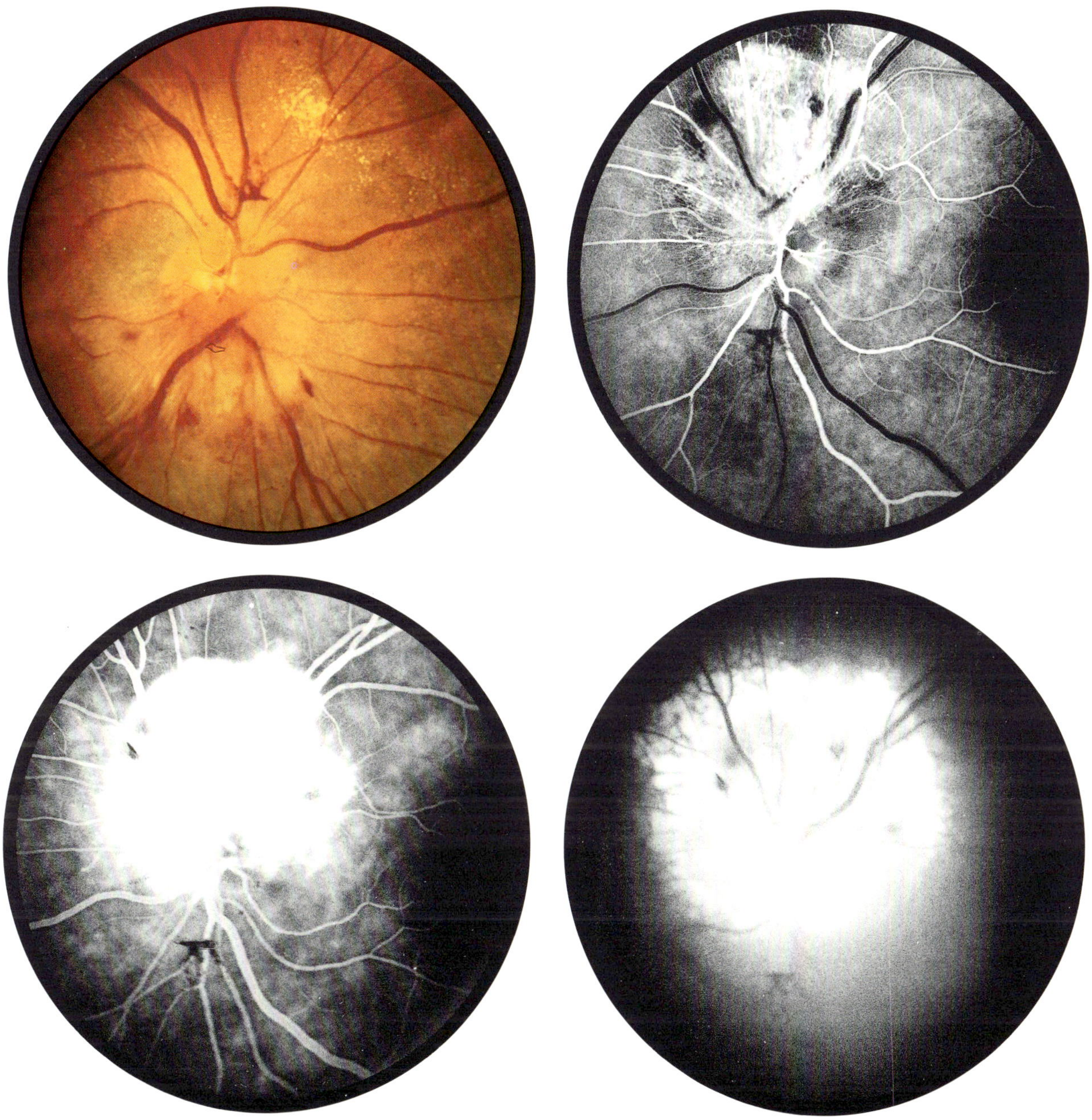

A C

B D

Figure 25.17. *A*, color photo of a juxtapapillary angioma involving the disc, with fluorescein leaks, is classified as a diffuse type. *B*, arteriovenous phase angiogram of a diffuse type of juxtapapillary angioma during the early filling phases, showing the filling of the capillary system. *C*, venous phase angiogram of the same lesion shows a greater hyperfluorescence due to complete filling of the capillary system with leakage into the surrounding tissue. *D*, late phase angiogram showing a persistent hyperfluorescence due to fluorescein within the lesion itself and the fluorescein has leaked into the vitreous cavity overlying and surrounding the lesion.

Figure 25.16. *A*, arterial phase angiogram of the afferent vessel filling a large retinal angioma in a patient with angiomatosis retinae. This is a peripheral diffuse (unencapsulated) lesion. *B*, slightly later in the study showing the efferent vessel with a more hyperfluorescent angioma due to the complete filling. *C*, late phase angiogram showing little fluorescein in the large afferent and efferent vessels with marked leakage, resulting in fluorescence of the vitreous cavity itself.

Table 25.5. Retina and disc lesions

Lesion	Fluorescence		
	Early	Mid	Late
Capillary Hemangioma	Hyper	Hyper	Hyper
Cavernous Hemangioma	Hyper	Hyper	Hyper
Racemose Angioma	Hyper	Hyper	Hyper
Astrocytoma	Hypo	Hyper	Hyper
Retinoblastoma	Hyper	Hyper	Hyper
Melanocytoma	Hypo	Hypo	Hypo

A

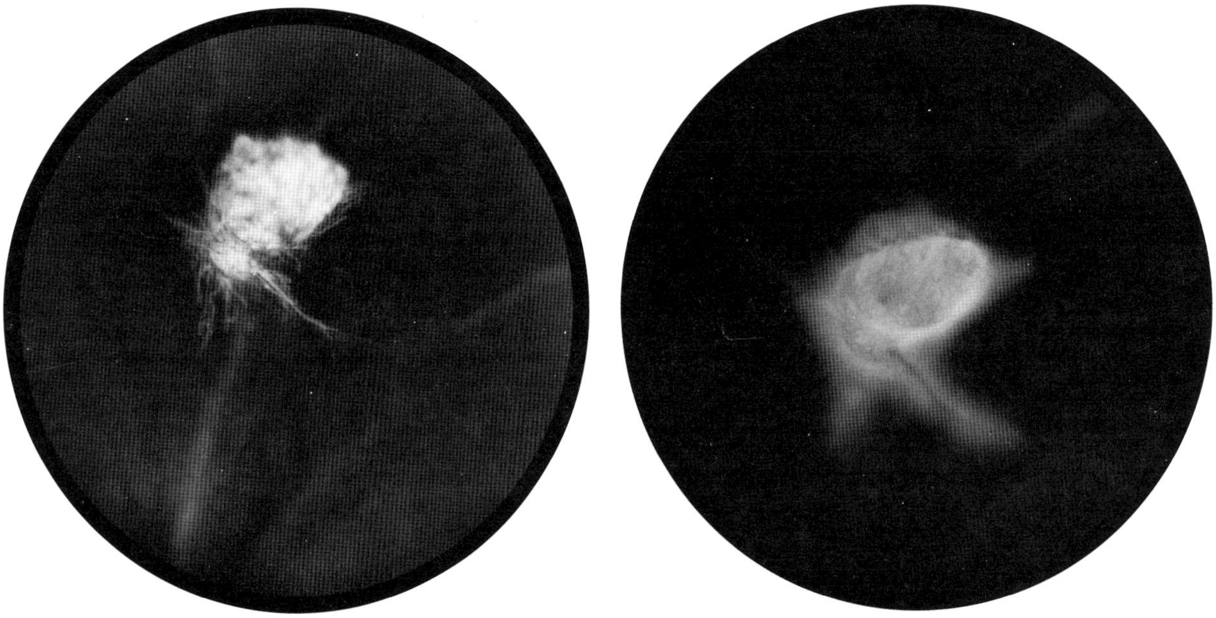

B

Figure 25.18. *A*, the clinical fluorescein angiographic appearance of a free-floating angioma within the vitreous cavity during the early phases showing the afferent feeding vessels and the lesion itself filling with fluorescein. *B*, late phase angiogram showing complete filling of the tumor and leakage into the vitreous and surrounding area.

A

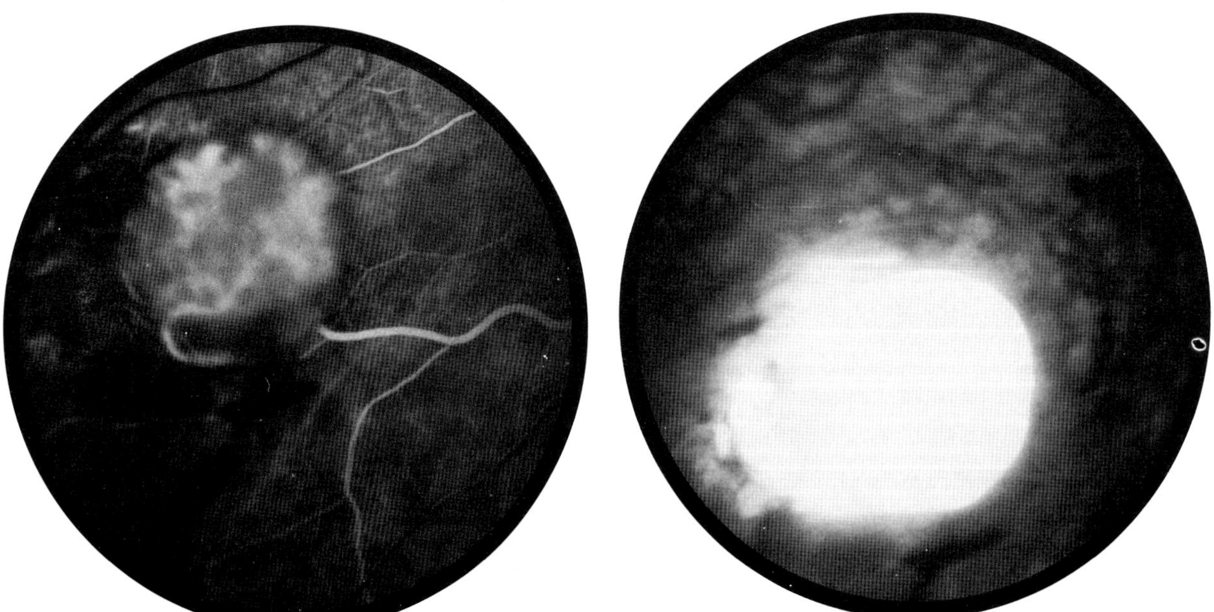

B

Figure 25.19. *A*, arterial phase angiogram of a peripheral encapsulated type of angioma showing the hyperfluorescence of the lesion itself due to capillaries filling with dye. *B*, late phase angiogram showing a persistent hyperfluorescence due to fluorescein retained within the lesion, but there appears to be little if any leakage from the lesion itself.

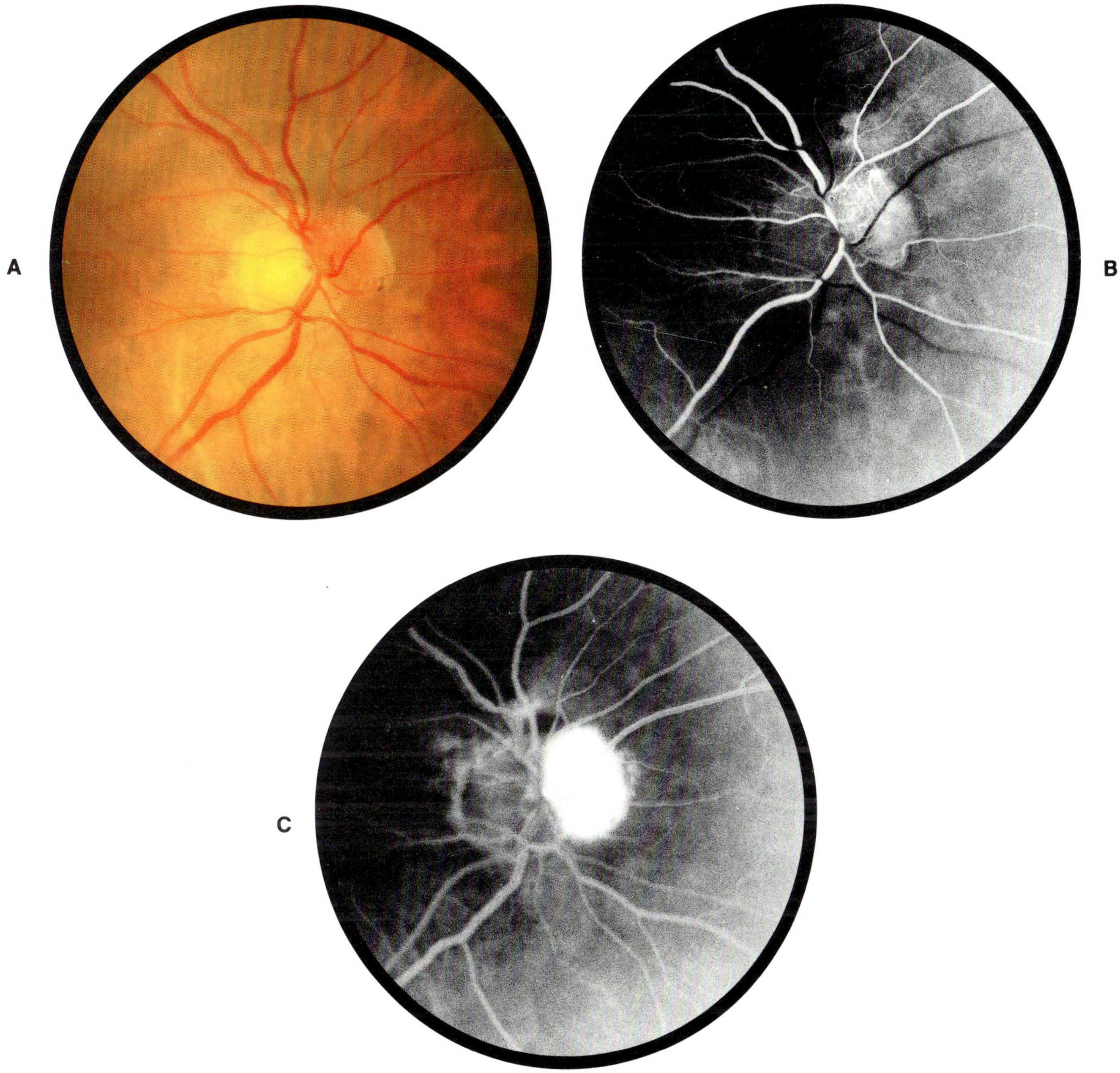

Figure 25.20. *A*, color photo of a juxtapapillary angioma at the disc, which when studied with fluorescein does not leak and is classified as an encapsulated type. *B*, arterial phase angiogram of an encapsulated juxtapapillary angioma showing diffuse filling of the capillary system within the angioma (see Fig. 25.11 *A*). *C*, late phase angiogram showing a greater hyperfluorescence due to persistence of dye within the capillary system with essentially no leakage into the vitreous or surrounding tissue.

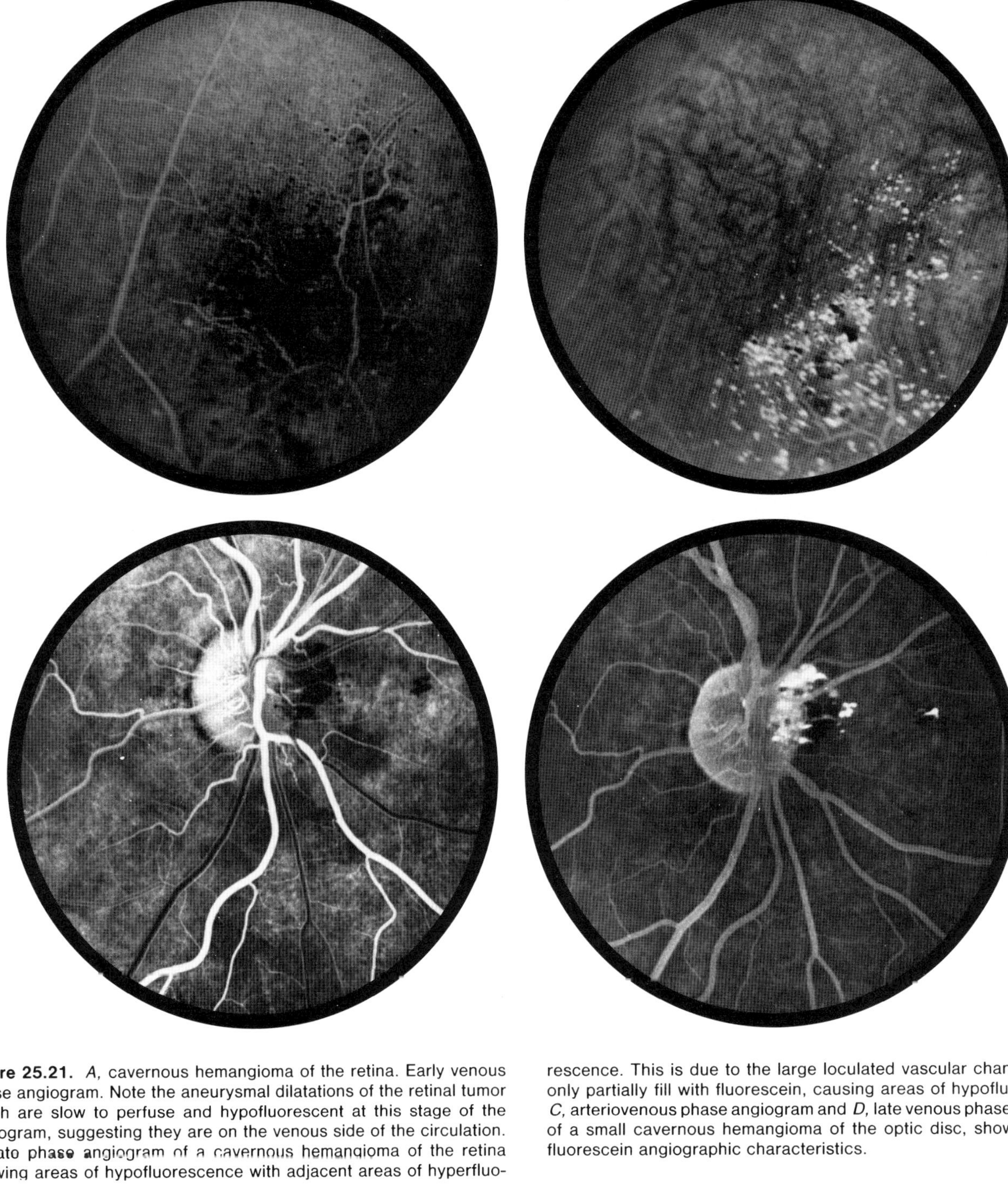

Figure 25.21. *A,* cavernous hemangioma of the retina. Early venous phase angiogram. Note the aneurysmal dilatations of the retinal tumor which are slow to perfuse and hypofluorescent at this stage of the angiogram, suggesting they are on the venous side of the circulation. *B,* late phase angiogram of a cavernous hemangioma of the retina showing areas of hypofluorescence with adjacent areas of hyperfluorescence. This is due to the large loculated vascular channels which only partially fill with fluorescein, causing areas of hypofluorescence. *C,* arteriovenous phase angiogram and *D,* late venous phase angiogram of a small cavernous hemangioma of the optic disc, showing similar fluorescein angiographic characteristics.

CAVERNOUS HEMANGIOMAS

Cavernous hemangiomas of the retina and optic nerve are rare tumors that appear as dark grape-like projections from the surface of the retina. They vary in size from a few vascular clusters to larger lesions with multiple aneurysmally dilated vascular tumefactions. Intraretinal and subretinal exudation are not associated with this lesion although occasionally vitreous hemorrhage can occur. There is a familial tendency, and these lesions may occur in association with intracranial and cutaneous hemangiomas. Growth potential is negligible in these tumors. Histopathologically, they represent clusters of thin-walled dilated blood vessels that replace the normal architecture of the inner portion of the retina or optic nerve head.

The fluorescein angiogram indicates that these aneurysmal dilatations are usually off the mainstream of flow and, therefore, do not begin to fluoresce immediately, suggesting a venous origin (Fig. 25.21*A*). They gradually fill and retain the dye for long periods and, thus, are fluorescent in the very late phases of the study when the fluorescein is not seen elsewhere in the fundus (Fig. 25.21, *B* through *D*).

RACEMOSE ANGIOMA

The racemose angioma is a retinal tumor which consists of a congenital retinal arteriovenous malformation limited to either the whole or one portion of the retina. These vascular malformations have a familial tendency and they are usually unilateral. The involved vessels are dilated, tortuous, and more numerous than in the normal eye. Visual function is usually normal, and spontaneous hemorrhages rarely occur. When these arteriovenous anomalies are associated with brain lesions, they are referred to as part of the Wyburn-Mason syndrome.

With fluorescein, the arteriovenous shunts are clearly outlined by the very rapid transit of dye, but there is no leakage into the surrounding retina (Fig. 25.22).

A

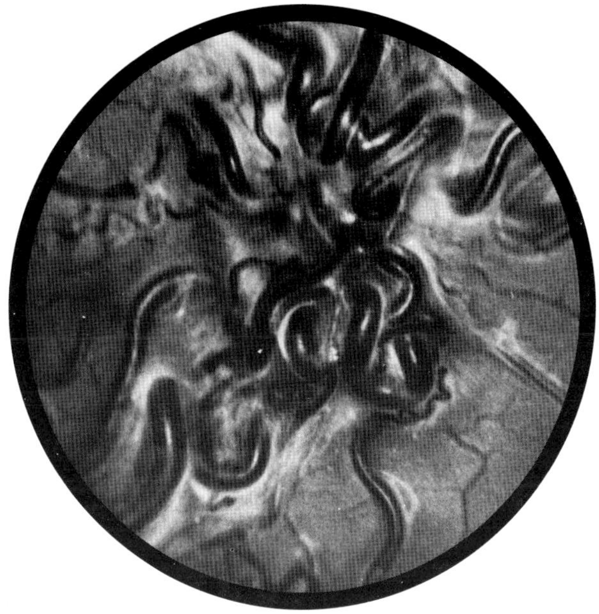

B

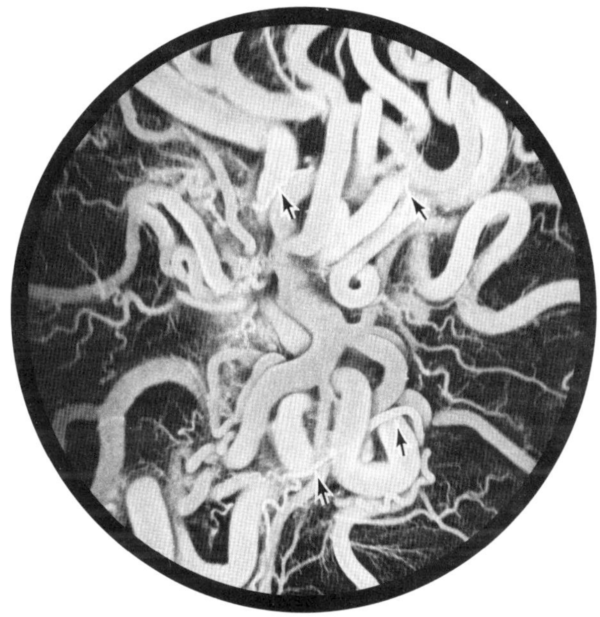

C

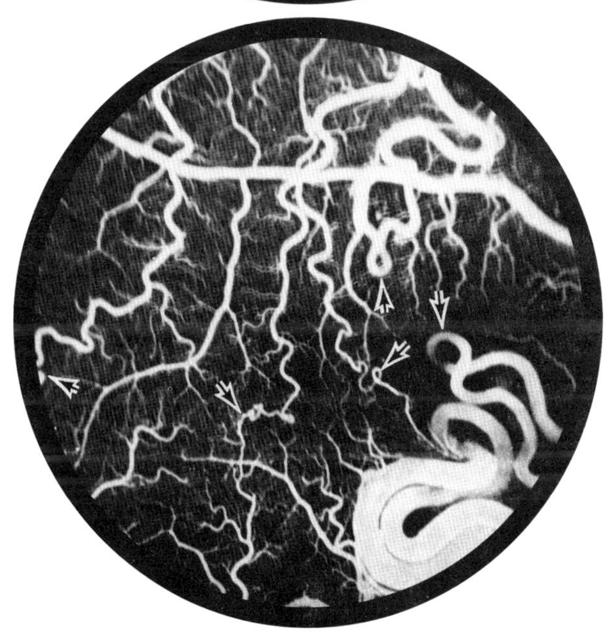

Figure 25.22. Racemose angioma. *A*, ophthalmoscopic photograph. Note the dilated retinal artery and veins originating at the optic nerve. *B*, late venous phase angiogram. This represents large dilated hiflow shunts and smaller recirculating arteriovenous shunts (*arrows*). *C*, same patient, more peripheral retina. Note the variably sized multiple arteriovenous shunts (*arrows*).

ASTROCYTIC HAMARTOMAS

Astrocytic hamartomas are retinal lesions typically seen in patients who have tuberous sclerosis. The tumors occur in the retina or at the disc and appear as whitish, spherical, elevated lesions with well delineated margins and occasional mulberry appearance. They are frequently multiple, are highly vascularized, usually with an extremely negligible growth potential. Histopathologically, these tumors are composed of astrocytes. They also contain sclerotic nodules that show considerable overgrowth of glial cells as well as immature embryonic cells and calcific degeneration.

These lesions during the very early phases of the fluorescein study, usually show a relative hypofluorescence blocking the background choroidal fluorescence (Figs. 25.23*A* and 25.24*A*). As the retinal circulation fills, the capillaries within the lesion begin to fill with fluorescein and eventually leak to stain the tumor, which continues to fluoresce in the late phases of the study (Figs. 25.23, *B* and *C*, and 25.24, *B* and *C*).

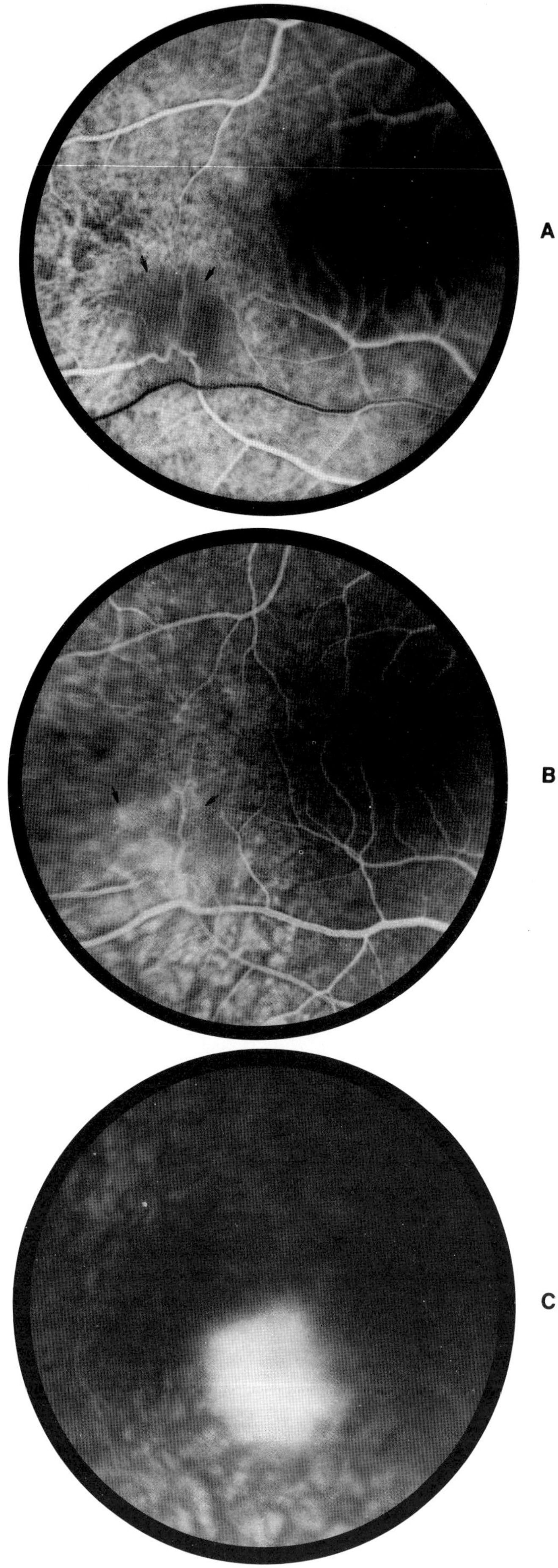

Figure 25.23. *A*, arteriovenous phase angiogram of a peripheral astrocytoma. This is an early filling phase of the study showing that the lesion itself blocks the background fluorescence at this stage (*arrows*). *B*, slightly later in the study during the venous phase of the retinal circulation showing a very subtle hyperfluorescence (*arrows*) due to filling of the lesion with dye. *C*, the very late phases of the study showing a persistent hyperfluorescence due to fluorescein retained in this highly vascular astrocytic tumor.

RETINOBLASTOMA

Retinoblastoma is the most common intraocular tumor in childhood. The average age at diagnosis is approximately 18 months, although the disease is sometimes evident at birth or in a patient who is considerably older. It is transmitted as an irregular dominant trait with incomplete penetrance. It occurs bilaterally in approximately 30% of the patients, with no sex or race predilection. The tumors grow in either an endophytic or exophytic pattern. The endophatic retinal mass usually has a cauliflower appearance with scattered tumor nodules along the inner retinal surface and in the vitreous. In the exophytic form there is marked prominence to the vasculature of the tumor. As the tumor grows, multiple secondary complications ensue including: rubeosis iridis, hypopyon, cataracts, hyphema, and glaucoma. Histopathologically, these tumors are composed of undifferentiated neuroblastic cells, with hypochromic nuclei, scanty cytoplasm, and rosette formation.

A

B

C

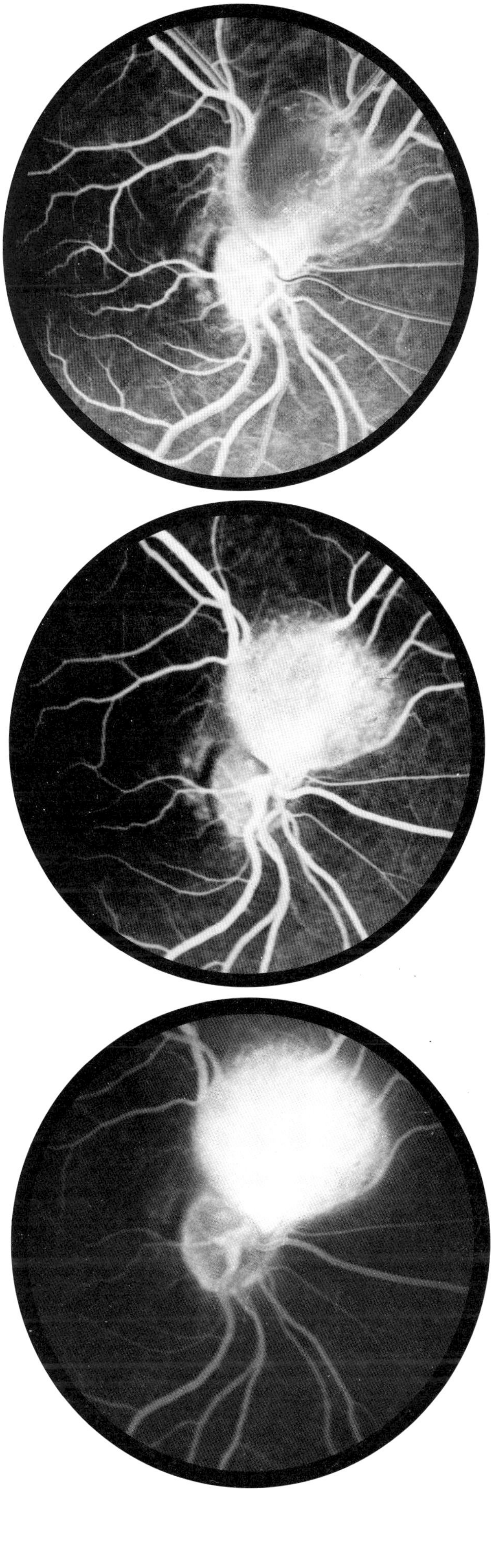

Figure 25.24. *A*, arteriovenous phase angiogram of an astrocytoma of the disc showing the early filling of the lesion. *B*, early venous phase angiogram showing the complete filling of the capillary system within the lesion causing an increased hyperfluorescence. *C*, late venous phase angiogram showing a greater degree of hyperfluorescence which persists in the very late phases of the study.

During the very early phases of the fluorescein angiogram vascular hyperfluorescence is evident from the large vessels which course throughout this cellular tumor. The rest of the tumor substance remains relatively hypofluorescent at this stage of the angiogram (Fig. 25.25*A*). During the capillary transition and venous drainage phase of the retinal circulation, the capillaries of the tumor fill and a subtle diffuse hyperfluorescence from the tumor tissue itself begins to develop (Fig. 25.25*B*). As the study continues, there is leakage from the tumor vasculature causing an increasing hyperfluorescence. Thus, the dye-stained tumor is markedly hyperfluorescent in the late phases of the study (Fig. 25.25*C*). It is interesting to note that the large vessels which at first were hyperfluorescent are now hypofluorescent. This results from the extravascular concentration of dye being greater than the intravascular concentration.

MELANOCYTOMA OF THE OPTIC NERVE

Melanocytomas are pigmentary tumors of the optic nerve. They vary in size from ¼ disc diameter to much larger lesions extending into the overlying vitreous and adjacent choroid. There is a predilection for these tumors to occur more frequently in pigmented individuals. The visual acuity is usually not affected; however, there may be field defects corresponding to the location of the lesion. Growth potential is usually negligible, although some lesions change in size and this is evident clinically. Histopathologically, these tumors are composed of melanocytes found near the region of the lamina cribrosa.

Because of the heavily pigmented cells, this lesion hypofluoresces early and remains hypofluorescent throughout the entire fluorescein angiogram (Fig. 25.26). This is due to blockage of the background and surrounding fluorescence. Occasionally the tumor's vasculature may be superficial and partially evident on the angiogram.

This chapter has reviewed some of the significant clinical features of the more important intraocular tumors that may affect the macula. The fluorescein angiographic characteristics were discussed with correlation to the histopathology. The patterns seen are not specific or diagnostic of any of these entities. Combining the fluorescein angiographic evaluation with the clinical examination provides the ophthalmologist with a better understanding of the underlying histopathology and enhanced diagnostic capability of these tumors.

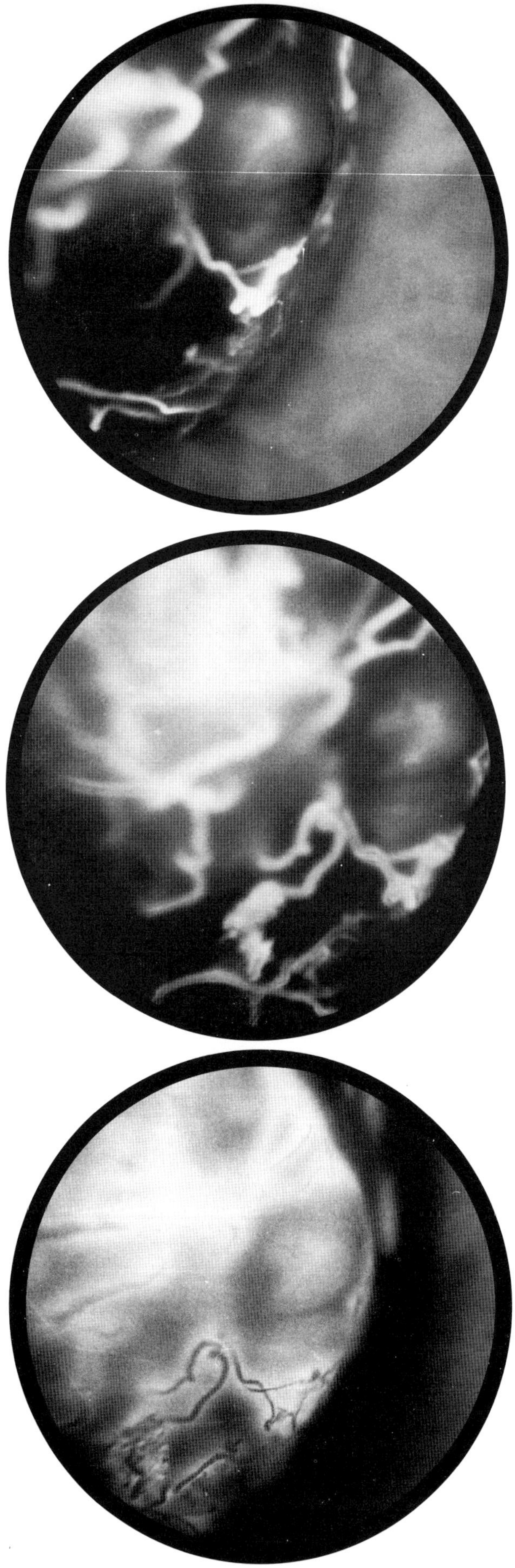

A

B

C

Figure 25.25. *A*, the clinical fluorescein angiographic appearance of a retinoblastoma during the early phases showing that the tumor itself is hypofluorescent but the vessels that course through the tumor fill with fluorescein. *B*, a slightly later phase of the same lesion showing that the vessels begin to leak fluorescein into the surrounding tumor tissue. *C*, late phase angiogram of the same study. The fluorescein is now more concentrated in the surrounding extravascular tissue of the tumor, but there is little fluorescein within the vessels themselves.

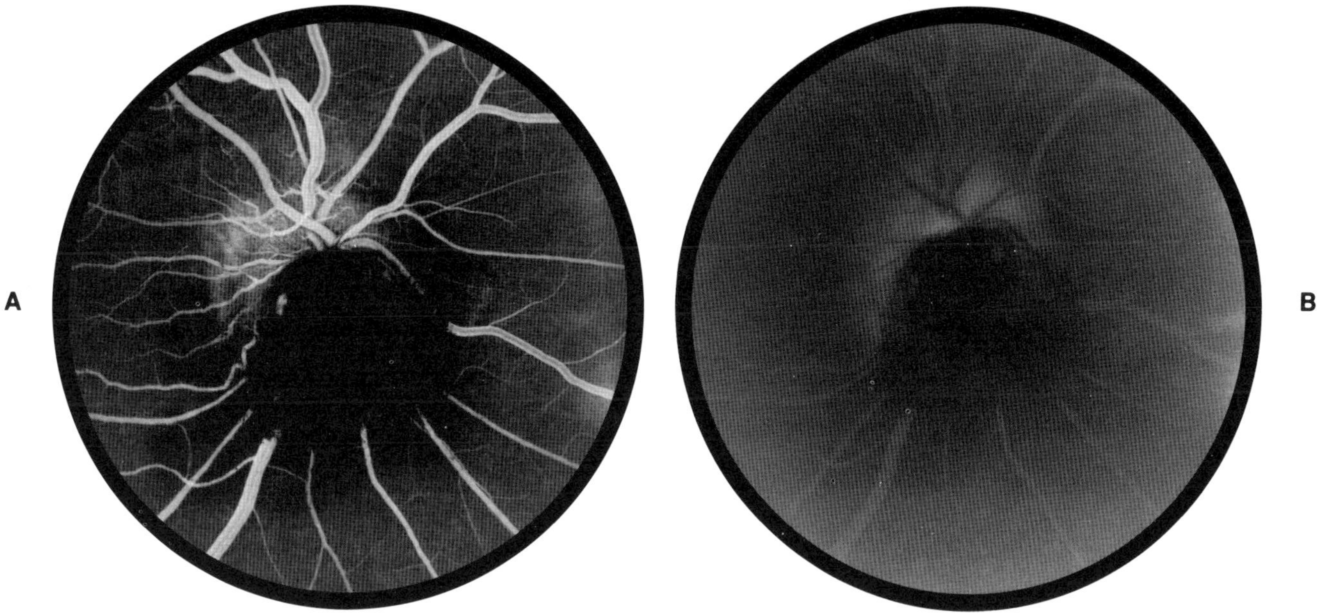

Figure 25.26. *A*, the early appearance of the melanocytoma of the optic nerve head showing the hypofluorescence due to blockage of the background and surrounding choroidal fluorescence from the heavily pigmented solid tumor itself. *B*, the late phase angiogram of the same patient showing a persistence in the hypofluorescence due to blockage from the heavily pigmented tumor tissue.

Suggested Readings

Archer, D.B., Deutman, A., Ernest, J.T., and Krill, A.E.: Arteriovenous communications of the retina. *Am J Ophthalmol, 75:* 224, 1973.

Bedford, M.A., Bedotto, C., and MacFaul, P.A.: Retinoblastoma: a study of 139 cases. Brit J Ophthalmol, 55: 19, 1971.

Davies, W.S., and Thumin, M.: Cavernous hemangioma of the optic disc and retina. *Trans Am Acad Ophthalmol Otolaryngol, 60:* 217, 1956.

Duke, J.R., and Maumenee, A.E.: An unusual tumor of the retinal pigment epithelium in an eye with early open-angle glaucoma. *Am J Ophthalmol, 47:* 311, 1959.

Edwards, W.C., Layden, W.E., and Macdonald, R., Jr.: Fluorescein angiography of malignant melanoma of the choroid. *Am J Ophthalmol, 68:* 797, 1969.

Fair, J.R.: Tumors of the retinal pigment epithelium. *Am J Ophthalmol, 45:* 495, 1958.

Flindall, R.J., and Gass, J.D.M.: A histopathologic fluorescein angiographic correlative study of malignant melanomas of the choroid. *Can J Ophthalmol, 6:* 258, 1971.

Ganley, J.P., and Comstock, G.W.: Benign nevi and malignant melanomas of the choroid. *Am J Ophthalmol, 76:* 19, 1973.

Gass, J.D.: Differential Diagnosis of Intraocular Tumors. C.V. Mosby, St. Louis, 1974.

Gass, J.D.M.: A fluorescein angiographic study of macular dysfunction secondary to retinal vascular disease. V. Retinal telangiectasis. *Arch Ophthalmol, 80:* 592, 1968.

Gass, J.D.M: Cavernous hemangioma of the retina—a neuro-oculo-cutaneous syndrome. *Am J Ophthalmol, 71:* 799, 1971.

Gass, J.D.M: Fluorescein angiography: an aid in the differential diagnosis of intraocular tumors. *Int Ophthalmol Clin, 12* (1): 85, 1972.

Gass, J.D.M., Sever, R.J., Sparks, D., and Goren, J.: A combined technique of fluorescein funduscopy and angiography of the eye. *Arch Ophthalmol, 78:* 455, 1967.

Hogan, M.M., and Zimmerman, L.E. (eds.): Ophthalmic Pathology, 2nd ed., W.B. Saunders, Philadelphia, 1963, p. 413.

Jones, I.S., and Cleasby, G.W.: Hemangioma of the choroid: a clinicopathologic analysis. *Am J Ophthalmol, 48:* 612, 1959.

Kuwabara, T., and Aiello, L.: Leukemic miliary nodules in the retina. *Arch Ophthalmol, 72:* 494, 1964.

MacLean, A.L., and Maumenee, A.E.: Hemangioma of the choroid. *Am J Ophthalmol, 50:* 3, 1960.

Naumann, G.O.H., Hellner, K., and Naumann, L.R.: Pigmented nevi of the choroid. Clinical study of secondary changes in the overlying tissues. *Trans Am Acad Ophthalmol Otolaryngol, 75:* 110, 1971.

Norton, E.W.D., and Gutman, F.: Fluorescein angiography and hemangiomas of the choroid. *Arch Ophthalmol, 78:* 121, 1967.

Novotny, H.R., and Alvis, D.L.: A method of photographing fluorescence in circulating blood in the human retina. *Circulation, 24:* 82, 1961.

Oosterhuis, J. A., and Rubinstein, K.: Haemangioma at the optic disc. *Ophthalmologica, 164:* 362, 1972.

Oosterhuis, J.A., and van Waveren, C.W.: Fluorescein photography in malignant melanoma. *Ophthalmologica, 156:* 101, 1968.

Pettit, T.H., Barton, A., Foos, R.Y., and Christensen, R.E.: Fluorescein angiography of choroidal melanomas. *Arch Ophthalmol, 83:* 27, 1970.

Redler, L.D., and Ellsworth, R.M.: Prognostic importance of choroidal invasion in retinoblastoma. *Arch Ophtahlmol, 90:* 294, 1973.

Reese, A.B.: Tumors of the Eye, 3rd ed., Harper & Row, New York, 1976.

Reese, A.B., and Jones, I.S.: Benign melanomas of the retinal pigment epithelium. *Am J Ophthalmol, 42:* 207, 1956.

Rones, B., and Zimmerman, L.E.: The production of heterochromia and glaucoma by diffuse malignant melanoma of the iris. *Trans Am Acad Ophthalmol Otolaryngol, 61:* 447, 1957.

Schatz, H., Burton, T., Yannuzzi, L., and Rabb, M.: Interpretation of Fundus Fluorescein Angiography, C.V. Mosby, St. Louis, 1978.

Shields, J.A., and Federman, J.L.: Malignant melanoma of the uvea. *In* Malignant Melanoma, ed. by W.H. Clark, L.I. Goldman, and M.J. Mastrangelo, Grune & Stratton, New York, in press.

Smith, J.L., David, N.J., Hart, L.M., Levenson, D.S., and Tillett, C.W.: Hemangioma of the choroid. Fluorescein photography and photocoagulation. *Arch Ophthalmol, 69:* 51, 1963.

Snyder, W.B., Allen, L., and Frazier, O.: Fluorescence angiography of ocular tumors. *Trans Am Acad Ophthalmol Otolaryngol, 71:* 820, 1967.

Wessing, A.: Fluorescein Angiography of the Retina, C.V. Mosby, St. Louis, 1969.

Wolter, J.R., Schut, A.L., and Martonyi, C.L.: Hemangioma-like clinical appearance of a collar-button melanoma caused by the strangulation effect of Bruch's membrane. *Am J Ophthalmol, 76:* 730, 1973.

Wyburn-Mason, R.: Arteriovenous aneurysm of mid-brain and retina, facial naevi and mental changes. *Brain, 66:* 163, 1943.

Yanoff, M., and Fine, B.S.: Ocular Pathology: A Text and Atlas, Harper & Row, New York, 1975.

Yanoff, M., and Zimmerman, L.E.: Histogenesis of malignant melanomas of the uvea. III. The relationship of congenital ocular melanocytosis and neurofibromatosis to uveal melanomas. *Arch Ophthalmol, 77:* 331, 1967.

Zimmerman, L.E.: Problems in the diagnosis of malignant melanomas of the choroid and ciliary body. *Am J Ophthalmol, 75:* 917, 1973.

CHAPTER 26

Trauma

Kurt A. Gitter, M.D., Lawrence A. Yannuzzi, M.D., and Howard Schatz, M.D.

Trauma to the eye, whether mechanical or nonmechanical, penetrating or nonpenetrating, direct or indirect, may affect any one or all of the tissues of the eye. This discussion of ocular trauma will concentrate predominantly on nonpenetrating injuries of the posterior pole, especially the retina, choroid, and retinal pigment epithelium in the macular zone.

Nonmechanical Injuries

Nonmechanical thermal injuries to the macula can be produced by solar, photocoagulation, cryo, diathermy, and high intensity ultrasonic energy.

SOLAR

Sun eclipses have long been known to produce ocular scotomata and/or permanent loss of central vision [1] and were already recognized during the time of Plato and Socrates. Solar burns can occur after sun gazing (apart from an eclipse) when practiced for therapeutic or religious purposes [1], or when under the influence of drugs [2]. This condition is more often seen in young people (perhaps due to greater transmissibility of the lens) or due to a desire for experimentation, more vivid in the young.

Affected patients often present with greater symptomatology than objective ophthalmoscopic findings. Patients complain of after-images, photophobia, metamorphopsia, and a dense scotoma usually within 24 hours, which often lasts for weeks to months and may be permanent. The objective retinal findings vary from normal to macular edema, to the presence of small, oval, white parafoveal spots surrounded by a zone of mottled pigmentation (Fig. 26.1). Visual prognosis, although variable, most frequently improves within 2 months with subsequent diminution of the central or paracentral scotomas.

Recently, Tso and LaPiana [3] studied the clinical, angiographic, and histopathologic effects of sun gazing in human eyes. Their fascinating study was performed on three eyes with ocular malignancies prior to enucleation and revealed retinal pigment epithelial changes (loss of melanin granules) histopathologically without affecting the overlying retina. Furthermore, they demonstrated delayed macular photostress tests and angiographic evidence of RPE changes (confirmed by histopathology) in all three eyes without clinical evidence of visual compromise [3].

A

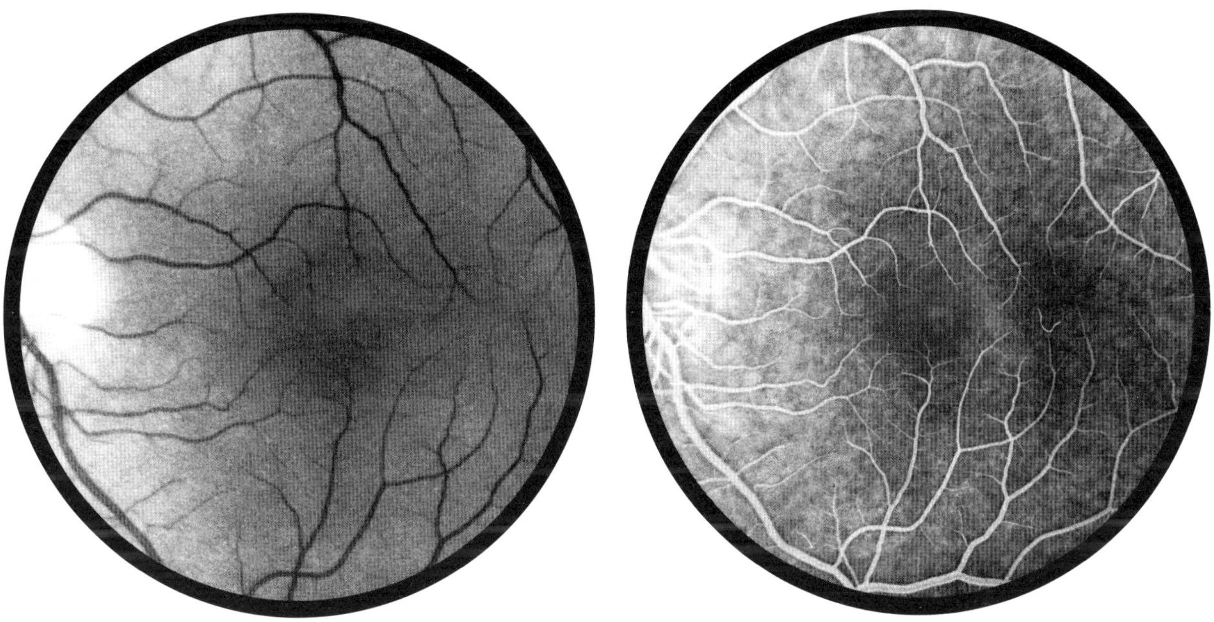

B

Figure 26.1. Solar retinopathy *A*, ophthalmoscopic photograph showing small circumscribed retinal pigment epithelial changes in the juxtafoveal position. *B*, arteriovenous phase angiogram showing minimal hyperfluorescence from choroidal transmission (pigment epithelial window defect) at the site of the lesion secondary to atrophy of the pigment epithelium.

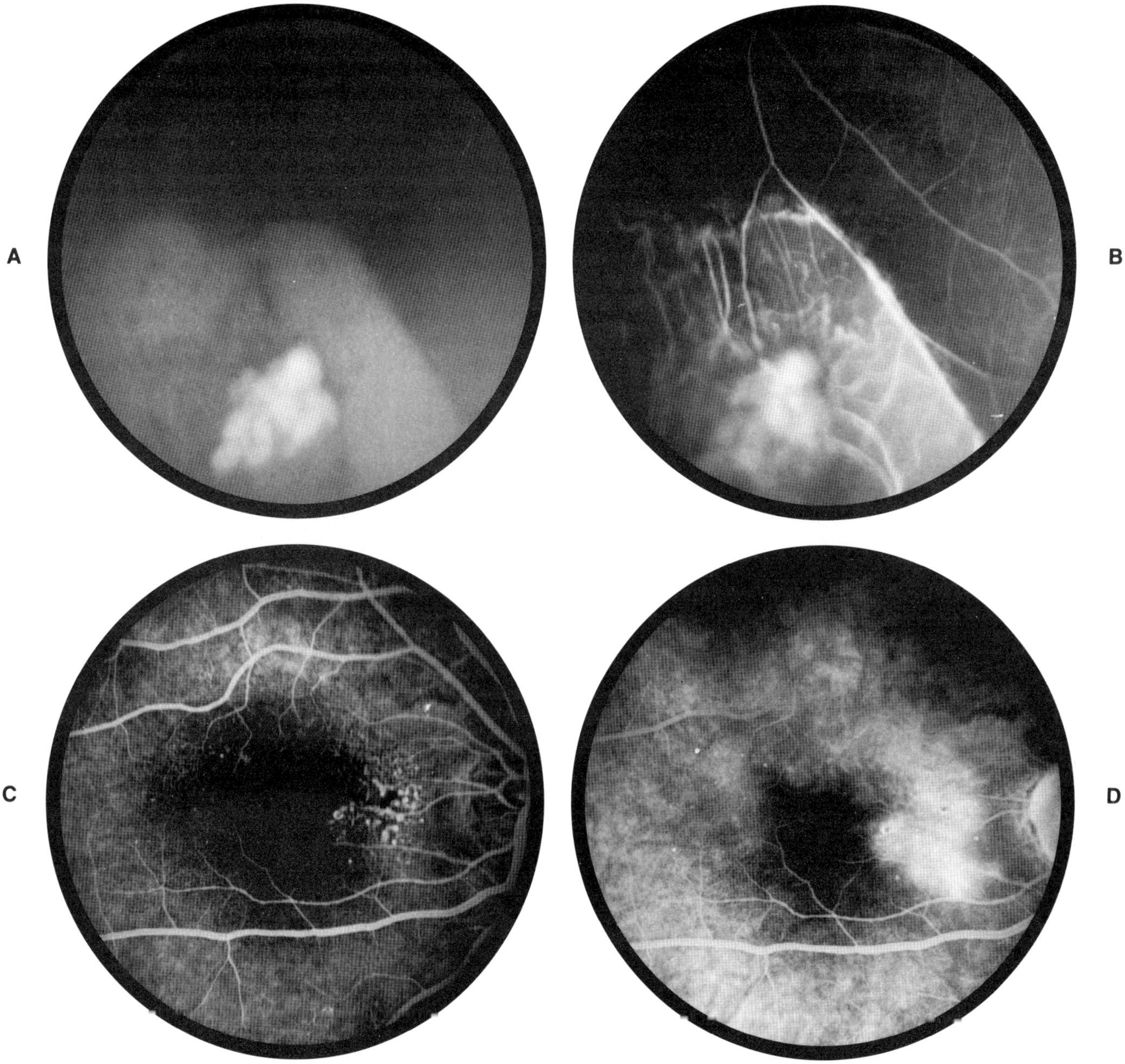

Figure 26.2. Radiation retinopathy. *A*, ophthalmoscopic photograph showing the peripheral remnant of a regressed retinoblastoma, which had been treated with 9,000 R 18 years before. *B*, early venous phase angiogram of same patient, showing leakage from the lesion. *C*, early venous phase angiogram of same patient, showing patchy areas of capillary nonperfusion and telangiectasia in the macula. *D*, late venous phase angiogram showing dye leakage from the localized telangiectasia.

PHOTOCOAGULATION, DIATHERMY, AND CRYO

Thermal injury (similar to solar burns) can be produced by diathermy, light, laser, and cryo coagulation. Light photocoagulation was first employed clinically by Meyer-Schwickerath [4] in 1949 with the development of xenon arc photocoagulation. Laser and cryo also produce similar retinal and retinal pigment epithelial effects. Diathermy, long used for the creation of chorioretinal scarring and adhesion, has been known to create preretinal macular fibrosis or pucker. Likewise, pucker can occur in xenon arc and, less commonly, secondary to laser photocoagulation. Macular pigmentary migration can occur in cases of peripheral cryoretinopexy as described by Sudarsky and Yannuzzi [5].

Ultrasound energy is also capable of thermal injury to the retina and choroid in high intensity doses. Purnell [6], and Karlin [7] have independently demonstrated ultrasonic effects on the retina: the former in affecting movement of the retina in eyes with retinal detachment, and the latter in creating chorioretinal lesions. These changes are only possible with extremely high intensity energy levels (much greater than employed clinically for diagnostic or therapeutic purpose, i.e., phakoemulsification).

RADIATION RETINOPATHY

Radiation retinopathy can produce papillitis, retinal pigment epithelial atrophy, retinal telangiectasia, capillary nonperfusion, exudates and microaneurysms, and neovascularization of the retina [8]. The clinical appearance can mimic localized areas of diabetic retinopathy.

The predominant effects are on the retinal vascular endothelium and are usually delayed with a variable latent period. Radiation retinopathy is rarely seen with small doses under 6,000 rad, but the development of retinopathy is extremely variable and depends on factors such as the type of radiation employed and the proximity of the radiation source. Clinically, radiation retinopathy has been seen in eyes treated for retinoblastoma (Fig. 26.2) and in some eyes that have received cobalt plaque radiation for choroidal melanoma. Radiation retinopathy can also occur following radiation therapy for paranasal and orbital tumors.

The differential diagnosis of radiation retinopathy includes all causes of segmental or isolated patchy areas of nonperfusion and new vessel formation, i.e., retinal telangiectasia, tributary branch vein occlusion, early Coats' disease or Leber's miliary aneurysms, retinal cavernous hemangioma, Eales', sarcoid, blood dyscrasia, hemoglobinopathies, and most importantly, diabetic retinopathy.

TOXIC

Chloroquine and phenothiazine derivatives (i.e., Thorazine, Mellaril) affect predominantly the retinal pigment epithelium. The former drug produces a characteristic bull's eye angiographic appearance surrounding the fovea with destruction of retinal pigment epithelium. The phenothiazine derivatives produce their toxic effects by primarily affecting the choriocapillaris with resultant change in the pigment epithelium and neurosensory retina as demonstrated clearly by Davidorf [9].

HEMORRHAGE

Macular hemorrhage from nonmechanical injury may occur with posterior vitreous detachment and can also be seen following any Valsalva maneuver (Fig. 26.3). The latter cause can produce intraretinal and, occasionally, preretinal hemorrhage of varying size. When the hemorrhage is small and not in the fovea, the patient can be asymptomatic. These hemorrhages mostly clear in a short period (days to weeks) with return of good vision.

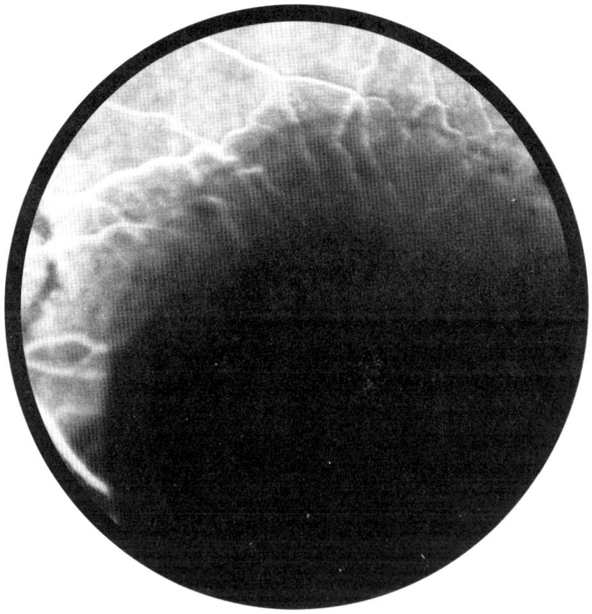

Figure 26.3. Valsalva hemorrhage. Arteriovenous fluorescein angiogram showing hypofluorescence from a massive preretinal hemorrhage in a 28-year-old female, following a sustained Valsalva maneuver.

Mechanical Injuries (Nonpenetrating)

The mechanical force of direct, nonpenetrating, blunt trauma to the eye sets up concussion waves which may produce anatomic disruption and concussion necrosis of ocular tissue. In the posterior segment, these changes can affect the retina, pigment epithelium, and choroid.

EFFECTS ON THE RETINA

Edema

Berlin's edema or commotio-retinae is seen in eyes sustaining blunt nonpenetrating injury (Fig. 26.4). Visual acuity is directly affected and is caused by vasospastic changes in the arteriolar vessels producing transitory exudations of intracellular retinal edema fluid. When studied angiographically, these eyes appear normal or, occasionally, hypofluorescent due to blockage of choroidal fluorescence by the retinal edema.

The clinical appearance is characteristic with the retina appearing cloudy white and the foveal reflex conspicuously red. Although vision is initially usually markedly disturbed, it rapidly improves and, in most instances, returns to normal within several days to a week. Rarely, however, macular edema can persist and lead to cyst and/or hole formation. These traumatic macular holes are usually full thickness and are associated with permanent decreased central visual acuity and a very low incidence of associated retinal detachment (Fig. 26.5).

Hemorrhage

Hemorrhages secondary to blunt trauma can occur in many anatomic positions and can be choroidal, sub-RPE, retinal, preretinal, and intraretinal. Retinal hemorrhages can occur beneath the internal limiting membrane or subhyaloid space or in the superficial (flame-shaped hemorrhages in the nerve fiber layer) and deep retinal layers (dot and blot hemorrhages).

Retinal Tears

Retinal tears, disinsertions, and detachments are all noted following traumas. Disinsertions occur in the superonasal quadrant following contusion in contrast to inferotemporal quadrant dialysis seen congenitally in young males.

A

B

C

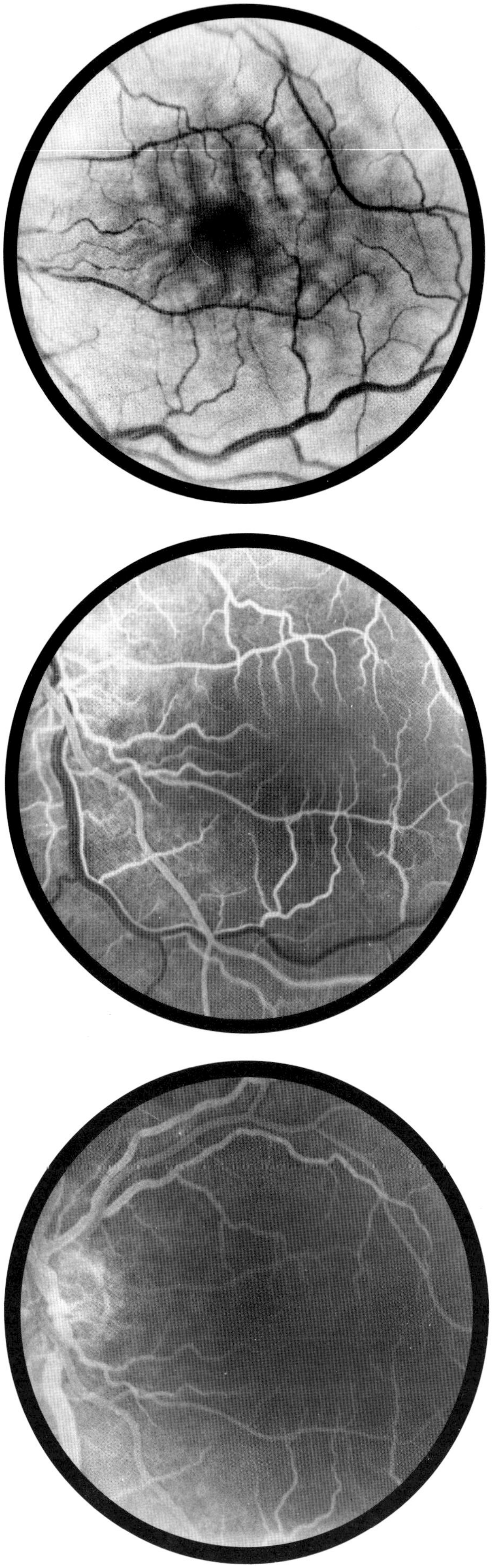

Figure 26.4. Berlin's edema. *A*, ophthalmoscopic photograph. Note the multiple areas of cloudy white disturbance in the macula surrounding a prominent foveal reflex. *B*, arterial phase angiogram, and *C*, late venous phase angiogram showing no filling defect or late leakage.

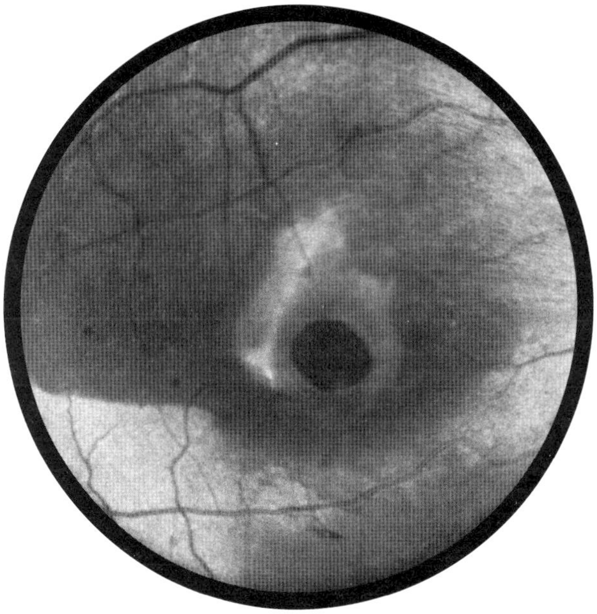

Figure 26.5. Macular hole. Ophthalmoscopic photograph with posterior retinal detachment and hemorrhage.

Purtscher's Retinopathy

Purtscher's retinopathy is an uncommon manifestation of severe indirect trauma affecting distant portions of the body, i.e., chest compression. Diffuse, multiple, whitish, oval, retinal lesions are seen in the posterior pole, which according to Paul Henkind, M.D. (personal communication) are always in the peripapillary radial capillary bed and represent cotton wool spots or ischemic infarcts. The angiographic findings confirm intraretinal microangiopathy with vascular permeability changes and dye leakage [10] (Fig. 26.6). Visual acuity is variable, but can be moderately to markedly reduced. Recovery is slow, but gradual (over weeks to months), and vision usually returns to normal.

Although initially thought to be associated with fat emboli, Purtscher's retinopathy occurs without other evidence of fat embolization and may represent a more marked vasospastic effect on the retinal arteriolar circulation than Berlin's edema. The sequence of events in Purtcher's retinopathy may represent the effects of a Valsalva maneuver followed by a crushing chest injury which forces blood into precapillary arteries with resultant damage to the endothelium secondary to vascular congestion. This produces occlusive phenomenon with resultant hemorrhage and cotton wool spots. Kelley [10] correctly advocates angiographic evaluation of eyes with reduced vision and chest injuries which can sometimes show abnormalities in the vascular permeability despite a normal fundus appearance.

A

B

C

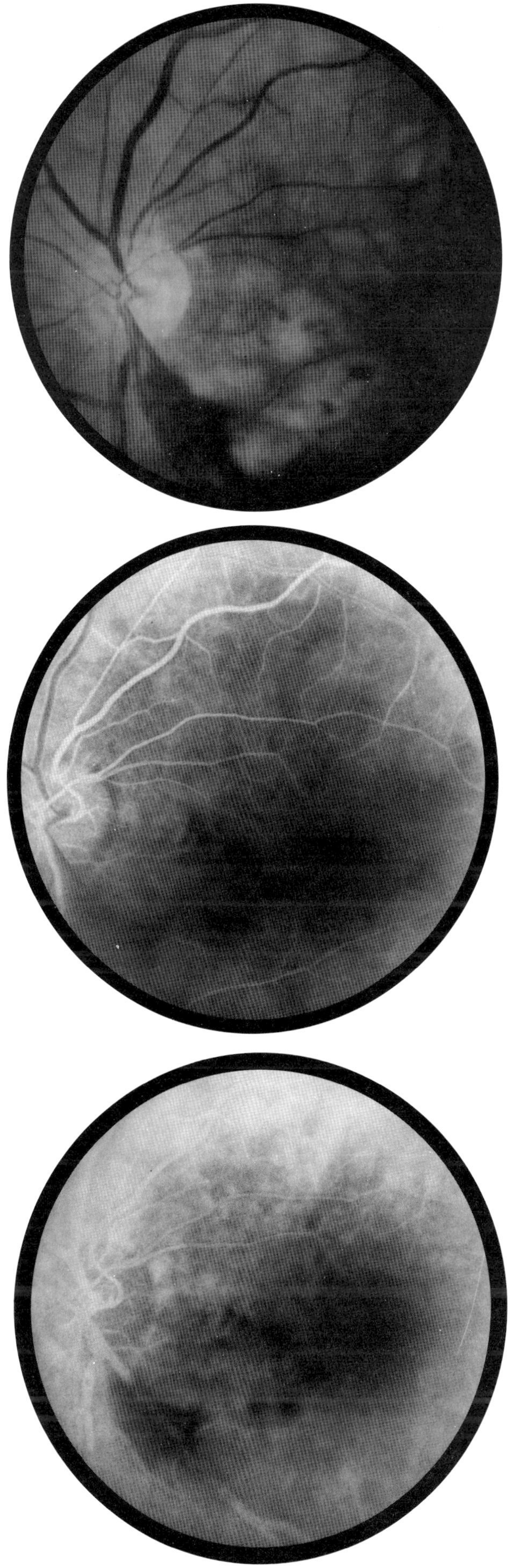

Figure 26.6. Purtscher's retinopathy. *A*, ophthalmoscopic photograph showing hemorrhage and exudate in the macula. *B*, arteriovenous phase angiogram, and *C*, late venous phase angiogram showing hypofluorescence.

EFFECTS ON CHOROID AND RETINAL PIGMENT EPITHELIUM

Blunt injury also has significant effects on the choroid and RPE. Changes in these tissues vary from minor RPE atrophic changes to marked effects on the RPE with production of a "pseudoretinitis pigmentosa" picture with bone spicules and total dispersion of the retinal pigment epithelium (Fig. 26.7).

Traumatic lesions of the pigment epithelium may be isolated to the region of the disc, macula, or periphery, or be more widespread. RPE atrophic changes can progress for several years following the initial insult with enlarging zones of atrophy and pigment dispersion developing with time. Often there is corresponding visual field cut due to loss of the photoceptors, but the nerve fibers appear to remain intact.

The most marked effect of trauma on the RPE is seen in "retinitis sclopetaria" [11, 12], a condition associated with choroidal rupture, hemorrhage, fibrosis with a proliferative scar, and marked RPE changes. This unusual occurrence is seen when a missile of high velocity, i.e., bullet, passes adjacent to the globe without penetration (Fig. 26.8).

CHOROIDAL RUPTURE

Choroidal rupture is another frequent finding in eyes with severe blunt trauma and occurs due to contrecoup force without global penetration. This lesion is really a rupture of Bruch's membrane with a disruption of the continuity of the choroid, choriocapillaris, and pigment epithelium. The lesion is linear or crescent-shaped and most frequently concentric to the disc, but occasionally traverses the macular vertically. These eyes initially present with a hemorrhagic detachment of the retinal pigment epithelium and bleeding in the choroid, sub-RPE, and/or retina. Occasionally, breakthrough of hemorrhage occurs into the vitreous cavity. Often these ruptures are noted initially, but occasionally cannot be identified until the hemorrhage is resorbed [13]. Fluorescein angiography is helpful in defining these ruptures which are sometimes partially obscured by blood. Angiography shows early hyperfluorescence and late staining of the scar. Eyes with choroidal ruptures must also be carefully followed for life as subretinal neovascular membranes can develop many years after the original trauma and produce sensory retinal detachments with visual decline (in one of the authors' (KAG) experience, 26 years after initial trauma). These are subretinal neovascular membranes potentially treatable by argon laser photocoagulation [14] (Fig. 26.9).

HYPOTONY MACULOPATHY

This lesion, associated with retinal and choroidal folds running temporally through the macula from disc, is seen in prolonged hypotony secondary to ciliary body shutdown or to a penetrating wound with loss of intraocular pressure.

A

B

C

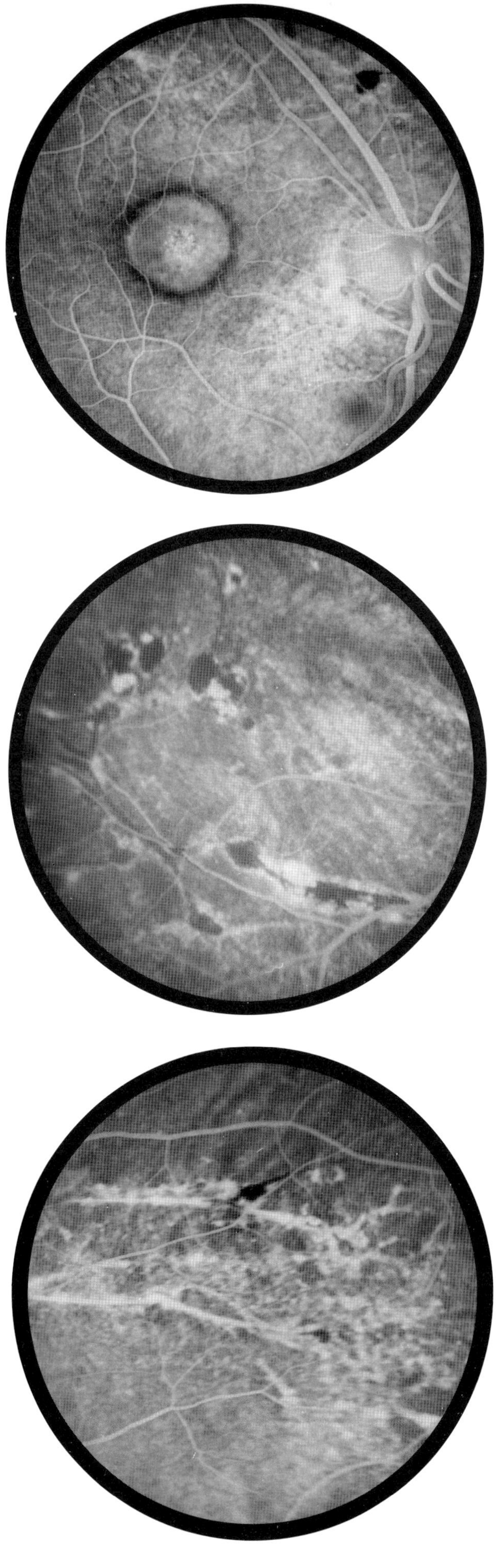

Figure 26.7. Traumatic pigment epitheliopathy, pseudoretinitis pigmentosa, and macular hole. *A,* venous phase angiogram. Note the macular hole and scattered retinal pigment epithelial disturbance. *B,* temporal retina, and *C,* nasal retina, showing retinal pigment epithelial changes of atrophy and pigment proliferation.

A

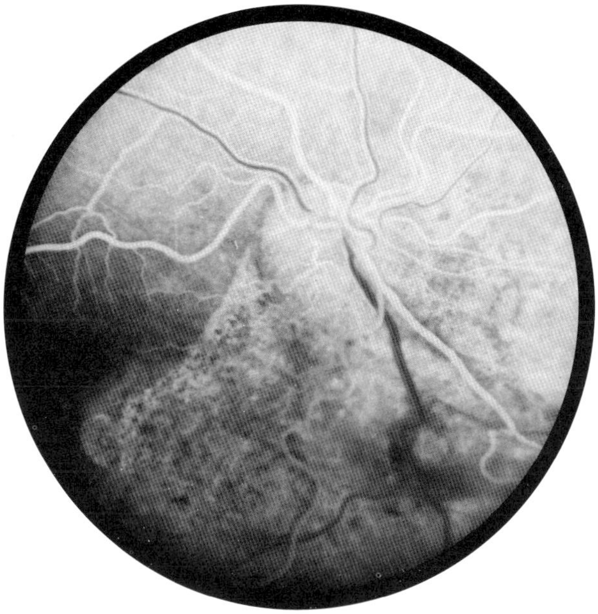

B

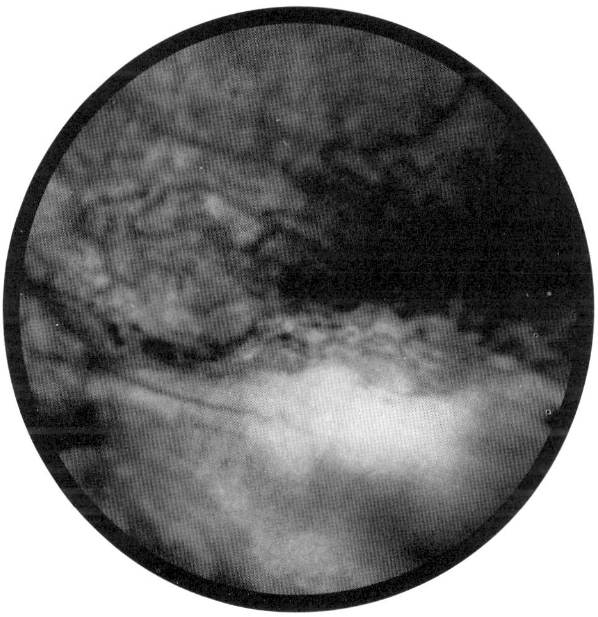

Figure 26.8. Retinitis sclopetaria. *A,* fluorescein angiogram showing the effects of missile (bullet) injury to the orbit without ocular penetration. Note the presence of marked retinal pigment epithelial changes in the macula and inferior to the disc. *B,* late phase angiogram showing the proliferative scar extending intravitreally in the inferonasal quadrant.

A

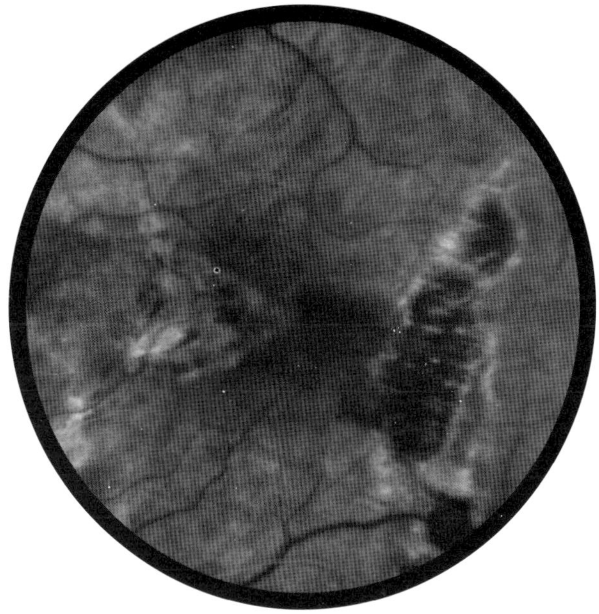

B

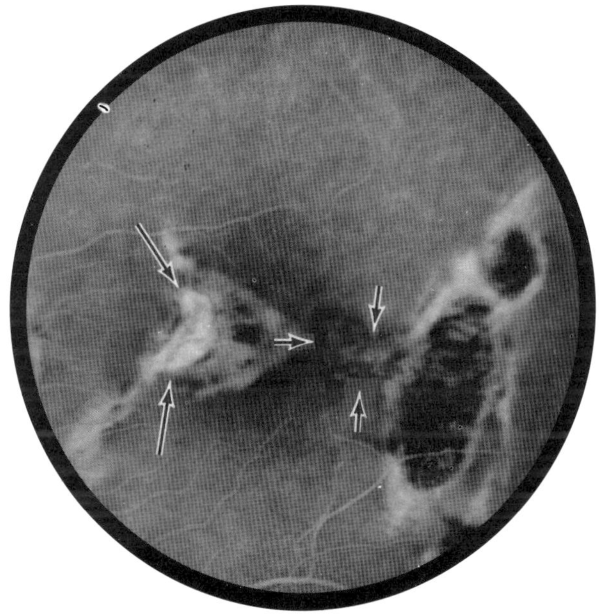

C

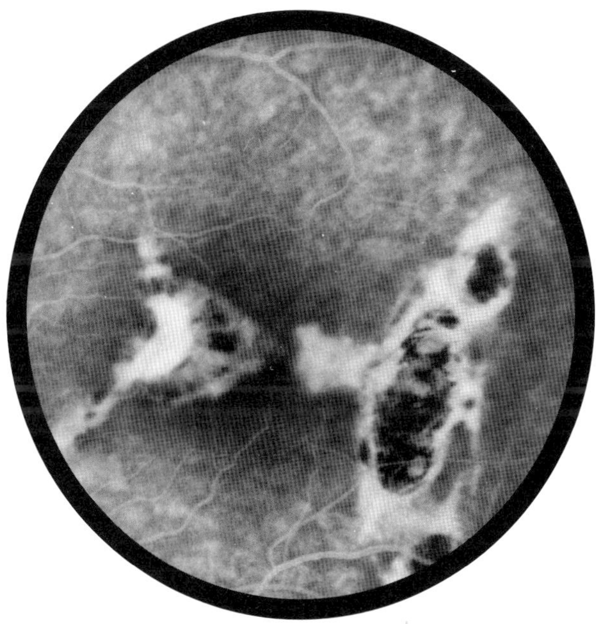

Figure 26.9. Choroidal rupture with subretinal neovascular complex, 26 years after the initial injury. *A,* choroidal filling phase angiogram. Note the large heavily pigmented choroidal rupture in the temporal macula and the smaller one adjacent and concentric to the disc margin. *B,* early venous phase angiogram. Note the lacy hyperfluorescence (*surrounded by a dark zone*) adjacent to and continuous with the large choroidal rupture from a recent fibrovascular network (*small arrows*) and an older disciform scar adjacent to the smaller rupture (*large arrows*). *C,* late phase angiogram showing staining of the disciform scar and pooling into the subsensory space from the subretinal neovascularization. Traumatic rupture of the choroid may become associated with subretinal neovascularization many years after the initial injury.

Underlying Disease States Affected by Trauma

Many ocular diseases are affected by external trauma. All of these clinical entities can have spontaneous hemorrhage, but due to the nature of their pathology, these eyes are more vulnerable to trauma. These diseases include peripheral retinal abnormalities such as lattice degeneration with holes and peripheral retinal tears. Hereditary dystrophies such as juvenile retinoschisis can be affected by trauma. Vitreous hemorrhage can occur from tearing of a retinal vessel involved in a peripheral schisis cavity. One of the authors (KAG) has also documented trauma triggering hemorrhage in a 9-year-old white male with Best's heredomacular vitelliform degeneration and subretinal neovascular membrane formation.

Retinal vascular occlusive diseases are associated with retinal and preretinal telangiectasia and neovascularization. These diseases such as Coats', Eales', and sickle cell hemoglobinopathy can likewise develop vitreous hemorrhage from shearing and blowout of these abnormal vessels following blunt trauma.

In the posterior pole, two important precursors of traumatic macular hemorrhage are angioid streaks and preexisting choroidal ruptures. Both conditions predipose toward the development of choroidal vascular proliferation through breaks in Bruch's membrane. Other diseases associated with subretinal neovascularization are also more vulnerable and susceptible to hemorrhage following blunt injury. It is, therefore, logical that these patients avoid severe trauma, wear safety lenses, and avoid contact sports.

References

1. Duke-Elder, S., and MacFaul, P.A. (eds.): System of Ophthalmology, vol. 14: Injuries, C. V. Mosby, St. Louis, 1972, p. 888.
2. Schatz, H., and Mendelblatt, F.: Solar retinopathy from sungazing under the influence of LSD. *Brit J Ophthalmol, 57:* 270, 1973.
3. Tso, M.O.M., and LaPiana, F.G.: Human fovea after sungazing. *Trans Am Acad Ophthalmol Otolaryngol, 79:* 788, 1975.
4. Meyer-Schwickerath G.: Light Coagulation, C. V. Mosby, St. Louis, 1960.
5. Sudarsky, R.D. and Yannuzzi, L.A.: Cryomarcation lines and pigment migration after retinal cryosurgery. *Arch Ophthalmol, 83:* 395, 1970.
6. Purnell, E., and Sokollu, A.: An evaluation of time-amplitude sonography in ocular diagnosis. *Am J Ophthalmol, 54:* 1103, 1962.
7. Karlin, D. B., and Lazar, M.: Experimental ultrasound in retinal detachment surgery. *In* Ophthalmic Ultrasound (Proceedings of the 1968 International Congress of Ultrasonography in Ophthalmology), ed. by K.A. Gitter and A.H. Keeney, C. V. Mosby, St. Louis, 1969, p. 343.
8. Chee, P.H.Y.: Radiation retinopathy. *Am J Ophthalmol, 66:* 860, 1968.
9. Davidorf, F.H.: Thioridazine pigmentary retinopathy. *Arch Ophthalmol, 90:* 251, 1973.
10. Kelley, J.S.: Purtscher's retinopathy related to chest compression by safety belts. *Am J Ophthalmol, 74:* 278, 1972.
11. Nover, A.: The Ocular Fundus: Methods of Examination and Typical Findings, 2nd ed. Lea & Febiger, Philadelphia, 1966, p. 130.
12. Richards, R.D., West, C.E., and Meisels, A.A.: Chorioretinitis sclopetaria. *Am J Ophthalmol, 66:* 852, 1968.
13. Gitter, K.A., Slusher, M., and Justice, J., Jr.: Traumatic hemorrhagic detachment of the retinal pigment epithelium. *Arch Ophthalmol, 79:* 729, 1968.
14. Fuller, B., and Gitter, K.A.: Traumatic choroidal rupture with late serous detachment of macula. Report of successful argon laser treatment. *Arch Ophthalmol, 89:* 354, 1973.

CHAPTER 27

Toxoplasmosis and Toxocariasis

Conrad L. Giles, M.D., and G. Richard O'Connor, M.D.

Ocular Toxoplasmosis

Toxoplasmosis is a rather common cause of inflammatory lesions of the fundus, accounting for between 30 and 50% of all posterior uveitis [1, 2]. The disease can destroy visually important structures of the eye; therefore, it is important that the ophthalmologist appreciate its disastrous potential for the patient, and be able to recognize its lesions.

SIGNS AND SYMPTOMS

The earliest symptoms noted by the patient generally are floating spots and blurred vision. Usually there is no inflammation of the anterior segment and the patient shows a white, comfortable-looking eye at the onset of the disease. In the early stages of the disease, the visual acuity is good unless the lesion affects the macula, the papillomacular bundle, or the optic nerve head. Examination by direct and indirect ophthalmoscopy and slit-lamp biomicroscopy usually reveals vitreous opacities. A whitish-yellow, slightly raised, fuzzy retinal lesion usually can be seen. The lesions occur in the posterior pole more often than elsewhere in the fundus, and, occasionally, are immediately adjacent to the optic nerve head, where they sometimes may be mistaken for primary optic neuritis (papillitis).

The characteristic lesion is an exudative focal retinitis (Fig. 27.1). The anterior layers of the retina often are the selected site for the multiplication of the causative organism, *Toxoplasma gondii.* In this predilection of the organism, toxoplasmosis differs from many other forms of chorioretinitis in which the choroid, rather than the retina, is primarily affected. Nevertheless, there is also a deep retinal form of ocular toxoplasmosis. The lesion does not cloud the vitreous early in the course of the disease. Moreover, the patient does not notice floating spots until the organism involves the anterior layers of the retina and the posterior hyaloid membrane [3].

A

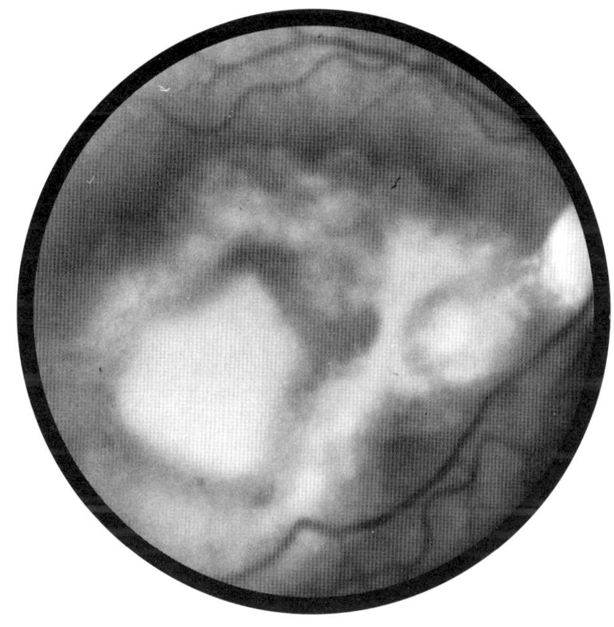

B

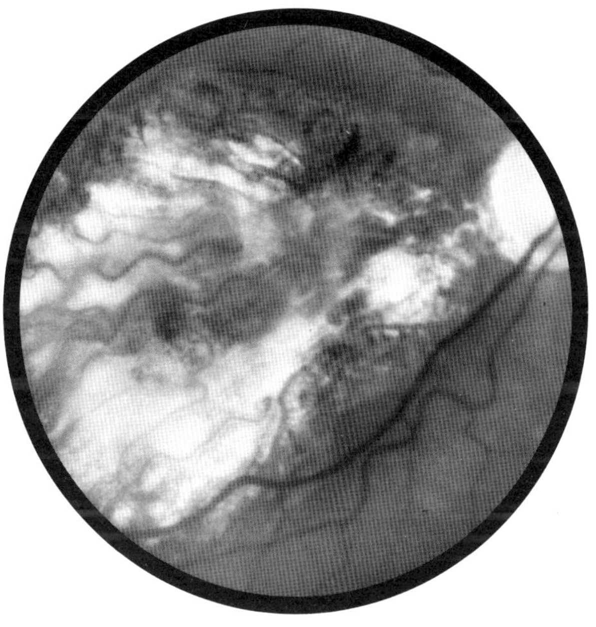

Figure 27.1. Retinochoroiditis and vitritis. *A*, ophthalmoscopic photograph. Note the huge, whitish-yellow, slightly raised, fuzzy retinal lesion in the macula in this 4-year-old female. There is also an overlying cellular reaction in the vitreous obscuring fundus details. *B*, ophthalmoscopic photograph, 2 years later. The retinal lesion has healed leaving an atrophic scar with scattered areas of pigmentation, atrophy of the retinal pigment epithelium and choriocapillaris, and baring of the sclera.

DIAGNOSIS

Ocular toxoplasmosis is diagnosed by the characteristic fundus lesion (focal necrotizing retinochoroiditis), the presence of the anti-*Toxoplasma* antibodies in the patient's serum, and by reasonable exclusion, after considering differential diagnoses, of other infectious diseases that might cause necrotizing lesions of the fundus [4]. These include, principally, syphilis, cytomegalovirus infection, fungus infection, and tuberculosis.

The Sabin-Feldman dye test is most often used to detect serum antibodies, but the dye test has been replaced in many laboratories by the hemagglutination test or the indirect fluorescent antibody test. All of these tests provide approximately the same information, but it should be noted that the serum titers of any of these tests may be *extremely low* in patients who have ocular toxoplasmosis but no other signs of the disease [5]. *Any* titer of serum antibodies is significant when the patient has a fundus lesion that is compatible with that of ocular toxoplasmosis.

Tests on the aqueous humor have been used to confirm the presence of toxoplasmosis in doubtful cases. Such tests are most significant when the titer of antibodies in the aqueous humor is higher than in the serum. In such cases, it must be shown that the titer of antibodies per milligram of γ-globulin is higher in the aqueous than in the serum. When this can be proved, it indicates that there is local formation of specific anti-*Toxoplasma* antibodies in the uveal tract, and this, indeed may be diagnostic.

PATHOGENESIS

The organism that causes toxoplasmosis is *Toxoplasma gondii,* now known to be an intestinal parasite of the cat [6]. The oöcysts of the organism are shed in cat feces, and the latter may be ingested by rodents or birds that can serve as reservoirs or intermediate hosts of the parasite. Insect vectors also may transmit *Toxoplasma* from cat feces to man's foods or to herbivorous animals whose flesh man eats [7]. Humans probably acquire the parasite most frequently by the ingestion of raw or undercooked meat, and many infections probably could be prevented by the avoidance of steak tartare or other similar foods.

When *Toxoplasma* reaches the retina and multiplies, it causes highly destructive reactions that rupture the cells. The organisms released by this process invade new, previously intact retinal cells in the vicinity, and the latter are also soon destroyed. The human body attempts to defend itself against the onslaught by sending lymphocytes, plasma cells, and macrophages to the site of the retinal lesion. These cellular elements arrange themselves as a "zonal granuloma" in the retina, an area of central necrosis being surrounded by lamellae of lymphocytes, plasma cells, and occasionally giant cells. Sometimes the necrosis is so severe as to cause infiltration by polymorphonuclear leukocytes [8, 9].

Toxoplasma appears to grow best in central nervous system tissue and in the retina. It is not known whether this represents a special tropism or whether these tissues are somehow less well defended than other tissues of the body. It has been shown that *Toxoplasma* often persists in the brain and the retina long after other organs of the body have rid themselves of the parasite.

The congenital form of the disease is best understood. A woman who acquires *Toxoplasma* infection during pregnancy is likely to transmit the disease to the fetus. The organism invades the placental barrier and may attack many organs of the fetus. The fetal brain and the eyes are especially susceptible to damage, particularly during the first 90 days of gestation. Babies infected by congenital toxoplasmosis are often born with well healed retinal scars, indicating that the disease has run its course *in utero* (Fig. 27.2). In later life such persons may show recurrences of toxoplasmic retinochoroiditis. Many investigators believe that virtually all ocular toxoplasmosis represents early or late recurrence of congenital disease.

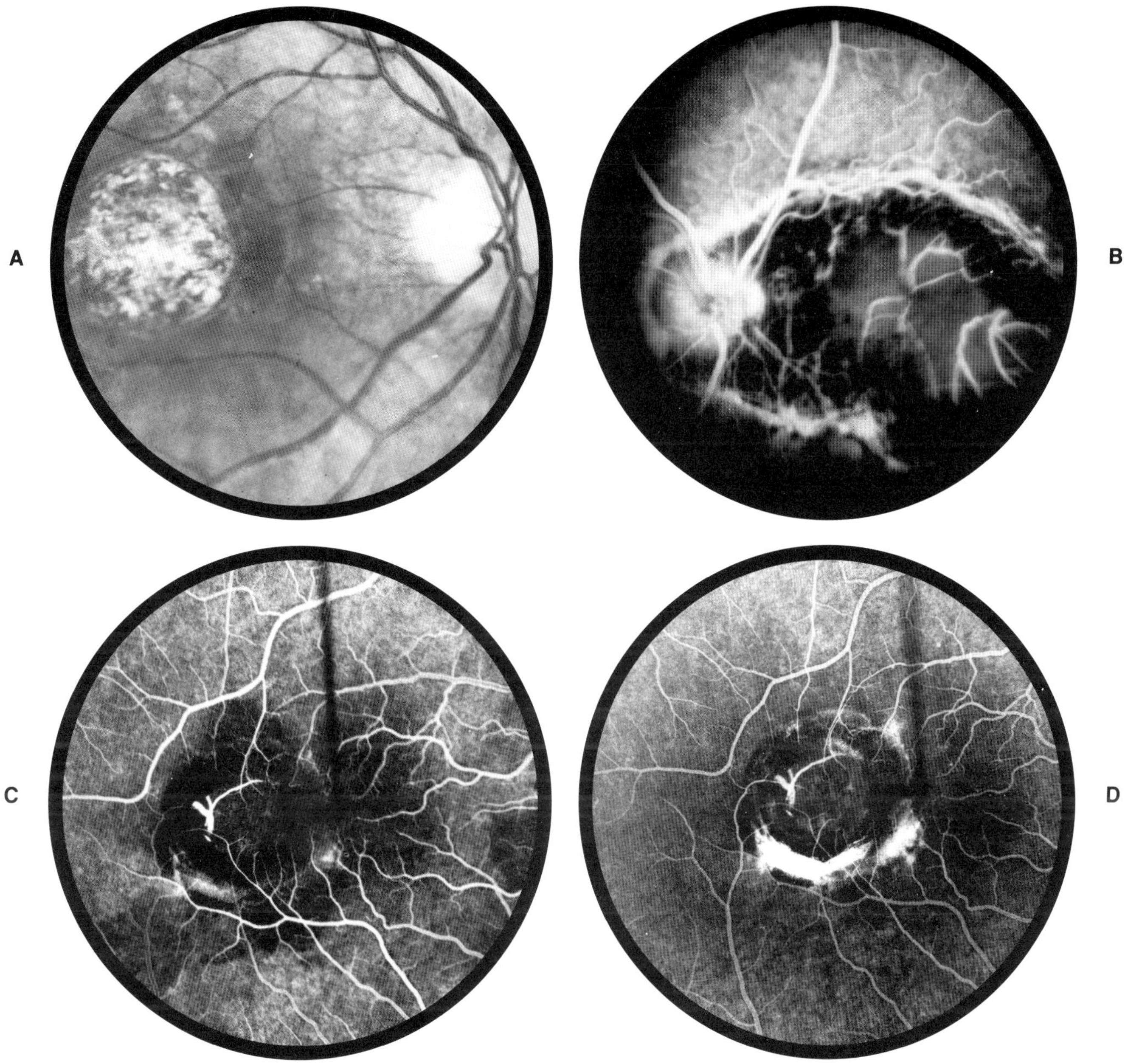

Figure 27.2. Presumed congenital toxoplasmosis. *A,* ophthalmoscopic photograph. Note the atrophic circumscribed macular scar. Similar pigmentary changes were noted in the peripheral fundus of both eyes. *B,* venous phase fluorescein angiogram on a child with a large peripapillary and macular atrophic scar. Note the absence of the ground glass hyperfluorescence within the central portion of the scar, indicative of an absence or reduction in the choriocapillaris. Larger choroidal vessels are seen to course through the lesion. Hyperfluorescence at the margin of the scar is produced by staining of the visible sclera from intact adjacent choriocapillaris. *C,* arteriovenous phase, and *D,* late venous phase of a 6-year-old patient with an atrophic scar and a visual acuity of 20/20 because of sparing of the fovea as indicated by the fixation target. A large choroidal vessel visible within the scar shows no evidence of leakage. Some retinal vessels, arterioles and particularly venules communicate with the subretinal scar. There is late staining of visible sclera and scar.

COURSE

Usually, the retinal lesions heal leaving atrophic spots with exuberant pigmentation around the edges (Figs. 27.1*B* and 27.3). The healing occurs from 3 weeks to 12 months, depending upon the virulence of the infecting organism, the competence of the patient's immunologic defense system, and the extent of the hypersensitivity response. With healing of the lesions, the vitreous usually clears and good visual acuity is restored only when the macula (or its neuronal connections to the optic nerve) has not been affected. Rarely, the severity of the exudative reaction in the vitreous during the active phase of the lesions will cause tearing of the retina from contracting strands of organized vitreous and eventuate in retinal detachment.

The patient generally remains free of symptoms until a recurrent lesion develops several months or even years after the initial attack. Recurrent lesions appear most often at sites immediately adjacent to former lesions and are known as "satellites" (Fig. 27.4). The patients notes reappearance of floating spots or blurred vision. Recurrences are believed to be caused by the breakdown of *Toxoplasma* cysts in the retina. These cysts, containing masses of dormant or metabolically depressed parasites, rupture into the retinal tissues releasing viable organisms and a considerable amount of antigen. It is thought that some of the organisms invade retinal cells, causing additional retinal necrosis. Hypersensitivity reactions in a previously sensitized patient also may occur at this time, and may account for the highly exudative reaction in the lesion as well as the perivasculitis that often develops adjacent to the recurrent retinal lesion. Retinal vascular ischemia, sensory retinal detachment, subretinal neovascularization, retinal phlebitis, and papillitis may accompany recurrent lesions (Fig. 27.5).

Recurrent lesions in the fundus often are accompanied or followed by an intense reaction in the anterior segment of the eye. This reaction is characterized by redness, pain, and photophobia. Slit-lamp examination shows the signs of acute granulomatous uveitis with "mutton fat" keratic precipitates on the cornea, numerous cells and flare in the anterior chamber, iris nodules, hyperemia of the iris, and posterior synechia formation. Sometimes there is also an acute rise of intraocular pressure [10].

Anterior uveitis occasionally appears at a time when only a minor recurrence can be seen in the fundus. Since proliferative organisms have never been found in the anterior segment, it is believed that the release of minute amounts of antigen of *Toxoplasma* in the posterior segment may trigger the anterior uveitis, as a strictly hypersensitivity or autoimmune reaction.

A

B

C

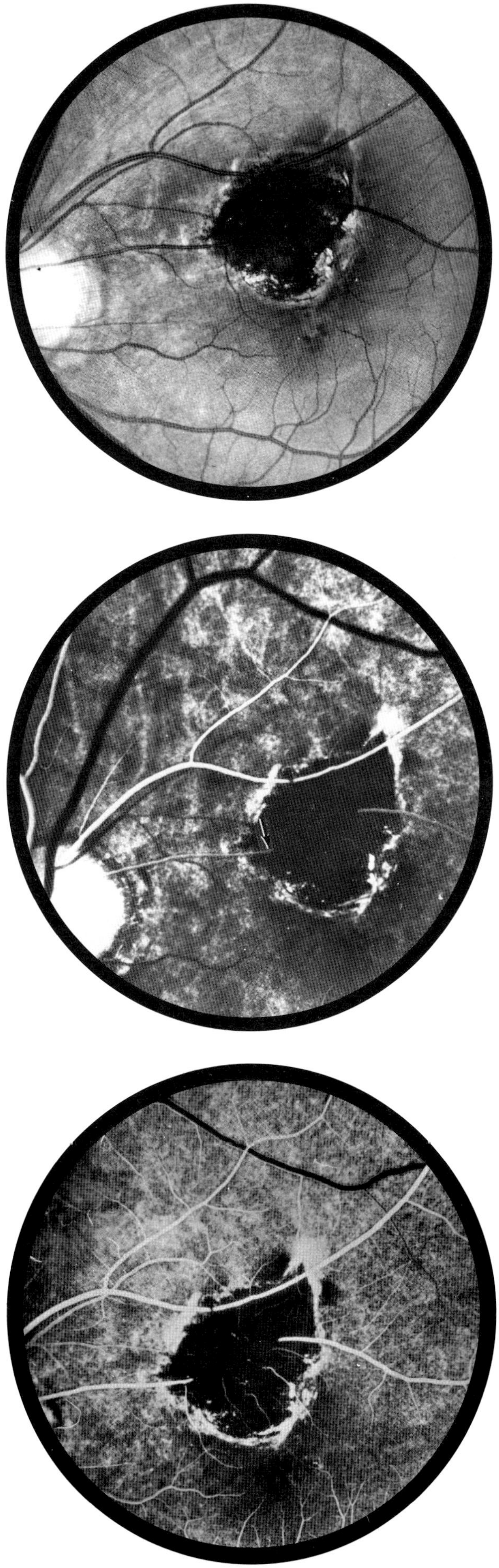

Figure 27.3. Healed pigmentary chorioretinitic scar presumed to be caused by ocular toxoplasmosis. *A*, ophthalmoscopic photograph with a dense pigmentary scar in the macular region, presumed to be due to ocular toxoplasmosis. *B*, arterial phase angiogram. The pigmented toxoplasmosis lesion is hyperfluorescent. Note that a segment of the superior temporal retinal artery disappears as it emerges into the scar (*arrows*) and reappears at its opposite end to perfuse the more distal retina. *C*, arteriovenous phase angiogram. Several small branches of the superior temporal vein also enter the chorioretinal scar to drain the healed lesion. A number of second order retinal vessels, which are branches of the major arteriole, emerge from the center of the scar. Some of the vascular channels may represent retinochoroidal anastomoses. The margins of the scar hyperfluoresce because of atrophy of the pigment epithelium and staining of visible sclera.

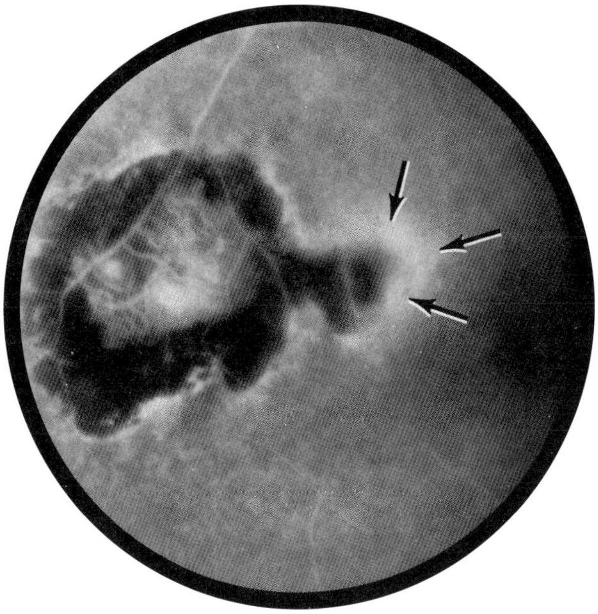

Figure 27.4. Fluorescein angiogram of recurrent retinitis at the site of old chorioretinal scars presumed to be caused by ocular toxoplasmosis. On the venous phase angiogram note the geographic area of hypofluorescence at the site of a pigmentary scar in the temporal macula. Centrally the large choroidal vessels are visible. An area of hyperfluorescence is noted (*arrows*) at the site of recurrent retinitis or "satellite" lesion. Such lesions appear most often immediately adjacent to former lesions many months or years after the initial attack.

A

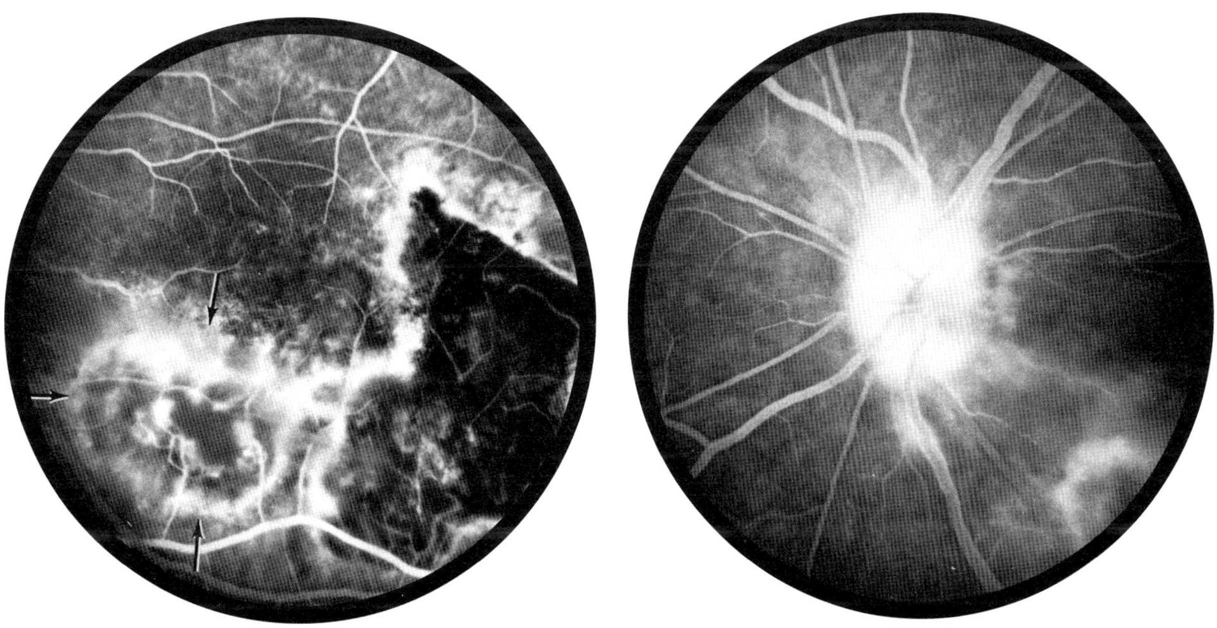

B

Figure 27.5. Fluorescein angiograms of recurrent retinitis in presumed ocular toxoplasmosis. *A*, early venous phase angiogram. Note the satellite lesion adjacent to an old chorioretinal scar (*arrows*). Retinal vascular nonperfusion is present within the area of active retinitis. These vessels are also permeable, showing evidence of leakage as they stain the scar. The old scar is predominantly hypofluorescent and shows multiple retinochoroidal anastomoses. *B*, late phase angiogram. An active papillitis and retinal phlebitis is present seen as late hyperfluorescence with staining of the disc and adjacent peripapillary veins. In addition to the retinal ischemia, phlebitis, and papillitis, sensory retinal detachments and subretinal neovascularization may also complicate lesions of toxoplasmosis retinochoroiditis.

TREATMENT

The standard treatment for ocular toxoplasmosis consists of pyrimethamine (Daraprim) and sulfonamide therapy. The drugs are given orally, with a loading dose of 150 mg pyrimethamine, followed by from 25–50 mg daily for 6 weeks. A loading dose of 2 g of triple sulfas or sulfadiazine is followed by 1g doses of the same medication four times a day for 6 weeks. Concomitant use of folinic aid, 3mg doses three times a week, generally prevents leukopenia and thrombocytopenia that could result from pyrimethamine therapy, but the leukocyte and platelet count must be monitored on at least a weekly basis throughout the course of therapy.

Results of therapy with pyrimethanime and sulfonamides are disappointing or not reliable in regards to old massive lesions of the fundus that have been present for several months [10]. For this reason new drugs such as clindamycin are being investigated for their efficacy by both oral and subconjunctival routes. Agents such as chlortetracycline hydrochloride and spiramycin also may have some efficacy, but they are not generally used in the United States.

Corticosteroids must be used not only with great caution, but strictly with the concomitant administration of antimicrobial agents [11]. Oral ingestion of corticosteroids may be in dosages of from 80–100 mg prednisone to quell acute inflammatory lesions that threaten the destruction of the macula or optic nerve. Periocular injections of depot corticosteroids should be *avoided* because such materials, administered by this route, may be immunosuppressive and may result in uncontrollable proliferation of the organism.

Agents that augment the efficiency of macrophages or of lymphocyte macrophage interactions eventually may prove useful in controlling this disease. Such agents as levamisole hydrochloride and "transfer factor" are undergoing experimental trials.

Light coagulation therapy [12] and cryotherapy [13] each have had limited success, although with these modalities overly vigorous treatment has resulted in ophthalmic disasters, and neither therapy invariably has prevented recurrences.

Ocular Toxocariasis

For several decades the systemic signs and symptoms of the larva migrans syndrome in children have been well defined, but only recently have the ocular manifestations become known [14–18]. The frequency of the ocular manifestations is still a controversial subject. Although toxocariasis has been seen in enucleated globes of 2% of children less than 15-years-old [19], some authorities cite an incidence as high as 10% in children with uveal and retinal inflammatory disease [20].

SIGNS AND SYMPTOMS

Toxocariasis primarily produces three recognizable ocular syndromes, occurring in different age groups: chronic endophthalmitis, localized granuloma, peripheral granuloma.

(1) Chronic endophthalmitis

This syndrome typically affects children between the ages of 2 and 9 years. The disorder almost always is unilateral and is associated with exudation that fills the vitreous cavity, and a cyclitic membrane. Pain, photophobia, increased lacrimation, severely decreased vision, and an acutely inflamed globe are present.

(2) Localized granuloma

Children between the ages of 6 and 14 years most frequently exhibit single localized granulomas as the manifestation of toxocariasis. The lesion may be present in the macula or in the peripapillary region; it is white, from 1–2 disc diameters in size, is elevated, and is localized in the retina. Little reaction is associated with the granuloma; the eye generally is quiet; and decreased vision usually is the only presenting symptom. Exotropia may be present along with the central visual loss, but when the granuloma does not affect the macula, the patient may be entirely asymptomatic. The granuloma in the macula may resemble a disciform scar with hemorrhagic detachment, and subretinal neovascularization (Fig. 27.6). In the juxtapapillary region it may mimic an optic nerve lesion (Fig. 27.7). Retinal-choroidal anastomoses usually originating from retinal venule may develop in the healed scar.

(3) Peripheral granuloma

Patients between ages of 6 and 40 years may exhibit peripheral granuloma formation. The peripheral hemispheric mass is associated with dense connective tissue strands in the vitreous cavity, which may connect to the disc. Usually, there are no acute inflammatory signs. The traction on the macula frequently results in heterotopia; with the extraocular muscle deviation depending on the direction of the macular tug. Vision usually is significantly decreased.

Localized vitreous abscess, papillitis [21], pars planitis [22] development of preretinal tubes, and preretinal and vitreous hemorrhages also have been reported.

A B C D

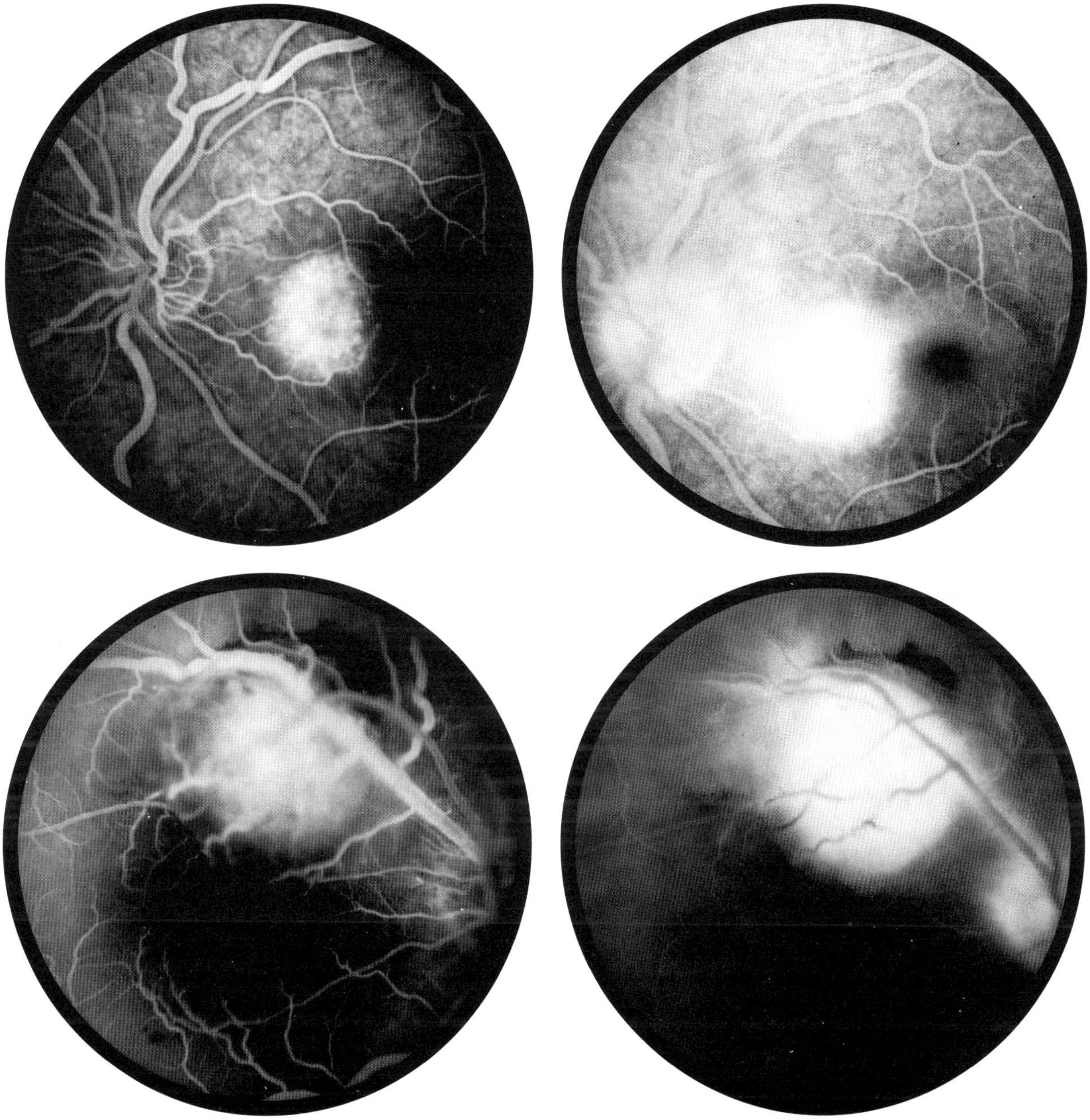

Figure 27.6. Presumed acute intraocular toxocariasis. *A*, late venous phase angiogram of a 13-year-old boy. Note the subretinal leakage at the site of the localized exudative lesion in the nasal macula. *B*, late phase angiogram of same patient. Late pooling beneath the subsensory retina and mild staining of the optic nerve is noted. *C*, late venous phase angiogram on a 22-year-old male with a hemorrhagic detachment of the macula. Note the hypofluorescence above the superior temporal arcade from subretinal hemorrhage and the hyperfluorescence subretinally from the associated subretinal neovascularization. *D*, late phase angiogram. There is marked late hyperfluorescence subretinally from staining of the scar and pooling into the subretinal space. A retinal phlebitis, evident as staining on the walls of the vessels and minimal staining of the optic nerve, also accompanies this lesion. The presence of a monocular localized, subretinal exudative lesion in the macula or a disciform scar in a child with no other evidence of ocular disese suggests the possibility of intraocular toxocariasis.

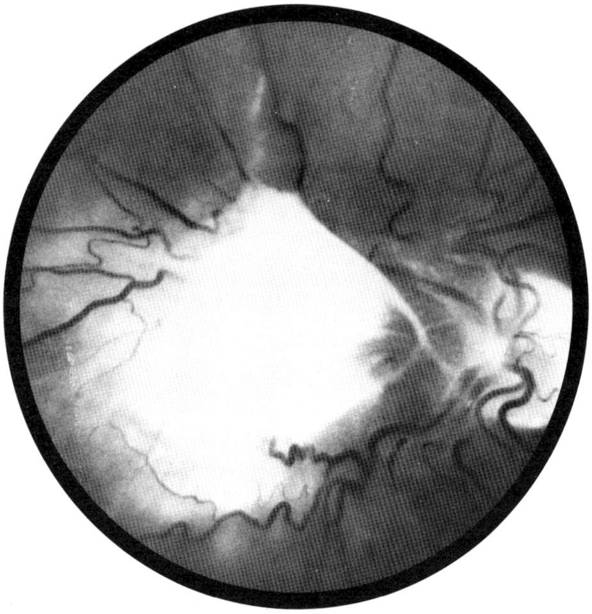

A

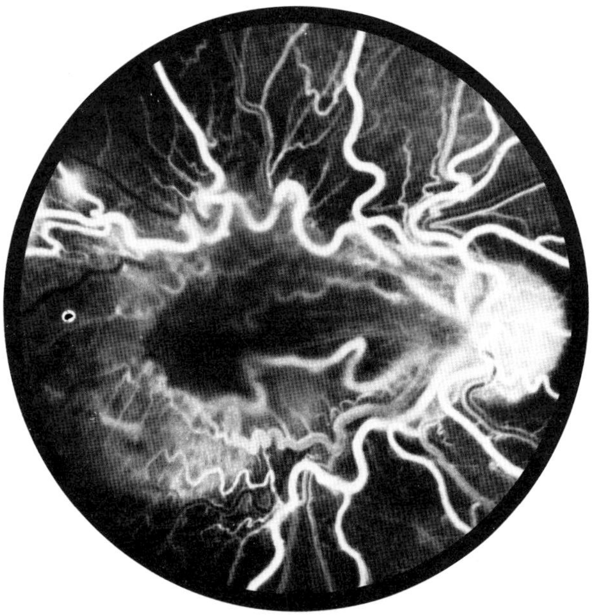

B

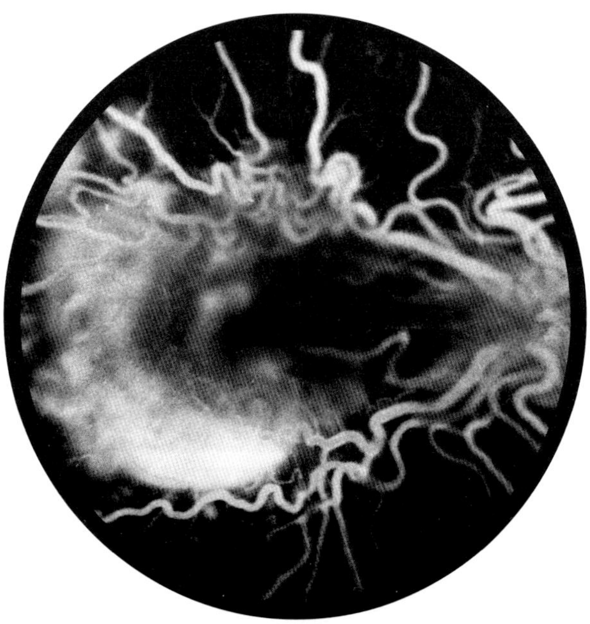

C

Figure 27.7. Presumed healed intraocular toxocariasis. *A,* ophthalmoscopic photograph of a 7-year-old male revealing elevated yellowish chorioretinal mass extending from the temporal aspect of the disc through the macular region, associated with retinal vascular tortuosity, prominent and preretinal membrane change. *B,* arteriovenous phase angiogram, same patient. Note accentuation of the marked retinal tortuosity and blockage of some retinal vessels by scar. Some of the retinal vessels communicate with the scar. *C,* late venous phase angiogram, same patient. Note dye leakage within and around the scar from some of its abnormal vessels. (Courtesy of Maurice Rabb, M.D.) *D,* ophthalmoscopic photograph of a 24-year-old female with a history of intraocular inflammation in childhood. Note the subretinal yellowish-white gliotic scar just above the disc. It is associated with a vitreoretinal interface disturbance, radiating retinal folds toward the macula and dilated, tortuous retinal vessels. *E,* arterial phase angiogram, same patient. Note the marked prominence and tortuosity of the retinal circulation in the region of the preretinal membrane formation. *F,* arteriovenous phase angiogram same patient. There is a delay in the filling of the large venule directly above the optic nerve. Its adjacent tributary is already fluorescing. Multiple venous-to-venous collaterals extend from this vein toward the optic nerve head (short arrows). A similar venous-to-venous anastomosis extends from a branch of the superior temporal vein toward the optic nerve head (*long arrows*). *G,* note the staining of the subretinal juxtapapillary scar. The anastomotic connections between the superior venule and the disc do not leak, indicating that they are collaterals rather than neovascularized vessels. In this juxtapapillary, subretinal, monocular tumor, obstruction of the superior branch of the superior temporal vein resulted in compensatory venous-to-venous collaterals which course through the scar. Patients with intraocular toxocariasis may present with a variety of clinical pictures which include an optic nerve tumor. These lesions may be associated with retinal choroidal or retinal-to-retinal venous anastomoses.

D

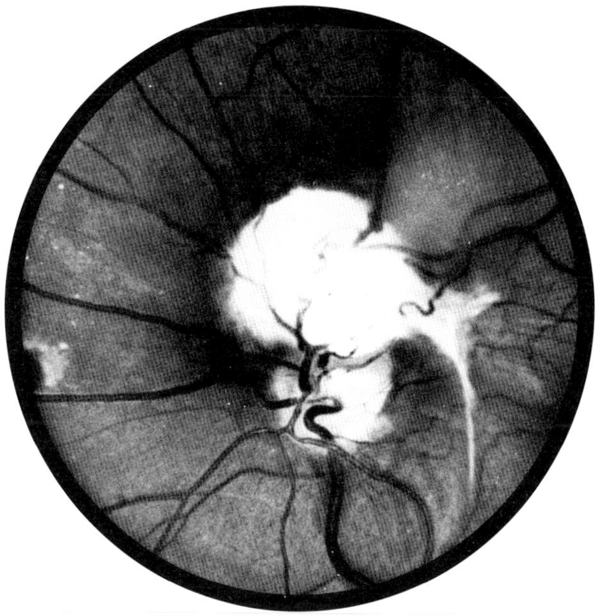

E

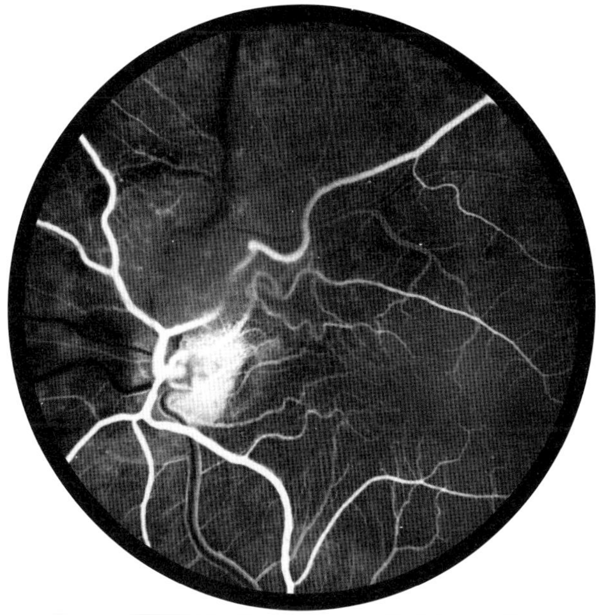

F

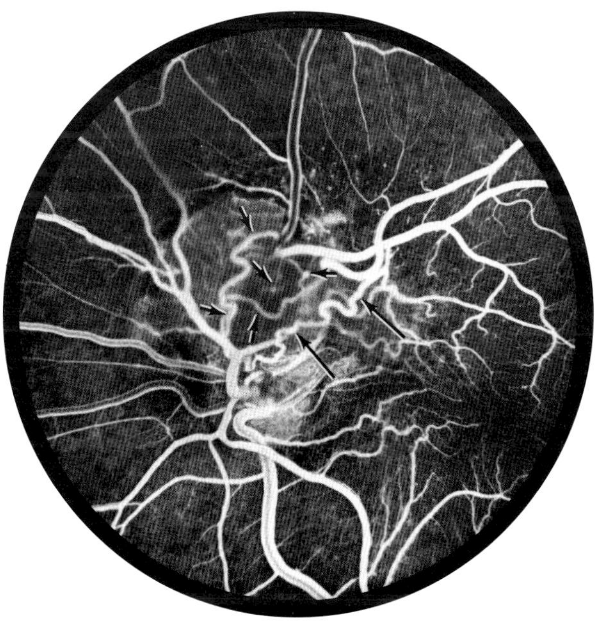

G

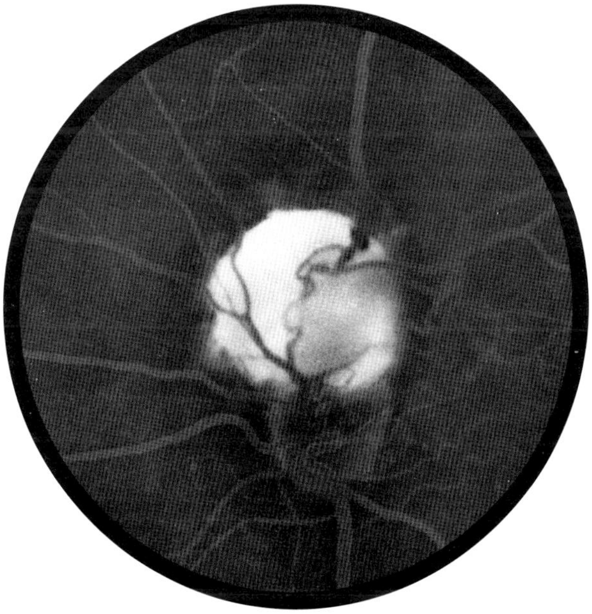

DIAGNOSIS

Confirmation by laboratory tests short of histopathologic corroboration of the clinical picture is not possible. The currently employed serologic and available skin testing material is of little value in establishing a diagnosis; although eosinophilia (3–12%) may be present early in the course of the syndrome, it seldom is present at the time of ocular involvement. The recent development of the enzyme linked immunosorbant agglutination (ELISA) serologic test for *Toxocara* holds some promise for additional laboratory help with the diagnosis. Presently, however, the ophthalmologist must diagnose the entity on the basis of the fairly characteristic clinical picture without the aid of confirming laboratory results of tests.

PATHOGENESIS

Toxocara canis and *Toxocara cati* are the organisms that produce the lesions of toxocariasis in humans. *Toxocara cati,* however, has not been isolated from an eye [23]. The *Toxocara canis* larva is 20 μ in diameter and 250 μ long. In transverse section, the appearance is of a refractile cuticle with lateral spines and two excretory columns, whereas longitudinal sections show a central tube surrounded by rows of small body nuclei.

In a world filled with dogs and cats there are infinite chances for human exposure to the ova of *Toxocara.* Although dirt-eating youngsters are the group most susceptible to the infection, the ability for the *Toxocara canis* and *Toxocara cati* ova to survive in the soil and to contaminate vegetation makes every human a potential reservoir for this disease.

Once ingested by man, the ova pass into the intestinal tract where they produce larvae. The larvae invade the wall of the intestine, penetrate the intestinal blood vessels, and are carried by the portal system to the liver where eosinophilic granulomas form. Some of the larvae survive, invade the lung, and are then distributed throughout the body. Because of the larval predilection for tissue of the central nervous system, it is not surprising that growth progresses in the retina [2]. The larva produces retinal tracks with hemorrhages, as well as subretinal tube formation [25], but the basic granulomatous lesion is caused by the response to larval death. The resulting eosinophilic granuloma consists of epithelioid cells, foreign body giant cells, fibrin, lymphocytes, and many eosinophils.

COURSE

Chronic endophthalmitis due to *Toxocara* usually results in destruction of the globe, which frequently is enucleated because of the clinical similarity to retinoblastoma. Both peripheral and central granuloma formation frequently are inactive and nonprogressive. Movement of the nematode is accompanied by retinal edema, with hemorrhage, a rarely reported phenomenon.

TREATMENT

In active disease, when live, motile larvae are present, care must be taken to avoid the use of agents that will kill the parasite and initiate an inflammatory response. Thiabendazole, an anthelmintic, should be used only when there is danger that the live worm will enter the macula. Periocular and systemic administration of corticosteroids, therefore, is the primary treatment of the active inflammatory response associated with the various forms of toxocariasis.

References

1. Jacobs, L., Naquin, H., Hoover, R., and Woods, A.C.: A comparison of the toxoplasmin skin tests, the Sabin-Feldman dye tests, and the complement fixation tests for toxoplasmosis in various forms of uveitis. *Bull Johns Hopkins Hosp, 99:* 1, 1956.
2. Woods, A.C.: Modern concepts of the etiology of uveitis. *Am J Ophthalmol, 50:* 1170, 1960.
3. Friedmann, C.T., and Knox, D.L.: Variations in active toxoplasmic retinochoroiditis. *Arch Ophthalmol, 81:* 481, 1969.
4. Frenkel, J.K.: Pathogenesis of toxoplasmosis with a consideration of cyst rupture in *Besnoitia* infection. *Surv Ophthalmol, 6:* 799, 1961.
5. Zscheile, F.P.: Recurrent toxoplasmic retinitis with weakly positive methylene blue dye test. *Arch Ophthalmol, 71:* 645, 1964.
6. Work, K., and Hutchinson, W.M.: A new cystic form of *Toxoplasma gondii. Acta Pathol Microbiol Scand, 75:* 191, 1969.
7. Wallace, G.D.: Experimental transmission of *Toxoplasma gondii* by filthflies. *Am J Trop Med Hyg, 20:* 411, 1971.
8. O'Connor, G.R.: Ocular toxoplasmosis. *Jpn J Ophthalmol, 19:* 1, 1975.
9. Perkins, E.S.: Ocular toxoplasmosis. *Brit J Ophthalmol, 57:* 1, 1973.
10. O'Connor, G.R.: Manifestations and management of ocular toxoplasmosis. *Bull N Y Acad Med, 50:* 192, 1974.
11. O'Connor, G.R., and Frenkel, J.K.: Dangers of steroid treatment in toxoplasmosis: periocular injections and systemic therapy. *Arch Ophthalmol, 94:* 213, 1976.
12. Spalter, H.F., Campbell, C.J., Noyori, K.S., Rittler, M.C., and Koester, C.J.: Prophylactic photocoagulation of recurrent toxoplasmic retinochoroiditis: a preliminary report. *Arch Ophthalmol, 75:* 21, 1966.
13. Dobbie, J.G.: Cryotherapy in the management of *Toxoplasma* retinochoroiditis. *Trans Am Acad Ophthalmol Otolaryngol, 72:* 364, 1968.
14. Ashton, N.: Larval granulomatosis of the retina due to *Toxocara. Brit J Ophthalmol, 44:* 129, 1960.
15. Wilder, H.C.: Nematode endophthalmitis. *Trans Am Acad Ophthalmol Otolaryngol, 55:* 99, 1950.
16. Beaver, P.C., Snyder, C.H., Carrera, G.M., Dent, J.H., and Lafferty, J.W.: Chronic eosinophilia due to visceral larve migrans: report of three cases. *Pediatrics, 9:* 7, 1952.
17. Nichols, R.L.: The etiology of visceral larva migrans. I. Diagnostic morphology of infective second-stage *Toxocara* larvae. *J Parasitol, 42:* 349, 1956.
18. Irvine, W.C., and Irvine, A.R., Jr.: Nematode endophthalmitis: *Toxocara canis*: report of one case. *Am J Ophthalmol, 47:* (part II) 185, 1959.
19. Leopold, I.H.: Is the dog really man's best friend? *Am J Ophthalmol, 59:* 717, 1965.
20. Perkins, E.S.: Patterns of uveitis in children. *Brit J Ophthalmol, 50:* 169, 1966.
21. Bird, A.C., Smith, J.L., and Curtin, V.T.: Nematode optic neuritis. *Am J Ophthalmol, 69:* 72, 1970.
22. Hogan, M.J., Kimura, S.J., and Spencer, W.H.: Visceral larva migrans and peripheral retinitis. *JAMA, 194:* 1345, 1965.
23. Brown, D.H.: Ocular *Toxocara canis.* II. Clinical review. *J Pediatr Ophthalmol, 7:* 182, 1970.
24. Ashton, N.: *Toxocara canis* and the eye. *In* Corneo-plastic Surgery, Proceedings of the Second International Corneo-Plastic Surgery Conference, ed. by P.V. Rycroft, p. 579, Pergamon Press, Oxford, 1969.
25. O'Connor, P.R.: Viceral larva migrans of the eye: subretinal tube formation. *Arch Ophthalmol, 88:* 526, 1972.

CHAPTER 28

Pars Planitis, Vogt-Koyanagi-Harada Syndrome, and Behçet's Disease

Stephen J. Ryan, M.D.

Pars Planitis

Intraocular inflammation is frequently accompanied by cystoid macular edema. Perhaps one of the most common inflammatory conditions with this association is the so-called pars planitis syndrome. This descriptive term and its related semantic problems have been oft debated and are the subject of some confusion. This same syndrome was termed "peripheral uveitis" by Schepens and Brockhurst [1–5]. Welch, *et al.* [6] provided a thorough descriptive name, but their abbreviated designation pars planitis has been adopted by many, while Hogan repopularized the term "chronic cyclitis" [7–9].

In his original description, Fuchs [10] described "chronic cyclitis" as a low-grade intraocular inflammation with minimal anterior chamber reaction and many vitreous opacities, but a quiet, external eye. Duke-Elder [11] emphasized the benign nature of the inflammation and added the findings of macular edema and retinal detachment. The exudate over the ora serrata-pars plana area inferiorly is characteristic. While exudate over the pars plana may be seen in other conditions such as sarcoidosis and other inflammations, it is typical of this entity.

The clinical constellation of cystoid maculopathy, disc edema, and vitreous cells is shared by "bird-shot choroidopathy" [12], senile "vitritis," and other intraocular inflammations in addition to pars planitis. Thus, pars planitis represents a syndrome and clinical constellation. Numerous uveitis surveys have failed to reveal any etiology for this syndrome. A great debate has raged as to whether this is primarily an inflammation of the ciliary body; whether, in fact, this is a "uveitis" primarily; or whether this is some disorder primarily of the vitreous or other parts of the eye.

The prognosis for vision correlates more with the severity rather than the duration of the inflammation. Smith, *et al.* [13] surveyed 100 patients with 173 involved eyes; and with good follow up, determined that 73% maintained 20/50 or better vision. They concluded that the visual prognosis is good despite the long course of most cases of chronic cyclitis. Cataracts are the most common complication, occurring in 76 eyes (42%) of those cases followed [13]. The great majority of these cases, however, tolerated cataract surgery extremely well. Cystoid macular edema proved to be the major cause of persistent decreased vision. Twenty-eight percent experienced severe macular involvement which accounted for their decreased vision [13].

Cystoid maculopathy is a very common accompaniment of pars planitis and frequently accounts for the gradual onset of blurred vision and can account for metamorphopsia and the appearance of a scotoma (Fig. 28.1). The leakage frequently occurs not only from the perifoveal capillary net, but also from many capillaries throughout the posterior pole and the disc. In this long-standing chronic inflammation, as in any case of long-standing cystoid maculopathy, irreversible changes can occur.

Treatment is directed toward the maculopathy. The most effective anti-inflammatory regimen seems to be corticosteroids. These can either be administered systemically as prednisone with the complications and side effects of long-term systemic steroid therapy or can be administered in a retrobulbar fashion with the complications related to repeated retrobulbar steroids.

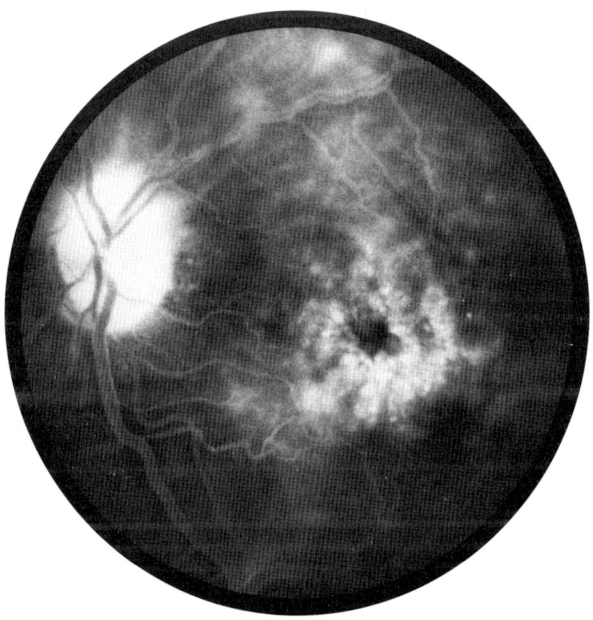

Figure 28.1. Late phase fluorescein angiogram in pars planitis. Note the intraretinal cystoid macular edema and more widespread intraretinal leakage from capillaries elsewhere in the posterior pole. Disc leakage, which often accompanies intraocular inflammation, is also evident.

Indomethacin has been employed but, as with other antiprostiglandins, questionable results have been noted. Antimetabolites have been used with varying success by different groups [14]. Cyclocryotherapy has been advocated by some ophthalmologists in refractory cases. Fortunately, however, it tends to be a self-limited condition with retention of good vision. Of those patients with significant maculopathy, the majority seem to respond to steroid therapy.

Related conditions include senile vitritis with some characteristics of the syndrome such as an otherwise quiet eye with intraocular inflammation and associated cystoid maculopathy, but without the pars plana exudate. Bird-shot choroidopathy also does not have pars plana exudates, but does have intraocular inflammation, a quiet eye, and may have cystoid maculopathy [12].

Vogt-Koyanagi-Harada Syndrome

Vogt-Koyanagi-Harada syndrome (VKH) is one of the uveomeningitides characterized by a granulomatous pan uveitis with central nervous system manifestations and depigmentation of the skin and hair [15]. This was initially described in 1892 by Hutchinson and in 1906 by Vogt [16] as bilateral uveitis with poliosis and alopecia. In 1926, Harada [17] described bilateral posterior uveitis with inferior exudative detachments and pleocytosis and lymphocytes in the cerebrospinal fluid. In 1929, Koyanagi [18] reviewed the syndrome with headache, fever, bilateral uveitis, dysacousia, poliosis, alopecia, and vitiligo. It would seem now to be apparent that there is no basis for a rigid distinction between Harada and Vogt-Koyanagi, but rather, that these are part of one syndrome—VKH [19].

The ocular findings in VKH include severe involvement of the anterior segment in 50% of cases reported in the United States [19]. The diffuse anterior uveitis can lead to synechiae and seclusion of the pupil with secondary glaucoma, cataract, and phthisis. The characteristic hallmark of the syndrome, however, is the exudative detachments, particularly inferiorly with 3+ vitreous opacities, with or without retinal hemorrhages, disc edema, and changes in the choroid. Disc hyperemia rather than optic neuritis can frequently be associated. Fluorescein angiography demonstrates a leakage of fluorescein from the choroid into the subpigment epithelial and subsensory retinal spaces (Fig. 28.2). The retinal vessels in most cases are normal. The optic disc most frequently reveals clinical hyperemia and leakage. The reattached retina demonstrates widespread pigmentary abnormalities throughout the fundus. This clumping of pigment leads to alternating areas of hyper- and hypopigmentation. Characteristic subretinal white spots occur more frequently in the periphery. These have been felt to be subretinal precipitates, but some may also represent areas of localized atrophy. Hemorrhagic macular detachment secondary to subretinal neovascularization has been reported as a manifestation of VKH [20].

The systemic associations include the central nervous system manifestations; i.e., headaches, loss of appetite with nausea and vomiting in association with seizures, coma, hemiparesis, psychosis, nystagmus, ataxia, the laboratory findings in the cerebrospinal fluid of lymphocytes, as well as an abnormal EEG.

Fifty percent of patients exhibit transient deafness and tinnitus. A frequent accompaniment is vitiligo, but most frequently, poliosis or alopecia will be associated. The course is one of gradual settling of the retina over a 6-month period with the diffuse pigmentary alterations in the fundus and occasionally iris depigmentation as well. Vision will usually return to normal within 1 year, but in some cases may remain decreased, particularly if there are microcystic macular changes at the macula.

Histopathologic studies have demonstrated a localized granulomatous response with epithelioid cells containing granules surrounded by plasma cells and lymphocytes. There can be marked proliferation of the retinal pigment epithelium [2]. The iris inflammation is nonspecific, containing lymphocytes and plasma cells without epithelioid cells. The choriocapillaris has been noted to be involved with VKH and classically is not involved in sympathetic ophthalmia.

The etiology of VKH is unknown and remains open for speculation. It is natural to suspect an infectious etiology because of its self-limiting nature and acute onset. There have been numerous studies in which animals have been injected with cerebrospinal fluid, vitreous, and subretinal fluid from VKH patients. Sugiura claimed to have isolated a virus from four to eight blind passages in mice. Schlaegel reported eosinophilic inclusions in subretinal fluid, but this has not been confirmed.

An allergic therapy has considered a possible role for uveal pigment as an allergen. Hypothalamic involvement has been suggested by some. The prognosis for visual acuity has varied with the experience of different authors.

Systemic steroids in high doses are the accepted form of therapy. Shimizu and other Japanese authors have noted a very good success rate.

The relation to sympathetic ophthalmia has always been particularly intriguing [22, 23]. All of the systemic manifestations of VKH have been seen in sympathetic ophthalmia. Histopathologically, there is a similar appearance, including Dalen-Fuchs' nodules. Likewise, there may be a favorable response to steroids as noted. However, the history and findings will clearly allow one to differentiate these findings.

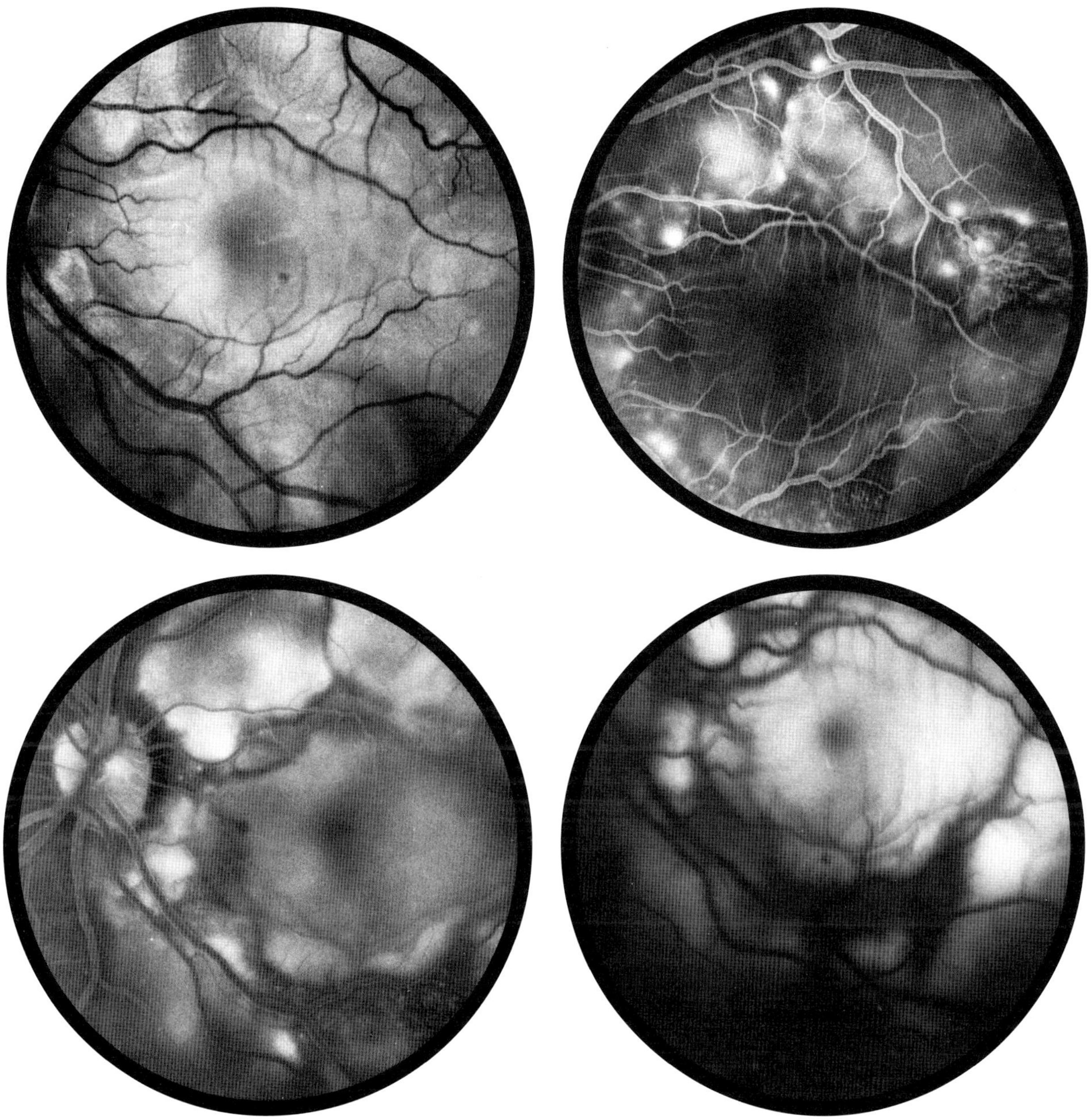

A B C D

Figure 28.2. Vogt-Koyanagi-Harada's syndrome. *A,* ophthalmoscopic photograph. Note the multiple pigment epithelial detachments beneath an overlying bullous retinal detachment. *B,* early venous phase angiogram. Note the numerous pigment epithelial leaks frequently located at the margins of the retinal pigment epithelial detachments, but also present in intervening spaces where pigment epithelium is flat. A faint hyperfluorescence is evident beneath the larger pigment epithelial detachments as dye slowly pools into the turbid subpigment epithelial space. *C,* late venous phase angiogram documenting clearly defined and well demarcated borders of the multiple pigment epithelial detachments which are filled with dye. *D,* late phase angiogram, as in *C.*

A B

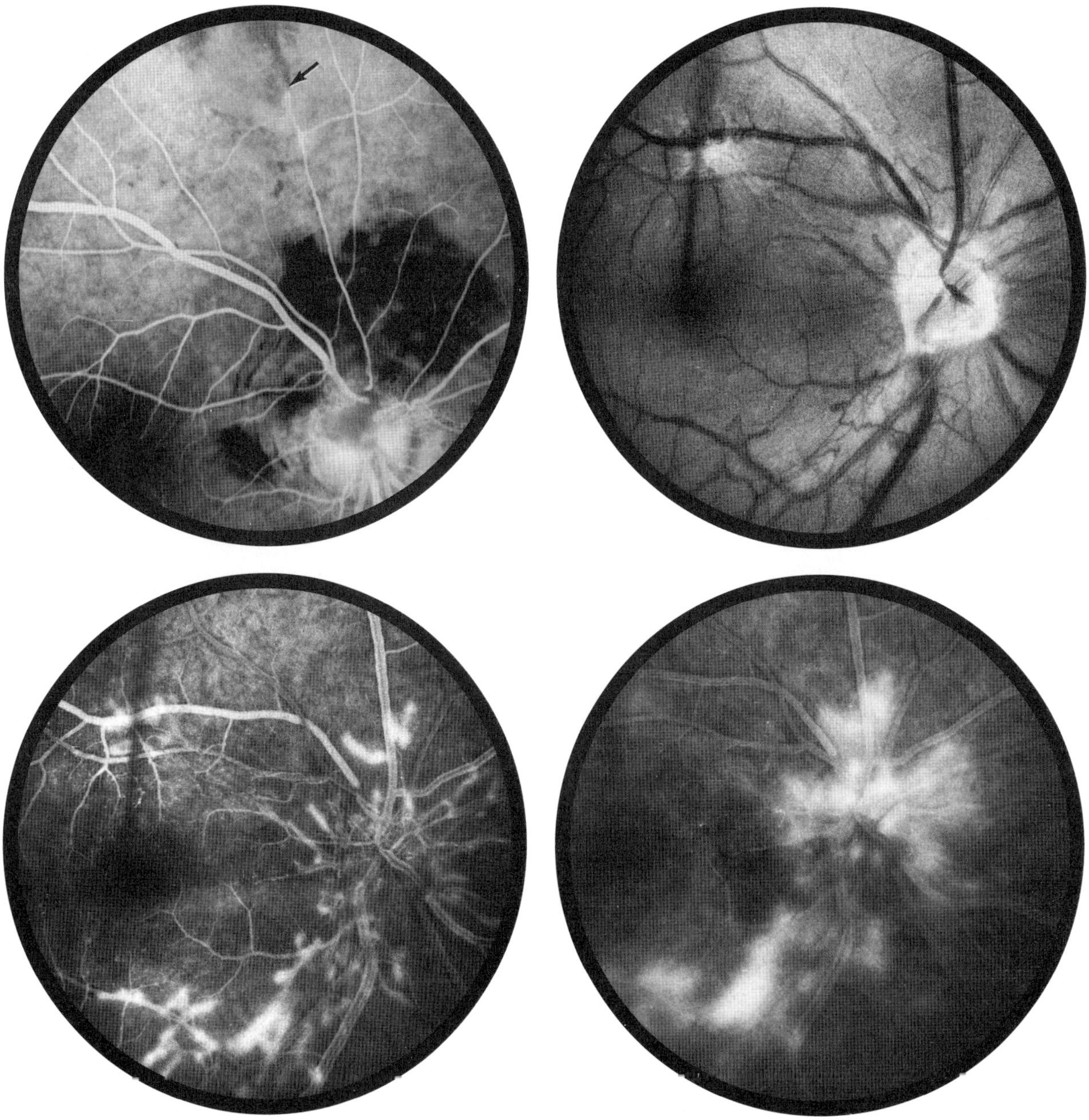

C D

Figure 28.3. Vascular occlusive changes in Behçet's disease. *A*, early venous phase angiogram. Note the hypofluorescence in the juxtapapillary area secondary to choroidal ischemia associated with vasoobliterative change in the superotemporal quadrant. Second order retinal capillaries are absent in this area and a tributary venule has occluded (*arrow*). This 26-year-old male eventually developed bilateral vaso-obliterative disease associated with genital and oral ulcers. *B*, ophthalmoscopic photo of patient with Behçet's disease. Note the retinal vascular proliferation and tortuosity surrounding the disc and along the retinal vascular arcades. A preretinal membrane is also present along the course of superotemporal arcade. *C*, late venous phase angiogram. Note the hypofluorescence at the site of preretinal and papillary neovascularization. *D*, late phase angiogram. Note the late hyperfluorescence from pooling of the dye into the vitreous. There is also widespread cystoid macular and retinal edema.

Behcet's Disease

Behçet emphasized the association of intraocular inflammation with hypopyon and ulceration of the genitalia and mouth as a distinct syndrome. It is of historical interest that Hippocrates had described this disorder in the 5th century B.C. [15]. It is most commonly encountered in the Middle East, the Mediterranean countries, and Japan. It characteristically occurs in the third decade and effects males more than females. The recurrent nature of this disorder is such that four to five attacks per year may occur for 20 years or more. It is characteristic for the eyes to become involved after the oral, mucosal, and genital ulcerations are present [24].

Acute anterior uveitis with hypopyon is the classic ocular presentation. However, cystoid macular edema with retinal periphlebitis and periarteritis as an occlusive vasculitis are frequently associated (Fig. 28.3). Retinal hemorrhage as well as vitreous hemorrhage can be associated. A significant number of patients also develop optic neuritis and atrophy. Most authors have emphasized the severity of this disease, i.e., going on to blindness of one or both eyes with phthisis or glaucoma, frequently the end result.

The systemic associations include the very large painful ulcers with a characteristic yellow necrotic base that can involve the gums, palate, pharynx, esophagus, and the tongue. The genital ulcerations characteristically involve the scrotum in the male and the labia minora in the female. Erythema nodosum may be the presenting dermatologic sign in the disorder. The observation that puncture of the skin may lead to a papule or pustule has been noted by many. Arthropathy, thrombophlebitis, and central nervous disorder, chiefly, involvement of the brainstem and cranial nerves [25], may accompany Behçet's syndrome.

The course is characterized by a series of progressive recurrences. While the disease may completely recede some 20 years or more after onset, it can also be accompanied by blindness at that stage [26]. The average resolution is 10–14 days; as might be expected, resolution would occur more slowly for the vitreous and posterior involvement. Fundus changes may occur before the appearance of iridocyclitis.

Mononuclear perivasculitis of the uvea and retina is the histopathologic hallmark of this disease. The retina may be detached and exhibit widespread hemorrhage. The optic nerve may be invaded with inflammatory cells. A polymorphonuclear response can be observed in the iris, anterior chamber, and vitreous [21, 27].

The etiology of Behçet's syndrome remains speculative. The fibrinoid degeneration observed has led to its consideration as a collagen disease. The possibility of an allergic or immunologic etiology has been considered by many [28, 29]. A possible viral etiology has, likewise, been the subject of much speculation and study [30, 31]. There is no satisfactory therapy available in this most difficult condition [33–35]. The role and efficacy of steroids remain debatable.

References

1. Schepens, C.L.: Examination of the ora serrata region: its clinical significance. *Acta XVI Consilium Ophthalmologica, 2:* 1384, 1950.
2. Brockhurst, R.J., Schepens, C.L., and Okamura, I.D.: Uveitis: I. Gonioscopy. *Am J Ophthalmol, 42:* 545, 1956.
3. Brockhurst, R.J., Schepens, C.L., and Okamura, I.D.: Uveitis: II. Peripheral uveitis: clinical description, complications, and differential diagnosis. *Am J Ophthalmol, 49:* 1257, 1960.
4. Brockhurst, R.J., Schepens, C.L., and Okamura, I.D.: Uveitis: III. Peripheral uveitis: pathogenesis, etiology, and treatment. *Am J Ophthalmol, 51:* 19, 1961.
5. Brockhurst, R.J., and Schepens, C.L.: Uveitis: IV. Peripheral uveitis: the complication of retinal detachment. *Arch Ophthalmol, 80:* 747, 1968.
6. Welch, R.B., Maumenee, A.E., and Wahlen, H.E.: Peripheral posterior segment inflammation, vitreous opacities, and edema of the posterior pole: pars planitis. *Arch Ophthalmol, 64:* 540, 1960.
7. Hogan, M.J., and Kimura, S.J.: Cyclitis and peripheral chorioretinitis. *Arch Ophthalmol, 66:* 667, 1961.
8. Hogan, M.J., Kimura, S.J., and O'Connor, G.R.: Peripheral retinitis and chronic cyclitis in children. *Trans Ophthalmol Soc U K, 85:* 39, 1965.
9. Kimura, S.J., and Hogan, M.J.: Chronic cyclitis. *Arch Ophthalmol, 71:* 193, 1964.
10. Fuchs, E.: Textbook of Ophthalmology, J. B. Lippincott, Philadelphia, 1908, p. 381.
11. Duke-Elder, S.: Textbook of Ophthalmology, Vol. 3: Diseases of the Inner Eye, C. V. Mosby, St. Louis, 1941.
12. Ryan, S.J., and Maumenee, A.E.: "Bird shot" choroidopathy, In preparation.
13. Smith, R.E., Godfrey, W.A., and Kimura, S.J.: Chronic cyclitis: I. Course and visual progress. *Trans Am Acad Ophthalmol Otolaryngol, 77:* 760, 1973.
14. Schlaegel, T.F.: Personal communication.
15. Duke-Elder, S.: System of Ophthalmology, Vol. 9: Diseases of the Uveal Tract, C. V. Mosby, St. Louis, 1966, pp. 359, 373.
16. Vogt, A.: Frühzeitiges Ergrauen der Zilien und Bemerkungen über den sogenannten plötzlichen Eintritt dieser Veränderung. *Klin Monatsbl Augenheilkd, 44:* 228, 1906.
17. Harada, E.: Bilateral exudative uveitis and pleocytosis of the cerebrospinal fluid. *Acta Soc Ophthalmol Jpn, 30:* 356, 1926.
18. Koyanagi, Y.: Dysakusis, Alopecia, und Poliosis bei schwerer Uveitis nach Traumatischen Ursprungs. *Klin Monatsbl Augenheilkd, 82:* 194, 1929.
19. Cowper, A.R.: Harada's disease and Vogt-Koyanagi syndrome. *Arch Ophthalmol, 45:* 367, 1951.
20. Carlson, M.R., and Kerman, B.M.: Hemorrhagic macular detachment in the Vogt-Koyanagi-Harada's syndrome. *Am J Ophthalmol, 84:* 632, 1977.
21. Hogan, M.J., and Zimmerman, L.E. (eds.): Ophthalmic Pathology, W. B. Saunders, Philadelphia, 1962, p. 406.
22. Hodgkinson, C.P.: Vogt-Koyanagi-Harada syndrome. *Henry Ford Med Bull, 9:* 543, 1961.
23. Wong, V.G., Anderson, R., and O'Brien, P.J.: Sympathetic ophthalmia and lymphocyte transformation. *Am J Ophthalmol, 72:* 960, 1971.
24. Dowling, G.B.: Behçet's disease. *Proc Roy Soc Med, 54:* 101, 1961.
25. Schotland, D.L., Wolf, S.M., White, H.H., and Dubin, H.V.: Neurologic aspects of Behçet's disease: case report and review of the literature. *Am J Med, 34:* 544, 1963.
26. Mamo, J.G.: The rate of visual loss in Behçet's disease. *Arch Ophthalmol, 84:* 451, 1970.
27. Winter, F.C., and Yukins, R.E.: The ocular pathology of Behçet's disease. *Am J Ophthalmol, 62:* 257, 1966.
28. Pearson, C.M., Waksman, B.H., and Sharp, J.T.: Studies of arthritis and other lesions induced in rats by injection of mycobacterial adjuvant. V. Changes affecting the skin and mucous membranes. Comparison of the experimental process with human disease. *J Exp Med, 113:* 485, 1961.
29. Shimizu, T., Katsuta, Y., and Oshima, Y.: Immunological studies on Behçet's syndrome. *Ann Rheum Dis, 24:* 494, 1965.
30. Sezer, F.N.: The isolation of a virus as the cause of Behçet's disease. *Am J Ophthalmol, 36:* 301, 1953.
31. Sezer, F.N.: Further investigations on the virus of Behçet's disease. *Am J Ophthalmol, 41:* 41, 1956.
32. Mortada, A., and Imam, I.Z.E.: Virus aetiology of Behçet's syndrome. *Brit J Ophthalmol, 48:* 250, 1964.
33. Kalbian, V.V., and Challis, M.T.: Behçet's disease: report of twelve cases with three manifesting as papilledema. *Am J Med, 49:* 823, 1970.
34. Wong, V.G.: Immunosuppressive therapy of ocular inflammatory diseases. *Arch Ophthalmol, 81:* 628, 1969.
35. Mamo, J.G., and Azzam, S.A.: Treatment of Behçet's disease with chlorambucil. *Arch Ophthalmol, 84:* 446, 1970.

PART V

Photocoagulation Therapy of Macular Disease

CHAPTER 29

Indications and Contraindications for Photocoagulation Therapy

Howard Schatz, M.D., Kurt A. Gitter, M.D., and Lawrence A. Yannuzzi, M.D.

The most important consideration in the treatment of macular disease is the viability of the fovea. Laser treatment is contraindicated for a fovea which has been irreversibly damaged but may be indicated for an abnormal but salvable fovea.

This chapter discusses the indications and contraindications for laser photocoagulation treatment of macular disease.

Indications for Laser Treatment

In the evaluation of an abnormal macula for possible argon laser photocoagulation, one must consider the specific histopathology of the macula as well as the potential reversibility of the abnormality either by natural history, laser or other means. There are three major changes occurring in the macula that may cause visual reduction by affecting the fovea and which may be reversible by laser. These changes are: (1) *fluid,* either in the substance of the retina or beneath it; (2) *exudate,* which has recently been deposited in the fovea or is threatening to do so; and (3) *neovascularization,* which is either on the surface of the retina or is growing from the retina into the vitreous, or neovascularization under the retina from proliferation of the choriocapillaris through Bruch's membrane, as occurs in macular degenerative and other diseases.

Each of these manifestations may reduce the vision. However, each change may be treatable with laser in order to arrest the progression of the disease and maintain vision, or to eliminate the abnormality and improve vision.

These three major changes occurring in the macula and affecting vision are outlined and discussed in the following section on indications for laser treatment of macular disease.

Indications for laser treatment of macular disease

- I. Fluid
  - (A) In retina (edema)
  - (B) Under retina
    - (1) Sensory retinal detachment
    - (2) Pigment epithelial detachment
- II. Exudate
  - (A) Foveal (recent)
  - (B) Threatening fovea
- III. Neovascularization
  - (A) Retinal and preretinal
  - (B) Subretinal

FLUID

Fluid in the Retina

Fluid in the retina (retinal edema), caused by leaking retinal vessels, will reduce vision when the perifoveal, capillary net, or macular retinal vessels leak fluid into the fovea and cause foveal edema. When the leakage is massive and involves all or most of the blood vessels of the macula, sufficient photocoagulation to cause resolution of the edema would be too intense and, therefore, too destructive to be of benefit. However, when the edema is localized, such as in certain cases of background diabetic retinopathy, branch vein occlusion or macular telangiectasia, laser therapy may be directed to the specific leaking areas without damage to the remainder of the macula. Resolution of the edema may occur and result in either an improvement of visual function or the prevention of further visual reduction.

Laser therapy is applicable in certain forms of nonproliferative diabetic retinopathy when vision is reduced to less than 20/50; the fluorescein angiogram will indicate the areas of retinal vascular leakage causing the foveal edema. The angiogram may also demonstrate that the foveal capillary net is intact. If it is not intact, i.e., if there is capillary nonperfusion involving the foveal capillary net, the visual reduction is probably irreversible and, therefore, treatment would be useless. For treatment to be effective and to cause resolution of the edema, it must be directed to the areas of retinal vascular leakage.

With branch vein occlusion, the leakage usually includes a portion of the perifoveal capillary net, in addition to the remainder of the macula that is involved in the occlusion. However, unless treatment to the abnormal portion of the perifoveal capillary net can be accomplished, treatment is useless. Treating only the remainder of the macular vessels without treating the leaking perifoveal capillary net will cause resolution of the macular edema without any change in the foveal edema; vision will, therefore, be unchanged. Treatment of the perifoveal capillary net is potentially hazardous and should be done with utmost caution (Fig. 29.1).

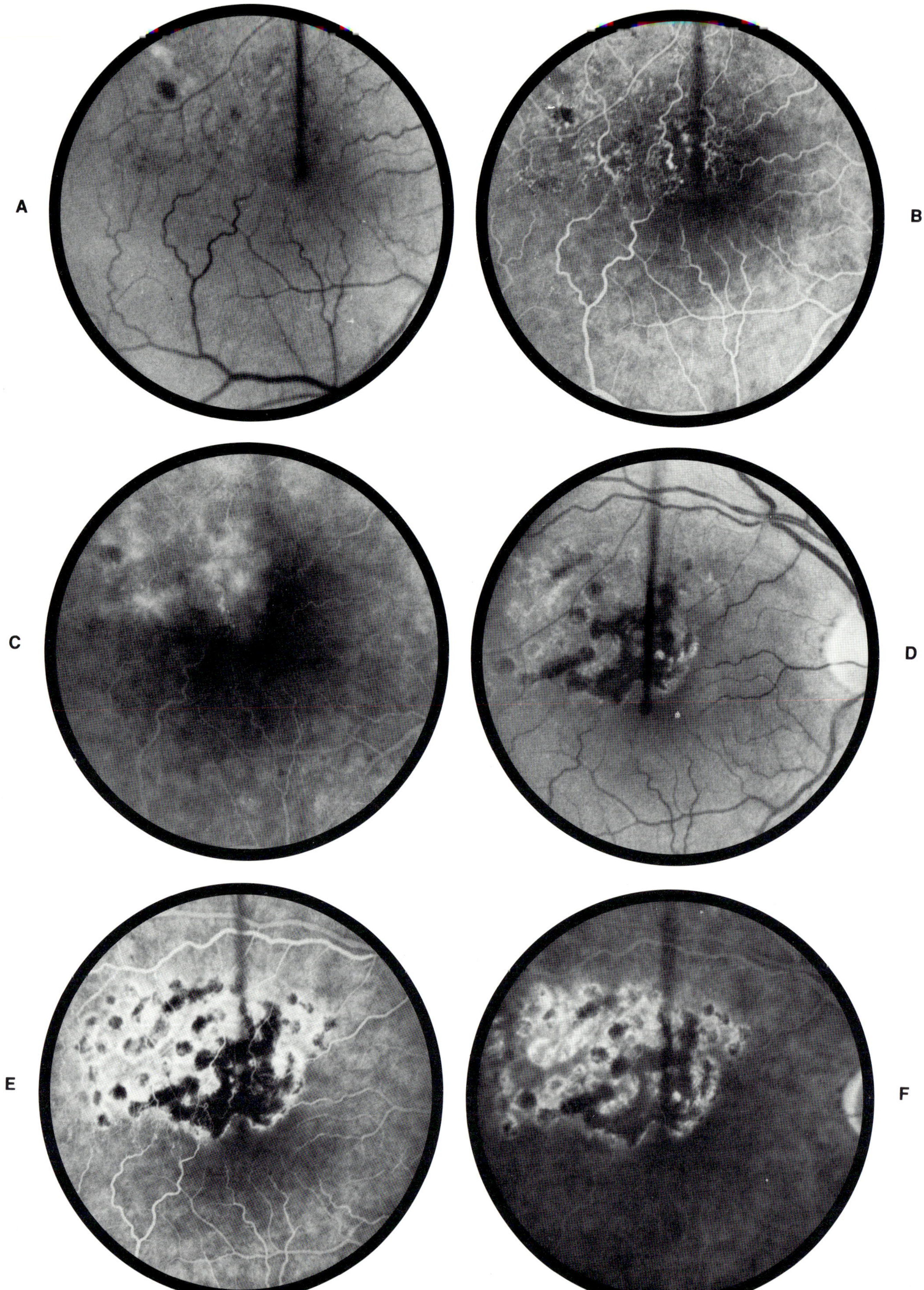

Figure 29.1

Fluid under the Retina

Deposition of fluid under the retina refers to a separation of the rods and cones from the pigment epithelium (a sensory retinal detachment) or separation of the pigment epithelium from Bruch's membrane (a pigment epithelial detachment).

Sensory retinal detachment

Any disease that causes detachment of the sensory retina of the macula results in reduction of central vision. There are many causes of sensory retinal detachment in the macula; one of the most common is central serous chorioretinopathy. Other choroidal diseases such as inflammation, tumors, subretinal neovascularization, and various retinal vascular diseases can cause sensory retinal detachment.

In central serous chorioretinopathy, leakage of fluid under the detached retina usually comes from the choriocapillaris through Bruch's membrane and through a single break in the pigment epithelium. This point of leakage can be sealed with laser and, thus, affect a reattachment of the sensory retina (Fig. 29.2). The indications for treatment of central serous chorioretinopathy are still not completely defined. It has been shown that the disease is resolved more quickly with treatment in comparison with the natural history. Some feel that the shorter duration of the disease with treatment produces better visual results, although no study has supported this impression. Although treatment is only infrequently recommended it is the general feeling among most ophthalmologists that the sooner the sensory retina is reattached, the better the ultimate visual result.

Figure 29.1. Branch vein occlusion with retinal edema, pre- and postoperative argon laser photocoagulation. *A*, ophthalmoscopic photograph of the right macula shows dilated and tortuous retinal vessels above and below the horizontal raphe. A few hemorrhages are also present. *B*, early venous phase angiogram shows that the dilated retinal vessels above the horizontal raphe are apparent along with a dilated superior portion of the perifoveal capillary net. A few areas of capillary nonperfusion are also present between these dilated vessels. *C*, late phase angiogram shows hyperfluorescence of the fovea and superior macula, indicating retinal edema. *D*, ophthalmoscopic photograph of the same patient, 12 weeks after argon laser photocoagulation. Note the pigmentation encircling the upper border of the fovea. *E*, arteriovenous phase angiogram shows hypofluorescence due to blockage by the pigmentation. There is some hyperfluorescence due to choroidal transmission (window defect) associated with the laser lesions. There is no significant retinal vascular dilation. *F*, late phase angiogram shows staining around the edges of the laser lesions, with no significant retinal edema. This patient had a branch vein occlusion with reduced vision secondary to dilated retinal vessels, which were leaking and causing foveal edema. Argon laser photocoagulation was directed to the dilated leaking retinal capillary bed; this treatment resulted in resolution of the edema and improvement of visual acuity.

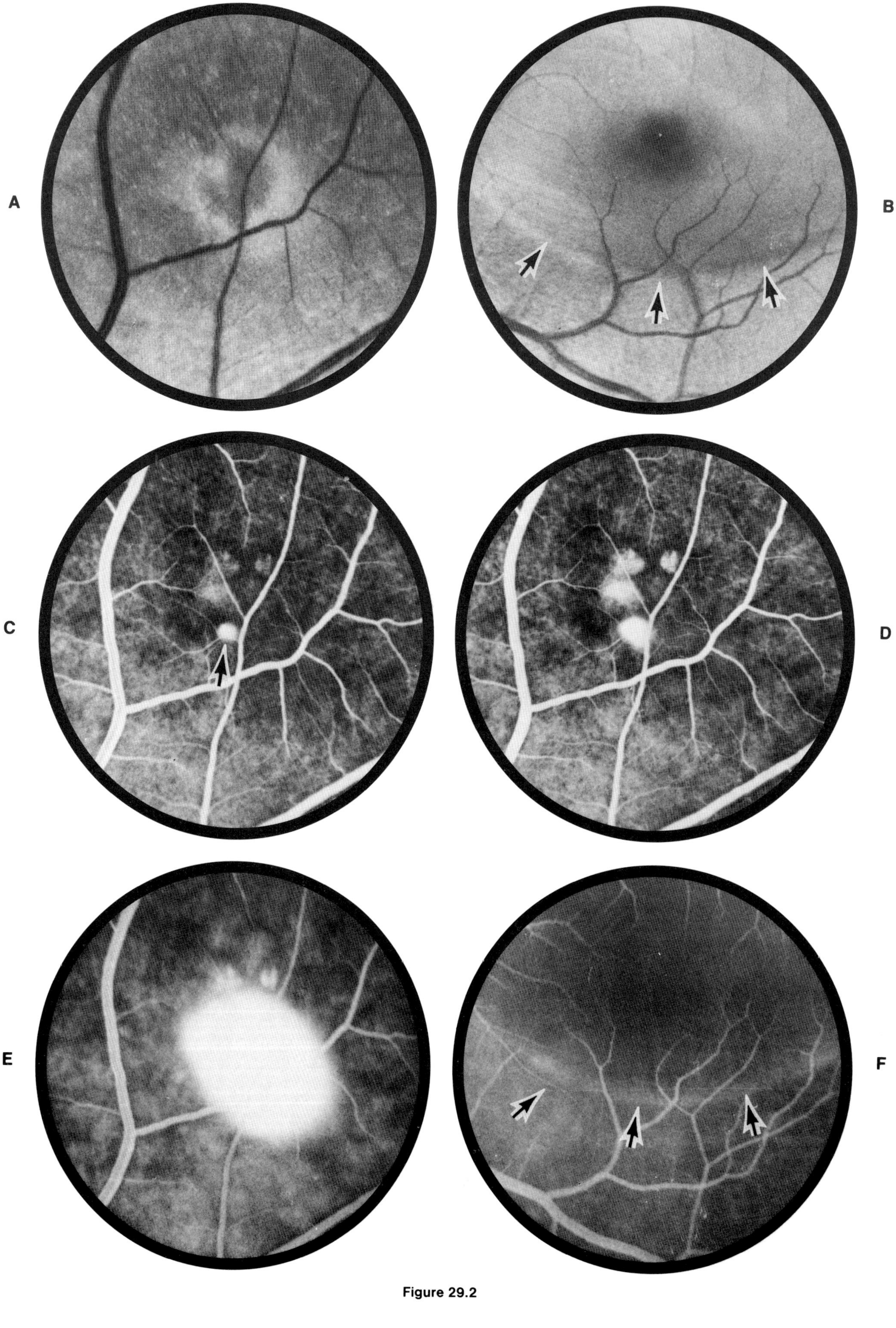

Figure 29.2

G

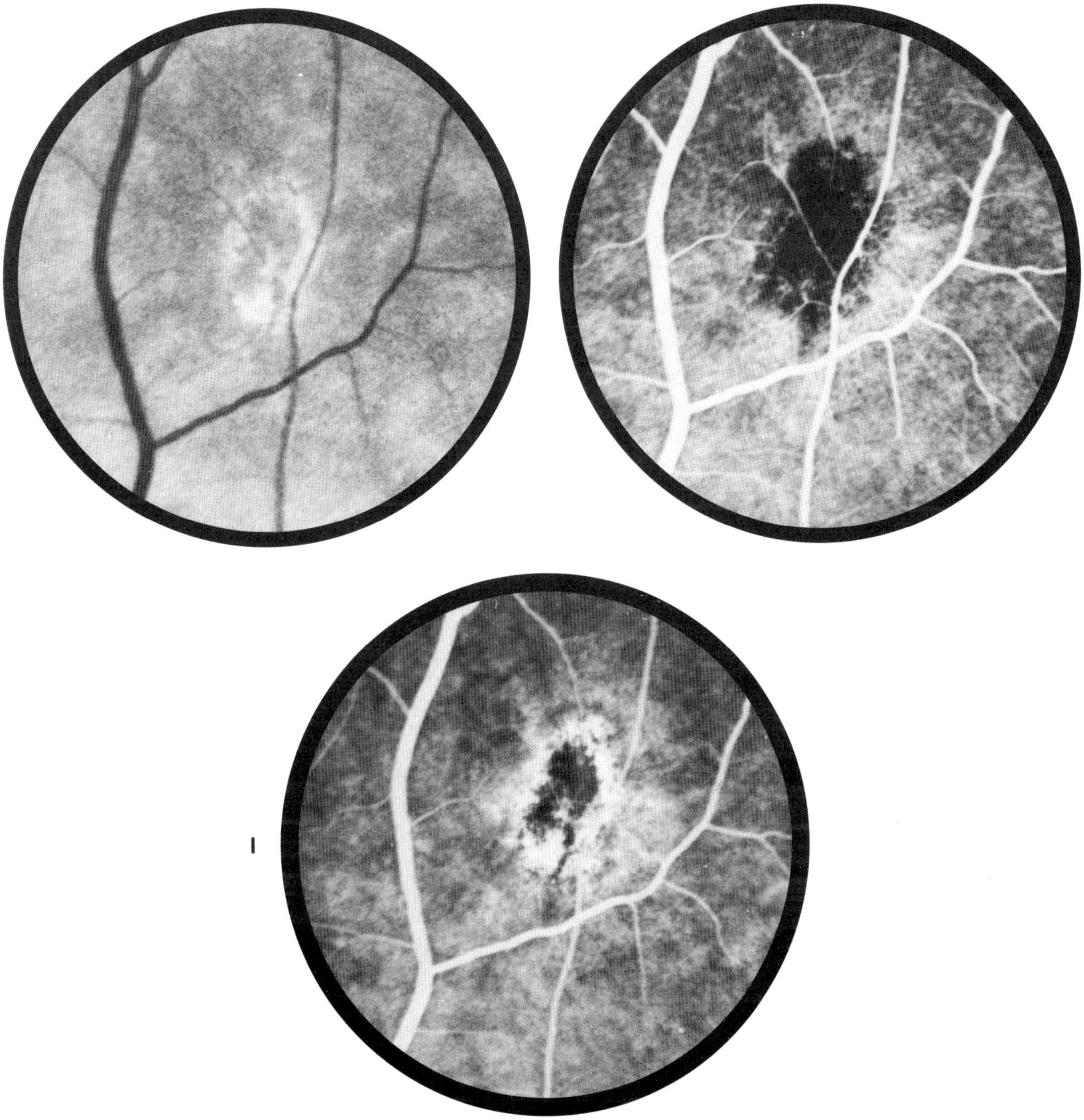

H

I

Figure 29.2—*continued*

Figure 29.2. Central serous chorioretinopathy (Pre- and postoperative argon laser photocoagulation). *A,* ophthalmoscopic photograph superior to the left macula shows an irregular pigment epithelial lesion. *B,* ophthalmoscopic photograph of the same eye shows a large sensory retinal detachment with clearly demarcated inferior edges (*arrows*). *C,* early venous phase angiogram shows a hyperfluorescent spot superior to the macula (*arrow*), with additional areas of hyperfluorescence superior to it. *D,* late venous phase shows increased hyperfluorescence of the primary spot. The other fluorescent spots have also increased in intensity but not in size. *E,* late venous phase angiogram. The primary spot has increased in size and is leaking fluorescein under the detached sensory retina. *F,* the lower edge of the detached sensory retina is demarcated by fluorescence (*arrows*). *G,* ophthalmoscopic photograph of the same area superior to the left macula, 2 weeks after argon laser photocoagulation, shows very fine pigmentation. On examination, the overlying sensory retina was found to be flat. *H,* early venous phase angiogram. The area treated with laser shows hypofluorescence without evidence of leakage. *I,* late venous phase angiogram shows some hyperfluorescent staining around the edges of the laser lesion, with no leakage into a fluid space. This patient had central serous chorioretinopathy with a pigment epithelial leak above the left macula, which resulted in a large detachment of the sensory retina involving the macula. Argon laser photocoagulation directed to the leak far above the macula resulted in complete reattachment of the sensory retina within 2 weeks.

However, in central serous chorioretinopathy, when the pigment epithelial leak is in or near the fovea, treatment should not be performed because of the risk of permanent foveal damage. The damage may result either from an inadvertent foveal laser burn or the development of subretinal neovascularization due to excessive absorption of laser energy in the more heavily pigmented pigment epithelium in the fovea and xanthopyll pigment in the outer retinal layers of the fovea.

In other causes of sensory retinal detachment in which the leakage is remote to the fovea but the secondary sensory retinal detachment includes the fovea, the lesion may be treated in order to resolve the detachment and, thus, stabilize or improve vision. An example of this is choroidal hemangioma that may occur in the macular region but may also exclude the fovea (Fig. 29.3). In such cases the overlying sensory retinal detachment often extends well beyond the hemangioma and may include the fovea. Treatment of the hemangioma will cause reattachment of the sensory retina and return of central vision when the fovea becomes reattached.

Pigment epithelial detachment

Vision will not be significantly affected when a pigment epithelial detachment affects the macular area without involving the fovea, and if there is no secondary sensory retinal detachment. When the pigment epithelial detachment includes the fovea but the sensory retina remains attached, vision still may not be significantly affected (Fig. 29.4). Pigment epithelial detachments of this type usually occur in patients under 50 and are rarely a problem in terms of visual reduction. However, when a pigment epithelial detachment affects the elderly patient as part of the maculopathy of aging (involutional macular degeneration) the overlying sensory retina is often detached and vision is therefore reduced.

Reduction of vision may occur secondary to degenerative changes of the pigment epithelium and overlying retina even when the sensory retina is not detached. In these cases argon laser photocoagulation may cause reattachment of the pigment epithelium and possible stabilization of vision.

Laser photocoagulation spots should be directed to a broad area over the pigment epithelial detachment, avoiding the foveal zone. Reattachment of the entire pigment epithelial detachment can be thus accomplished (Fig. 29.5). In some cases we have tried to punch a small hole with a 50-μ laser spot in the detached pigment epithelium, very distant from the fovea, in order to allow the subpigment epithelial fluid to leak out under the sensory retina. In these cases the pigment epithelium usually reattaches and the fluid slowly resolves from under the sensory retina. This treatment does not accomplish complete reattachment in every case.

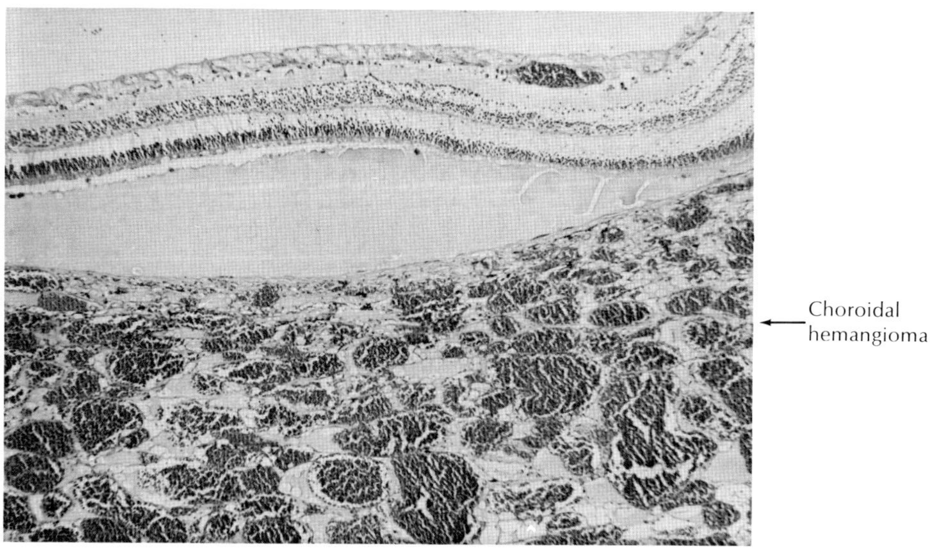

Figure 29.3. Choroidal hemangioma with an overlying secondary sensory retinal detachment. (From H. Schatz, T. Burton, L. Yannuzzi and M. Rabb: Interpretation of Fundus Fluorescein Angiography, © 1978, C.V. Mosby Co., St. Louis; reprinted with permission.)

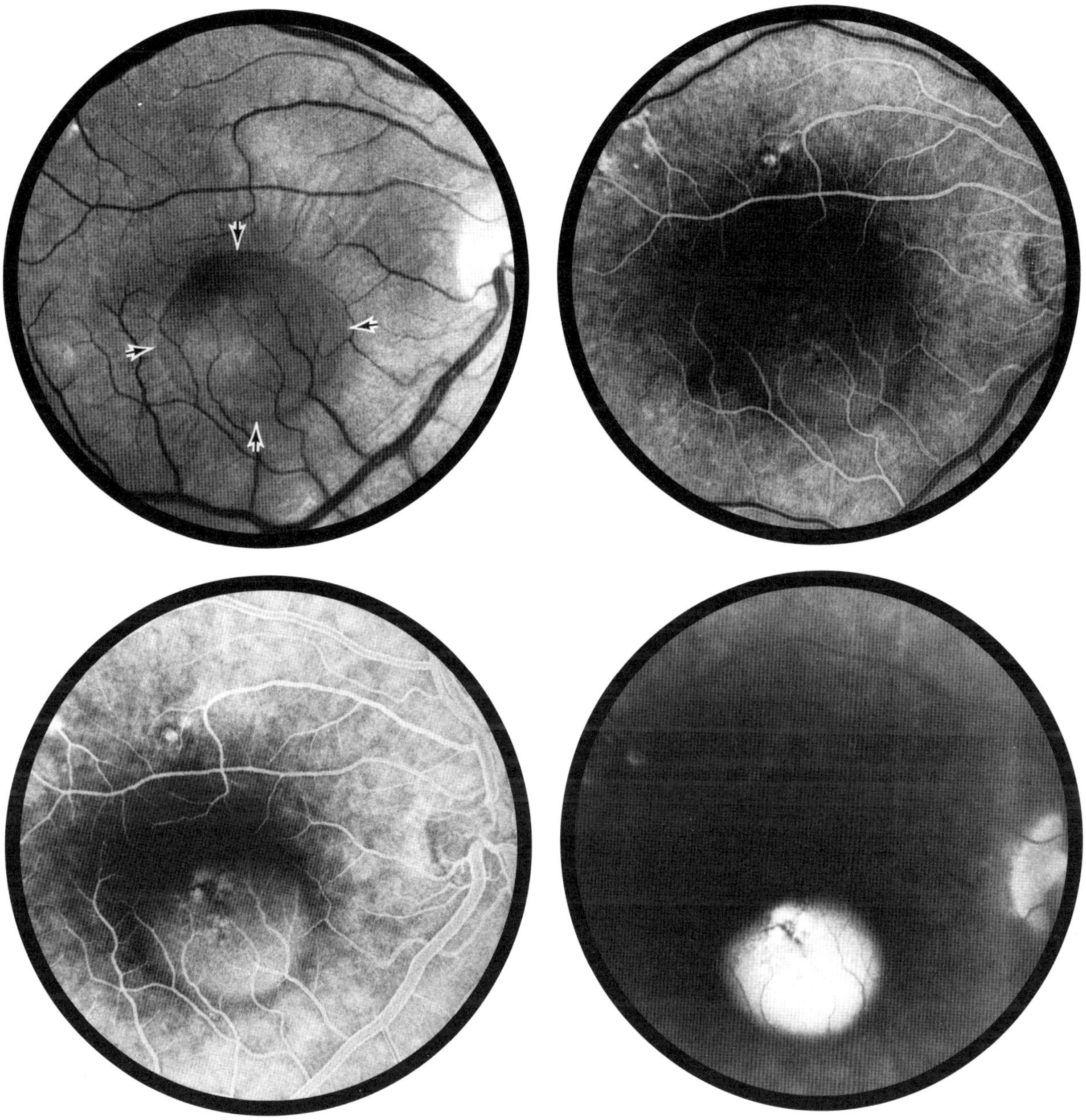

A B C D

Figure 29.4. Pigment epithelial detachment. *A,* ophthalmoscopic photograph of the right macula shows a 1½ disc diameter-sized pigment epithelial detachment (*surrounded by arrows*). *B,* arteriovenous phase angiogram. The detachment shows slight hyperfluorescence. *C,* early venous phase angiogram shows the pigment epithelial detachment beginning to increase in intensity but not in size. Patchy hypofluorescence on the surface of the detachment is due to pigment epithelial proliferation. *D,* late phase angiogram. The pigment epithelial detachment is completely fluorescent while remaining the same size throughout the angiogram. This patient's pigment epithelial detachment involved the macula with no sensory detachment and with vision of 20/20. Treatment was not necessary. (From H. Schatz, T. Burton, L. Yannuzzi and M. Rabb: Interpretation of Fundus Fluorescein Angiography, © 1978, C.V. Mosby Co., St. Louis; reprinted with permission.)

Figure 29.5. Pigment epithelial detachment (pre- and postoperative argon laser photocoagulation). *A*, ophthalmoscopic photograph of the left macula. There is a pigment epithelial detachment involving the central macular region (*arrows*). Drusen surround the detachment. *B*, early venous phase angiogram. The detachment hyperfluoresces slightly with the fluid of the detachment partially blocking choroidal fluorescence. *C*, late phase angiogram shows further hyperfluorescence from pooling beneath the detachment. *D*, ophthalmoscopic photograph of the same patient, 8 weeks after argon laser photocoagulation. The left macula is flat with no detachment. Laser lesions are present in the macula along with some scarring of the pigment epithelium. *E*, early venous phase angiogram shows laser lesions in a horseshoe pattern surrounding the macula. *F*, late venous phase angiogram. The laser lesions stain slightly with no evidence of pooling. This patient had reduced vision due to a long-standing pigment epithelial detachment associated with confluent drusen. Argon laser photocoagulation resulted in reattachment of the pigment epithelium and improvement in vision.

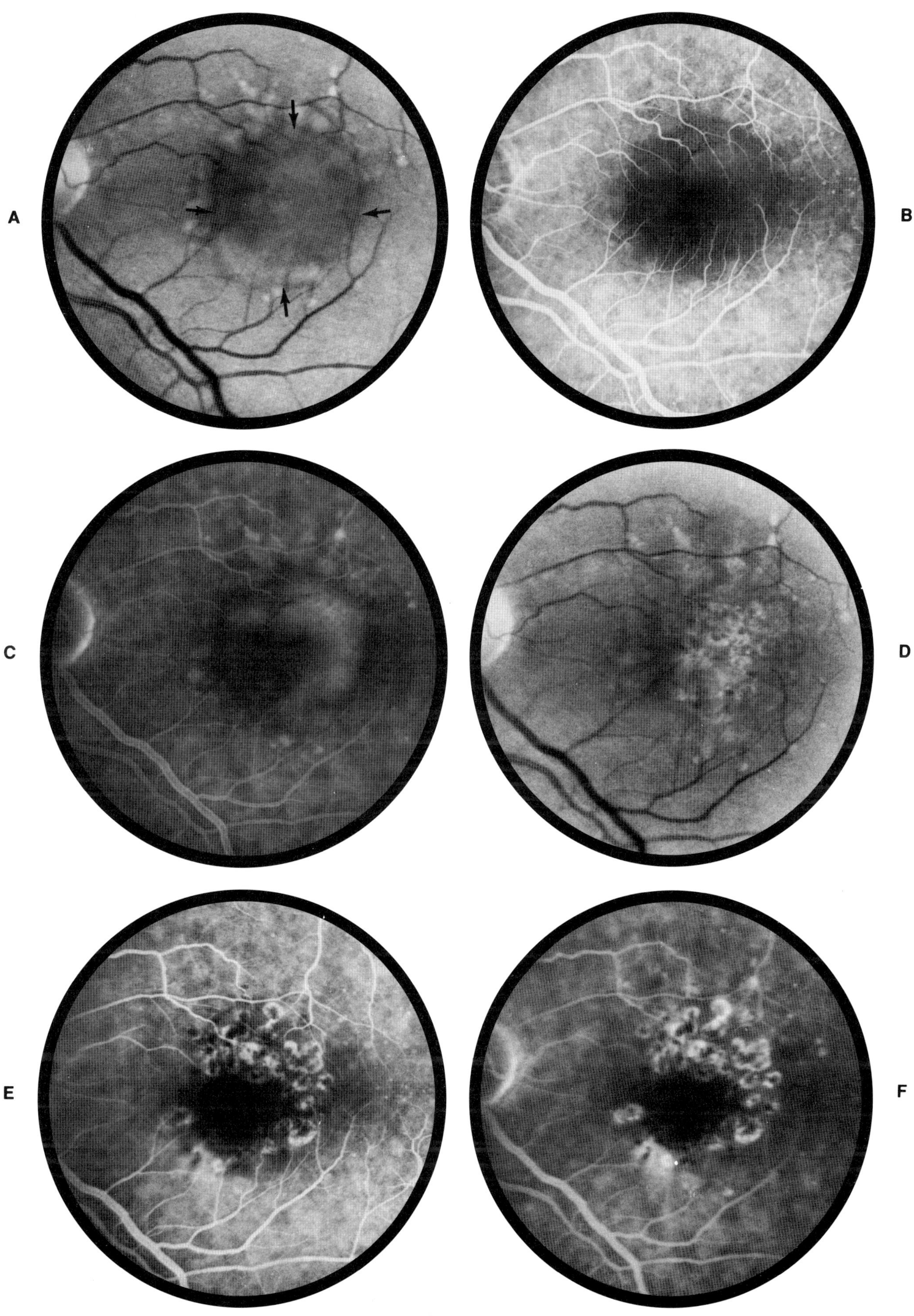

Figure 29.5

EXUDATE

This section discusses the presence of lipid exudate in the retina, secondary to retinal vascular disease, and the indications for laser photocoagulation to resolve the exudate.

Foveal (recent)

When leaking retinal blood vessels deposit lipid exudate in the fovea, vision will be reduced (Fig. 29.6). A number of retinal vascular leaking diseases may cause this problem such as diabetic retinopathy, branch vein occlusion, telangiectasia, and arterial macroaneurysm. Any other retinal vascular occlusive disease that tends to result in leaking retinal vessels may also cause the deposition of lipid exudate in the retina.

When exudate involves the fovea (for more than a few months), the fovea is usually permanently destroyed. (Longstanding foveal exudate will be discussed later in this chapter.) However, if the exudate has been recently deposited in the fovea, laser therapy may be directed to the leaking retinal vessels to affect resolution; in some cases this will result in a return of central vision.

Figure 29.6. Foveal exudates secondary to nonproliferative diabetic retinopathy. *A,* ophthalmoscopic photograph. Note the heavy lipid exudation in the macula. *B,* early venous phase angiogram. There is multifocal hyperfluorescence predominantly in the superior temporal macula, corresponding to dilated retinal capillaries and microaneurysms. *C,* late intraretinal leakage from these vessels can be seen in the late venous phase angiogram. (From H. Schatz, T. Burton, L. Yannuzzi, and M. Rabb: Interpretation of Fundus Fluorescein Angiography, © 1978, C.V. Mosby Co., St. Louis; all reprinted with permission.) *D,* ten weeks after argon laser photocoagulation, ophthalmoscopic photograph showed pigmentary laser burns (*arrows*) and resolution of lipid. *E,* early venous phase angiogram. Laser burns are hypofluorescent and the abnormal vessels are no longer evident. *F,* late phase angiogram shows only staining of the margins of the laser burns. With the resolution of the edema and lipid exudate, the visual acuity improved from a preoperative level of 20/100 to 20/20.

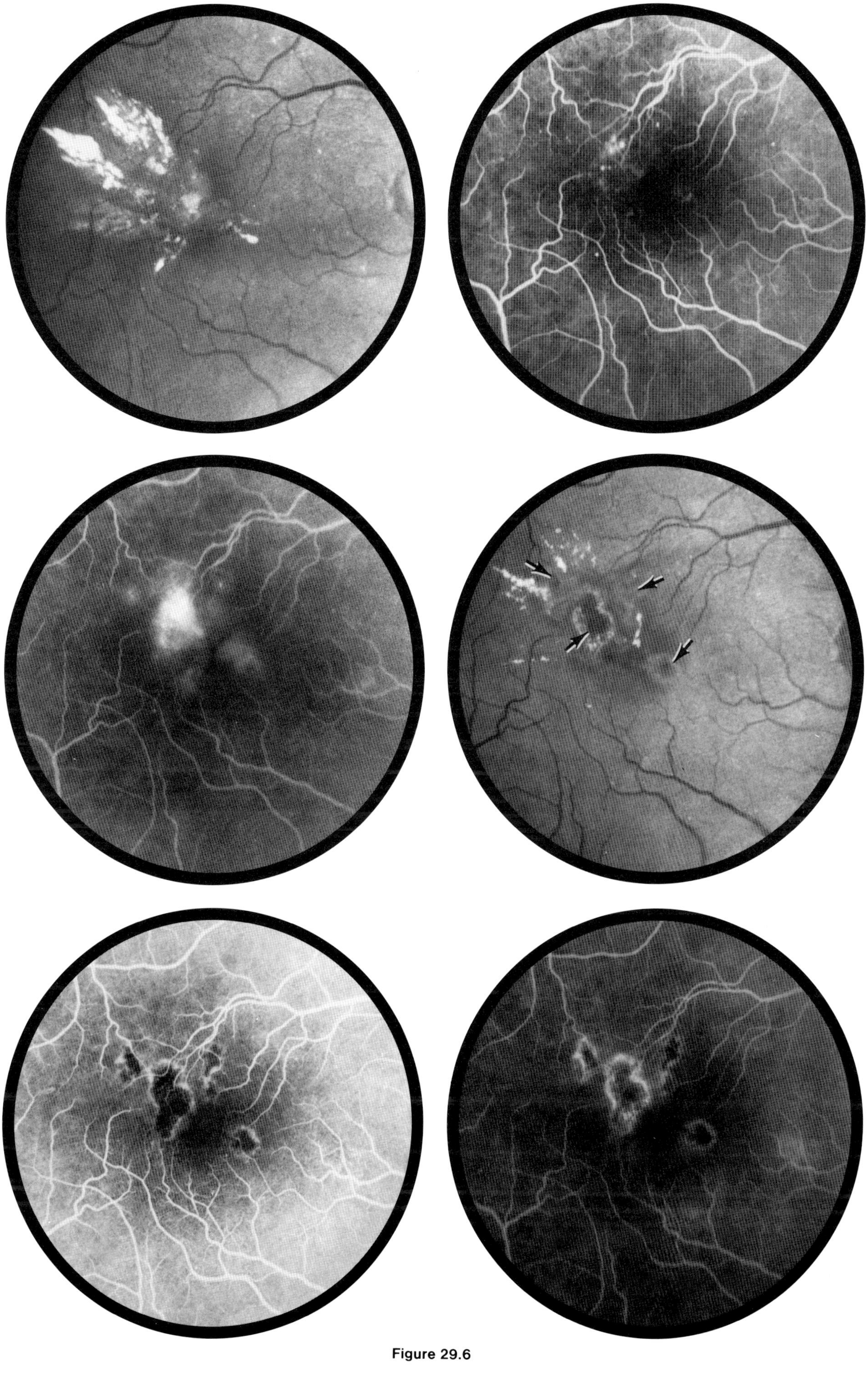

A B C D E F

Figure 29.6

Threatening Fovea

An indication for laser treatment occurs when a circinate ring begins to form but is not yet complete and its completion would involve the fovea. Vision in such patients may be excellent, even 20/20, but if the lipid deposition increases upon successive follow-up examinations, and threatens to include the fovea, treatment should be considered (Fig. 29.7). Laser treatment is directed to the leaking retinal vessels causing the deposition of exudate. Adequate laser energy will stop the retinal vascular leakage and cause resolution of the exudate. Immediately after treatment, the exudate may increase because the edematous retina within the circinate ring begins to resorb most of the components of the edema; the remaining exudate that was in solution in the edema cannot be resolved by the retinal blood vessels and, therefore, precipitates. Thus, an increase in exudate a few weeks or a month after laser therapy may be a sign of resolution. The fluorescein angiogram should be repeated 4–6 weeks after laser surgery to see whether vascular leak-

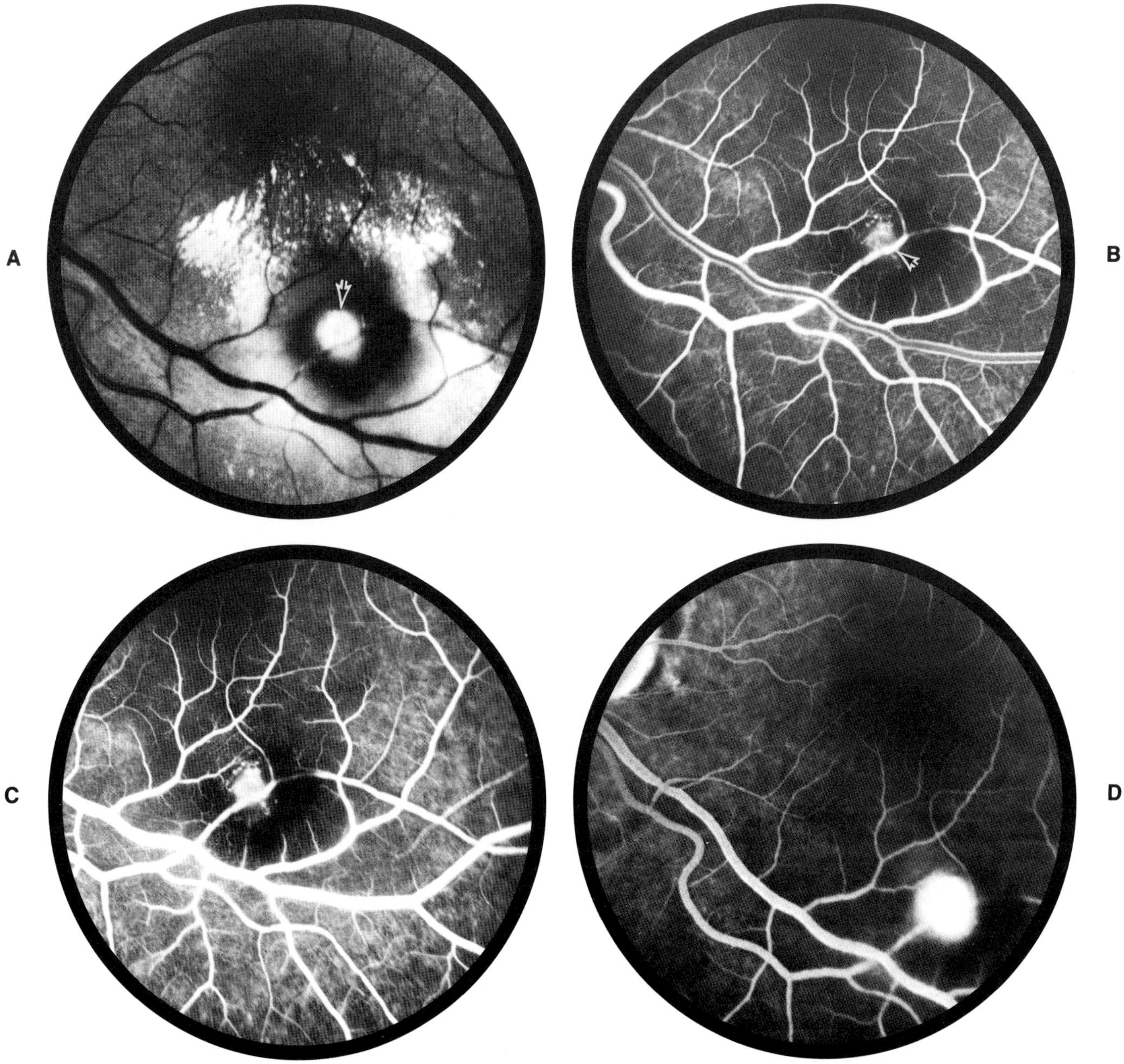

Figure 29.7. Arterial macroaneurysm with circinate exudate threatening fovea. *A,* ophthalmoscopic photograph of the left macula shows hemorrhage associated with an arterial macroaneurysm (*arrow*). A circinate ring of exudate accumulated around the aneurysm is caused by leakage. Successive examinations showed increasing deposition of exudate in the fovea. *B,* arteriovenous phase angiogram. The aneurysm fluoresces (an arrow points to the arteriole out of which the macroaneurysm developed). *C,* early venous phase angiogram shows increased hyperfluorescence of the aneurysm. *D,* late venous phase shows marked hyperfluorescence of the retina that surrounds the aneurysm, indicating leakage from it. Leakage from aneurysm caused a large amount of retinal edema along with encircling circinate exudate, which threatened the fovea. This patient was later treated with argon laser photocoagulation which resulted in resolution of the edema and exudate. (From H. Schatz, T. Burton, L. Yannuzzi, and M. Rabb: Interpretation of Fundus Fluorescein Angiography, © 1978, C.V. Mosby Co., St. Louis; all reprinted with permission.)

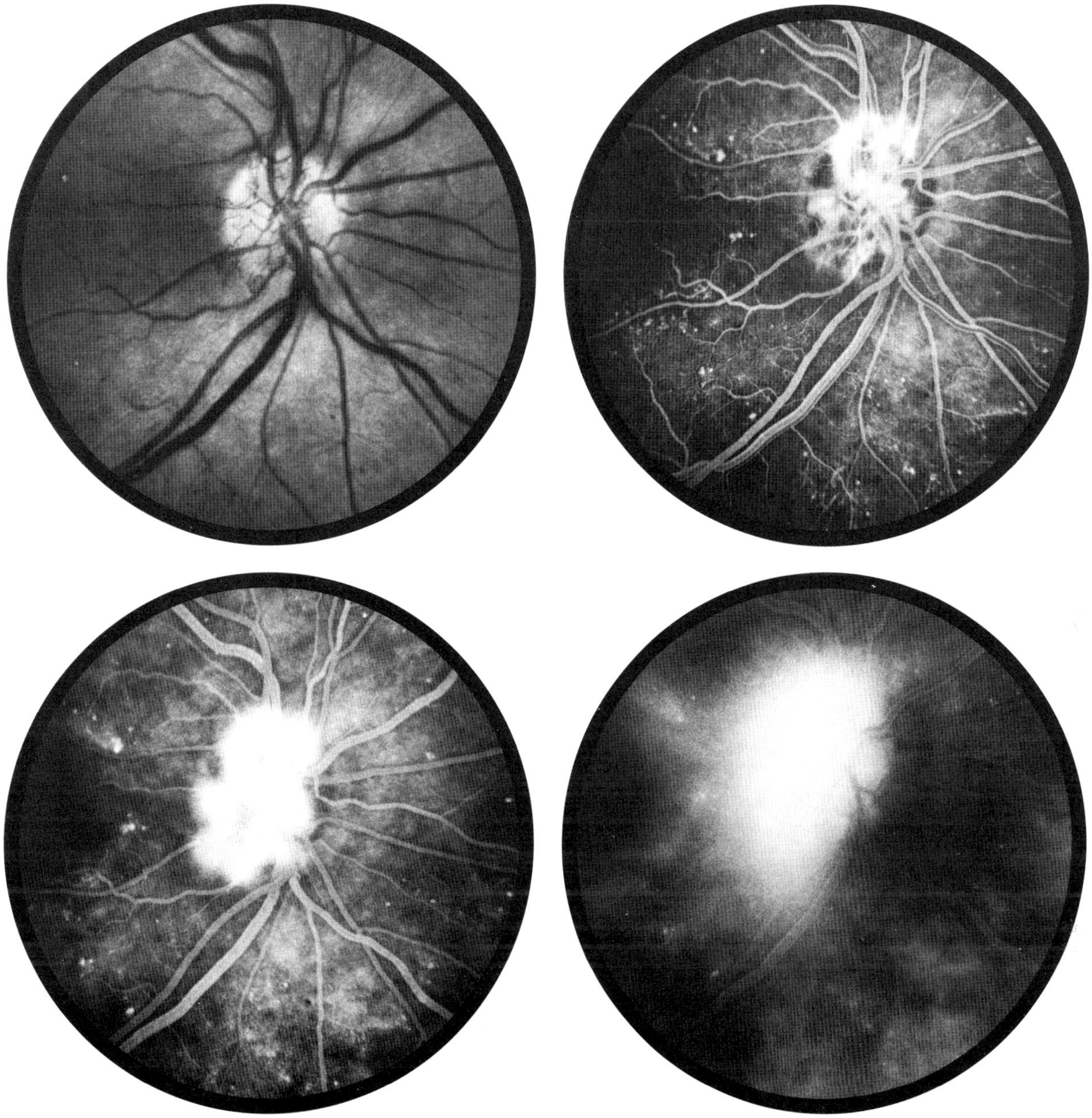

Figure 29.8. Disc neovascularization secondary to diabetic retinopathy. *A*, ophthalmoscopic photograph of the right disc shows fine, lacy blood vessels emanating from the optic nerve head into the vitreous and onto the surface of the retina. *B*, arteriovenous phase angiogram shows neovascularization on the disc with marked hyperfluorescence. Scattered microaneurysms and areas of capillary nonperfusion are also present in the posterior pole. *C*, disc neovascularization shows fluorescein leakage in the late venous phase angiogram. *D*, late phase angiogram. There is marked vitreous hyperfluorescence caused by heavy leakage from the disc neovascularization. (From H. Schatz, T. Burton, L. Yannuzzi and M. Rabb: Interpretation of Fundus Fluorescein Angiography, © 1978, C.V. Mosby Co., St. Louis; all reprinted with permission.)

age is continuing. If the leakage has stopped, no further therapy is necessary. The exudate is removed by a cellular response (macrophages) and resolution may take 6 months or even a year after laser treatment.

Exudate that does not enter or even threaten the fovea should not be considered for treatment. For example, if there is a circinate ring of exudate superior to the optic nerve head caused by retinal vascular leakage in this area, this exudate will not affect central vision and, therefore, no treatment is necessary. Patients who have any kind of nonmacular exudate should be taught to test the vision in each eye every day and report immediately any visual reduction, indicating that the macula may be involved.

NEOVASCULARIZATION

Retinal and Preretinal Neovascularization

Although retinal and preretinal neovascularization are not, strictly speaking, diseases of the macula, they may have a profound effect on central vision by causing vitreous hemorrhage and retinal traction detachment. Many conditions cause retinal neovascularization including diabetic retinopathy (Fig. 29.8), branch vein occlusion (Fig. 29.9), Eales' disease, sickle cell disease (Fig. 29.10), sarcoidosis, intraocular inflammation, radiation retinopathy, and others. Their common factor, with the exception of certain inflammatory conditions, is occlusion of the retinal vessels.

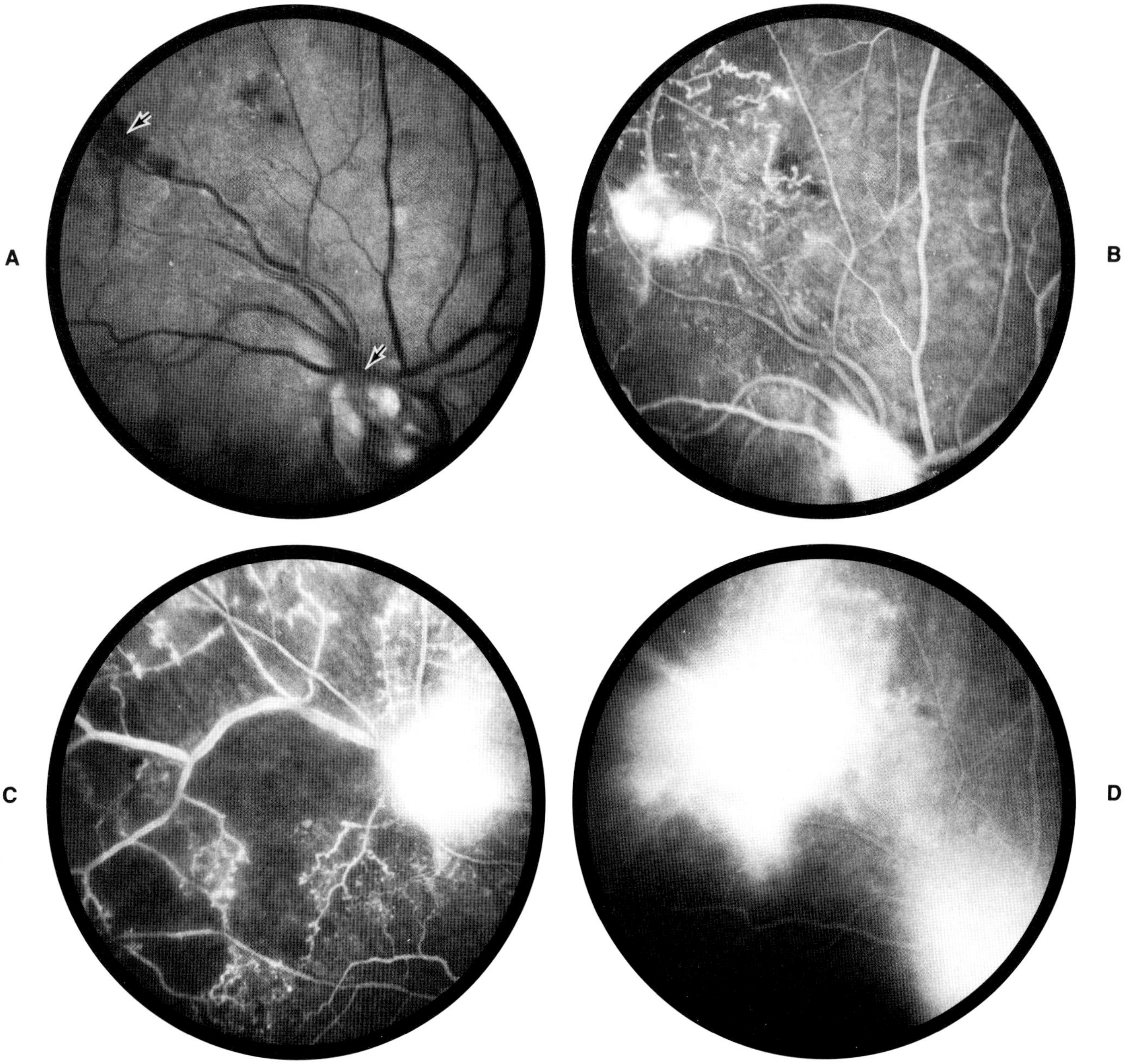

Figure 29.9. Branch vein occlusion with neovascularization on the disc and in the posterior pole. *A,* ophthalmoscopic photograph shows neovascularization on the disc and along the superior temporal arcade above the macula (*arrows*) in this patient with antecedent branch vein occlusion. *B,* early venous phase angiogram shows delayed filling of the superotemporal vein. The capillary bed feeding into this vein is dilated and telangiectatic. There is also leakage from the neovascularization. *C,* late venous phase angiogram shows a huge area of capillary nonperfusion and dilation and tortuosity of the capillary bed, which is still patent. The neovascularization leaks markedly. *D,* late phase angiogram shows profuse leakage from both neovascular fronds. In this patient, a modified (quadrantic) panretinal laser photocoagulation was directed to the retina involved by the occluded vein. The neovascularization which was not treated, completely resolved 2 months after the treatment. (From H. Schatz, T. Burton, L. Yannuzzi, and M. Rabb: Interpretation of Fundus Fluorescein Angiography, © 1978, C.V. Mosby Co., St. Louis; all reprinted with permission.)

Some conditions including retrolental fibroplasia, leukemia, and anemia, cause neovascularization exclusively in the periphery.

The current accepted method of treatment involves obliteration of the occluded retina using the panretinal photocoagulation technique. In diabetic retinopathy the entire retina, with the exception of the large areas of the macular arcade and the periphery beyond the equator, is treated with large spot sizes (usually 500 μ) in fairly close proximity but without direct treatment to the neovascularization. This treatment results in resolution of the neovascularization in a vast majority of patients and greatly reduces the threat of blindness from vitreous hemorrhage. In patients with branch vein occlusion and neovascularization, photocoagulation directed to the occluded quadrants with no direct treatment to the new vessels will usually cause resolution of the neovascularization.

Inflammatory conditions such as Behçet's disease and other intraocular inflammations can produce retinal and disc neovascularization. The usual method of treatment is to attempt to curb the inflammation with either steroids, chlorambucil, or other drugs. Photocoagulation treatment has not proved to be of definite benefit in these conditions.

A

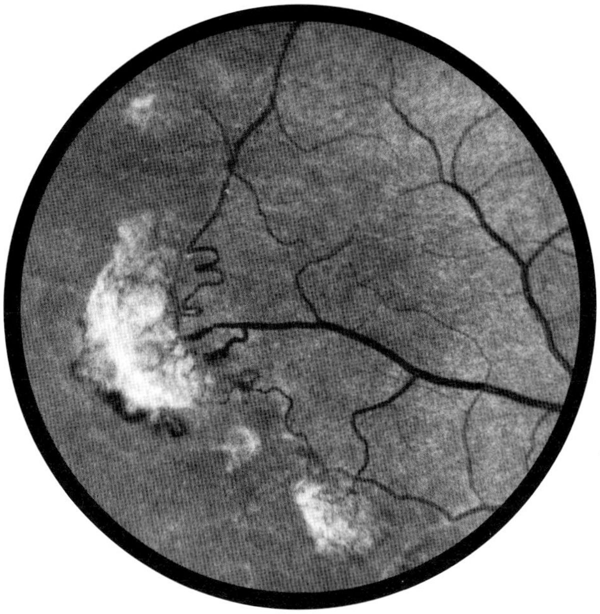

B

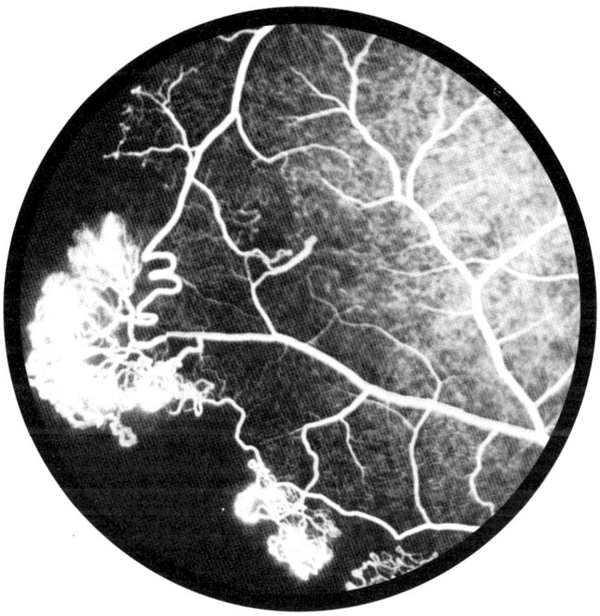

C

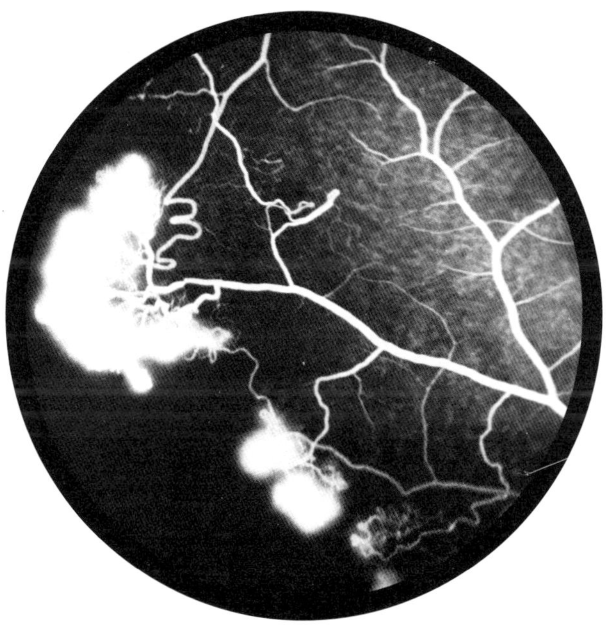

Figure 29.10. Peripheral neovascularization associated with sickle SC retinopathy. *A,* ophthalmoscopic photograph of the far periphery of the right fundus shows neovascularization and associated fibrosis. *B,* early venous phase angiogram shows the neovascular tissue (sea fan) filling with fluorescein. The retina, peripheral to the neovascularization, is nonperfused and hypofluorescent. *C,* late venous phase angiogram shows the neovascularization leaking fluorescein into the vitreous. Argon laser photocoagulation was performed and resulted in obliteration of the neovascularization. (From H. Schatz, T. Burton, L. Yannuzzi and M. Rabb: Interpretation of Fundus Fluorescein Angiography, © 1978, C.V. Mosby Co., St. Louis; all reprinted with permission.)

Subretinal Neovascularization

As previously discussed, there are many causes of subretinal neovascularization. The pathogenesis involves a proliferation of capillaries from the choriocapillaris under the pigment epithelium through a break in Bruch's membrane. These new blood vessels leak fluid and blood causing serous and hemorrhagic detachment of both the pigment epithelium and sensory retina, and eventual reduction of vision. Fluid may also leak into the overlying retina causing cystoid edema and retinal exudate.

Associated with the new blood vessels, fibrous tissue proliferates, developing into a fibrous disciform scar which replaces the blood vessels.

When subretinal neovascularization involves the macular area, the fovea is often involved either by hemorrhage, fluid under the sensory retina, or cystoid edema. The vessels may grow and permanently reduce vision by direct involvement of the fovea. Whenever the macula contains subretinal neovascularization and the fovea is free of the new blood vessels, laser treatment may be beneficial. Argon laser photocoagulation treatment should be directed to the entire patch of subretinal neovascularization, while avoiding the fovea (Figs. 29.11 through 29.14). If all the blood vessels cannot be treated because some are too close to or involve the fovea, or if hemorrhage partially obscures them, treatment is contraindicated (Fig. 29.15). If the subretinal neovascularization involves an area distal to the macula and the resultant fluid and hemorrhage do not involve the macula or the fovea, treatment is not indicated, although the patient should be carefully followed.

In summary, fluid in or under the retina, lipid exudate in the fovea or threatening it, retinal or subretinal neovascularization, may cause visual reduction and each may be reversible by laser.

A

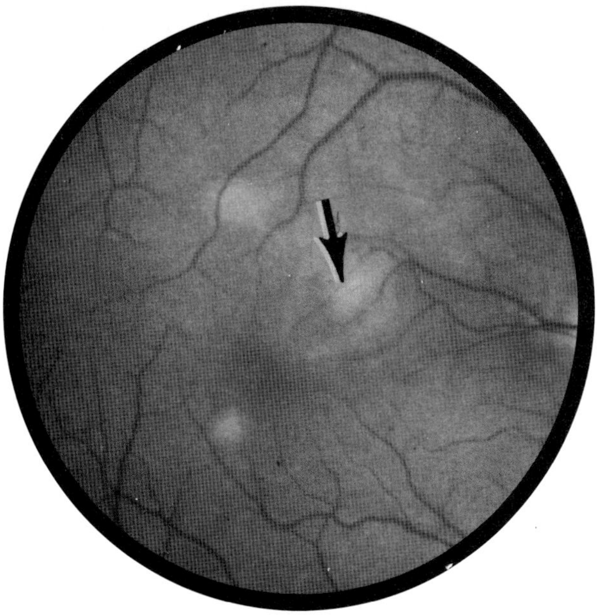

B

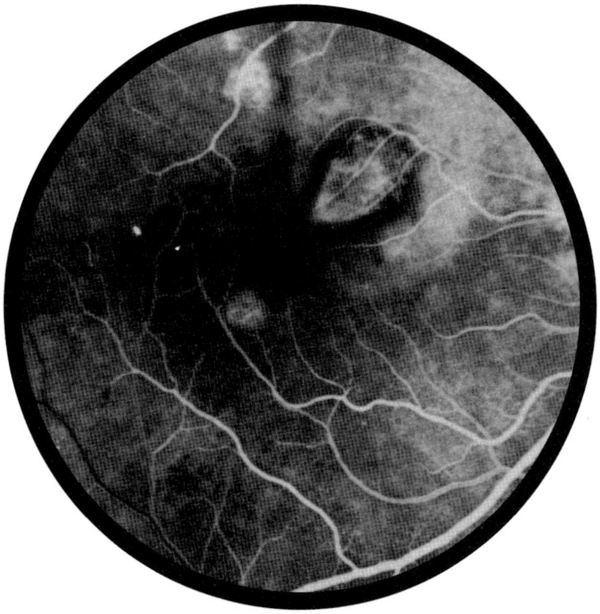

C

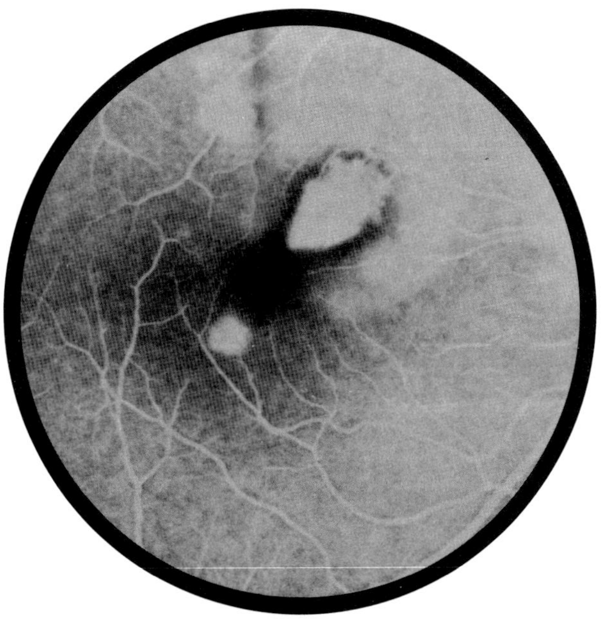

Figure 29.11. Subretinal neovascularization associated with histoplasmosis. (Pre- and postoperative argon laser photocoagulation). *A,* ophthalmoscopic photograph of the right macula. There is a localized sensory retinal detachment secondary to a dirty gray membrane (*arrow*) representing subretinal neovascularization located just superonasal to the fovea. A few "histo spots" are also present above and below the macula. *B,* arterial phase angiogram shows the subretinal neovascular membrane superotemporal to the fovea with a surrounding pigmented ring. *C,* arteriovenous phase angiogram showing the subretinal neovascular membrane leaking fluorescein. *D,* late phase angiogram shows the subretinal neovascular membrane leaking fluorescein under the detached sensory retina. *E,* ophthalmoscopic photograph of the same patient, one week after argon laser photocoagulation, shows the slightly edematous treated lesion. The fovea appears uninvolved. *F,* arteriovenous phase angiogram shows the hypofluorescent treated lesion with a hyperfluorescent margin around it. *G,* late phase angiogram shows that the lesion stains in its central portion and around its edges from the laser burns. There is no evidence of persistent neovascularization or detachment. This patient had reduced vision due to a sensory retinal detachment secondary to subretinal neovascularization. Laser photocoagulation was directed to the subretinal neovascularization; 2 months later the vision had improved to 20/30.

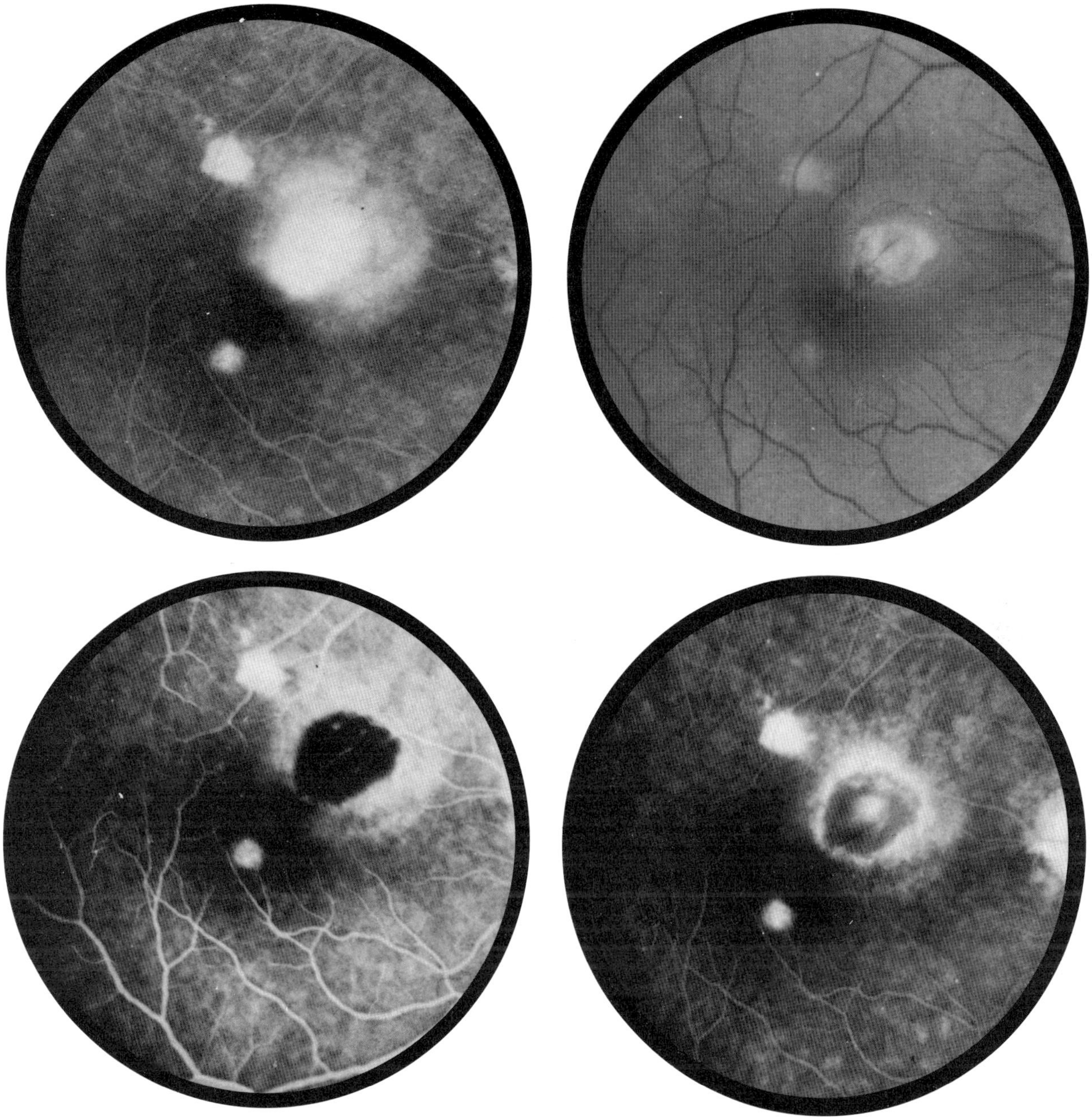

D E F G

Figure 29.11—*continued*

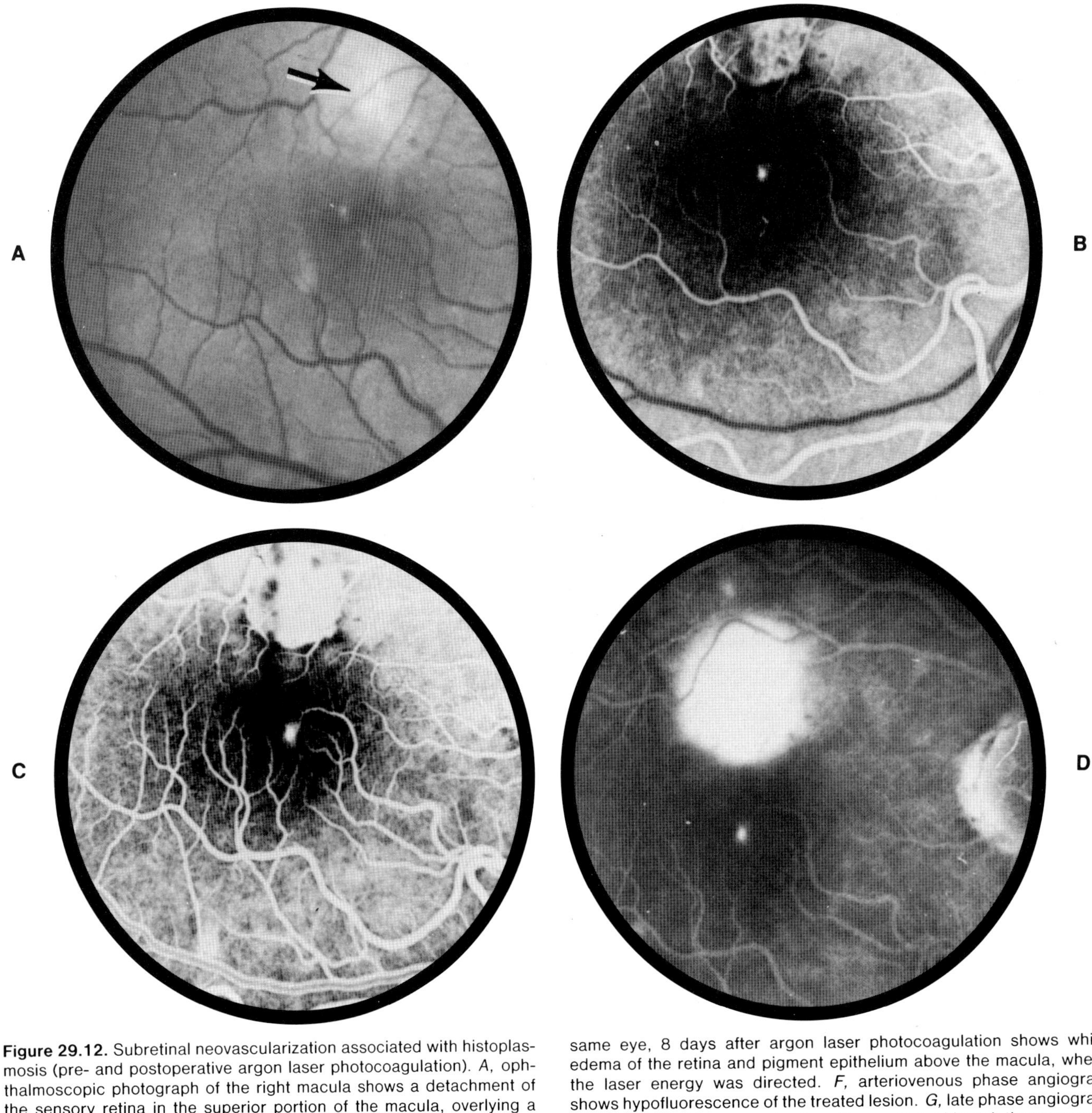

Figure 29.12. Subretinal neovascularization associated with histoplasmosis (pre- and postoperative argon laser photocoagulation). *A*, ophthalmoscopic photograph of the right macula shows a detachment of the sensory retina in the superior portion of the macula, overlying a grayish subretinal disturbance (*arrow*). *B*, arterial phase angiogram shows subretinal neovascularization above the macula. A small "histo spot" is located just below the fovea. *C*, arteriovenous phase shows early leakage of subretinal neovascularization. *D*, late phase angiogram shows marked leakage from the subretinal neovascularization under the sensory retinal detachment. *E*, ophthalmoscopic photograph of the same eye, 8 days after argon laser photocoagulation shows white edema of the retina and pigment epithelium above the macula, where the laser energy was directed. *F*, arteriovenous phase angiogram shows hypofluorescence of the treated lesion. *G*, late phase angiogram shows that the lesion remains hypofluorescent, although the surrounding rim is hyperfluorescent. Six weeks following argon laser photocoagulation to the subretinal neovascularization. The macula was flat and dry. The visual acuity had improved to 20/20 from a pretreatment level of 20/50.

E

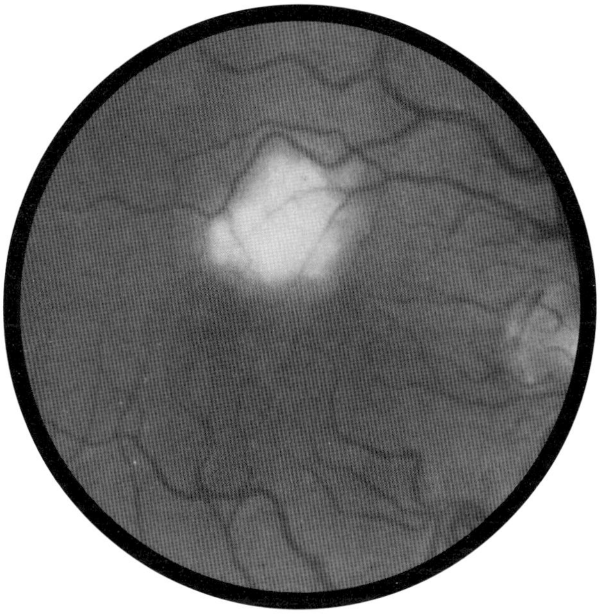

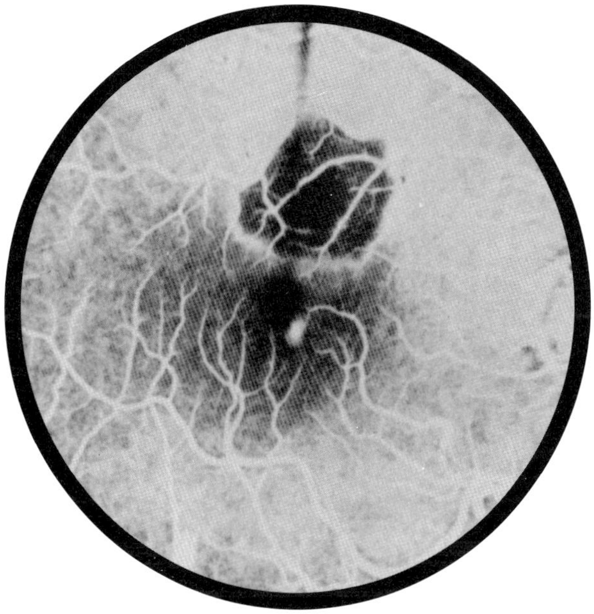

F

G

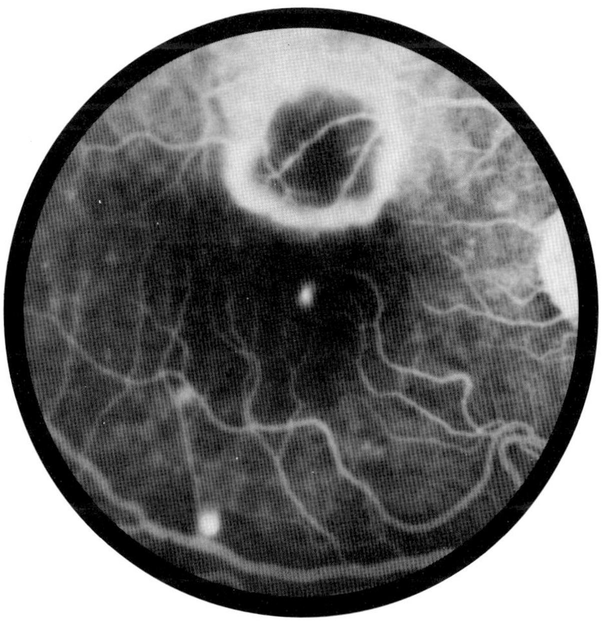

Figure 29.12—*continued*

Figure 29.13. Subretinal neovascularization secondary to high myopia (pre- and postoperative argon laser photocoagulation). *A,* ophthalmoscopic photograph of the left fundus shows hyperpigmentation in the center of the macula (Fuchs' spot). A small spot of hemorrhage is located superonasal to the fovea (*arrow*). *B,* early venous phase angiogram shows a small amount of hyperfluorescence superonasal to the fovea, which represents a small tuft of subretinal neovascularization. *C,* late phase shows leakage from the subretinal neovascularization. *D,* ophthalmoscopic photograph of the same eye, 4 weeks after argon laser photocoagulation, shows that the macula is completely flat and dry with a laser lesion located superotemporal to the fovea. *E,* early venous phase angiogram shows no abnormal fluorescence. *F,* late phase angiogram shows hypofluorescence of the laser lesion with hyperfluorescence of its margins. This patient had a small tuft of subretinal neovascularization associated with high myopia. Laser treatment caused resolution of the subretinal neovascularization, resulting in 20/25 visual acuity.

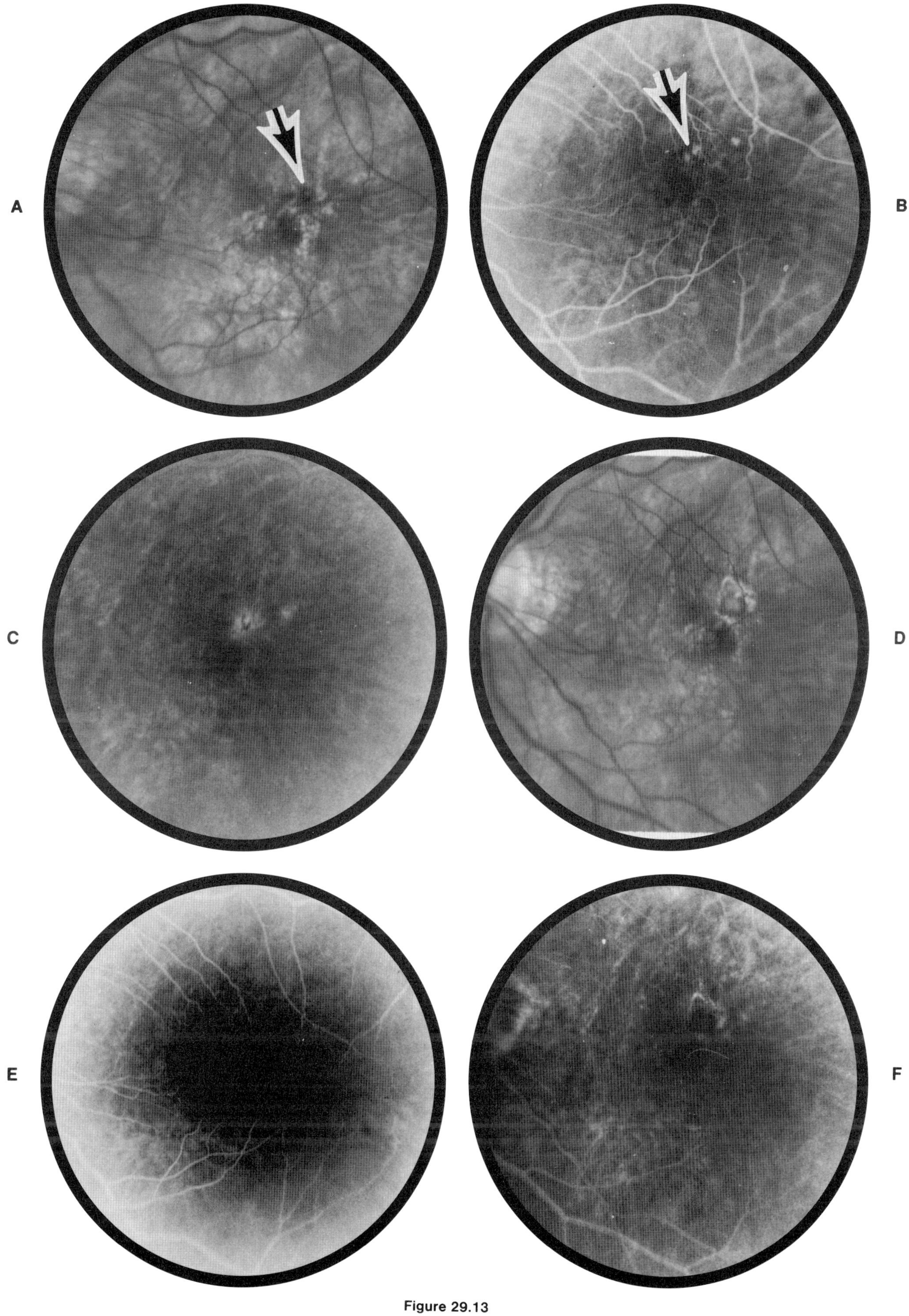

Figure 29.13

Figure 29.14. Four patches of subretinal neovascularization associated with histoplasmosis (pre- and postoperative argon laser photocoagulation). *A*, ophthalmoscopic photograph of the macula shows four patches of gray discoloration surrounding the fovea. *B*, early venous phase angiogram shows irregular hyperfluorescence surrounded by a pigment ring at the site of each patch of neovascularization. *C*, late phase angiogram shows the four patches leaking fluorescein. The most temporal lesion is leaking least, while the other three lesions (two above the macula and one below) are leaking fluid under the sensory retina, as demonstrated by the fuzzy edges. *D*, ophthalmoscopic photograph of the same eye, 6 days after argon laser photocoagulation, shows white edema of the pigment epithelium and retina caused by the laser treatment. *E*, early venous phase shows that the treated areas are hypofluorescent. *F*, late phase angiogram shows staining of the lasered lesions but no persistence of neovascularization. The fovea (*arrow*) was flat and dry. This patient's vision remained 20/25 postoperatively.

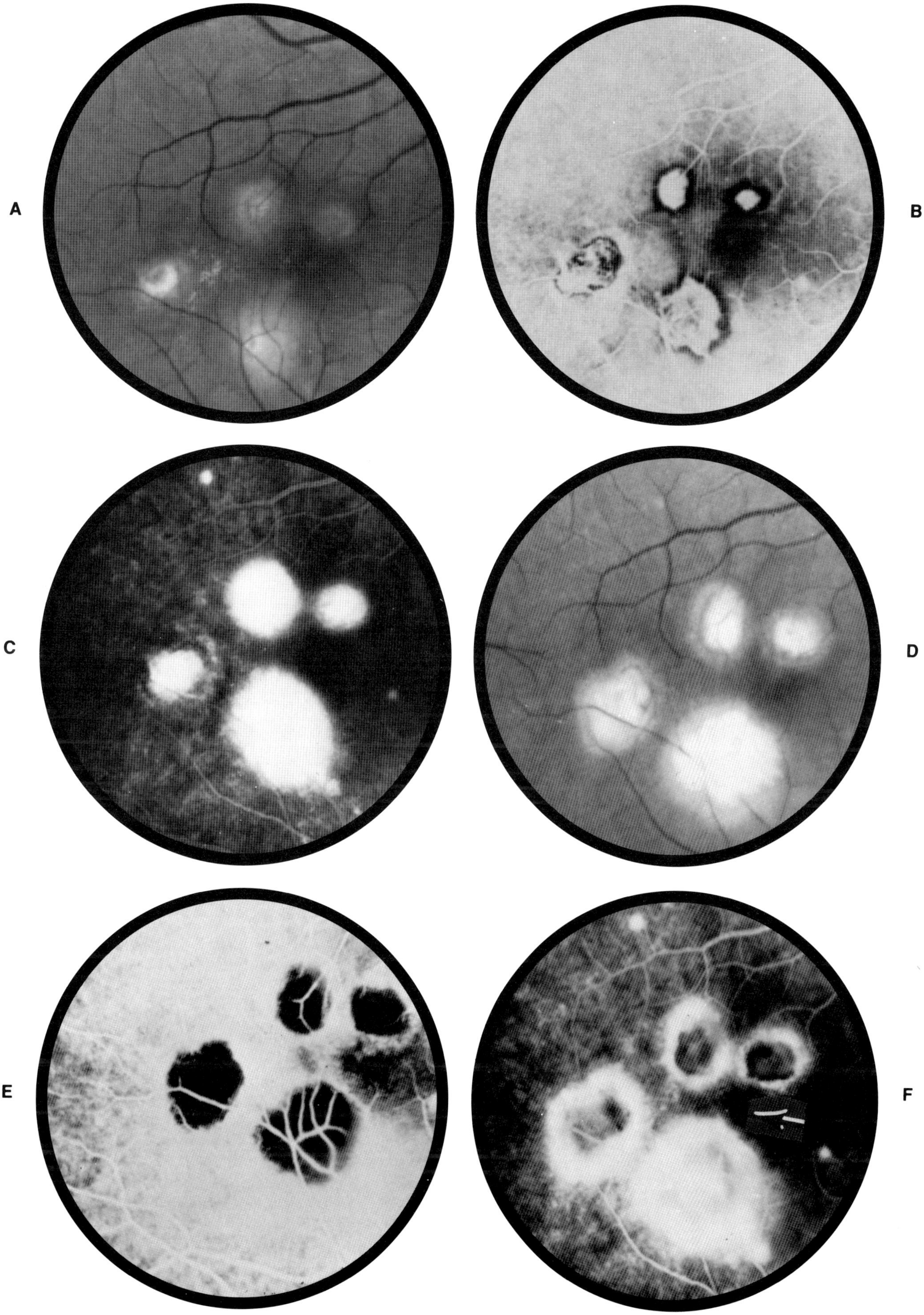

Figure 29.14

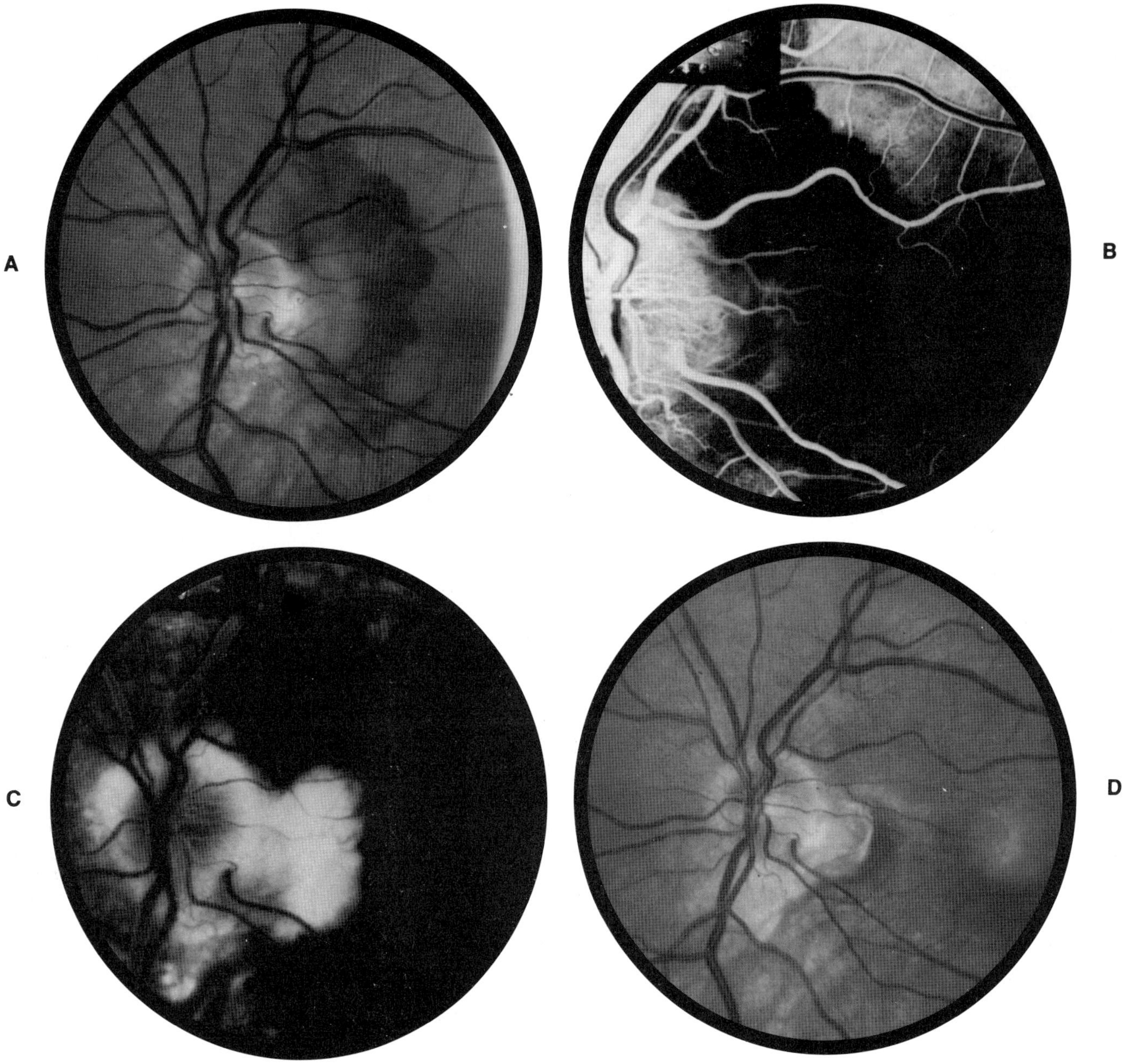

Figure 29.15. Peripapillary subretinal neovascularization with hemorrhage. *A*, ophthalmoscopic photograph of the macula shows a dirty gray membrane surrounded by subretinal hemorrhage just temporal to the disc. *B*, arteriovenous phase angiogram shows hyperfluorescence of the area temporal to the disc. In a large area above and below the papillomacular bundle, the hemorrhage blocks fluorescence. *C*, late phase angiogram shows hyperfluorescent leakage under the detached sensory retina. *D*, ophthalmoscopic photograph of the same eye, 1 year later, shows a small disciform scar temporal to the disc, with resolution of hemorrhage and fluid. This patient had peripapillary subretinal neovascularization with subretinal hemorrhage and sensory retinal detachment, causing reduced vision. The entire patch of subretinal neovascularization could not be seen due to obscuration by hemorrhage; therefore, the subretinal neovascularization was not treated. The patient was followed, the hemorhage cleared, and the subretinal neovascularization resolved into a small disciform scar. The sensory retina reattached and vision returned to 20/20.

Contraindications

When one wishes to evaluate a macula for possible argon laser photocoagulation treatment, one must consider the viability not only of the macula, but also specifically of the fovea. If the fovea has been irreversibly damaged, central visual acuity will be irrevocably reduced and, therefore, laser photocoagulation treatment will most likely not be indicated.

There are eight important pathologic changes occurring in the macula which cause a permanent reduction in vision by irreversibly damaging the fovea. In the following section on contraindications for laser treatment these eight major changes will be outlined and discussed.

Contraindications for Laser Treatment of Macular Disease:

(1) Dry, flat, atrophic changes
(2) Foveal subretinal neovascularization
(3) Foveal scar
(4) Foveal exudate (long-standing)
(5) Cystoid macular edema
(6) Macular hole
(7) Preretinal, membrane formation
(8) Foveal capillary nonperfusion

DRY, FLAT, ATROPHIC CHANGES

Atrophy of the pigment epithelium in the fovea irreversibly damages the rods and cones and, therefore, irreversibly reduces the central visual acuity. Atrophy of the pigment epithelium may occur with various conditions, i.e., maculopathy of aging (involutional macular degeneration), various hereditary maculopathies, trauma, pigment epithelial atrophy caused by certain drugs, or old inflammatory conditions.

When the pigment epithelium is atrophied, the choriocapillaris often also undergoes atrophy. One form of this atrophy is central areolar choroidal atrophy which is a nonspecific pathologic tissue response to various stimuli (e.g., various hereditary and aging maculopathies). The absence of the pigment epithelium and choriocapillaris appears as a well demarcated, usually oval or round zone of atrophy in the macula, often involving the fovea.

In the conditions causing atrophy, the fluorescein angiogram will demonstrate choroidal transmitted fluorescence (pigment epithelial window defect) in the fovea if the choriocapillaris is still intact. When the choriocapillaris has also been lost, the large choroidal vessels coursing through the fovea will be seen both ophthalmoscopically and angioscopically.

In all the conditions in which the pigment epithelium is atrophied in the fovea, vision will be irreversibly reduced. This finding often constitutes a contraindication to laser treatment for the specific macular disease causing the atrophy (Figs. 29.16 and 29.17).

A

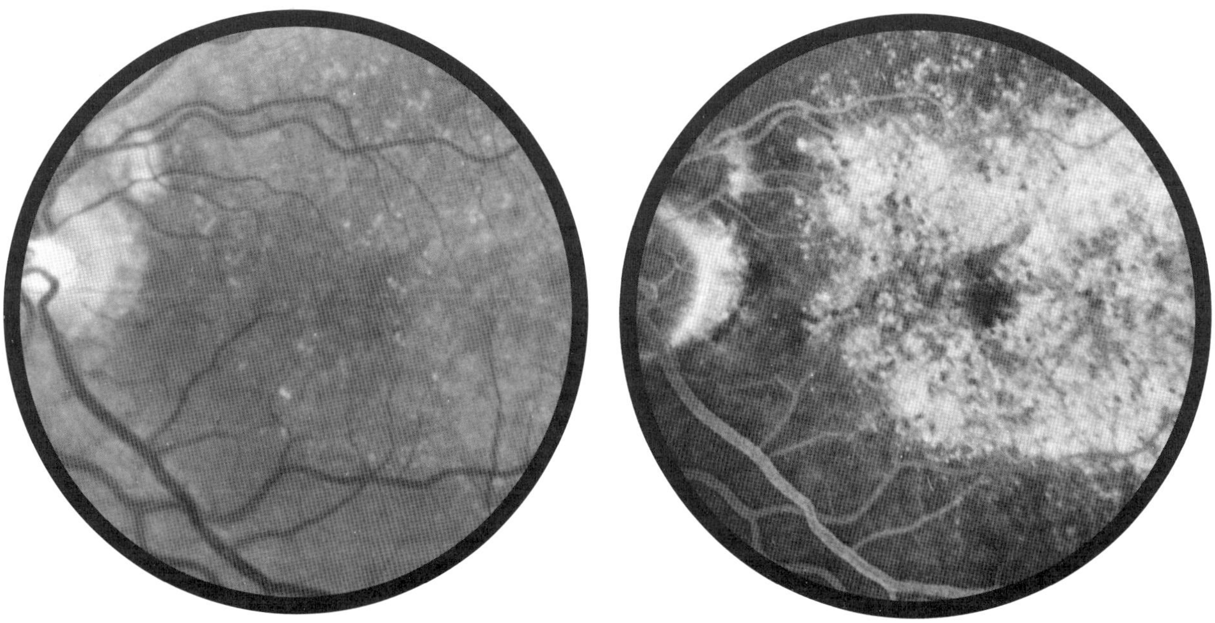

B

Figure 29.16. Macular pigment epithelial atrophy. *A*, ophthalmoscopic photograph of the left macula shows many drusen and depigmentation of most of the central macular area. *B*, late venous phase angiogram demonstrates widespread patchy hyperfluorescence from choroidal transmission (pigment epithelial window defect). There is a small amount of pigment clumping in the central macula.

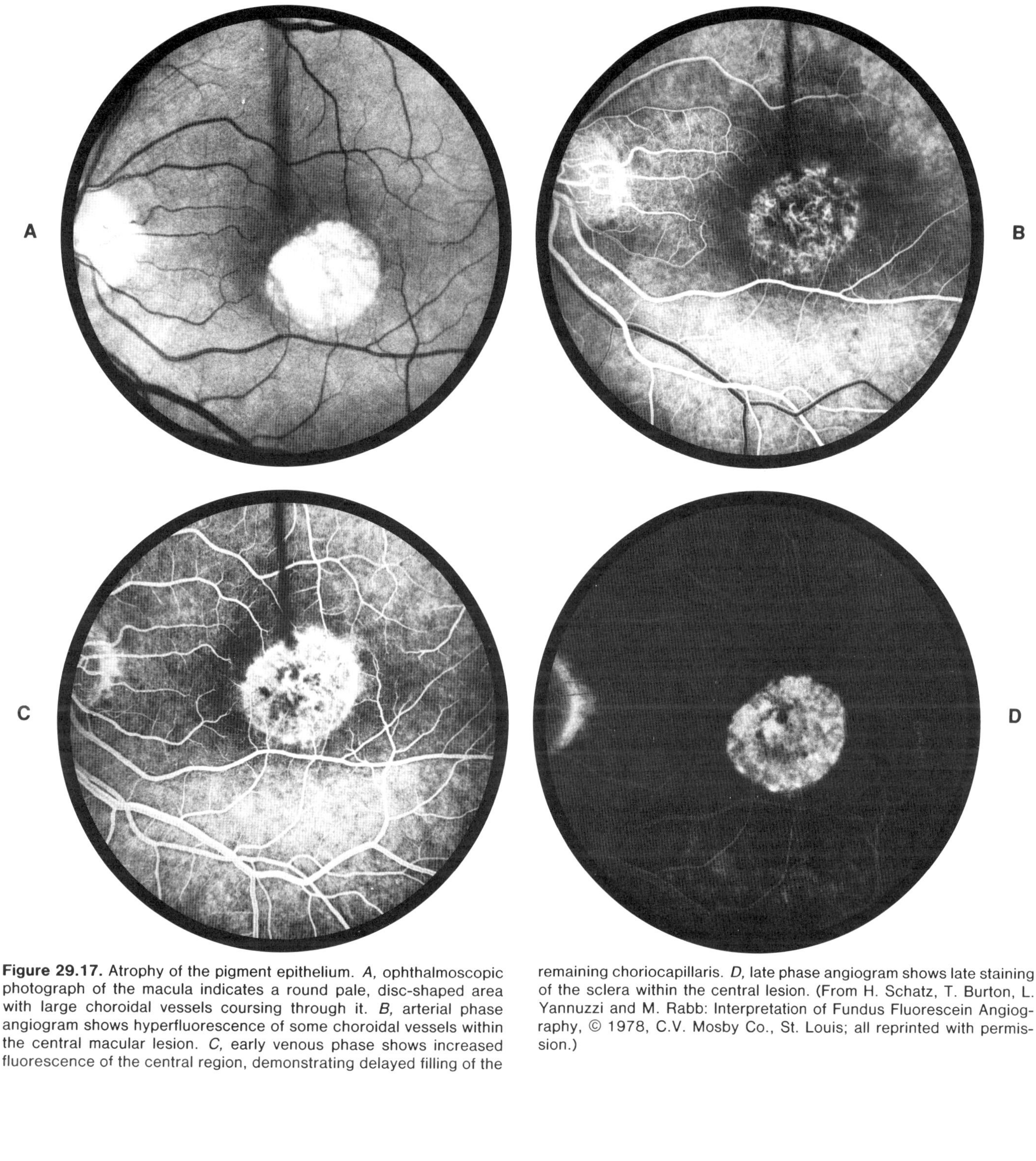

Figure 29.17. Atrophy of the pigment epithelium. *A*, ophthalmoscopic photograph of the macula indicates a round pale, disc-shaped area with large choroidal vessels coursing through it. *B*, arterial phase angiogram shows hyperfluorescence of some choroidal vessels within the central macular lesion. *C*, early venous phase shows increased fluorescence of the central region, demonstrating delayed filling of the remaining choriocapillaris. *D*, late phase angiogram shows late staining of the sclera within the central lesion. (From H. Schatz, T. Burton, L. Yannuzzi and M. Rabb: Interpretation of Fundus Fluorescein Angiography, © 1978, C.V. Mosby Co., St. Louis; all reprinted with permission.)

FOVEAL SUBRETINAL NEOVASCULARIZATION

Foveal subretinal neovascularization, regardless of the cause, constitutes a firm contraindication to laser treatment, since the foveal pigment epithelium and rods and cones are also irreversibly damaged or will be soon after the development of subretinal neovascularization. The subretinal neovascularization, although small in size, is not treatable if it involves the central foveal area (Fig. 29.18). Proposals have been made to treat small foveal subretinal neovascularization in order to prevent extension into the remainder of the macula. Since the specific degree of progression of subretinal neovascularization is unpredictable, there is no indication for treatment if the fovea is involved. Treatment would have to include the surrounding area which constitutes the best visual portion of the patient's remaining macula. Some have proposed treating the extrafoveal (nonfoveal) portion of a subretinal neovascularization, which also involves the fovea. Treatment of most of the subretinal neovascular membrane, leaving even a small part of it remaining, makes little sense because further growth can be expected, perhaps even at an accelerated rate, known as "fertilization." The entire subretinal neovascularization must be treated or none of it. Therefore, if the fovea is involved, the subretinal neovascular membrane cannot be treated.

Figure 29.18. Foveal subretinal neovascularization in presumed ocular histoplasmosis. *A*, ophthalmoscopic photograph of the macula shows a small gray membrane in the center of the fovea (*arrow*). *B*, early venous phase angiogram shows a tiny hyperfluorescent lesion corresponding to the membrane. A diagnosis of a small patch of subretinal neovascularization was made; it was not treated due to its proximity to the fovea. *C*, ophthalmoscopic photograph of the same eye, 6 months later, shows a macular detachment secondary to a large subretinal membrane (*arrow*) associated with hemorrhage. Peripapillary chorioretinal atrophy is also evident. *D*, arteriovenous phase angiogram. The subretinal neovascular membrane is hyperfluorescent. *E*, late phase angiogram shows hyperfluorescence, not only under the detached sensory retina, but also within the cystoid spaces of the overlying detached sensory retina. This patient's subretinal neovascularization began as a small tuft in the fovea and, left untreated, increased in size to overtake and completely encompass the central macular area.

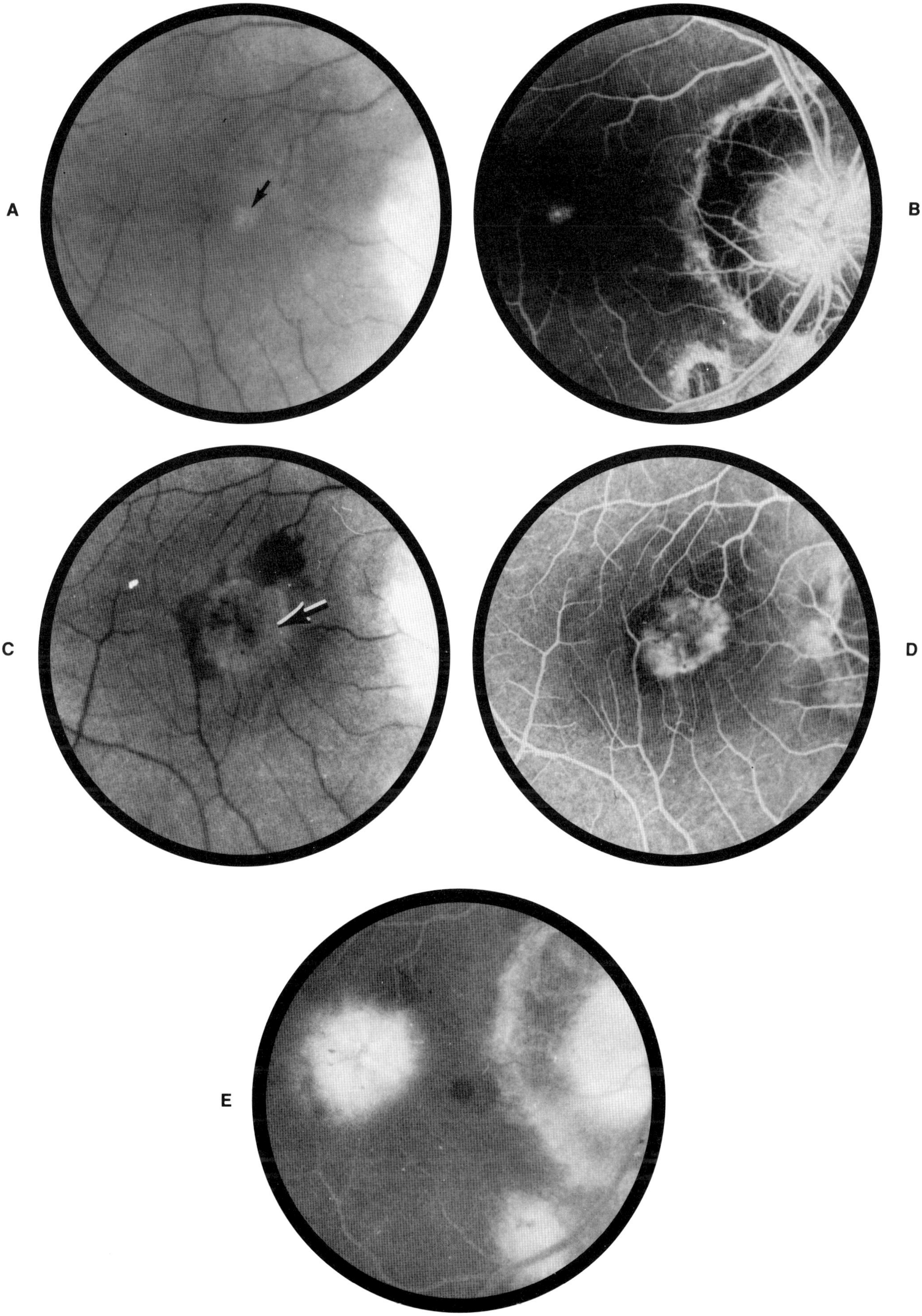

Figure 29.18

A 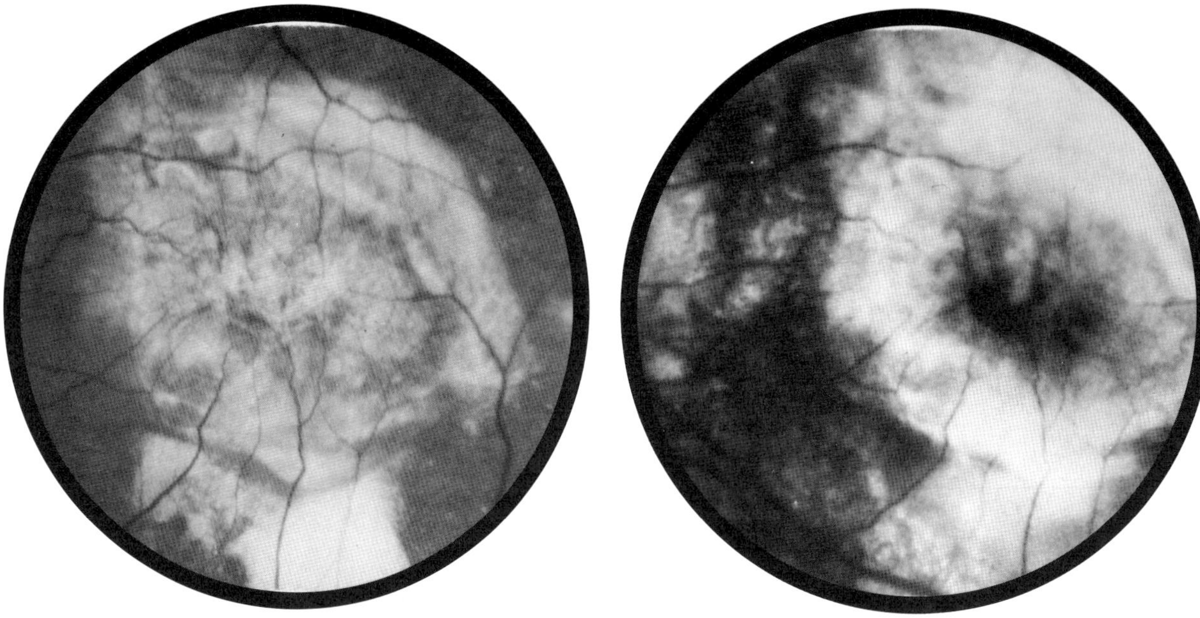 B

Figure 29.19. Foveal scar. *A*, ophthalmoscopic photograph of the left macula shows a large disciform scar involving most of the macular area. *B*, late phase angiogram shows staining of the scar tissue.

A 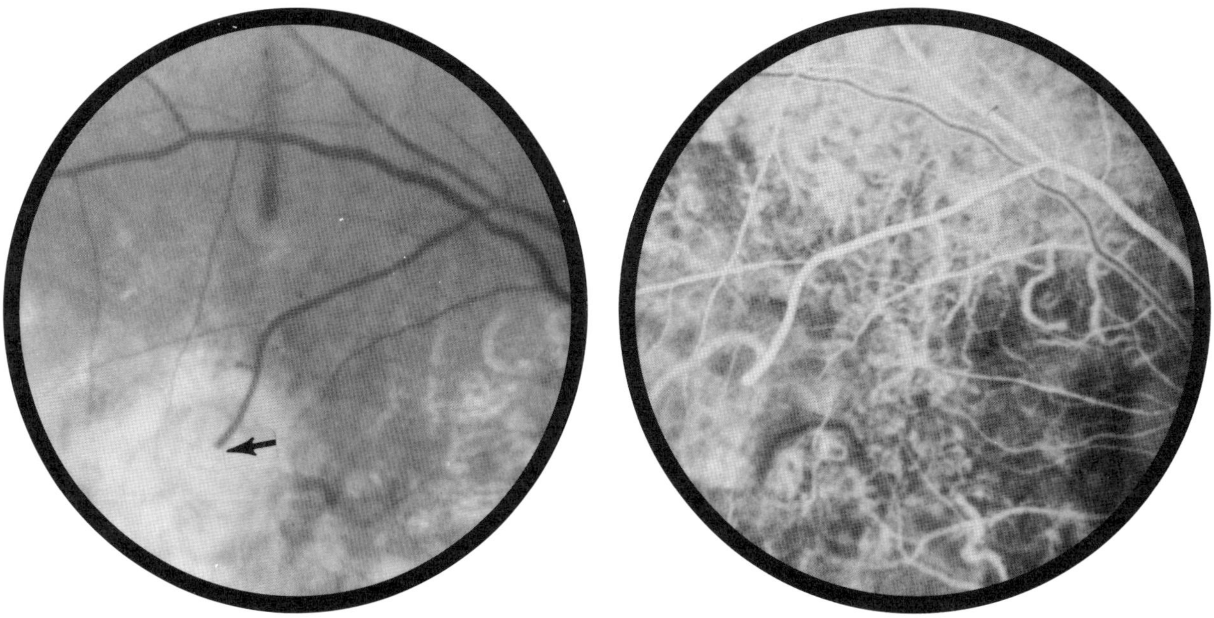 B

Figure 29.20. Macular scar with retinal-choroidal anastomoses. *A*, ophthalmoscopic photograph of the right macula shows a retinal vessel dipping down into a disciform macular scar (*arrows*). *B*, arteriovenous phase angiogram demonstrates a connection between this retinal vessel and a vessel within the disciform lesion.

FOVEAL SCAR

Scar formation involving the fovea includes loss of the foveal rods and cones and, therefore, indicates irreversible reduction of vision. Foveal subretinal neovascularization leads to scar formation since the new vessels are followed by fibrous tissue (Figs. 29.19 and 29.20). Scar can also occur secondary to inflammatory conditions or other pathologic factors (Fig. 29.21). Scar is usually indicative of a quiescent or "healed" pathologic state with little chance of progression, although re-exacerbation of the disease process may occur with further fresh subretinal neovascular membrane formation, or inflammation. Additionally, fibrotic tissue can neither be resolved with laser nor can the tissue damage be reversed. Fibrotic scar may be very slight and small, it may be a part of a huge disciform process (Figs. 29.19, and 29.20), or it may represent any one of a number of various changes along this continuum. However, in each case, irreversible loss of vision and contraindications for laser treatment are the rule.

FOVEAL EXUDATE (LONG-STANDING)

Hard (lipid) exudate involving the fovea often rapidly causes irreversible damage due to a macrophagic and gliotic response within the retina. Hard exudate deposition may occur with various retinal vascular diseases involving the macula, such as diabetic retinopathy or branch vein occlusion. In addition to macular retinal vascular diseases, peripheral retinal vascular diseases such as Coats' disease (peripheral telangiectasia) or von Hippel's disease (retinal angioma) may cause lipid deposition in the macula. Lipid deposition may also occur with various optic nerve diseases such as severe inflammation or severe hypertensive retinal vasculopathy. Additionally, subretinal neovascularization may cause an exudative response resulting in deposition of lipid exudate in the fovea.

Regardless of the cause, lipid deposition remaining in the fovea for more than a few months causes irreversible damage from the macrophagic response. Although laser treatment may cause resolution of the exudate in some of these diseases, return of central vision will not occur because of irreversible structural damage. This is true for macular, optic nerve, or peripheral causes of foveal-macular exudate. Therefore, we do not recommend using laser treatment for cases which involve only long-standing foveal exudate.

A

B

C

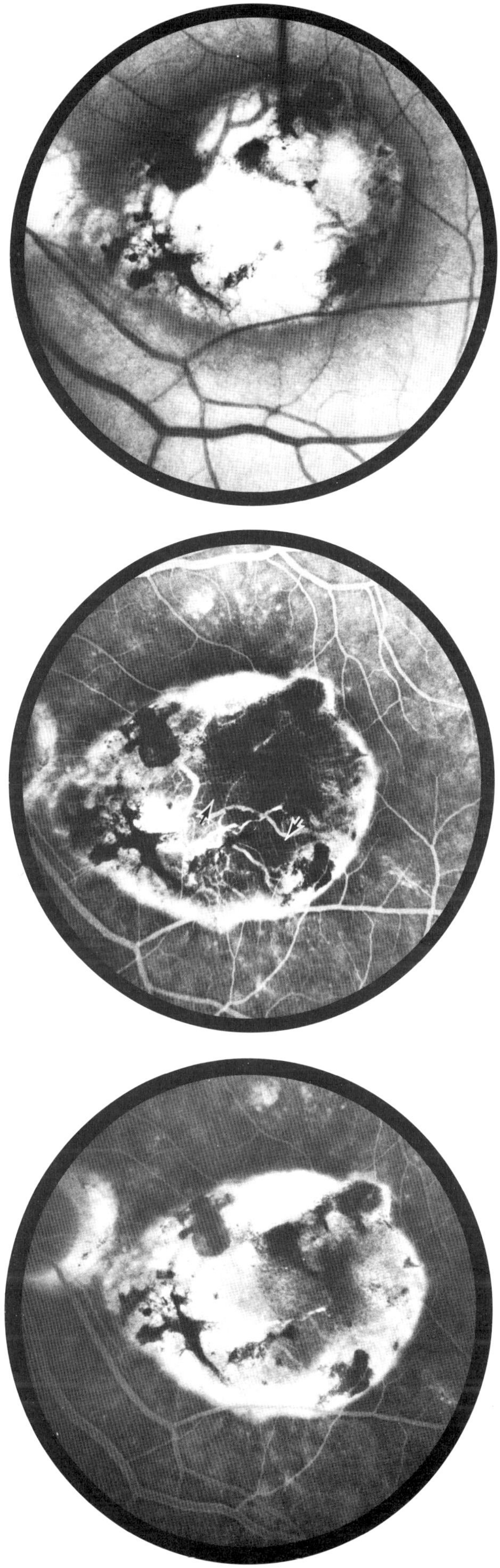

Figure 29.21. Macular scar. *A,* ophthalmoscopic photograph of the macula demonstrates an atrophic scar with patches of pigment epithelial hyperplasia. Large choroidal vessels can be seen coursing through some portions of the scar. *B,* early venous phase angiogram shows hyperfluorescence of the edges around the scar, indicating some remaining choriocapillaris. Hypofluorescence within the mass of the scar is due to hyperpigmentation and loss of choriocapillaris (*arrows*). *C,* late phase angiogram shows hyperfluorescence due to staining of scar tissue and sclera. This patient had toxoplasmic chorioretinitis which resulted in the atrophic macular scar. (From H. Schatz, T. Burton, L. Yannuzzi, and M. Rabb: Interpretation of Fundus Fluorescein Angiography, © 1978, C.V. Mosby Co., St. Louis; all reprinted with permission.)

CYSTOID MACULAR EDEMA

There are many conditions causing cystoid macular edema; i.e., retinal vascular leaking disease, inflammations causing leakage of the retinal vessels in the macula, subretinal neovascularization, choroidal inflammation, and tumors. Most cases of cystoid macular edema are not reversible by argon laser photocoagulation. If the entire perifoveal capillary net is leaking, such as in aphakic cystoid macular edema, or in certain cases of iridocyclitis (Fig. 29.22), the delivery of laser energy, adjacent to and completely around the center of the fovea, would cause severe central visual field defect. There is also a significant risk of misplacement of the laser into the fovea with this type of treatment.

In some cases of retinal vascular leaking disease, the cystoid edema affects only one portion of the macula and, although there may be a foveal cyst generated from leakage of the focal area, treatment of this area of leakage to resolve the edema may be possible (Fig. 29.23).

Occasionally, the retinal vessels adjacent to the fovea-wide leak, with spill-over of the edema fluid into the fovea causing foveal cystoid edema and resultant reduction in vision. In these cases, the extrafoveal leaking retinal vessels may be treated in order to cause resolution of the edema. However, most cases of cystoid macular edema are not amenable to laser photocoagulation treatment because of the foveal or perifoveal source of the leaking fluid (Fig. 29.24).

A

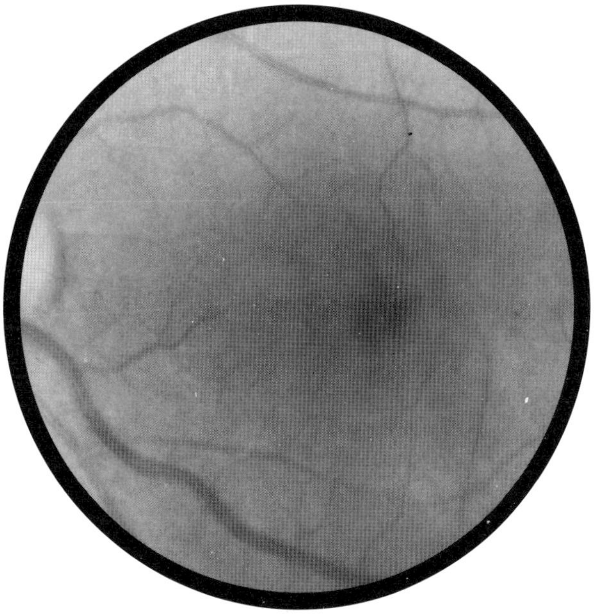

B

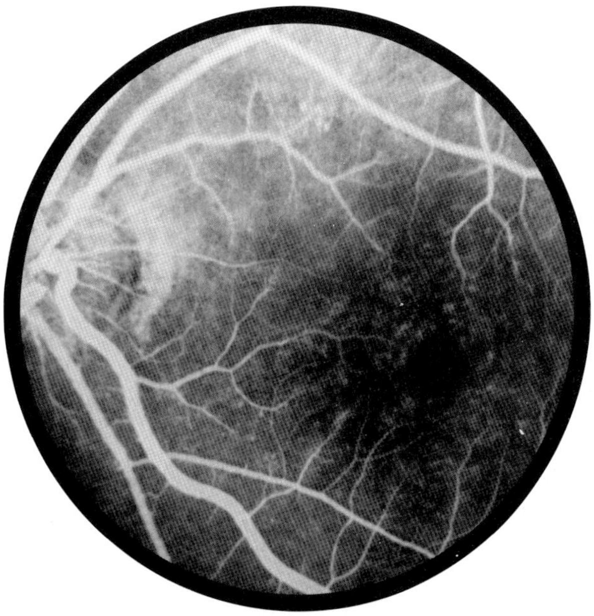

C

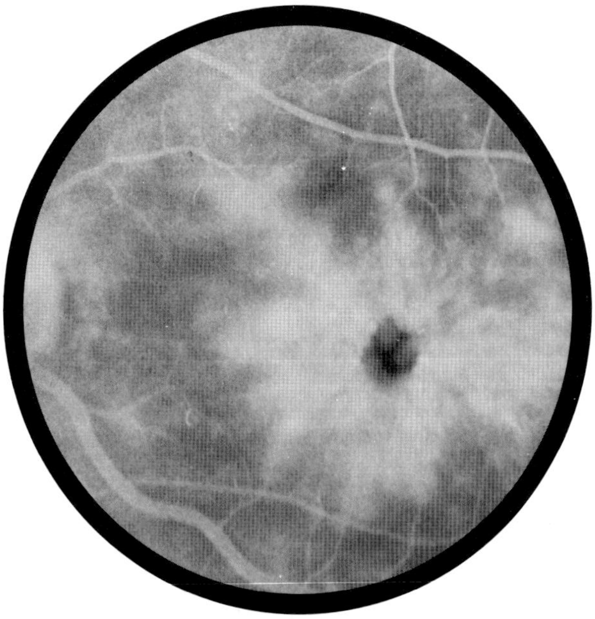

Figure 29.22. Cystoid macular edema secondary to intraocular inflammation. *A*, ophthalmoscopic photograph of the macula demonstrates edema of the retina. *B*, early venous phase angiogram shows dilation of the retinal vascular capillary bed in the macula. *C*, late phase angiogram demonstrates marked cystoid macular edema.

Figure 29.23. Cystoid macular edema secondary to branch vein occlusion (pre- and postoperative argon laser photocoagulation). *A*, ophthalmoscopic photograph of the right disc and macula shows retinal edema above the macula, dilated retinal vessels, and hemorrhages. *B*, early venous phase angiogram shows areas of capillary nonperfusion (superotemporal to the macula) and a dilated retinal vasculature. *C*, late phase angiogram shows marked leakage from the retinal vessels into the retina with resultant cystoid edema. A central foveal cyst is apparent (*arrow*). *D*, ophthalmoscopic photograph of the same patient, two months after argon laser photocoagulation, shows reduced edema and pigmentation in the superior portion of the fovea. *E*, venous phase angiogram shows the absence of retinal vascular dilation in the treated portion of the fovea. The untreated superior area demonstrates dilated leaking retinal vessels. *F*, late phase angiogram shows the fovea to be dry, with some staining around the laser lesions. The untreated superior macula still shows retinal edema. The perifoveal capillary net and vessels in the superior portion of the fovea were treated with argon laser photocoagulation. The edema and cystoid change of the fovea were then resolved, and the patient's vision improved.

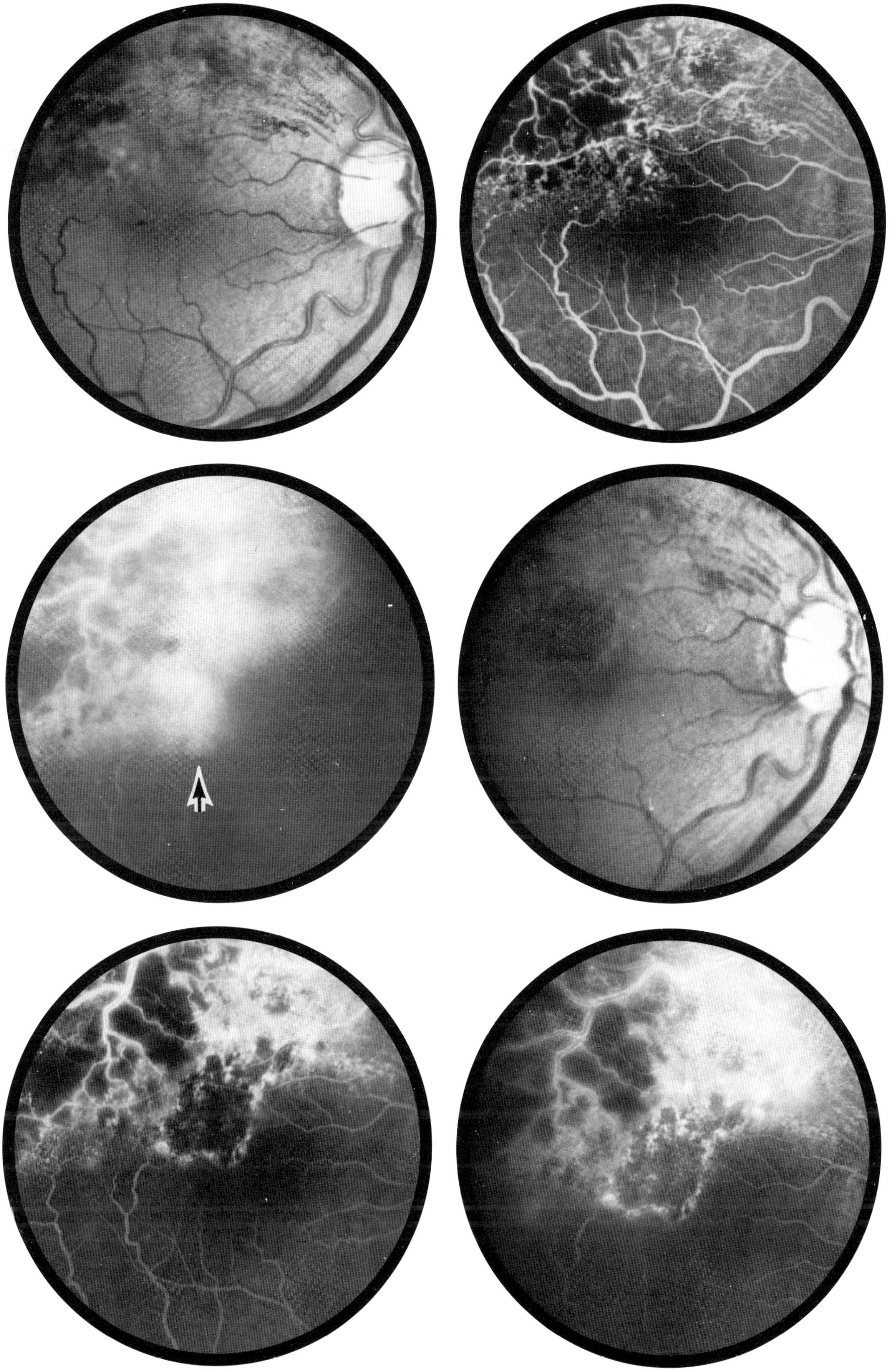

Figure 29.23

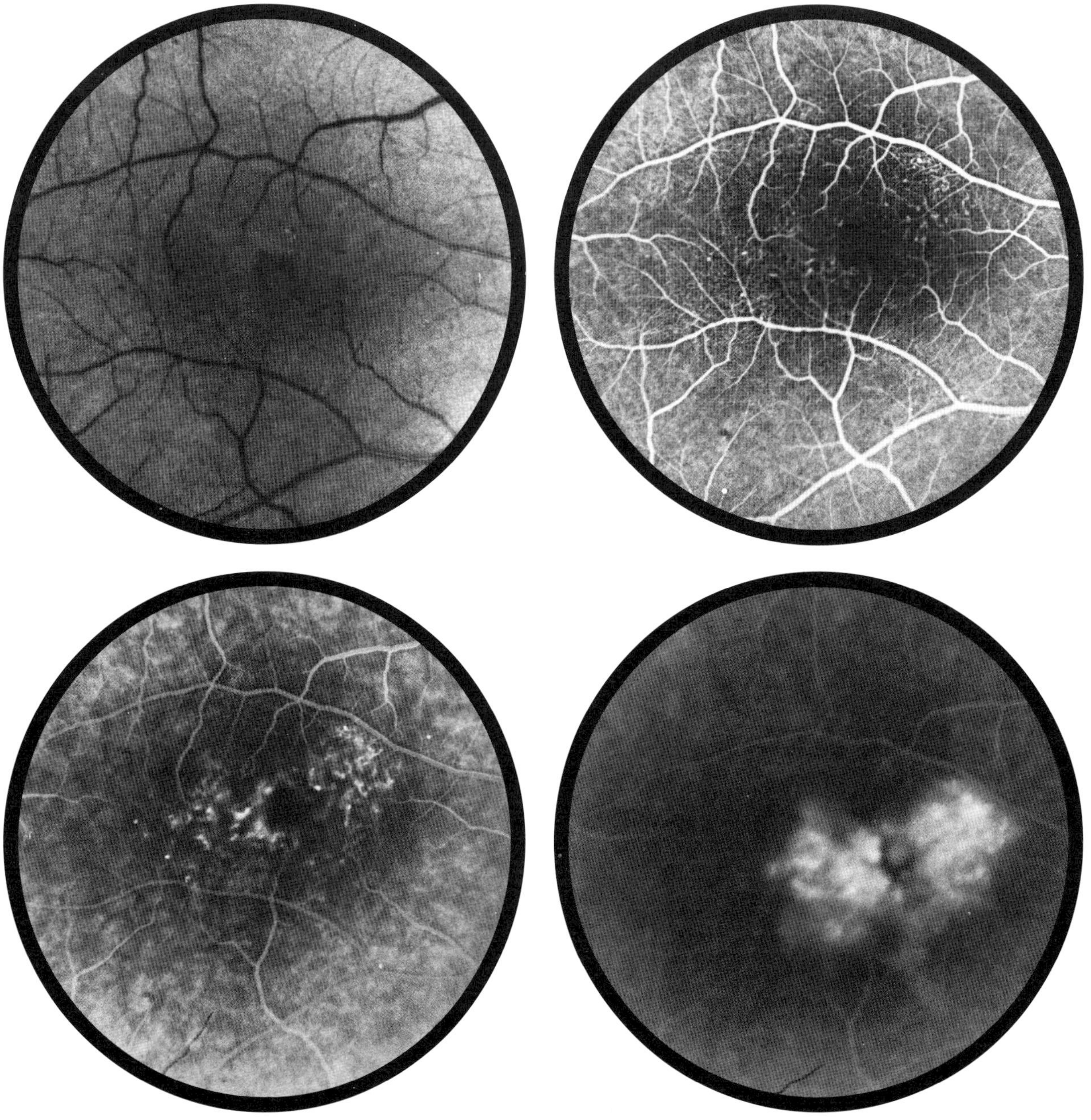

A B C D

Figure 29.24. Macular telangiectasia with cystoid macular edema. *A*, ophthalmoscopic photograph of the macula shows edema and numerous microaneurysms. *B*, early venous phase angiogram shows dilated capillaries in the center of the macula. *C*, late venous phase angiogram shows leakage from the dilated macular vessels. *D*, late phase angiogram shows marked cystoid edema in the central area of the macula. Laser photocoagulation therapy is not helpful in this type of case since the entire capillary bed of the fovea must be treated in order to resolve the edema. (From H. Schatz, T. Burton, L. Yannuzzi and M. Rabb: Interpretation of Fundus Fluorescein Angiography, © 1978, C.V. Mosby Co., St. Louis; all reprinted with permission.)

MACULAR HOLE

There are many causes of macular hole including: aging, trauma, myopia, and long-standing cystoid edema. A macular hole is nearly always foveal and, therefore, irreversible in terms of the return of central vision (Fig. 29.25). The risk of retinal detachment from a complete "through-and-through" macular hole is rare, although this can happen in certain cases of high myopia and trauma. The concept of performing laser treatment in order to seal the surrounding retinal edges of a macular hole is probably not valid. Additionally, there is no indication for laser treatment of a lamellar hole in which the inner portion of the retina is gone leaving only outer retinal elements, as laser can neither halt the development of a through-and-through macular hole nor can it improve the situation in any way (Fig. 29.26).

A

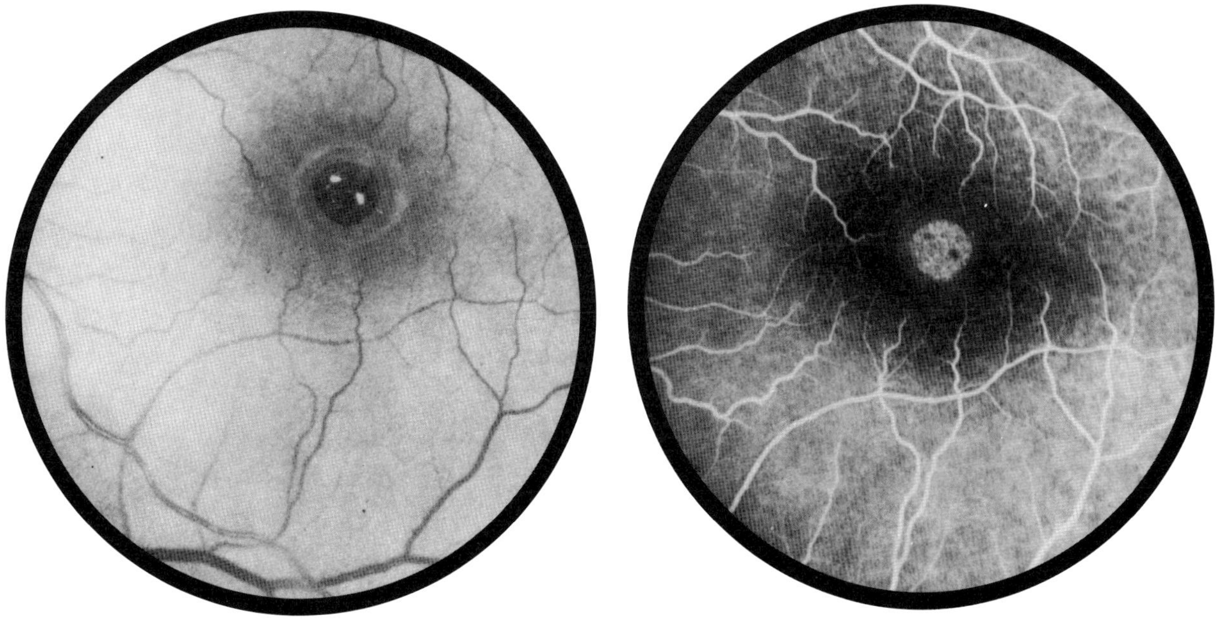

B

Figure 29.25. Macular hole. *A*, ophthalmoscopic photograph of the left macula demonstrates a "through-and-through" macular hole, with small yellow lesions within the hole at the level of the pigment epithelium. The retinal edges around the hole are elevated. *B*, angiogram demonstrates pigment epithelial window defect corresponding to macular hole. The two yellow lesions block fluorescence and correspond to macrophages.

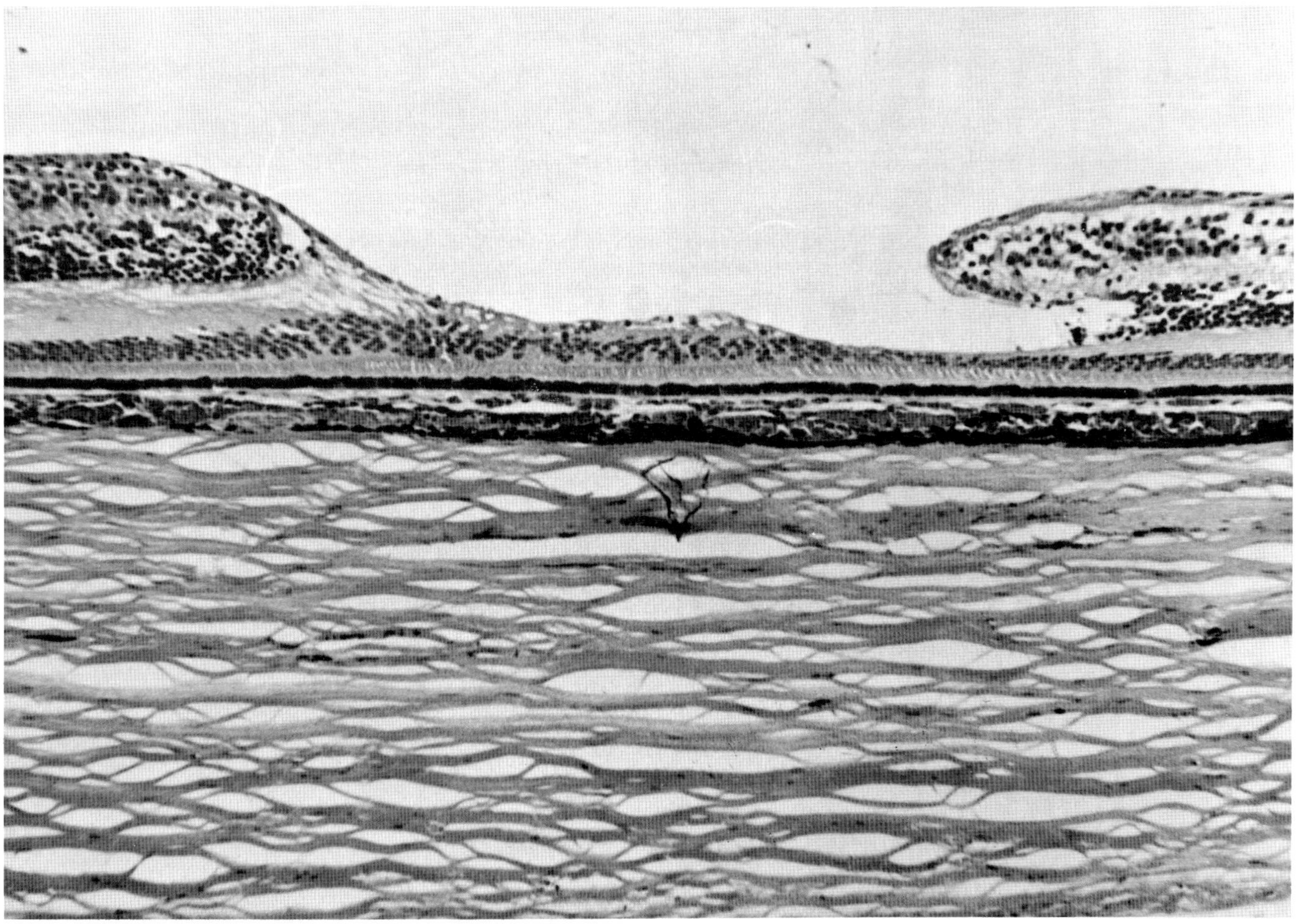

Figure 29.26. Lamellar macular hole. The inner layers of the retina are absent. The rods and cones and a portion of the outer nuclear layer remain. (From H. Schatz, T. Burton, L. Yannuzzi and M. Rabb: Interpretation of Fundus Fluorescein Angiography, © 1978, C.V. Mosby Co., St. Louis; all reprinted with permission.)

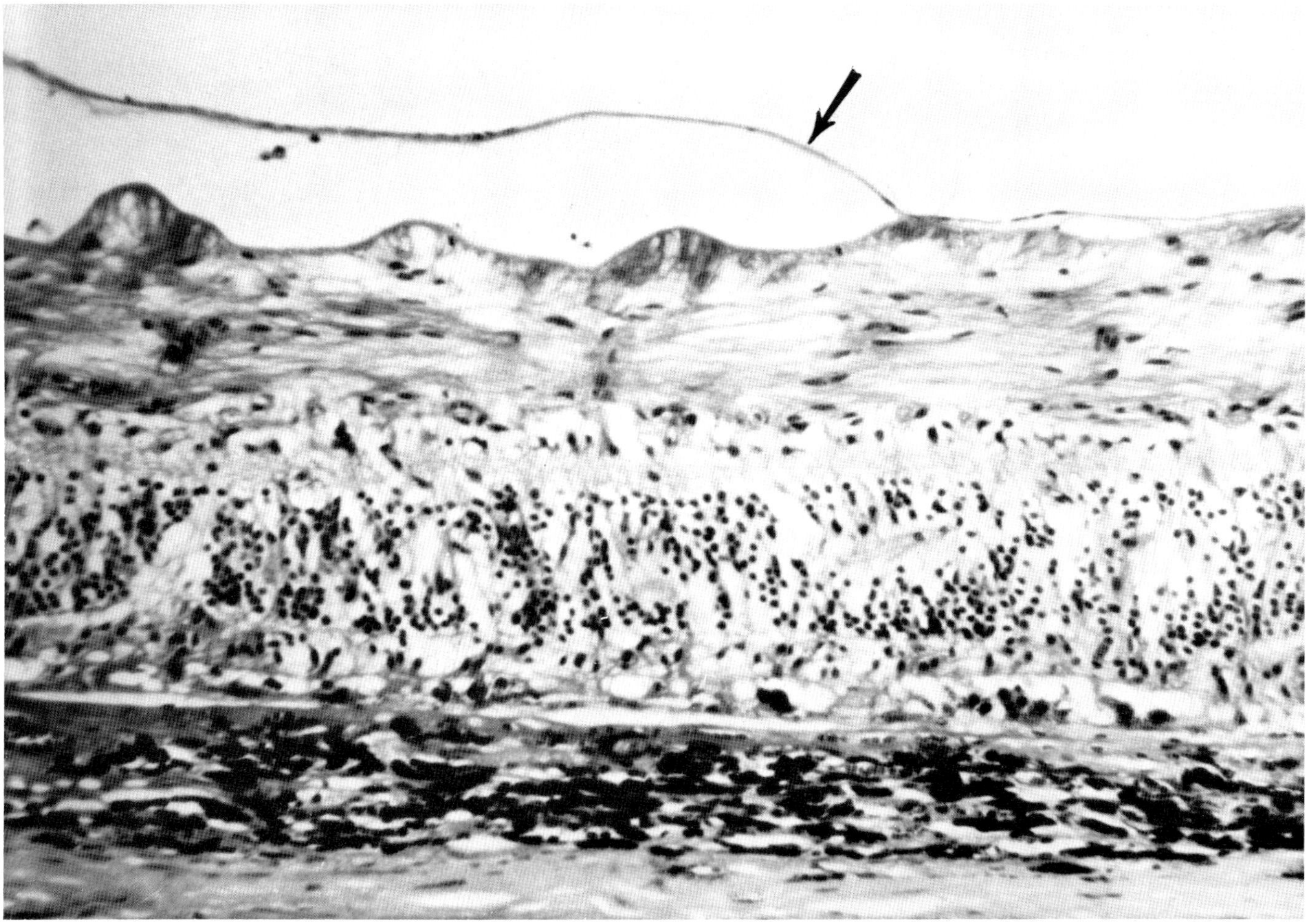

Figure 29.27. Preretinal gliosis (epiretinal membrane). Note the fine glial membrane on the surface of the retina (*arrow*) causing folding of the inner retina. (From H. Schatz, T. Burton, L. Yannuzzi, and M. Rabb: Interpretation of Fundus Fluorescein Angiography, © 1978, C.V. Mosby Co., St. Louis; all reprinted with permission.)

A

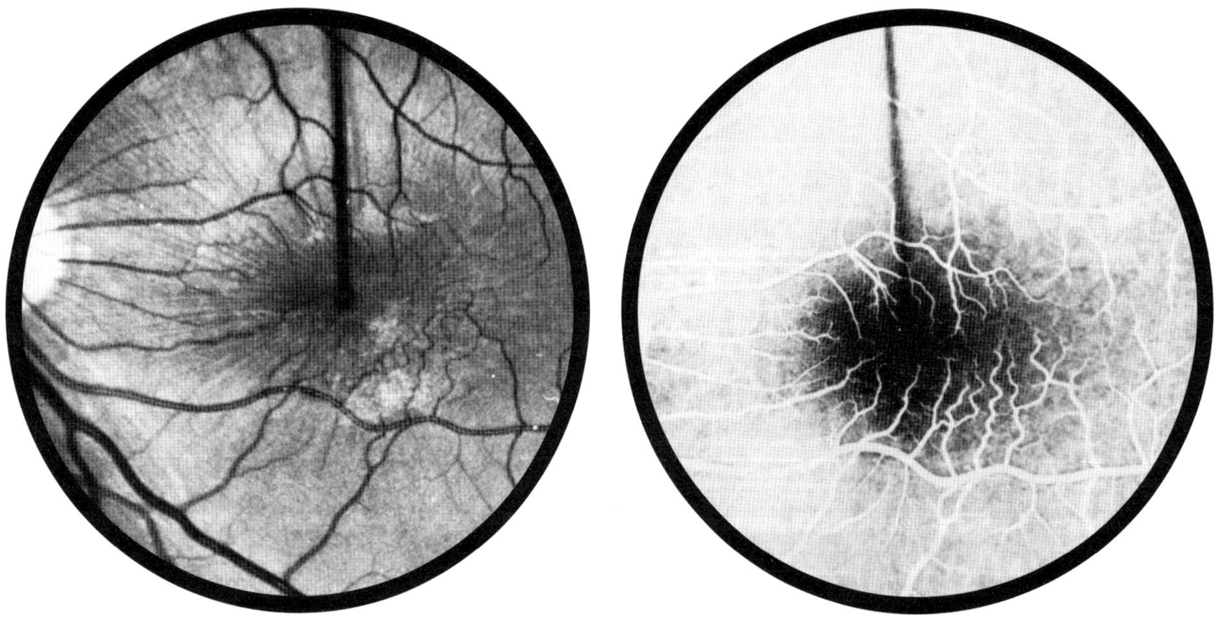

B

Figure 29.28. Preretinal membrane formation. *A,* ophthalmoscopic photograph shows wrinkling of the internal limiting membrane with surrounding retinal atriae. *B,* venous phase angiogram shows tortuosity and prominence of the retinal vessels, but no leakage.

PRERETINAL MEMBRANE FORMATION

Preretinal membrane formation, also known as epiretinal membrane, cellophane maculopathy, internal limiting membrane contraction, vitreoretinal innerface disease, surface wrinkling retinopathy, or macular gliosis, fibrosis, or pucker, is a fairly common maculopathy. In such cases a membrane, usually of glial or fibrous tissue, grows on the surface of the retina and causes distortion and folding of the retina by traction (Fig. 29.27). This is usually an idiopathic change seen in middle-aged and elderly patients and is often associated with posterior vitreous detachment and in some cases hypertension, or retinal vascular occlusive disease. More severe forms occur associated with retinal detachment or after cryo or laser photocoagulation treatment for peripheral retinal pathology.

The traction of the membrane stretches some retinal vessels and wrinkles others (Fig. 29.28). When severe traction occurs the retinal vessels may leak, resulting in retinal edema. This leakage can be demonstrated on fluorescein angiography (Fig. 29.29).

Laser photocoagulation treatment of the leaking retinal vessels in this condition is contraindicated because the heat of the laser may increase the traction on the retina by the membrane and thus further reduce vision. Additionally, it is the mechanical distortion of the retina, rather than the retinal edema, that reduces vision.

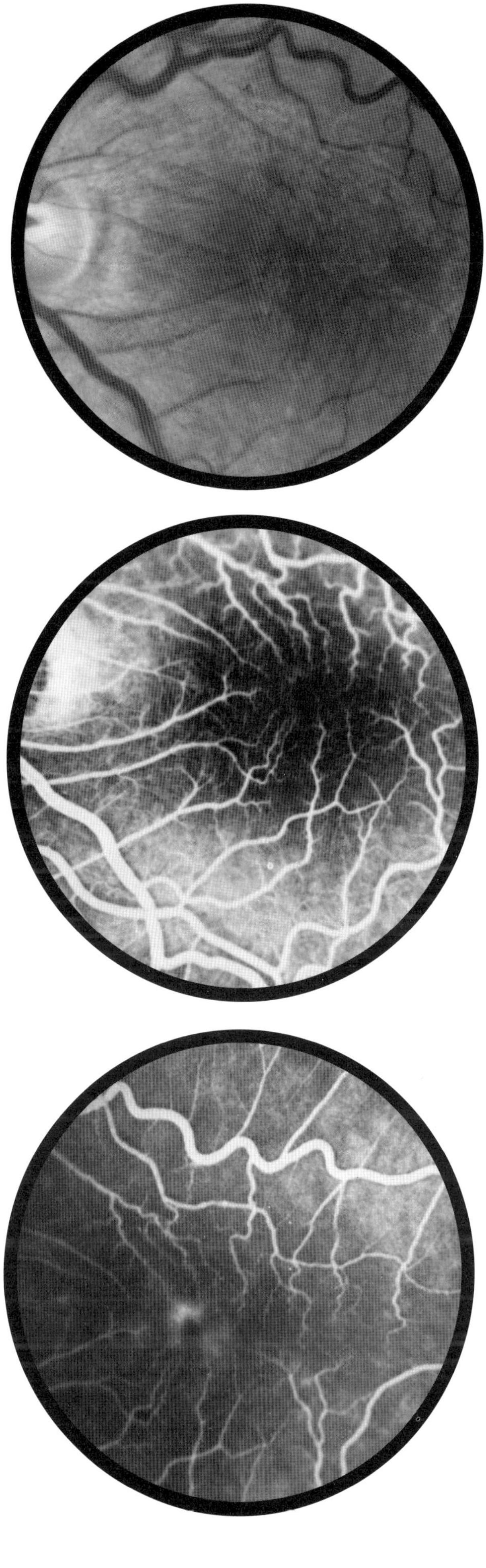

Figure 29.29. Preretinal membrane formation with retinal vascular leakage. *A*, a fine semi-translucent membrane is located on the surface of the retina. It is associated with prominence and tortuosity of the retinal vessels. *B*, early venous phase angiogram shows that the retinal vessels are tortuous and drawn close to the fovea. *C*, late venous phase angiogram shows leakage from the retinal vessels causing retinal edema.

A

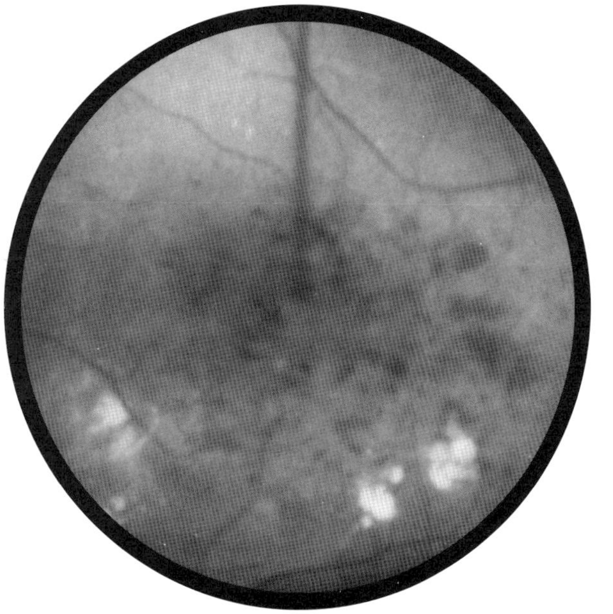

B

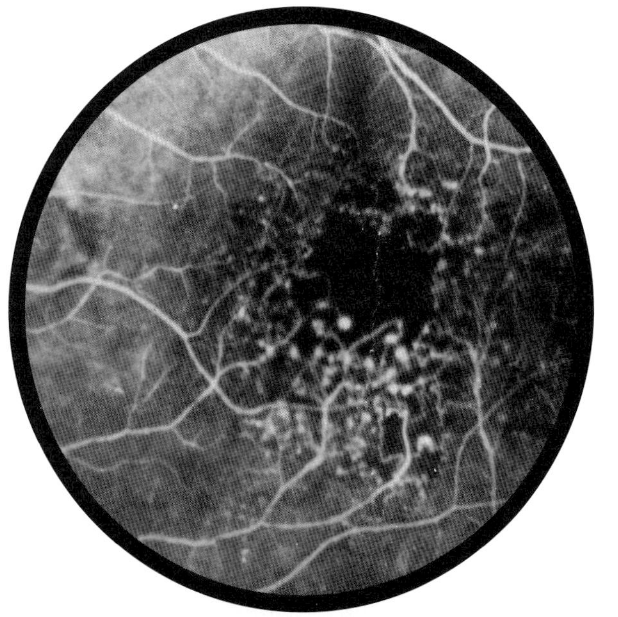

C

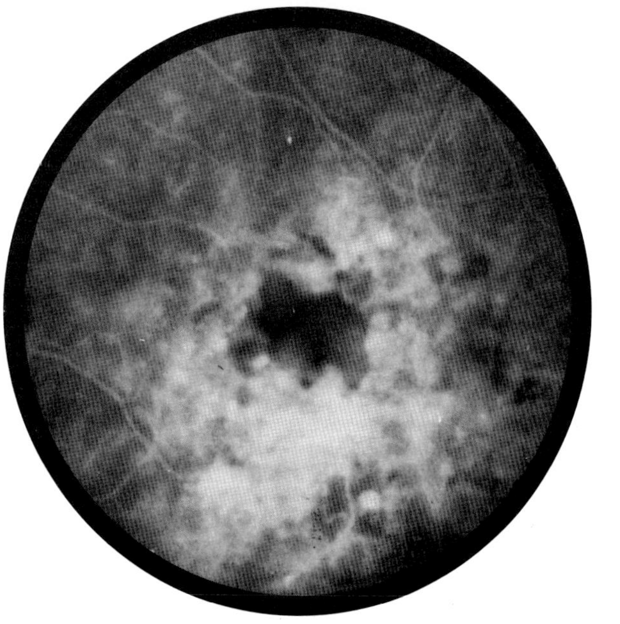

FOVEAL CAPILLARY NONPERFUSION

Various retinal vascular occlusive diseases can result in closure of the perifoveal capillaries. These conditions include: diabetic retinopathy, branch vein occlusion, radiation retinopathy, sickle cell disease, carotid stenosis, and other retinal vascular occlusive disorders (Fig. 29.30). When capillaries are occluded, retinal tissue fed by these capillaries is irreversibly destroyed. When the capillary nonperfusion includes the perifoveal capillary net nasal to the fovea (the papillomacular bundle), vision is usually irreversibly reduced. Laser treatment is fruitless in these cases. No other treatment is known to cause re-opening of the occluded capillaries. Occasionally, capillary nonperfusion includes other portions of the perifoveal capillary net such as the superior, inferior, or temporal areas, and in some of these cases, central vision may still be maintained.

A well resolved fluorescein angiogram is the best method of evaluating the perifoveal capillary net. The net varies with age, but it is usually 300–500 μ in diameter (approximately ¼ disc diameter). When the perifoveal capillary net is irregular or enlarged, occlusion of these vessels is thus indicated.

In summary, the prime consideration in the treatment of macular disease is the viability of the fovea. If the fovea is abnormal, or threatened by fluid, exudate, or neovascularization, yet still salvable or viable, an indication for laser therapy exists. On the other hand, if the fovea has been irreversibly damaged, from any one of a number of pathologic changes, there exists a final contraindication for any further treatment or consideration of laser photocoagulation.

SUGGESTED READINGS

Bird, A.C.: Recent advances in the treatment of senile disciform macular degeneration by photocoagulation. *Brit J Ophthalmol, 58:* 367, 1974.

Campbell, C.J., and Wise, G. N.: Photocoagulation therapy of branch vein obstructions. *Am J Ophthalmol, 75:* 28, 1973.

Diabetic Retinopathy Study Research Group: Preliminary report on effects of photocoagulation therapy. *Am J Ophthalmol, 81:* 383, 1976.

Gitter, K. A., and Cohen, G.: Photocoagulation of active and inactive lesions of presumed ocular histoplasmosis. *Am J Ophthalmol, 79:* 428, 1975.

Little, H.L.: Macular diseases: Classification and treatment with argon laser slit lamp photocoagulation. *Doc Ophthalmol, 1:* 35, 1973.

Patz, A., Maumenee, A.E., and Ryan, S.J.: Argon laser photocoagulation. *Trans Am Acad Ophthalmol Otolaryngol, 75:* 569, 1971.

Patz, A., Schatz, H., Berkow, J.W., *et al.*: Macular edema: an overlooked complication of diabetic retinopathy. *Trans Am Acad Ophthalmol Otolaryngol, 77:* 34, 1973.

Schatz, H., and Patz, A.: Exudative senile maculopathy. I. Results of argon laser treatment. *Arch Ophthalmol, 90:* 183, 1973.

Schatz, H., and Patz, A.: Exudative senile maculopathy. II. Complications of argon laser treatment. *Arch Ophthalmol, 90:* 197, 1973.

Schatz, H., and Patz, A.: Cystoid maculopathy in diabetics. *Arch Ophthalmol, 94:* 761, 1976.

Schatz, H., Yannuzzi, L., and Gitter, K.A.: Subretinal neovascularization masquerading as central serous retinopathy. *Trans Am Acad Ophthalmol Otolaryngol,* in press.

Zweng, H.C., Little, H.L., and Vassiliadis, A.: Argon Laser Photocoagulation, C.V. Mosby Co., St. Louis, 1977.

Figure 29.30. Capillary nonperfusion in retinal vascular occlusive disease. *A,* ophthalmoscopic photograph of the left macula demonstrates hemorrhage, exudate, and edema in the macula. *B,* early venous phase angiogram shows dilation of the retinal vascular bed in the macula. The perifoveal capillary net is enlarged and irregular in shape, indicating that portions of it are occluded. *C,* late phase angiogram shows leakage, indicating retinal edema.

CHAPTER 30

Complications of Photocoagulation Therapy

Francis A. L'Esperance, Jr., M.D.

Complications resulting from photocoagulation can occur relatively infrequently and assume little importance when the proper therapeutic approach is used. It must be noted that some complications cannot be avoided, but the great majority can be the result of improper diagnostic evaluation of the eye and faulty photocoagulation techniques. In the sections below, I will attempt to describe some of the complications that have occurred with argon laser, the principal light modality used in the photocoagulation treatment of macular disease, and to discuss them by anatomic area as listed below.

COMPLICATIONS OF ARGON LASER PHOTOCOAGULATION

LIDS/ADNEXA:	ECCHYMOSIS, MUSCLE PARESIS, RETROBULBAR HEMORRHAGE, SUBCONJUNCTIVAL HEMORRHAGE
CORNEA:	OPACIFICATION
IRIS:	SPHINCTER DAMAGE, CONTRACTION, RUPTURE
LENS:	OPACIFICATION
VITREOUS:	DENATURATION, CONTRACTION
RETINA:	HEMORRHAGE, CONTRACTURE, STRIAE, RECEPTOR LAYER DAMAGE NERVE FIBER LAYER DAMAGE
OPTIC NERVE:	NEURITIS (THERMAL AND ISCHEMIC) NERVE FIBER DAMAGE

External

Although argon laser photocoagulation can be accomplished with only topical anesthesia, a retrobulbar injection is occasionally required in certain patients. The proximity of the macular lesion to the fovea, the location of a tuft of neovascularization near a large retinal vessel, the use of xenon arc photocoagulation, or the inability of the patient to cooperate and maintain fixation have necessitated the use of an injection of 2% lidocaine in the retrobulbar space. In these cases, hemorrhages into the lids or the subconjunctival space can occur, and transient paresis of an extraocular muscle can be observed. No particular treatment for the subconjunctival hemorrhages or areas of ecchymoses in the lids is advocated.

Cornea

Perhaps the most important area to observe with the biomicroscopic portion of the argon laser photocoagulation instrument is the precorneal tear film prior to insertion of the contact lens. Defects in the epithelium, embedded foreign bodies, and opacities in the tear film, such as mascara, flecks of dust, and face powder can act as nidi for the conversion of light to heat energy when trapped beneath the contact lens. Corneal coagulations can be produced, and caution should be exercised in this regard. Stromal cauterization and opacification cannot usually occur, although the focus of the beam can inadvertently be brought close to the central cornea, with coagulation of that structure. Corneal burns have occurred during both retinal photocoagulation and anterior segment photocoagulation, but these have not proved to be significant problems. The endothelium of the cornea can be damaged easily, particularly when photocoagulation is used for anterior segment defects. An iris cyst closely approximated to the cornea may produce sufficient heat to damage the sensitive endothelium, particularly if blood clots or pigment deposits are located on the anterior cyst wall. The endothelium should be closely examined prior to photocoagulation to ascertain if there are any pigment clumps or cells on the endothelial surface that might absorb the incoming laser beam.

Iris

For the most part, the iris cannot be injured during the process of argon laser photocoagulation, unless the beam is quite eccentric to the visual axis and impinges on the pupillary border. In these cases, the iris sphincter can be damaged sufficiently to weaken the pupillary constrictive effect and cause some atrophy of the iris tissue. Hemorrhage from the iris usually does not occur with an accidental iris coagulation, unless a large amount of rubeosis iridis is present. Hemorrhages have occurred during iris photocoagulation during the procedure called photomydriasis, but these hemorrhages have cleared within several days. Atrophy of the iris stroma and pigment epithelium can occur if the iris is treated inadvertently, but this has not proved to be a problem.

Lens

It is extremely difficult to produce lenticular opacification by the use of argon laser energy. Cortical opacities in the lens can obstruct the laser beam sufficiently so that higher powers are necessary for proper retinal coagulation. If the argon laser beam is moved from the cortical lenticular wedge to a clear area in the lens, and the argon laser power is not reduced, it is conceivable that the full energy impacting on the retinal surface can cause retinal hemorrhages and disruption. It is most important to search, prior to the insertion of the contact lens, for pieces of blood, pigment, or other debris that have adhered to the posterior or anterior surface of the lens, in order that they might be avoided at the time of laser photocoagulation. The small absorbant particles can cause localized opacifications of the lens if sufficient energy is absorbed and converted to heat.

Vitreous

During the prephotocoagulation evaluation, the vitreous must be examined with particular care in order to locate clumps of pigment, blood or other debris that might absorb the incoming argon laser beam. Diffuse vitreous blood may absorb the argon beam and contribute to the degradation of the vitreous structure. Photocoagulation should not be attempted if the lesion to be photocoagulated cannot be seen well by direct ophthalmoscopy. Photocoagulation should be deferred until the vitreous body has cleared sufficiently for this observation, so that the possibility of vitreous traction is minimized.

In some cases, the vitreous traction on various layers and sections of the retina may be enhanced by argon laser photocoagulation. The vitreous must be very carefully evaluated, particularly with regard to its relationship with the retina. Tenting of the posterior portion of the anterior vitreous base, glial proliferation in the macular and perimacular region, wrinkling of the macular retina, plateauing of the distal aspect of the temporal vascular arcades, localized star-figure formation, and the configuration of the various types of vitreoretinal neovascularization should be evaluated with great care, since these signs may indicate early, and perhaps dangerous, vitreous traction. Argon laser photocoagulation should not be employed in these cases if the vitreous traction can be determined to be moderately severe, since retinal detachments, retinoschisis, or macular pucker can be produced by relatively small amounts of photocoagulation energy.

Retina

Hemorrhage from the small or large retinal vessels is perhaps the most common complication of argon laser photocoagulation. Choroidal hemorrhage has been seen following intense argon laser photocoagulations of high power density. The treatment of small nests of neovascularization in the retina has resulted in the occurrence of occasional hemorrhages, but these hemorrhages have never proved significant (Fig. 30.1). It has been recommended that larger spot sizes be used to minimize the problem of hemorrhages from areas of small-vessel surface neovascularization.

Retinal striae may occur when photocoagulation produces a large area of fibrous proliferation. This problem may not be important in the mid-peripheral zones but can be detrimental if the retinal striae involve the foveal or macular region.

In general, photocoagulation into the macular area should not approach within 500 μ of the central fovea, because heat may be transmitted to the pigment epithelium or choroid into the central foveolar region. If blood occurs underneath the retina in the foveal region, photocoagulation should not be attempted within 1,000 μ of the umbo, because of the distinct possibility that heat could easily be conducted to the foveolar zone through the blood layer. Preretinal clots and other areas of diffuse blood in the retrohyaloid space should also be avoided because of the localized production of heat and possibility of increased conduction of the heat to the macular and perifoveal zone (Fig. 30.2).

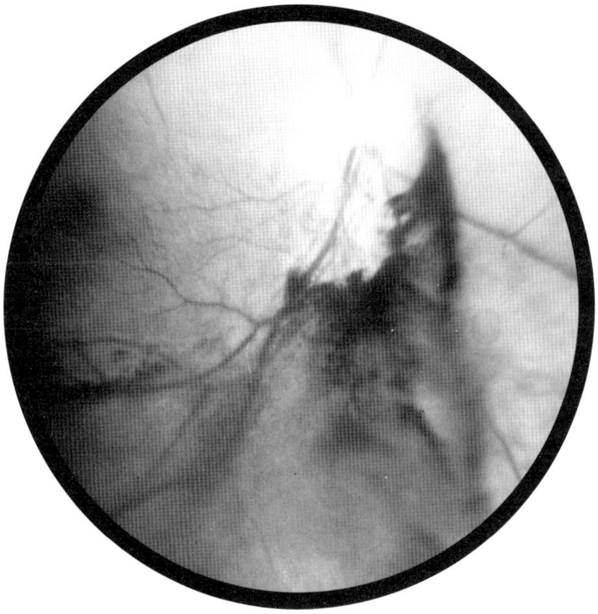

Figure 30.1. Preretinal hemorrhage from a nest of small epipapillary vessels immediately after photocoagulation.

Optic Nerve

The optic nerve is relatively resistant to argon laser photocoagulation but can be damaged by thermal abuse, ischemic insults, or an extremely high power density. Similar damage can occur when an attempt is made to photocoagulate a large vessel on the optic nerve head. As this vessel absorbs the argon laser beam, it can produce sufficient heat to cause coagulation necrosis of the nerve fiber layer. Damage can also occur to the optic nerve through the creation of ischemic optic neuritis. As a considerable amount of blood supplying the optic nerve comes from the surrounding choroidal vasculature, photocoagulation in the peripapillary region can reduce the blood supply sufficiently to cause a marked and devastating ischemia to the optic nerve. The third way that nerve fibers on the optic nerve head can be destroyed is through the inadvertent use of extremely small spot sizes with high power settings (Fig. 30.3). The power density thus created at the photocoagulation site is sufficient to disrupt the nerve fibers, regardless of the presence of any absorbing substance.

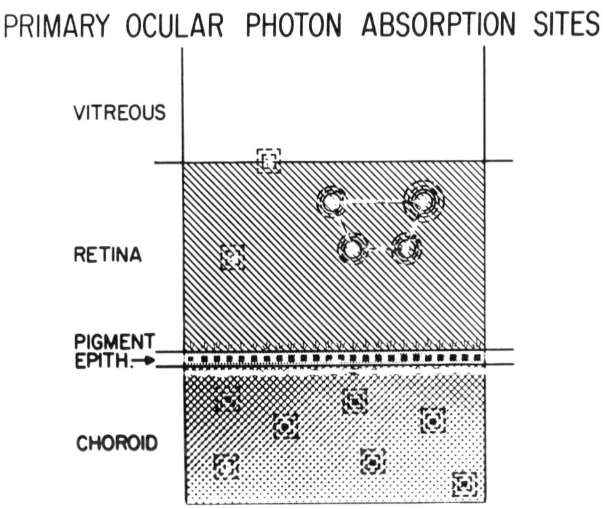

Figure 30.2. Diagram illustrating some zones of pigment accumulation, hemoglobin concentration, and other regions that can selectively absorb argon laser photocoagulation, with the production of heat foci.

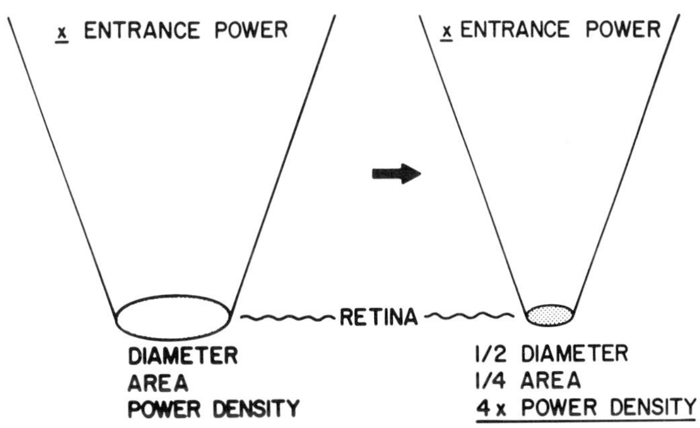

Figure 30.3. Diagram illustrating that a one-half reduction of the beam diameter on the retina produces a 4× power density increase. The power density should be maintained when reducing spot size by an appropriate reduction in entrance power.

In summary, the possible complications of photocoagulation can be generally divided into the three anatomic areas or portions of the globe. First, the macular region is extremely susceptible to various complications by the introduction of argon laser photocoagulation energy. Although I have never seen a foveal burn, I have observed some very close coagulations. Ophthalmologists should always be concerned with treating close to the foveal region in the inferior portion, since a very pronounced Bell's phenomenon could cause a streaked coagulation through the fovea if the exposure is longer than 0.10 second. Thermal diffusion can also be extremely important, with various compartmental defects, such as serous detachments of the pigment epithelium or serous or hemorrhagic detachments of the sensory retina (Fig. 30.4). In these cases, the heat generated at the coagulation site can be conducted effectively to the receptor elements in the nearby fovea, causing irreparable damage. Flecks of gliosis, hemorrhage, or pigment can also create foci that can generate sufficient quantities of heat to damage the nearby visual cells. Care must also be taken when moving from one section of the macula to another, where an inequality of edema, microcystic disease, pigment dispersion or proliferation, or atrophy of the vessels exist. The laser energy must be constantly tailored to the absorption potential of the proposed macular coagulation site. In addition, intense photocoagulations in the perimacular region or perifoveal region can obstruct the tiny terminal arterioles or venules in the macular region, causing hemodynamic alterations in that region, occlusion of the various choroidal arteriolar segments, partial retinal vein obstruction, increased production of microcystic disease in the macular zone, and an increase in the degree of preretinal fibrosis (Fig. 30.5).

Photocoagulation in the periphery of the retina must be applied cautiously and with great care. The vitreoretinal traction on the anterior vitreous base can be accentuated by widespread or intense treatment in that region. Direct photocoagulation to peripheral retinal neovascularization can produce transient choroidal ischemia or, more significantly, a choroidal hemorrhage with secondary choroidal-retinal-vitreal neovascularization. Pigment proliferation, preretinal gliosis, macular pucker, macular schisis, macular edema, as well as generalized degradation of the vitreous body can occur from widespread or intense peripheral photocoagulation.

The panretinal photocoagulation technique can also be responsible for massive choroidal effusions which can lead to relative closure of the trabecular meshwork and a situation that resembles an angle-closure glaucoma. Defects in the nerve fiber layer, with resultant visual field alterations, can occur from extensive panretinal photocoagulation, as with photocoagulation in any portion of the choroid and retina. The effect of peripheral photocoagulations on the macular region cannot be underestimated at any time.

The complications encountered with anterior segment photocoagulation have not been serious but must be avoided, if possible. Corneal burns, iris hemorrhage, the production of severe iritis, glaucoma, cataracts, and retinal coagulations have been reported but can be minimized, if not completely eliminated, by the proper photocoagulation approach to the particular disease.

Ocular photocoagulation, like many special procedures in the practice of medicine, is not without the potential for various types of complications. However, these complications are being reduced as photocoagulation is becoming safer, with the careful evaluation of the eye and the judicious use of this modality during treatment.

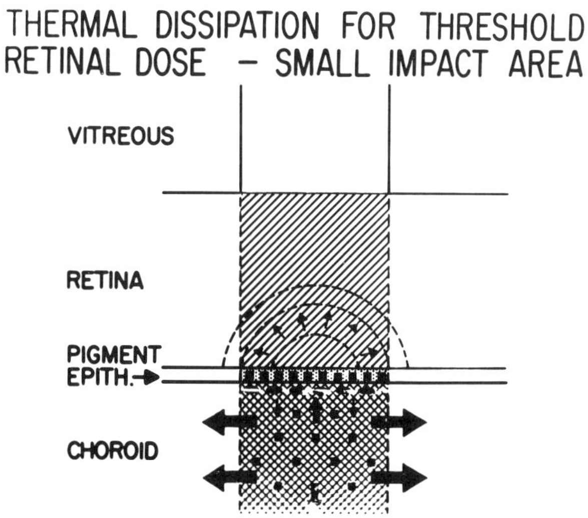

Figure 30.4. Diagram illustrating the conduction of heat from the pigment epithelial region to the surrounding choroid and retina. Thermal dissipation is less effective with larger spot sizes, and lower power densities should be employed.

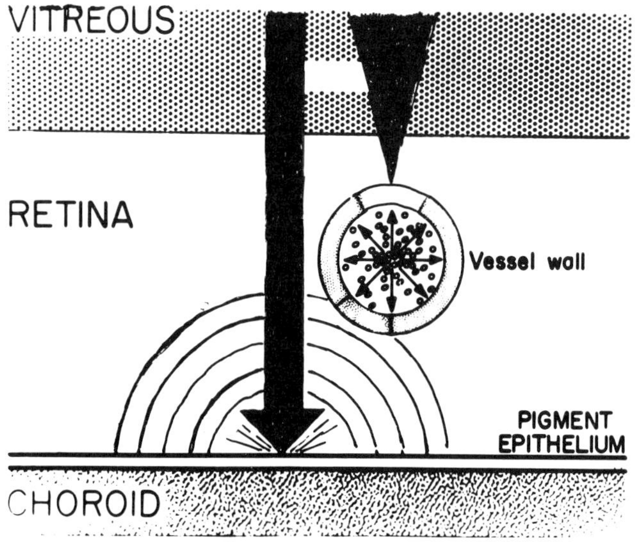

Figure 30.5. Diagram illustrating the methods of possible vascular rupture in the retina from heat produced at the pigment epithelial layer, or by the direct action of the laser beam on the superficial retinal vessel. Either mechanism may cause rupture or necrosis of the vessel wall, resulting in an intraretinal or preretinal hemorrhage.

Suggested Readings

Francois, J. (ed.): Symposium on Light Coagulation, Argon Laser and Xenon Arc, 1972. *Doc Ophthalmol, 1,* 1973.

L'Esperance, F.A.: Ocular Photocoagulation: A Stereoscopic Atlas, C.V. Mosby, St. Louis, 1976.

Zweng, H.C., et al.: Laser Photocoagulation and Retinal Angiography with Current Concepts in Retinal and Choroidal Diseases, C.V. Mosby, St. Louis, 1969.

CHAPTER 31

Evaluation of Photocoagulation Therapy

Thomas C. Burton, M.D.

The majority of studies involving photocoagulation management of various macular disorders have errors in design, limiting the value of the reports. How can the ophthalmologist determine the validity of such material? Each article should be examined carefully for deficiencies in the protocol (material and method). Common sources of errors occur in the following areas:

(1) Assessment of visual acuity,
(2) Selection of patients for treatment,
(3) Selection of control patients,
(4) Duration of observations,
(5) Technique of treatment,
(6) Criteria for determining change in visual acuity, and
(7) Statistical evaluation.

The purpose of this review is to discuss selected investigations on photocoagulation therapy of macular diseases and to illustrate some of the flaws which reduced the effectiveness and reliability of the reports.

Assessment of Visual Acuity

Because results following photocoagulation treatment are based primarily on the final central visual acuity, there should be an exact description of the methods used to determine visual function. Individual patient data may be excluded in the text and should be analyzed critically. For example, if no patients were observed to have visual acuities between 20/100 and 20/200, the Snellen chart must have been employed. Unfortunately, the Snellen system is inadequate to estimate visual acuity below 20/80. There is no accurate method to determine visual acuities of 20/200 or less; therefore, the observations on such patients should be discarded.

The Sloan chart [1] is superior to the Snellen chart for several reasons. The 10 recurring letters of the Sloan system have been determined to approximate the difficulty of the Landolt C test. Each line is 0.1 log units (26%) larger than the preceding line. Acuities of 20/125 and 20/160 can be ascertained. There are more characters for each level of vision. At 20/100 the Snellen chart has only two letters, while the Sloan chart has six.

To avoid bias by the therapist, all visual acuities should be recorded by a technician utilizing the same chart, distance, and lighting condition on each occasion.

In 1971 a group of investigators reported on xenon arc photocoagulation of 62 eyes in 54 patients with senile disciform macular degeneration [2]. The technique for determining visual acuity was not stated. Most notations were in the Snellen format, but nine patients were recorded as having finger counting vision at a variety of distances. Acuities were recorded at 10 different distances ranging from 6 inches to 25 feet. Thirty patients were tested preoperatively and postoperatively at different distances. Thirty patients had initial visual acuities of less than 20/200. The criterion for determining the change in visual acuity was not stated, but presumably was accepted as only a single line difference.

The authors concluded that the vision improved in 60% of the cases and became worse in 22%. If two lines difference had been selected as the criterion for detecting a change in visual acuity, then the number of patients demonstrating improvement would be only 29% (Table 31.1). If only patients with acuities of 20/200 or better are evaluated, then 41% are found to have decreased vision following treatment.

Selection of Patients for Treatment

In a report on the results of ruby laser photocoagulation of "vascular macular pathology" [3], many fundus lesions were not defined and classified accurately. Twenty-two of their patients were diagnosed as having central serous chorioretinopathy. Following treatment, five patients obtained poor visual results with two patients developing subretinal fibrosis. It is now well known that central serous chorioretinopathy has a 100% spontaneous remission rate with a low morbidity of 10–15%, usually in the form of a mild decrease in visual acuity.

Inadequate attention was directed to initial visual acuity, age, clinical appearance of the macula, and history of visual problems in the opposite eye. Five patients entered the study with visual acuities of 20/200 or less. Severe loss of vision is extremely rare in central serous chorioretinopathy. One patient with a small macular hemorrhage (which never occurs in central serous chorioretinopathy) was 62-years-old and had lost central vision in the fellow eye from a

Table 1. Xenon photocoagulation of senile macular degeneration[2]

Criterion for change in acuity	Final acuity compared to initial acuity		
	Same	Better	Worse
1 line	18%	60%	22%
2 lines	48%	29%	23%

disciform degeneration. The mean age of central serous chorioretinopathy patients is approximately 43 years. It is very uncommon for a patient with this disease to exceed 55 years of age [4].

Obviously some of the cases were misdiagnosed. The inclusion of senile disciform patients in the central serous chorioretinopathy group invalidated the conclusions drawn by the authors.

Selection of Control Patients

Despite increasing awareness of the value of well designed prospective studies with randomly selected control patients, most reports are accompanied by no control subjects at all, or by historical control patients at best. These "control patients" are usually derived from previously published data or from a group of similar appearing cases retrieved from the filing cabinets. The latter technique was employed in 1968 in reporting on xenon photocoagulation of the presumed ocular histoplasmosis syndrome [5]. Forty-seven patients were treated on 74 occasions. Curiously, the authors published the data for only 32 eyes. The comparison group of 49 control patients had received no treatment for undetermined reasons other than "lack of interest by them or their referring ophthalmologist" (Table 31.2).

All final visual acuities were displayed in a fashion implying that patients receiving photocoagulation had a better opportunity to achieve 20/15 vision (16% in the treatment group versus 6% in the control group). Had a more appropriate level of vision, such as 20/50, been chosen to indicate a satisfactory result, then the two groups would have been shown to be nearly identical (28% in the treatment group versus 31% in the control group).

In this study not all of the treated patients were reported. The control patients were not selected by chance alone from the same population over the same time interval. Many control patients were evaluated before photocoagulation was utilized for the treatment of histoplasmic choroiditis. Therefore, this group of patients of necessity was followed longer and could be predicted to have a poorer long-range prognosis. The control patients obtained during the photocoagulation period did not receive treatment for subjective reasons. These patients easily could represent a class in which poor results were anticipated.

Table 2. Xenon photocoagulation of histoplasmic choroditis[5]

Category	No. of patients	Final Visual Acuity	
		20/15	20/50 or better
Xenon	32	16% (5)	28% (9)
Control subjects	49	6% (3)	31% (15)

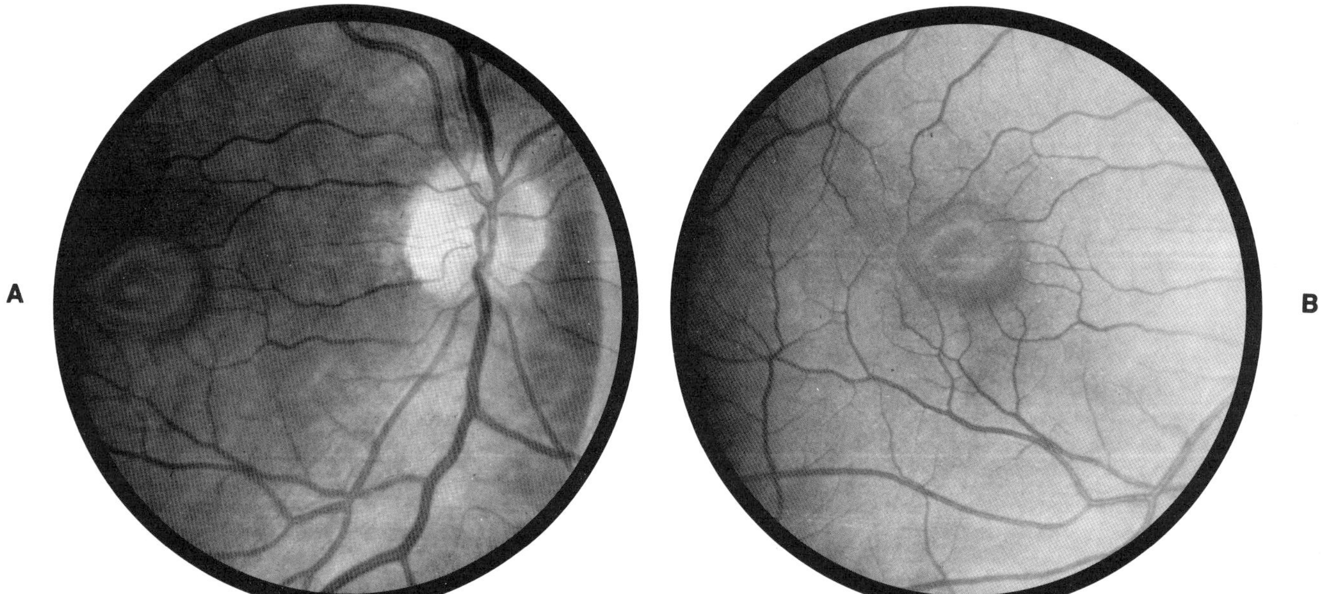

Figure 31.1. *A*, ophthalmoscopic photograph of right eye showing serous detachment of the retinal pigment epithelium in a 53-year-old man. Visual acuity was 20/25. *B*, ophthalmoscopic photograph of same patient, 2½ years later. Visual acuity remains 20/25.

Duration of Observations

In 1974 there was a report on argon laser photocoagulation in 81 patients with senile macular degeneration [6]. In the avascular group there was only one patient who lost a single line of visual acuity following treatment, while 15 of 24 patients improved. This investigation suffered from several errors including lack of randomized controls subjects, no standardized method for assessing visual acuity, insufficient criteria for establishing changes in visual acuity, recruitment of numerous patients with very poor initial acuity (35% with 20/200 or less) and no statistical consultation. The follow-up ranged from 6 months to 3 years with an average of 10 months. Given a disease with marked variation in expression and long natural course of progression, the follow-up in this study is obviously inadequate. The patients described in Figures 31.1 and 31.2 illustrate that all pigment epithelial detachments do not have a rapidly progressive downhill course.

In this study, the author placed considerable weight on the subjective observation of flattening of serous detachments of the retinal pigment epithelium. Assuming that accurate preoperative and postoperative refractions are performed, resolution of a pigment epithelial detachment is poorly correlated with an alteration of visual acuity. The patient described in Figure 31.3 demonstrates a serous retinal pigment epithelial detachment which was flattened by argon laser photocoagulation with long term stabilization of central visual acuity. A permanent paracentral scotoma occurred from treatment. A gradual atrophy of the pigment epithelium eventually caused a severe reduction in visual acuity. This patient would have been considered a success in any study with a follow-up of less than 3 years.

A

B

C

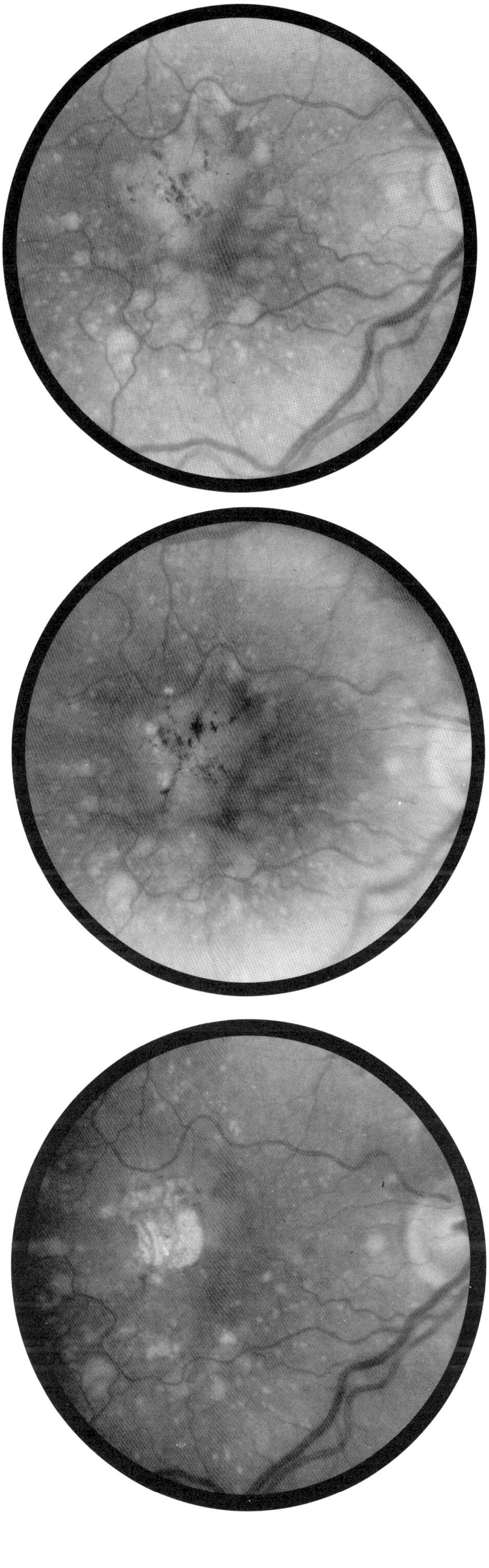

Figure 31.2. *A*, ophthalmoscopic photograph of right eye of a 77-year-old woman showing extensive drusen and irregularly outlined serous detachment of the retinal pigment epithelium. Overlying pigment disruption indicates chronic process. Visual acuity measured 20/25 with +4.50 sph. *B*, ophthalmoscopic photograph of same eye, 2½ years later, showing increased pigmentation. Visual acuity was 20/25. *C*, ophthalmoscopic photograph of same eye, 3½ years after initial examination, showing spontaneous flattening of retinal pigment epithelial detachment, calcified drusen, and areolar atrophy of pigment epithelium temporal to fovea. At age 81, the patient is asymptomatic with visual acuity corrected to 20.30 with +4.00 sph.

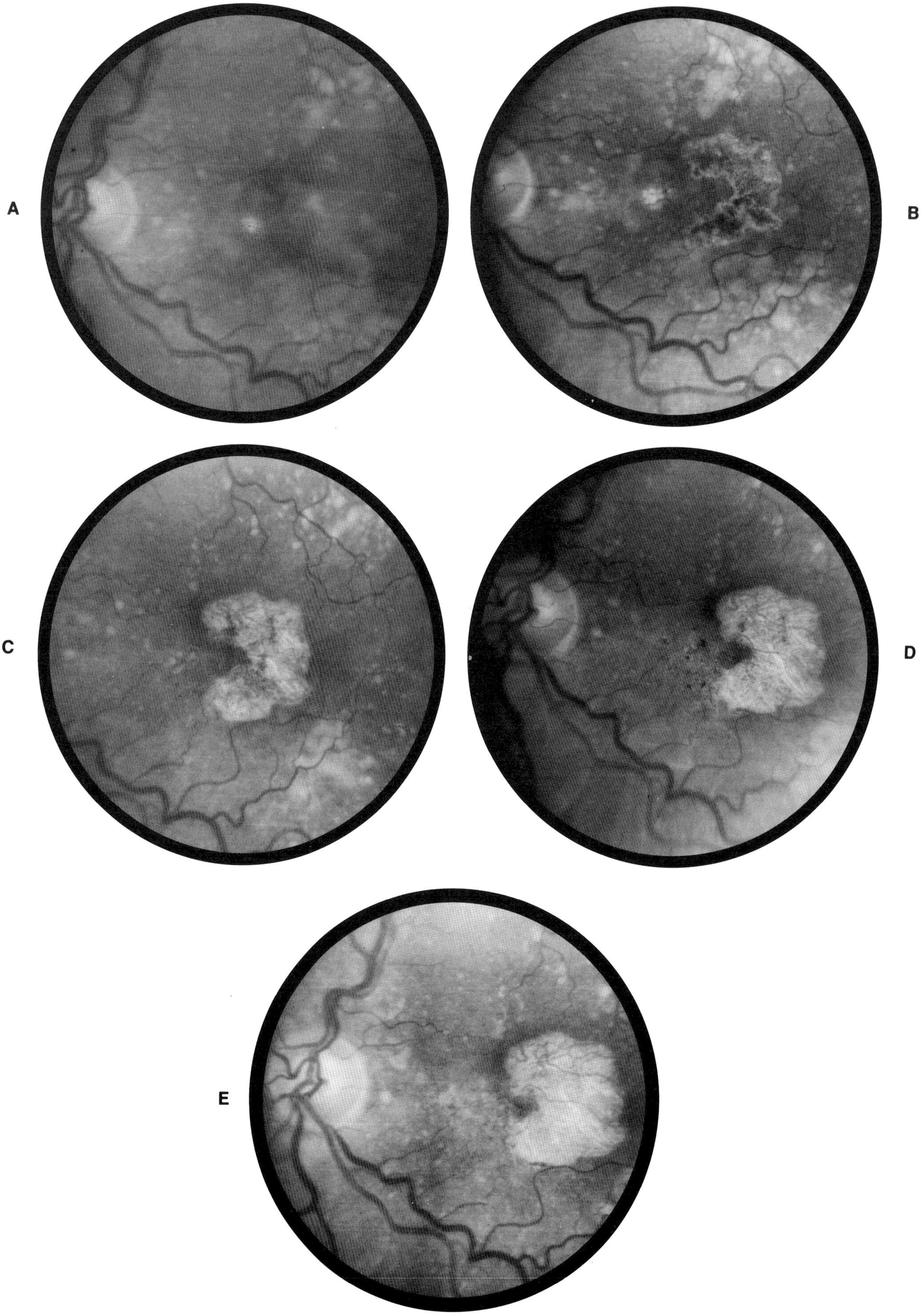

Figure 31.3

Technique of Treatment

Encouraged by a preliminary project suggesting that xenon photocoagulation was beneficial in the management of histoplasmic choroiditis, two investigators reported a prospective study accompanied by randomly selected control patients [7]. Based on a minimum change of two lines on the Sloan chart after 1 year of observation, there was no difference between the treatment and control groups.

At least three objections to the design of the investigation could be raised. First, fluorescein angiography was not performed on all patients to establish the exact location and extent of the subretinal vessels. Second, there was no clinical separation of patients dependent on the distance between the fovea and the nearest margin of the neovascular membrane. Last, the photocoagulation was applied with only sufficient intensity to produce a barely perceptible whitening of the retina. More recent experience indicates that photocoagulation must be very intense, resulting in complete opacification of the overlying retina, to be effective in obliterating subretinal vessels. Despite a well designed randomized study to reduce bias, the results must be questioned due to inadequate treatment.

Under the best conditions there is considerable variation in recording central visual acuity for a specific patient. A recent refraction, type of acuity chart, target contrast, ambient lighting, pupillary diameter, opacities of the media, cooperation of the patient, and diligence of the technician or physician are some of the determining factors. With scotomatous vision associated with macular degeneration, it seems unlikely that a single line change in visual acuity can be detected. With proper standardization of technique, it is possible that reliance can be placed on two or three lines of change in acuity.

In 1969 there was a report on the results of xenon photocoagulation in 89 patients with senile disciform degeneration [8]. Thirty-six patients were followed for less than 1 year. Sixty-three patients had an entry acuity of 20/200 or worse. Half the patients had acuities of 20/400 or worse. The authors contended that disciform macular degeneration ultimately progressed to a visual acuity below the 20/400 level. Based on this premise (for which there was no supporting data), they concluded that only 6% of the treated patients demonstrated progressive visual decline.

There were only 26 patients with initial acuities adequate to permit reliable serial measurements. If the criterion of two lines difference in visual acuity had been applied to this group, then 46% of the patients would have been shown to lose vision following treatment.

Statistical Evaluation

Comparisons by percentage can be very deceptive. Occasionally it is necessary for the reader to convert percentage back to simple numerical form for a clear perspective. An appropriate statistical test, such as the chi square test, should be performed whenever a group of treated patients is compared to any type of control group. To be statistically significant, there should be an indication that any reported differences could have occurred by chance alone with less than 5% probability. Ordinarily, this requires the assistance of a qualified statistician.

In a study in 1975 [9], 51 cases of retinal branch vein occlusion treated by argon laser were compared to the results in two previously published natural history studies (Table 31.3) [10, 11]. By implication, the treated patients and control patients were derived from similar populations. The authors then contended that their patients were selected to exclude those with good visual acuity. This automatically makes the treatment group different from the "control patients" and any subsequent comparison may not be valid.

The authors suggested that the percentages of patients achieving better than 20/40 vision and 20/50 to 20/100 vision were similar in all three studies. They concluded that significantly more untreated patients progressed to visual levels of 20/200 or worse. If the three independent studies consisted of similar patient material, then the conclusion is mathematically impossible. In other words, if the results in the 20/200 column are different, then one or both of the other groups must be different. Assuming the conclusion to be correct, that the only differences occurred in the 20/200 group, then the original populations were not comparable.

If the percentages of patients with 20/200 vision are converted to the original numbers, the differences among

Table 3. Argon laser photocoagulation of retinal branch vein occlusion

Group	No. of eyes	Final visual acuity			
		20/40 or better	20/50–20/100	20/200 or worse (No. of eyes)	
Treatment study [9]	51	50%	39%	11%	(6)
Natural history study [10]	43	53%	28%	19%	(8)
Natural history study [11]	40	60%	18%	23%	(9)

Figure 31.3. *A*, ophthalmoscopic photograph of left eye of 77-year-old patient described in Figure 31.2, showing drusen and irregular serous detachment of retinal pigment epithelium. Visual acuity was 20/40 with +3.25 sph. *B*, ophthalmoscopic photograph 6 weeks after application of argon laser. Crescent shaped scar spares fixation area and maculopapillary bundle. Retinal pigment epithelial detachment is completely flattened. Visual acuity was 20/40 with +3.00 sph. Patient was aware of paracentral scotoma and need for eccentric viewing when reading monocularly. *C*, ophthalmoscopic photograph, 1½ years after laser treatment, showing increased zone of pigment epithelial atrophy. Visual acuity was 20/40 with −3 sph. Patient was unable to see letters on the right side of acuity chart. *D*, ophthalmoscopic photograph, 2½ years after laser treatment showing progressively enlarging scar. Visual acuity had decreased to 20/60. *E*, ophthalmoscopic photograph, 3½ years after laser treatment. Gradual atrophy of pigment epithelium has included fixation area. No retinal pigment epithelial detachment or neurosensory detachment present. Visual acuity less than 20/200.

six, eight, and nine patients seem much less impressive. Further, if a chi square test had been performed, the apparent differences in the 20/200 column clearly would have been insignificant ($p > 0.05$).

In summary, photocoagulation has been utilized for the treatment of macular diseases for more than 20 years. During this time there has not been one single prospective study with randomly selected control patients, which proves that photocoagulation affects the visual prognosis of central serous chorioretinopathy, serous detachment of the retinal pigment epithelium, histoplasmic choroiditis, retinal branch vein occlusion, central retinal vein thrombosis, or exudative macular degeneration. Neither are there any studies showing this form of treatment to be especially harmful. Complications directly attributable to photocoagulation appear to be uncommon. It becomes necessary to weigh the risks of treatment against the speculative benefits.

The limitations of the value of preliminary trials, such as discussed in this review, point out the need for properly designed clinical research in macular diseases. There is no question that prospective studies with human volunteers are complicated and time consuming. Increasing patient awareness, government regulations, inadequate funding, human research committees, and informed consent all tend to depress investigative enthusiasm. Furthermore, many physicians, already convinced that photocoagulation is beneficial, find it difficult to withhold treatment from half the patients.

There are two important positive factors to be considered. First, all the previously discussed macular degenerations occur with sufficient frequency permitting a carefully controlled study to reach a conclusion within a few years. Second, most well informed patients are willing to join human research investigations in which therapy is allocated on a random basis.

It is time for photocoagulation treatment of macular disease to be submitted to valid tests. The efficacy of photocoagulation finally will be established. More important, the natural histories of acquired macular diseases will be documented accurately.

References

1. Sloan, L.L.: New test charts for the measurement of visual acuity at far and near distances. *Am J Ophthalmol, 48:* 807, 1959.
2. Cleasby, G.W., Fung, W.E., and Fiore, J.V., Jr.: Photocoagulation of exudative senile maculopathy. *Arch Ophthalmol, 85:* 18, 1971.
3. Wise, G.N., Campbell, C.J., Wendler, P.F., and Rittler, M.C.: Photocoagulation of vascular lesions of the macula. *Am J Ophthalmol, 66:* 452, 1968.
4. Burton, T.C.: Central serous retinopathy. *Curr Concepts Ophthalmol, 3:* 1, 1972.
5. Schlaegel, T.F., Jr., Cofield, D.D., Clark, G., and Weber, J.C.: Photocoagulation and other therapy for histoplasmic choroiditis. *Trans Am Acad Ophthalmol Otolaryngol, 72:* 355, 1968.
6. Bird, A.C.: Recent advances in the treatment of senile disciform macular degeneration by photocoagulation. *Brit J Ophthalmol, 58:* 367, 1974.
7. Watzke, R.C., and Leaverton, P.E.: Light coagulation in presumed histoplasmic choroiditis: a controlled clinical study. *Arch Ophthalmol, 86:* 127, 1971.
8. Jepson, C.N., and Wetzig, P.C.: Photocoagulation in disciform macular degeneration. *Am J Ophthalmol, 67:* 920, 1969.
9. Gitter, K.A., Cohen, G., and Baber, B. W.: Photocoagulation in venous occlusive disease. *Am J Ophthalmol, 79:* 578, 1975.
10. Michels, R. G., and Gass, J.D.M.: The natural course of retinal branch vein obstruction. *Trans Am Acad Ophthalmol Otolaryngol, 78:* 166, 1974.
11. Gutman, F.A., and Zegarra, H.: The natural course of temporal retinal branch vein occlusion. *Trans Am Acad Ophthalmol Otolaryngol, 78:* 178, 1974.

Index

R